Eponyms and Names in Obstetrics and Gynaecology

Third Edition

Eponyms and Names in Obstetrics and Gynaecology

Third Edition

Thomas F. Baskett

MB BCh BAO (The Queen's University of Belfast)
FRCS (C) FRCS (Ed) FRCOG FACOG DHMSA
Professor Emeritus, Department of Obstetrics and Gynaecology,
Dalhousie University, Halifax, Nova Scotia, Canada

CAMBRIDGE
UNIVERSITY PRESS

CAMBRIDGE
UNIVERSITY PRESS

University Printing House, Cambridge CB2 8BS, United Kingdom

One Liberty Plaza, 20th Floor, New York, NY 10006, USA

477 Williamstown Road, Port Melbourne, VIC 3207, Australia

314–321, 3rd Floor, Plot 3, Splendor Forum, Jasola District Centre, New Delhi – 110025, India

79 Anson Road, #06–04/06, Singapore 079906

Cambridge University Press is part of the University of Cambridge.

It furthers the University's mission by disseminating knowledge in the pursuit of education, learning, and research at the highest international levels of excellence.

www.cambridge.org
Information on this title: www.cambridge.org/9781108421706
DOI: 10.1017/9781108421706

First published by Royal College of Obstetricians and Gynaecologists 1996
Second edition published by Royal College of Obstetricians and Gynaecologists 2008
Third edition published by Cambridge University Press 2019

Printed in the United Kingdom by TJ International Ltd. Padstow Cornwall

A catalogue record for this publication is available from the British Library.

Library of Congress Cataloging-in-Publication Data
Names: Baskett, Thomas F., author.
Title: Eponyms and names in obstetrics and gynaecology / Thomas F. Baskett.
Other titles: On the shoulders of giants
Description: Third edition. | Cambridge, United Kingdom ; New York, NY : Cambridge University Press, 2019. | Preceded by On the shoulders of giants : eponyms and names in obstetrics and gynaecology / Thomas F. Baskett. 2nd ed. 2008. | Includes bibliographical references and index.
Identifiers: LCCN 2018034172 | ISBN 9781108421706 (hardback : alk. paper)
Subjects: | MESH: Eponyms | Obstetrics | Gynecology | Physicians | Biography
Classification: LCC RG45 | NLM WZ 112.5.O2 | DDC 618.1003–dc23
LC record available at https://lccn.loc.gov/2018034172

ISBN 978-1-108-42170-6 Hardback

....

Contents

Image Credits

Portraits

Aveling, von Baer, Baillie, Ballantyne, Barcroft, Barnes, Bartholin, Baudelocque, Blundell, Boivin, Bourgeois, Braun, Browne, Camper, Carus, Chamberlen, Chaussier, Cloquet, Clover, Colebrook, Cooper, Credé, Culpeper, Dale, Denman, Deventer, Duchenne, Duncan, Erb, von Euler, Exner, Fallopius, Farre, Fothergill, Fracastoro, de Graaf, Gregg, Harvey, Braxton Hicks, Hoboken, Holmes, Hunter, Kielland, Krukenberg, Lee, van Leeuwenhoek, Lever, Levret, Little, Lugol, Malpighi, Malthus, Martin, Mauriceau, Maygrier, McDowell, Mercier, Meyer, Morgagni, Müller, Murray, Naegele, Nihell, Ould, Paget, Paré, Pfannenstiel, Pinard, Portal, Read, Récamier, Rigby, Sänger, Santorini, Scarpa, Semmelweis, Sharp, Simpson, Sims, Smellie, Snow, Stopes, Tait, Tarnier, Waldeyer, Wassermann, Wells, White, Wolff, Zondek, are **courtesy of the Wellcome Collection CCBY**. Bard, Bergstrom, Champetier de Ribes, Cullen, Denonvilliers, Down, Joseph, Kelly, Kelsey, Klumpke, Kristeller, Neisser, Noeggerath, Porro, Scanzoni, Soranus, Stearns, Webster, Wharton, Williams are **courtesy of the National Library of Medicine**. Aldridge, Baldy, Caldwell, Channing, Craigin, Curtis, DeLee, Dickinson, Hanks, Hodge, Holmes, Hunner, Irving, Kimball, Keep, McCall, Meigs, Moloy, Pajot, Papanicolaou, Piper, Potter, Rubin, Skene, Smith, Spalding, Stein, Leventhal, Sturmdorf, Thoms, Tucker, du Vigneaud, Watkins, Wright are **courtesy of the American Gynecological and Obstetrical Society**. Blair-Bell, Döderlein, Donald A, Donald I, Green-Armytage, Haultain, Kerr, Novak, Steptoe and Edwards are **courtesy of the Royal College of Obstetricians and Gynaecologists**. Aburel, Barton, Basset, Brenner, Cochrane, Coombs, Cyprianus, McDonald, Potter, Smithells, Ramsey are **courtesy of Elsevier**. Arias-Stella, Aschheim, Asherman, Gräfenberg, Latzko, Le Fort, Madlener, Pincus, Schuchardt, Steinbüchel, Steiner, Tanner are **courtesy of Taylor and Francis**. Baird is **courtesy of the College of Life Sciences and Medicine, University of Aberdeen**. Apgar **is courtesy of the Wood Library-Museum of Anesthesiology**. Bovie, Bowen are **courtesy of the Boston Medical Library, Francis A. Countway Library of Medicine**. Call is **courtesy of the Bentley Historical Library, University of Michigan**. Campbell is **courtesy of the Royal Children's Hospital Archives, Melbourne**. Buford Word is **courtesy of UAB Archives, University of Alabama at Birmingham**. Clay is **courtesy of the University of Manchester**. Heaney is **courtesy of Rush University Medical Center Archives**. Kennedy is **courtesy of Rotunda Hospital, Dublin**. Houston, is **courtesy of the Royal College of Surgeons in Ireland**. Montgomery is **courtesy of the Royal College of Physicians of Ireland**. Moschcowitz is **courtesy of the Arthur H. Aufses Jr MD Archives, Mount Sinai Medical Center, New York**. Sheehan is **courtesy of the University of Liverpool**. Torpin is **courtesy of The Historical Collection and Archives, Robert B. Greenblatt, MD Library, Augusta University**. Voorhees and Hühner are **courtesy of the New York Academy of Medicine**. Hamlin, Mahfouz, Martius, Mettauer are **courtesy of RF Zacharin**. Logothetopoulos is **courtesy of Dr Aris Antsaklis, Athens**. Donné, O'Sullivan are **courtesy of the BMJ Publishing Group**. Foley, Hopkins are **courtesy of the William P Didusch Center for Urologic History**. Hart is **courtesy of the University of Toronto Archives**. Huntington is **courtesy of the Porter-Phelps-Huntington Foundation**. Kehrer is **courtesy of Universitätsbibliothek Heidelberg**. Marker is **courtesy of Roche, Palo Alto, California**. Palmer is **courtesy of the Journal of Reproductive Medicine**. Roberts is **courtesy of the Victoria Medical Society Archives**. Te Linde is **courtesy of Wolters Kluwer Health - Lippincott Williams & Wilkins**. Collip is **courtesy of the Thomas Fisher Rare Book Library, University of Toronto**. Litzmann, Michaelis, Semm are **courtesy of the Department of Obstetrics and Gynaecology,**

University Hospitals, Schleswig-Holstein, Kiel. Clarke is **courtesy of CA Clarke.** Barker is **courtesy of DJP Barker.** Mendelson is **courtesy of CL Mendelson.** Rubin A is **courtesy of Dr A Rubin, Philadelphia.** Veres is **courtesy of Dr Béla Molnár, Szeged, Hungary** and **Mrs Veres** for the photograph of her late husband, János Veres. Kegel is **courtesy of Dr Bob Shull, Texas A&M University, Health Science Center.** Behçet is **courtesy of Dr Cagatay Ustun, Ege University, Bornova, Turkey.** Gardner is **courtesy of Dr Dale Brown, Houston, Texas.** Marshall is **courtesy of Dr ED Vaughan, New York-Presbyterian Medical Center.** Hon is **courtesy of Dr EH Hon, California.** Sertoli is **courtesy of Dr Eugenio Beer, Omegna, Italy.** Bird is **courtesy of Dr GC Bird.** Wrigley is **courtesy of Dr Howard Pendleton, Vancouver, Canada.** Marchetti is **courtesy of Dr James Magovern, Georgetown University Medical Center, Washington DC.** Barr is **courtesy of Dr Robert Barr, London, Ontario.** Burch is **courtesy of Dr Robert Tosh, Nashville, Tennessee.** Maylard is **courtesy of Dr SD Slater and the Victoria Infirmary, Glasgow.** Menon, Shirodkar are **courtesy of Dr Subhash Naergolkar, Pune, India.** Bishop is **courtesy of Dr EH Bishop, North Carolina.** Friedman is **courtesy of Emanuel A Friedman.** Malmström is **courtesy of Eva Malmström.** Lippes is **courtesy of Jack Lippes MD.** Hulka is **courtesy of Jaroslav F Hulka MD.** Ferguson, JKW is **courtesy of JKW Ferguson.** Krantz is **courtesy of KE Krantz.** Filshie is **courtesy of Mr GM Filshie.** Moir is **courtesy of Professor David Barlow, University of Oxford.** Kleihauer is **courtesy of Professor Dr E Kleihauer, Germany.** Saling is **courtesy of Professor Dr E Saling.** Bracht is **courtesy of Professor Erich Saling, Berlin.** Smythe is **courtesy of Professor Gordon Stirrat, University of Bristol.** Macafee is **courtesy of Professor Graham Harley, Belfast.** Uchida is **courtesy of Professor Hitoo Nakano, Fukuoka, Japan.** Bevis is **courtesy of Professor James Drife, University of Leeds.** Kergaradec is **courtesy of Professor JHM Pinkerton, Belfast.** White is **courtesy of Professor John Hare, Joslin Diabetes Center, Boston.** Betke is **courtesy of Professor KH Betke, Germany.** Youssef **is courtesy of Professor Maher Mahran, Cairo, Egypt.** Løvset is **courtesy of Professor Per Bergsjø and** ***Acta Obstetrica Gynecologia Scandinavia*** **1982; 61: 193.** Philpott is **courtesy of Professor RH Philpott.** Liggins, Liley are **courtesy of Professor Sir Graham Liggins, New Zealand.** Caldeyro-Barcia is **courtesy of R Caldeyro-Barcia.** Cherney is **courtesy of the San Francisco Medical Society Bulletin.** Stroganoff is **courtesy of the USSR Ministry of Health.** McRoberts is **courtesy of WA McRoberts, Texas.** Zavanelli **is courtesy of WA Zavanelli.** Andrews is **courtesy of William C Andrews MD.** Vacca is **courtesy of Mrs Janet Vacca**, Rodeck is **courtesy of Dr Charles Rodeck**, Robson is **courtesy of Dr Michael Robson**, Pereyra is **courtesy of Dr Benson Harer, California.** Allen is **courtesy of PubMed.**

Other Images

External pelvimeter measuring Baudelocque's diameter, Post-partum medication orders for the Countess of Mornington and her infant son, the future Duke of Wellington, delivered by Fielding Ould are **courtesy of the Wellcome Collection CCBY.** Blond–Heidler saw, Braun hook, Diagram illustrating the Burns–Marshall manoeuvre for breech delivery, the original Chamberlen forceps, Chapman's forceps, Ian Donald scans his daughter, Caroline, Dusée's forceps, Gräfenberg rings, Kielland's forceps, Lippes loop, Malmström vacuum cup, Moir's kymographic tracing, Pinard stethoscope, Pugh's forceps, Spurs of ergot, Wrigley's forceps are **courtesy of the Royal College of Obstetricians and Gynaecologists.** Modified WHO partogram incorporating Philpott's principles is **courtesy of Professor RH Philpott.** Steptoe's and Edwards' report of the first successful case of in vitro fertilisation, Torpin's uterine packer, Willett's scalp forceps, Illustration of wooden model in Woods' paper describing the screw manoeuvre are **courtesy of Elsevier.** Ayres spatula, Cullen's sign, Plaque dedicated to Gordon, Jane Todd Crawford memorial, McDowell house, Novak curette, OmniCup vacuum extractor, JY Simpson's table. Smellie's tomb, Drew Smythe catheter, Steptoe's grave, Word catheter are **courtesy of TF Baskett.** Barton's forceps, Piper's forceps, Tarnier forceps, Tucker–McLane forceps are **courtesy of photos taken by TF Baskett at the Ralph Hale History Museum of the American College of Obstetricians and Gynecologists, Washington DC.**

About the Author

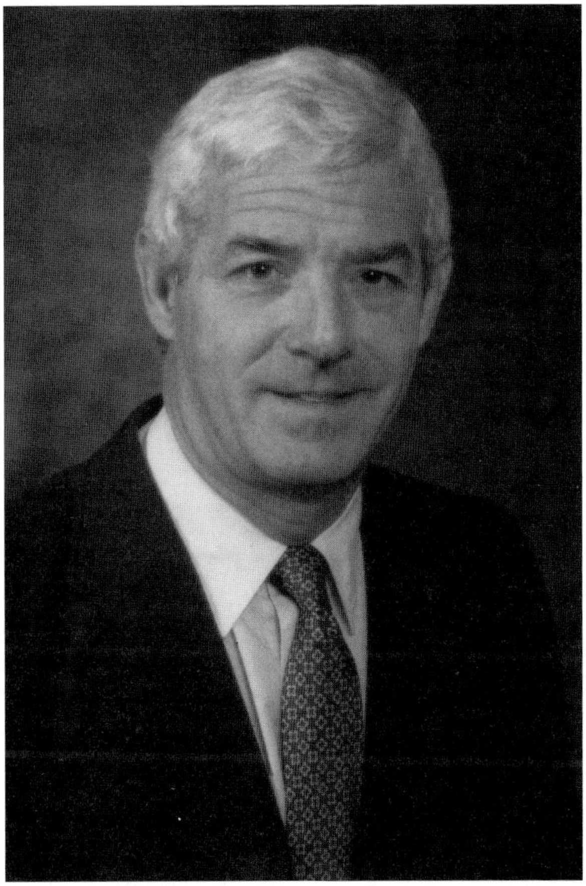

Tom Baskett was born during the Second World War in Belfast, Northern Ireland. He spent most of the first weeks of his life in a cot under a heavy dining room table during the air raids on the Belfast shipyards. He was later reassured they were not aiming specifically at him – thereby avoiding a diagnosis of neonatal post-traumatic stress disorder. His subsequent evacuation to the country made him an unwitting pioneer of perinatal outreach programmes.

Educated at Belfast Royal Academy and the Queen's University of Belfast, he received his school colours for rugby and athletics but no academic distinction. He claims that under modern admission criteria he would never gain entry to medical school; most people agree with him.

He qualified in medicine in 1964 and did six years postgraduate training in surgery, obstetrics and gynaecology and some general practice in Northern Ireland. He worked at the Royal Victoria, Royal Maternity and Belfast City hospitals.

As one of the three main export groups from Ireland – racehorses, nurses and doctors – he emigrated to Canada in 1970. He spent 10 years in Winnipeg and from there acted as a consultant in obstetrics and gynaecology to the Central Canadian Arctic, which he visited regularly. In 1980 he moved to Halifax.

In addition to his day and night job he has served as president of the Society of Obstetricians and Gynaecologists of Canada and the Canadian Gynaecological Society, examiner in obstetrics and gynaecology for the Royal College of Physicians and Surgeons of Canada and editor-in-chief of the *Journal of the Society of Obstetricians and Gynaecologists of Canada.*

Like grey hair, his interest in medical history has grown insidiously over the years. In 1997 he completed the Diploma in the History of Medicine from the Worshipful Society of Apothecaries of London (DHMSA) and was awarded the Maccabean Prize and the Osler Medal. He was the 2008 History Fellow of the American College of Obstetricians and Gynecologists.

Preface

Despite misguided attempts to discourage them, eponyms continue to enrich the language and literature of medicine. Few specialties have a longer or richer eponymous background than obstetrics and gynaecology. Eponyms add a human side to an increasingly technical profession in which both the providers and recipients of medical care continue to crave the human touch and are diminished by its absence. They also provide a practical shorthand for some complex clinical manoeuvres, syndromes and procedures. Eponyms represent the tradition and language of a specialty and acknowledge the contribution of pioneers. The purpose of this collection is to help perpetuate the names and provide an introductory profile of some of the founders in whose steps we follow. I have not confined myself to eponyms but have included other notable names in the development of the specialty. I have also added several from other specialties whose contributions are relevant to obstetrics and gynaecology.

In each case biographical data are provided and the eponym or work for which they are known is outlined with context. I have included quotations from the authors' original work that, in addition to the entertaining language of the different eras, provide a glimpse into their rationale and humanity. Where available, the original and related references are provided. I have included a bibliography of linked references to assist the reader wanting more detailed information on individual subjects. Since the first edition was published in 1996 I have added 80 names, along with additional information and images for the entries in the first two editions. There are now 391 names from 34 countries.

My own exposure to eponyms began when I was a medical student in the 1960s. In Hamilton Bailey's classic, *Demonstrations of Physical Signs in Clinical Surgery*, there were small footnotes describing some of the eponymous characters, which piqued my interest. It was not uncommon for consultants at ward rounds to ask, 'Who was so and so?' Legend around oral examination tactics had it that, towards the end of the oral, if you were asked about an eponym, you had either passed very well or failed utterly – either way it was better to go out with one's eponymous guns blazing!

A positive aspect of the study of eponymy is that it inevitably leads to a greater understanding of the evolution and relevance of the associated clinical event and is therefore both educational and entertaining, thereby fulfilling my favourite quote from Marshall McLuhan, the Canadian philosopher and sociologist: 'Anyone who tries to make a distinction between education and entertainment doesn't know the first thing about either'. I hope this third and final edition will be both.

T.F. Baskett
Halifax, Nova Scotia

Acknowledgements

The lifeblood of a work of this nature is the library and I am indebted to the libraries that I have used over the past 30 years: the WK Kellogg Health Sciences Library, Dalhousie University, Halifax, Nova Scotia; the Bay Jacobs History Library of the American College of Obstetricians and Gynecologists (ACOG), Washington DC; the United States National Library of Medicine, Bethesda, Maryland and four libraries in London: the British Library; the Royal College of Obstetricians and Gynaecologists (RCOG); the Royal Society of Medicine and the Wellcome Institute for the History of Medicine. In particular, I wish to acknowledge the assistance of Patricia Want, former Librarian at the RCOG and her successor, Lucy Reid. Debra Scarborough, History Librarian and Archivist at the ACOG History Library, has been extremely helpful in tracing biographical information from American sources. I am most grateful for her gracious co-operation and mastery of the archives. My thanks go to Dr Fritz Nagele of the University of Vienna, who guided me on a trip to historical sources in Vienna and also translated many papers.

A number of the subjects in this book kindly met my requests for information and photographs of themselves: DJS Barker, KH Betke, GC Bird, EH Bishop, R Caldeyro-Barcia, CA Clarke, RRA Coombs, JKW Ferguson, GM Filshie, EA Friedman, EHG Hon, JF Hulka, E Kleihauer, KE Krantz, GC Liggins, J Lippes, VF Marshall, WA McRoberts, CL Mendelson, K O'Driscoll, RH Philpott, MS Robson, CH Rodeck, A Rubin, E Saling and WA Zavanelli, I thank them for their courteous co-operation. Mrs Eva Malmström wrote most generously and provided me with details and a photograph of her late husband, Tage Malmström.

Many colleagues have generously responded to my enquiries about various subjects in this work: Dr S MacMillan, Aberdeen (Dugald Baird and Alexander Gordon); Dr Barbara Thompson, Aberdeen (Dugald Baird); Dr A Vacca, Brisbane (Geoffrey Bird); Dr C Ustun, Bornova, Turkey (Hulusi Behçet); Dr E Saling, Berlin (Erich Bracht and Hans Hinselmann); Dr RH Tosh, Nashville, Tennessee (John Burch); Dr R Kennison, Boston and Mr R Krupinski, Ann Arbor (Emma Call); Ms B Hewitt, Parkville, Australia (Kate Campbell); Dr AH Johnston, San Francisco (Leonid Cherney); Dr JW Goodwin, Toronto (Geoffrey Dawes); Dr D Brown, Houston, Texas (Herman Gardner); Dr RF Zacharin, Victoria, Australia (Reg and Catherine Hamlin); Dr AP Goldbloom, Toronto (Alfred Hart); Dr SW Campbell and Mr Bullington, Chicago and Dr MA Schellpfeffer, Kenosha, Wisconsin (Sproat Heaney); Dr JB Roche, Sydney (Ed Hon); Dr DH Morse, Los Angeles (Arnold Kegel); Professor JHM Pinkerton, Belfast (Jacques Kergaradec); Sir Graham Liggins, Auckland (William Liley);Dr Aris Antsaklis, Athens (Konstantinos Logothetopoulos); Professor P Bergsjø, Bergen and Professor O Larsen, Oslo (Jørgen Løvset); Dr TF Magovern, Washington DC (Andrew Marchetti); Dr ED Vaughan, New York (Victor Marshall); Dr A Mickal, New Orleans (Milton McCall); Dr S Nargolkar, Pune (Krishna Menon and Vithal Shirodkar); Dr AH Auffses, New York (Alexis Moschcowitz); Dr AD Browne, Dr L Lunney and M O'Doherty, Dublin (William Neville); Dr Benson Harer, California (Armand Pereyra); Dr E Beer, Omegna, Italy (Erico Sertoli); Dr E Vizza, Rome (Pier Spinelli); Dr A Kernbauer, Graz, Austria (Richard von Steinbüchel); Dr PJ Taylor, Vancouver (Patrick Steptoe); Ms L Westrick, Augusta, Georgia (Richard Torpin);

Professor H Nakano, Fukuoka, Japan (Hajime Uchida); Dr BG Molnár, Szeged, Hungary (János Veres); Dr B Ward, Charlottesville, Virginia (George White); Dr JW Hare, Boston (Priscilla White); Dr AM Hetzer, Hempstead, New York (Charles Wood); Mr T Pennycuff, Birmingham, Alabama (Buford Word); Ms MR Hanley, London and Dr HJ Pendleton, Vancouver (Arthur Wrigley); Dr Gamal Serour, Cairo (Abdel Youssef). Their willingness to seek out and provide me with vital information is greatly appreciated.

I am grateful to Nicholas Dunton and Cambridge University Press for the opportunity to publish this third edition.

As always, my deepest gratitude goes to my wife Yvette, who typed the new manuscript. With the three editions, we have worked on and off for 30 years on this project. It would not have happened without her.

A

Aburel, Eugen Bogdan (1899–1975)

Continuous Epidural Analgesia

The first report of single dose epidural local anaesthetic injection for pain relief in labour was in 1906 by Walter Stoeckel. In 1931, Eugen Aburel, a Romanian obstetrician working in Paris, presented the first description of a technique for continuous epidural analgesia in labour. His report before the Society of Obstetrics and Gynaecology of Paris was given on 12 January, 1931. After extensive research involving detailed dissection, Aburel concluded that the uterus had a double sensory innervation. To obviate the need for repeated injection, and in the absence of long-acting local anaesthetics, Aburel developed his technique by introducing a soft, flexible silk catheter through a needle into the epidural space, at either the caudal or lumbar level. The needle was withdrawn and the catheter left in place for subsequent injections of 0.5% cinchocaine. He experimented with other local anaesthetics but ultimately achieved his best results with 0.5% cinchocaine plus 1:100,000 adrenaline, which lasted for 3–5 hours.

Eugen Bogdan Aburel was born in Galatzi, Romania. His initial leaning was to a career in engineering, but he changed to medicine and graduated from Iassy University, Romania in 1923. He studied surgery and psychiatry before choosing obstetrics and gynaecology. In 1928 he went to Paris and combined clinical work in the Tarnier and Boucicant Hospitals with research in the physiology department of the Sorbonne. He returned to Romania in 1933 and was appointed professor of obstetrics and gynaecology at Iassy University in 1936. In 1945 he moved to the same chair at Bucharest University, which he held until his retirement in 1969. His academic output was prodigious, with over 700 publications. The limitation of these publications to Romanian and French journals, plus the lack of scientific exchange between east and west, meant that the pioneer work of Aburel was not fully acknowledged until the 1970s.

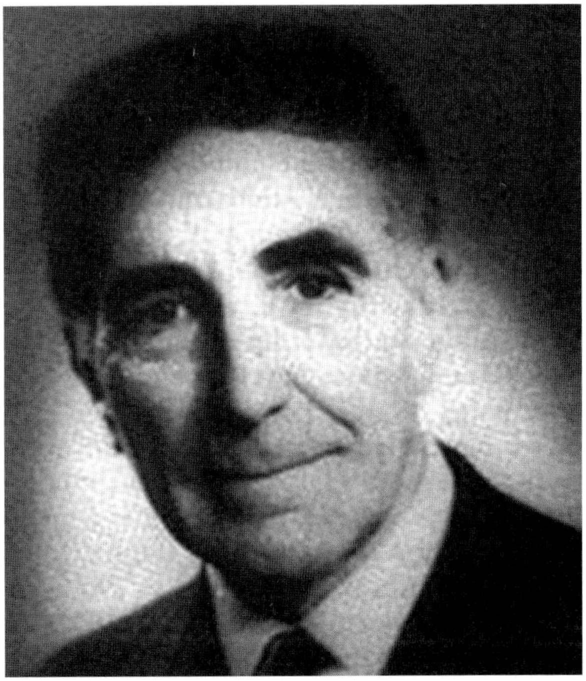

Eugen Bogdan Aburel

Selected Publications

Aburel E. La topographie et le mécanisme des douleurs de l'accouchement avant la période d'expulsion. *CR Soc Biol Paris* 1930; 103: 902–4.

Aburel E. L'anesthésie locale continue (prolongée) en obstetrique. *Bull Soc Obstét Gynéc Paris* 1931; 20: 35–7.

Bibliography References

5, 58, 59, 341, 430, 431, 584, 894, 1336, 1730.

Alcock, Benjamin (b. 1801)

Alcock's (Pudendal) Canal

The space within the pelvic (obturator) fascia that transmits the pudendal vessels and nerve was first described in detail by Benjamin Alcock in Robert Todd's *Cyclopaedia of Anatomy and Physiology*, which was published in six volumes between 1835 and 1859:

> *In a canal in the obturator fascia the artery (int pudendal) is contained through the posterior part of the third (perineal) muscle; by some it is maintained to be between the fascia and the muscle ... but this is not correct; the vessel being in the fascia, and not extreme (lateral) to it ...*

The description is often incorrectly attributed to the English apothecary and surgeon, Thomas Alcock.

Born in Kilkenny, Ireland, 'the son of a doctor, descended from a long line of doctors', Benjamin Alcock was a pupil of Abraham Colles and graduated from Dublin University. He taught anatomy in the private schools of medicine in Dublin from 1825 until his appointment, in 1849, as the first professor of anatomy at the new Queen's College in Cork. He was reputedly hot-tempered, and in 1853 a dispute arose between Alcock and the university over the interpretation of the Anatomy Act. Alcock resigned at the behest of the Lord Lieutenant of Ireland, who felt his position in the college 'was not beneficial, nor of good example'. After an unsuccessful petition to Queen Victoria, Alcock went to America. He was never heard of again.

Selected Publications

Alcock B. Iliac arteries. In: Todd RE (ed.) *Cyclopaedia of Anatomy and Physiology*. Vol. 2. London: Sherwood, Gilbert and Piper; 1836, p. 835.

Bibliography References

228, 946, 1085, 1137, 1138.

Aldridge, Albert Herman (1893–1983)

Aldridge Sling

Albert Herman Aldridge was born in Victor, New York on 19 July 1893. He was brought up on a farm, and after taking his undergraduate degree in science entered the medical school at the University of Syracuse and graduated MD in 1918. He served for two years as a medical officer at the United States Naval Hospital in Chelsea, Massachusetts. He then did one year as an obstetric resident at the Sloane Hospital for Women in New York, followed by two years as a gynaecology resident in the Women's Hospital in the state of New York. Thereafter he joined the staff of the Women's Hospital, from which he carried out a private practice of obstetrics and gynaecology for more than 50 years, ultimately retiring in 1977. He was surgeon-in-chief of the Women's Hospital from 1938 to 1955 and held the rank of professor of obstetrics and gynecology at the College of Physicians and Surgeons, Columbia University. In this position he built a strong training programme in obstetrics and gynaecology, although his main clinical interest was in operative gynaecology.

At a meeting of the New York Obstetrical Society on 10 March 1942, Aldridge presented his rationale for surgical relief of urinary stress incontinence using transplantation of rectus fascia. He began by stating, 'Unfortunately, we have not acquired either a complete knowledge of the anatomic structures in and about the female urethra or an entirely satisfactory explanation of the physiology of the delicate urethral sphincter mechanism which is responsible for the control of urination'. Aldridge declared that the standard vaginal repair procedures may not be successful, 'due not so much to faulty techniques as to the fact that there has been unusual destruction of the urethral sphincter muscles themselves and perhaps of their nerve and blood supply'. He then went on to review seven surgical techniques developed between 1910 and 1929: 'The purpose in all of these techniques was to prevent the escape of urine by providing external pressure on the urethra as a substitute for the normal sphincter mechanism which had been destroyed or was congenitally absent'. Aldridge felt that 'the good results claimed for all the techniques briefly described above have been attained through improved support for the urethra and partial urethral stricture'.

Aldridge described his own modification, which involved incising the fascial strips from the aponeurosis over the rectus and oblique muscles. These strips were mobilised from lateral to medial, and the strips were then pushed through the rectus muscles 2 cm from the midline. Through an anterior vaginal incision these strips were then sutured together to form a sling beneath the urethra. Aldridge outlined the merits of his operation as follows:

> *It seems fair to state that the new procedure which has been described has certain advantages over those previously recommended, in that: 1) It utilizes the rectus abdominus muscles which are always well developed and easily accessible. 2) It involves no displacement of the recti muscles or possible loss of function through damage to their nerve or blood supply. 3) It develops a fascial sling in a position and manner which provides additional support and external pressure to the urethra at the point where it is likely to be most effective, i.e., at the junction of the urethra and bladder and 4) it takes advantage of the favorable anatomic relationship of the recti muscles to the urethra. By utilizing the normal variation and position of these muscles, in response to changes of intra-abdominal pressure, compression of the urethral lumen is automatically increased at the exact times when it is most necessary in order to prevent leakage of urine.*

Held in high esteem for his innovation in gynaecological surgery and as a teacher, Aldridge was honoured in 1952 by the award of an honorary LLD degree from the University of Leeds in England. He became president of both the New York Obstetrical Society and the American Gynecological Society. Married for 55 years, he had two sons, one of whom became an obstetrician/gynaecologist and the other a poet. He retired to the gentler climate of Pinehurst, North Carolina and died there on 13 November 1983 in his ninety-first year.

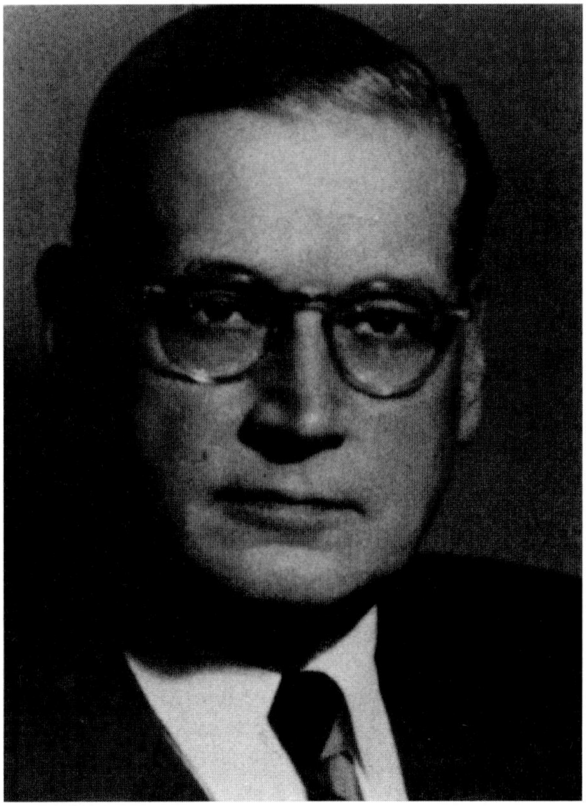

Albert Herman Aldridge

Selected Publications

Aldridge AH. Transplantation of fascia for relief of urinary stress incontinence. *Am J Obstet Gynecol* 1942; 44: 398–411.

Bibliography References

168, 443, 801, 1623.

Allen, Edgar (1892–1943)
Doisy, Edward Adelbert (1893–1986)
Oestrogen

The basic physiology of the female reproductive cycle slowly came to be understood in the early twentieth century through isolation of the hormones that governed the cycle. The word 'hormone' was first suggested in 1905 by Ernest Starling (1866–1927) for 'the active substances secreted into the blood stream . . . by the ductless or endocrine glands'.

As early as 1896, Emil Knauer (1867–1935), a Viennese gynaecologist, showed that the ovaries regulated female sexual maturity, when he transplanted mature ovaries into immature female rabbits and observed the rapid development of mature sex characteristics. He postulated that the mature ovary produced some sort of 'generative ferment' that was carried from the ovary via the blood stream.

In 1922, two young American scientists, Edgar Allen and Edward Doisy, working at the Washington School of Medicine in St Louis, noted that the injection of fluid from the ovarian follicle of sow's ovaries into ovariectomised mice produced the changes of a mature oestrus cycle. In their 1923 report they attributed this result to an 'ovarian hormone':

> *This hormone seems to be an efficient substitute for the endocrine function of the ovaries of the nonpregnant animal. It is probable that its alternate presence and absence in the circulation is sufficient to explain the mechanism of estrual phenomena in the genital tract in the absence of pregnancy . . . It is probable that this hormone is produced under the influence of maturing ova by their follicle cells. Since it is obtained from the ovaries of hogs and cattle and produces results in the mouse and rat, it is not species specific. It is probably produced in all ovaries as their ova mature, and therefore is probably common to all female animals.*

Following this work, they moved on, Allen to the University of Missouri and Doisy to St Louis University, but continued to collaborate. Doisy later isolated oestrone and oestradiol at about the same time as Adolf Butenandt (1903–1995) of Göttingen, Germany.

Edgar Allen was born in Canyon City, Colorado on 2 May 1892. He grew up in Providence, Rhode Island and received his education at Brown University. During the First World War he served in France with the Brown University Ambulance Unit. After his PhD in 1921 he was appointed to the department of anatomy at the Washington School of Medicine at St Louis, where he did his work with Doisy. In 1922 he became professor of anatomy at the University of Missouri and, in 1933, was appointed to the chair of anatomy at Yale University. His entire career was devoted to the study of ovarian hormones and their relationship to the reproductive cycle. He died of a heart attack on 3 February 1943, while on patrol with the United States Coast Guard off Long Island, New York.

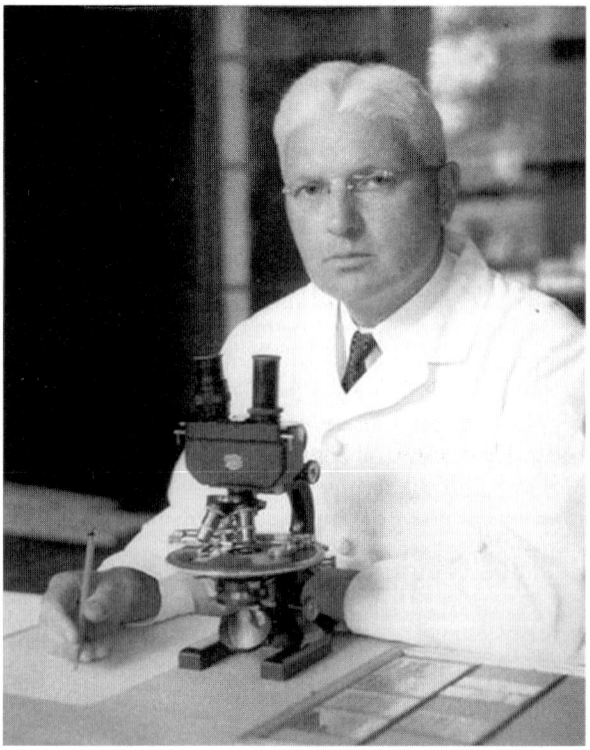

Edgar Allen

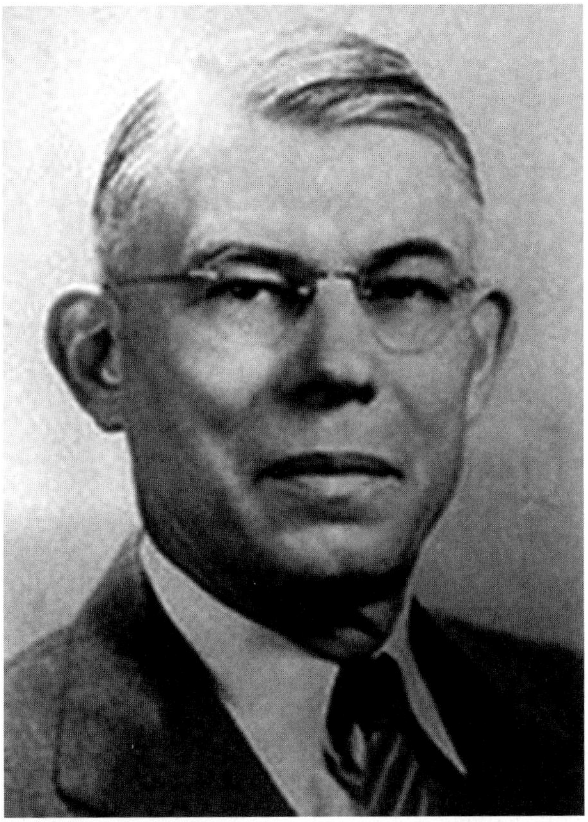
Edward Adelbert Doisy

Edward Adelbert Doisy was born on 13 November 1893 in the small town of Hume, Illinois, where as a youth he delivered papers and worked on a farm. His initial university education was at the University of Illinois and he later transferred to Harvard University, where he received his PhD in biochemistry in 1920. He was made professor of biochemistry at St Louis University in 1923 and remained there the rest of his professional life, becoming head of the department in 1924. He isolated vitamin K in 1939, for which he shared the Nobel Prize for physiology and medicine in 1943. He died on 23 October 1986 at the age of 92, having lived almost twice as long as his co-discoverer, Edgar Allen.

Selected Publications

Allen E, Doisy EA. An ovarian hormone: preliminary report on its localization, extraction and partial purification, and action in test animals. *JAMA* 1923; 81: 819–21.

Allen E, Doisy EA. The extraction and some properties of an ovarian hormone. *J Biol Chem* 1924; 61: 7–11.

Knauer E. Einige Versuche über Ovariantransplantation bei Kaninchen. *Zentralbl Gynäkol* 1896; 20: 524–8.

Bibliography References

314, 315, 317, 409, 559, 560, 600, 642, 717, 1031, 1166, 1480, 1485, 1486.

Apgar, Virginia (1909–1974)

Apgar Score

Virginia Apgar was born in Westfield, New Jersey on 7 June 1909. She graduated BA from Mount Holyoke College in Massachusetts in 1929, and four years later she received her MD from Columbia University College of Physicians and Surgeons in New York. The first four years of her medical career were spent as a surgical intern and resident at the Presbyterian Hospital in New York; she then switched to anaesthesia and served her residency at the Presbyterian Hospital, in the Wisconsin General Hospital in Madison and at the Bellevue Hospital in New York. In 1939, she was the second woman to take the diploma of the American Board of Anesthesiology. She was appointed to the Columbia Presbyterian Medical Center and, in 1949, was the first woman to receive a full professorship at Columbia University. During her 21 years as an anaesthetist she was said to have given 20,000 anaesthetics and to have provided analgesia for a similar number of women during delivery. It was at the Sloane Women's Hospital that she developed and applied the Apgar Score.

Apgar introduced a simple technique for newborn assessment based on systematic appraisal of five criteria: heart rate, respiration, reflex irritability, muscle tone and skin colour. Each of these signs was rated as

0, 1 or 2 and assessed at one minute of age. The total became the Apgar Score. In her introduction to the paper she wrote:

> *Resuscitation of infants at birth has been the subject of many articles. Seldom have there been such imaginative ideas, such enthusiasms, and dislikes, and such unscientific observations and study about one clinical picture . . . the poor quality and lack of precise data of the majority of papers concerned with infant resuscitation are interesting.*

A subsequent report, *Further Observations on the Newborn Scoring System*, was published by Apgar and her colleague Stanley James (1925–1994) 10 years later. This paper summarised the experience of eight years between 1952 and 1960 with newborn scoring in 27,715 live births. It confirmed the correlation of a poor score with neonatal mortality as well as the acid-base status of the newborn. They felt the main benefit of the scoring system was in the selection of infants for resuscitation:

> *The method has been found to be a valuable guide both in teaching and clinical practice in deciding which infants to resuscitate. By its use, delivery room personnel learn to observe several physical signs at once, evaluating them rapidly, and act accordingly.*

She developed this technique to ensure systematic and consistent appraisal of the newborn so that resuscitation would be instituted promptly if necessary. The simplicity of this evaluation has assured its universal adoption, and it has been said that 'every baby born is first seen through the eyes of Dr Virginia Apgar'.

In 1959, on her fiftieth birthday, she received the degree of master of public health from Johns Hopkins University. At this point, she joined the staff at the National Foundation March of Dimes, where she became head of the division of congenital malformations. By 1967, she was appointed director of the basic research department within the Foundation and the following year became vice-president for medical affairs. At the same time, she held an appointment as clinical professor of pediatrics in teratology at Cornell University Medical College. Her stature and energetic speaking schedule ensured that recognition and funding for research in birth defects increased considerably during her tenure at the Foundation.

The tributes paid to Virginia Apgar during her life and after her death provide a picture of a single, very energetic woman with a broad range of interests and talents. She was apparently a fast talker, fast walker and fast driver, claiming that her car tyres never wore out as they rarely touched the ground. She started flying lessons when she was 59 years old. Apgar was a considerable musician and played viola and cello in a string quartet in her home town of Teaneck, New Jersey and, occasionally, with the Teaneck Symphony. She was one of the founders of the Amateur Chamber Music Players and the Catgut Acoustical Society. Under the influence and tutelage of a former patient, Apgar became a skilled instrument maker. This began when the patient was convalescing in hospital and noticed that a shelf in the public phone booth was made of 'a fine well-seasoned piece of curly maple', which apparently had a good resonance to the drumming fingers. She felt it would make an ideal back of a viola and asked Apgar if she could arrange to have the shelf removed and replaced with another. In keeping with the standard mentality of hospital

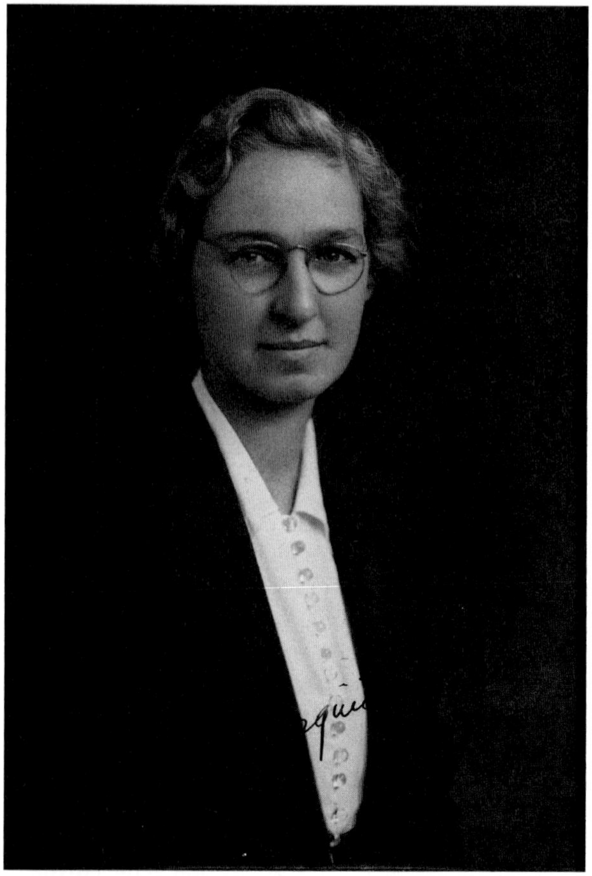

Virginia Apgar

administration they refused. Thus, late one night, Apgar and the patient, suitably equipped with carpentry tools, 'liberated' the shelf and replaced it with a piece of identically stained plywood. It was with this piece of wood that Apgar crafted her first viola under the guidance of her former patient. Over the years, she made three other string instruments, the last of which was finished by her tutor just after Apgar's death. Ultimately, the instruments – a cello, violin, viola and mezzo violin – were purchased by a group of paediatricians and donated to Columbia University College of Physicians and Surgeons.

On the twentieth anniversary of her death in 1994, a 20-cent stamp with Virginia Apgar's portrait was issued in the US Postal Service's Great Americans Series. That same year, at the American Academy of Pediatrics annual clinical meeting in Dallas, Texas, a quartet of paediatrician musicians played some of Apgar's favourite chamber music on the instruments she had crafted.

Virginia Apgar's newborn score is used almost universally. She claimed that her main reason for developing this method of early appraisal of the neonate was to redirect some of the attention from the mother to the newborn infant at a very critical stage when, if required, resuscitation efforts would yield great benefit. As she later said, 'I wanted to find a way to get doctors to pay attention to the baby'. Some have altered the wording and sequence of the five cardinal signs to produce the acronym APGAR: Appearance, Pulse, Grimace, Activity and Respiration.

Virginia Apgar died in her sleep on 7 August 1974. The memorial service held in her local church was attended by a mix of prominent medical and local people, including the local traffic policeman with whom she had so many encounters.

Selected Publications

Apgar V. A proposal for a new method of evaluation of the newborn infant. *Curr Res Anesth Analg* 1953; 32: 260–7.

Apgar V, James LS. Further observations of the newborn scoring system. *Am J Dis Child* 1962; 104: 419–28.

Bibliography References

84, 221, 222, 229, 272, 629, 639, 772, 911, 1105, 1163, 1202, 1265, 1431.

Arias-Stella, Javier (b. 1924)

Arias-Stella Reaction

In 1954 Javier Arias-Stella described atypical endometrial changes in association with early pregnancy. These consisted of marked hypertrophy of the secretory glands and hyperchromatic and pleomorphic nuclei with occasional atypical mitotic figures suggestive of early adenocarcinoma. He felt these cellular changes were due to hormonal production from trophoblastic tissue:

> *Secretory change, usually exaggerated, with simultaneous proliferative activity of variable degree and cellular enlargement, principally of the nuclei, are main histological features which occur in these areas displaying maximum change. When extreme secretory activity is combined with an equally great proliferative effect, one sees groups of glands with very vacuolated, foamy cells, which are practically without lumens. Here and there are cells with hypertrophic nuclei, sometimes monstrously enlarged and hyperchromatic. Usually these enlarged nuclei show variations in shape, some being lobulated or elongated while others assume more bizarre forms.*

Later, he and others emphasised the association of this pattern with ectopic pregnancy. In the days before sensitive hCG assays, ultrasound and laparoscopy, the finding of the Arias-Stella endometrial reaction without chorionic villi at uterine curettage was a diagnostic pointer to ectopic pregnancy. Subsequently it has been commonly found with intrauterine pregnancy and in response to pharmacological induction of ovulation. It was later pointed out that Somers Sturgis (1905–1991), working in the ovarian dysfunction clinic of the Massachusetts General Hospital, Boston, had described these endometrial changes in the 1930s.

Javier Arias-Stella, a pathologist from Lima, Peru, was born on 2 August 1924. He described his findings

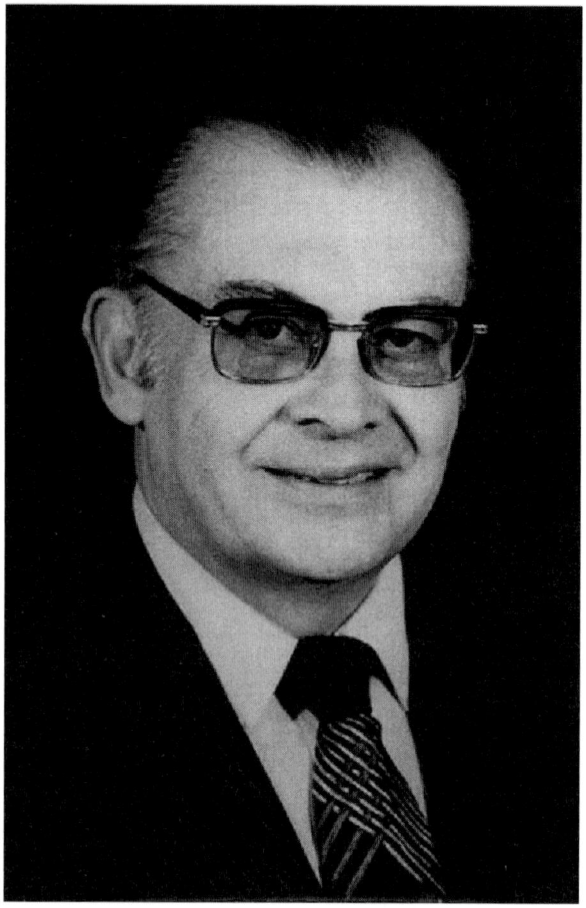

Javier Arias-Stella

while working as a Kellogg Foundation fellow in pathology at the Memorial Center for Cancer and Allied Diseases in New York. In 1962 he was appointed head of the department of pathology at the Peruvian University in Lima. He was later active in political life and was appointed minister of public health (1963), minister of foreign affairs (1980) and, in 1983, permanent representative of Peru to the United Nations.

Selected Publications

Arias-Stella J. Atypical endometrial changes associated with the presence of chorionic tissue. *Arch Pathol* 1954; 58: 112–28.

Arias-Stella J, Gutierrez J. Frecuencia y significado de las atipias endometriales en el embarazo ectopico. *Rev Lat Amer Anat Patol* 1957; 1: 81–7.

Sturgis SH. Duration of secretory activity in the glands of the decidua vera. *Am J Obstet Gynecol* 1938; 35: 752–61.

Sturgis SH. Arias-Stella phenomenon. *Am J Obstet Gynecol* 1973; 116: 589.

Bibliography References

968, 1413, 1480.

Aschheim, Selmar (1878–1965)
Zondek, Bernhard (1891–1966)

Aschheim–Zondek Pregnancy Test

For centuries physicians and quacks, sometimes one and the same, have made medical predictions from inspection of the urine. They were appropriately known as 'piss prophets', and one of the most common predictions was that of pregnancy. In 1928 Aschheim and Zondek, working at the Charité Hospital in Berlin, reported a sensitive and specific test for pregnancy based on a substance in the urine that stimulated the ovarian follicles of mice. They thought this was the gonadotrophic-stimulating substance produced by the anterior pituitary, which they had discovered earlier that year and called prolan. They believed there were two components to prolan: one governing follicle maturation (prolan A) and the other luteinisation (prolan B). These were later called follicle stimulating hormone (FSH) and luteinising hormone (LH).

The test consisted of injecting the first morning specimen of urine subcutaneously into 3- to 4-week-old mice. The test was positive if haemorrhagic ovarian follicles or corpora lutea developed after five days. The test was positive in 77 of 78 pregnant women, and there were only two false positive results in 198 controls. This level of sensitivity and specificity was a stunning development at the time. Understandably, but incorrectly, they attributed the reaction to the high output of anterior pituitary hormone in pregnancy:

> *We cannot demonstrate any specific substance for pregnancy, for the anterior pituitary hormone is produced in every organism. The only thing characteristic of pregnancy is the tremendous increase in the anterior pituitary hormone and its heavy excretion in the urine.*

Subsequently, other work showed the hormone responsible to be produced by the placenta and not the pituitary, so it was given the name human chorionic gonadotrophin (hCG).

Selmar Aschheim was born on 4 October, 1878 in Berlin, Germany. His medical studies were taken at the universities of Freiburg, Hamburg and Berlin. He practised obstetrics and gynaecology and also worked at the gynaecological pathology laboratory at the Charité Hospital in Berlin, where he was appointed director in 1912. It was here that he and Zondek carried out their work on the pituitary–ovarian relationship. He became a professor at the University of Berlin in 1931 but had to leave in 1936 when Hitler's influence became manifest. He moved to France, was granted citizenship and eventually became director of the laboratory in the Maternité in Paris. He died on 15 February 1965.

Bernhard Zondek was born on 29 July 1891 to a family of doctors in Wronke, Germany. He received his MD from the University of Berlin in 1918. He chose postgraduate work in obstetrics and

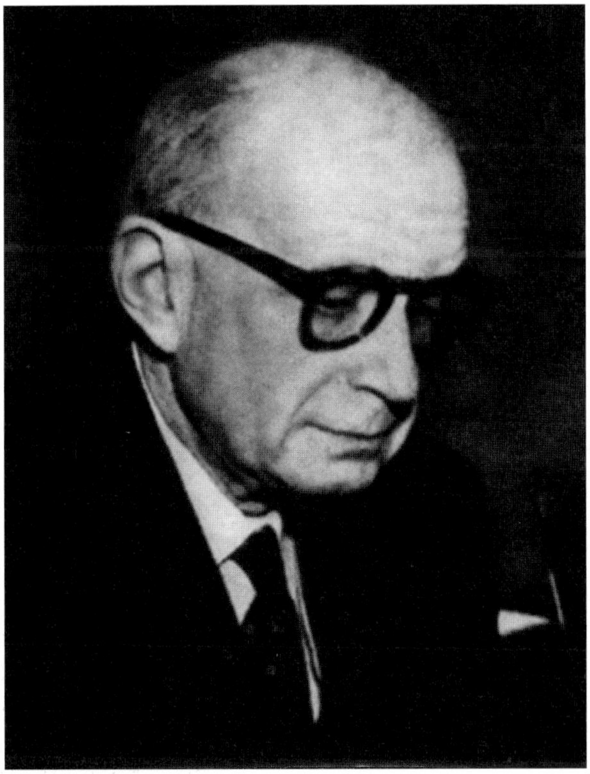

Selmar Aschheim

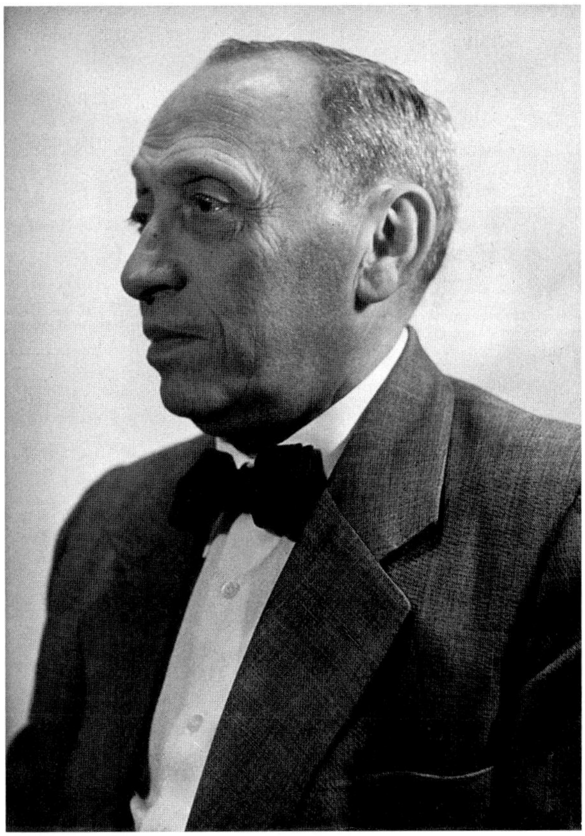

Bernhard Zondek

gynaecology, despite being discouraged by the professor owing to unimpressive marks in his final student examination on gynaecology. He later became a valued assistant to the same professor. In 1929 he was appointed chief of the department of obstetrics and gynaecology at the Berlin–Spandau Municipal Hospital. Hitler also caused Zondek's departure from Germany, and in 1933 he left for Stockholm, where he spent one year at the Biochemical Institute. In 1934 he emigrated to Israel and an appointment as professor of obstetrics and gynaecology and head of the hormone research laboratory at the Hebrew University–Hadassah Medical School in Jerusalem. He died on 8 November 1966.

Selected Publications

Aschheim S, Zondek B. Schwangerschaftsdiagnose aus dem Harn (durch Hormonnachweis). *Klin Wochenschr* 1928; 7: 8–9; 1404–11; 1453–7.

Bibliography References

549, 552, 734, 788, 1031, 1335, 1380, 1480, 1684, 1750.

Asherman, Joseph (1889–1968)

Asherman's Syndrome

Asherman's syndrome is described as amenorrhoea due to intrauterine adhesions following vigorous curettage, usually of the early pregnant or post-partum uterus:

> *This pathological reaction of the uterus is the outcome of a graver injury than usual, such as repeated or deep curettage for missed abortion . . . or as a result of a normal or even very slight injury when the uterus has been harmed by large-scale haemorrhage.*

In fact, Asherman's first report on the subject in 1948 did not describe endometrial destruction and adhesions as the cause of amenorrhoea. In a series of 29 cases treated between 1944 and 1946, he attributed the amenorrhoea to stenosis of the internal cervical os:

> *Following complicated labour or abortion a stenosis or blockage of the internal os of the cervix may occur under certain conditions, thus producing amenorrhoea. This amenorrhoea is not functional but organic; ovulation continues but the uterus does not react and the endometrium remains in a state of inactivity. Hormonal therapy is neither reasonable nor effective, whereas simple removal of the blockage is sufficient to restore menstruation to normal.*

Asherman felt that the stenosis was due not to fibrosis but to muscular contraction:

> *In our opinion, under certain conditions, the uterus reacts to curettage by tetanic contractions, which . . . may also continue so long as to become permanent . . . In the cases under consideration here, prolonged spastic stricture becomes organic in the course of time.*

The treatment was simple: the passage of a uterine sound through the internal os and dilatation up to Hegar 7–8. This successfully restored some degree of menstruation in 27 of the 29 cases, ten of whom achieved subsequent pregnancy, albeit with poor outcome in most. Because of the absence of haematometra in his and most other reported cases, Asherman felt that the endometrium remained 'quiescent' and was 'restored to activity as soon as the sound is introduced into the uterus'. He proposed the names 'amenorrhoea traumatica' or 'amenorrhoea atretica' to describe this condition.

In his subsequent report two years later, Asherman came closer to describing the pathological entity we now attribute to his name. Between 1948 and 1950 he collected 65 cases evaluated by hysterosalpingography and in these he correlated the findings of intrauterine adhesions with curettage: 'the regional obliteration of the uterine cavity, due to partial conglutination of the opposing uterine walls'. The menstrual pattern in these patients ranged from amenorrhoea to normal menstruation. For treatment he advocated hysterotomy and digital breakdown of the adhesions. He also speculated that hysteroscopy might become the treatment of choice (as it has):

> *Also, hysteroscopy, which has so often been mentioned in the literature and just as often discarded, may perhaps be of use for this purpose. If it were possible to see the adhesions and to loosen them instrumentally, using the eye as a guide, the ideal method would have been found.*

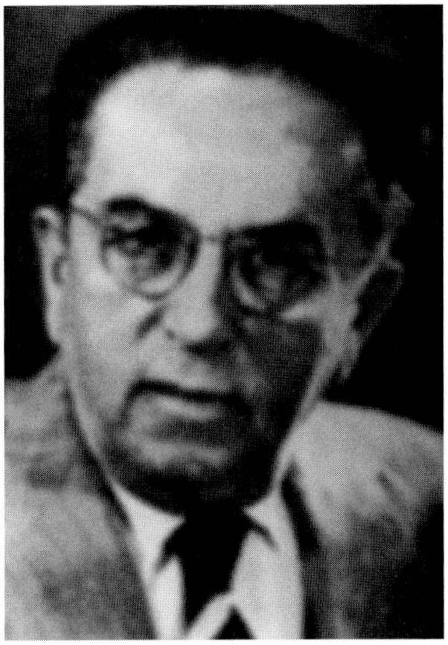

Joseph Asherman

Asherman was not the first to report the syndrome that bears his name. In 1894, Heinrich Fritsch (1844–1915) described a case of amenorrhoea associated with obliteration of the uterine cavity following vigorous uterine curettage for secondary post-partum haemorrhage. Two years before Asherman's original report, Stamer in Copenhagen reviewed the case reports in the literature and added 20 cases of his own, a fact acknowledged by Asherman in an addendum to his first paper.

Joseph Asherman was born on 11 September 1889 in Rosovice, Czechoslovakia and received his MD from Prague University in 1913. He emigrated to the part of Palestine that is now Israel in 1920 and worked in the department of obstetrics and gynaecology of the Hadassah Municipal Maternity Hospital, Tel Aviv. He was subsequently appointed director of the hospital, where he made many improvements, including the introduction of early post-partum mobilisation. Asherman developed the surgical management of vesicovaginal fistula, which meant that women no longer had to leave the country for treatment. As Head of the Advisory Council for Preventive Medicine he introduced welfare centres for impoverished pregnant women and their children. In the 1950s Asherman was appointed director of the 'Popular Sick Fund', a programme of the Hadassah Organisation that organised medical clinics for the poor. He was elected the first president of the Israeli Society of Obstetrics and Gynaecology in 1927. He retired in 1963 and died on 10 October 1968.

Selected Publications

Asherman JG. Amenorrhoea traumatica (atretica). *J Obstet Gynaecol Br Emp* 1948; 55: 23–30.

Asherman JG. Traumatic intra-uterine adhesions. *J Obstet Gynaecol Br Emp* 1950; 57: 892–6.

Fritsch H. Ein fall von volligem schwund der gebaumutterhohle nach Auskratzung. *Zentralbl Gynäkol* 1894; 52: 52–4.

Stamer S. Partial and total atresia of the uterus after excochleation. *Acta Obstet Gynecol Scand* 1946; 26: 263–97.

Bibliography References

2, 968, 1448, 1565.

Aveling, James Hobson (1828–1892)

Aveling's Repositor

Of the various mechanical contraptions used in an attempt to replace cases of chronic uterine inversion, the sigmoid repositor of Aveling proved to be the most successful. It consisted of a hard wooden cup fitted to the fundus of the inverted uterus with gentle continuous upward pressure provided by elastic bands attached to the end of sigmoid-shaped metal stems below and attached to a waist belt above. The belt was kept in place by shoulder braces. In Aveling's report on the subject he described 10 cases of chronic uterine inversion, cured by use of his repositor over intervals ranging from two months to nine years:

> *It was a case of obstinate chronic inversion, to be related more fully presently, which induced me to invent the sigmoid repositor . . . I had, in 1868, invented sigmoid*

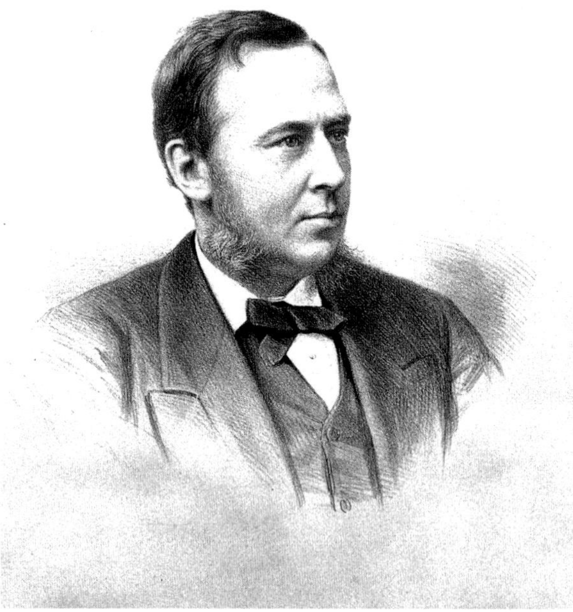

James Hobson Aveling

axis-traction forceps, ten years before those of Tarnier, which have the same form, and, remembering that the sigmoid shape of this forceps gave traction in the axis of the pelvic inlet, I came to the conclusion that axis-pushing in the same line might be effected by a repositor having the sigmoid form . . . My anticipations have been fulfilled in a most satisfactory and gratifying manner, for I shall now have the pleasure of relating ten cases of chronic inversion, which have been treated and cured by my sigmoid repositor.

Aveling also invented a simple device for direct blood transfusion from a donor. He carried this with him for eight years, 'until at length the opportunity for using it arrived'. The occasion, in 1872, was a woman with post-partum haemorrhage who was given about 250 ml of her coachman's blood. Aveling's device consisted of two silver canulae, inserted into the donor and recipient respectively and connected by rubber tubing with a compressible bulb in the middle.

James Hobson Aveling was born at Whittlesea, Cambridgeshire. He studied medicine at Aberdeen, winning the gold medal in anatomy. In 1856 he was appointed lecturer in midwifery and diseases of women and children in the Sheffield School of Medicine. In 1871 he moved to London and helped found the Chelsea Hospital for Women. It was said that part of his motivation was that, at 43, he was too old to accept a junior position and not old enough to obtain a senior appointment at an established London hospital. Thus, he founded his own eight-bed hospital.

Aveling was a considerable medical historian and wrote authoritatively on the origins of midwifery and forceps.

Selected Publications

Aveling JH. Immediate transfusion in England: seven cases, and the author's method of operating. *Obstet J Gr Brit Irel* 1873; 289: 311.

Aveling JH. A repositor for inversion of the uterus. *Trans Obstet Soc Lond* 1878; 20: 126–30.

Aveling JH. A lecture on inversion of the uterus: with ten cases successfully treated by the sigmoid repositor. *BMJ* 1886; 1: 475–81.

Bibliography References

42–48, 57, 155, 648, 721, 756, 1000, 1495, 1604.

Ayre, James Ernest (1910–1974)

Ayre's Spatula

James Ernest Ayre was born in the small town of Tilsonburg, Ontario on 29 July 1910. As a son of the manse and one of eight children he was raised in modest circumstances in Western Canada during the drought and depression. He graduated in medicine from the University of Alberta, Edmonton, in 1936. After a spell in rural general practice in Lethbridge, Alberta, he took training in obstetrics and gynaecology at the Royal Victoria Hospital, Montreal. He became lecturer at McGill University and director of the gynaecological cytology laboratory at the Royal Victoria Hospital. On three separate occasions he spent one week with George Papanicolaou, learning cytology techniques in his New York laboratory.

His main contribution was to refine the collection of cells from the cervix, initially pioneered by Papanicolaou. Ayre pointed out that directly scraping cells from the squamocolumnar junction, rather than aspirating exfoliated cells from the posterior vaginal fornix, produced a direct sample of well-preserved cells from the affected area improving the diagnostic interpretation. He designed a wooden spatula with different shaped ends to accommodate the variable architecture of the squamocolumnar junction and likened this technique to a surface biopsy:

> *Previous cytology smear techniques consisted of the aspiration of cells which had already been exfoliated. The spatula technique is a means of collecting the cells before their exfoliation. This is performed simply by utilizing a small spatula to scrape gently the surface of the tissues at the precise squamocolumnar junction ... This method permits selectivity of cells collected, so that a large concentration of squamous cells from this key point may be studied while they are still in an excellent state of preservation before they have become shrunken or degenerated.*

Ayre published his technique in both the academic and public sectors. The latter brought him into conflict with Montreal's medical and hospital establishments. In the academic world his work was praised, and he travelled and lectured widely. Ayre made a deliberate decision to put his message before the lay public, which in the 1940s was considered inappropriate by many in the medical establishment. His claim that cancer of the cervix could be prevented was not accepted: 'If every woman over the age of 20 took the cytology test once a year, advanced and incurable cases of uterine cancer would become a medical rarity'. This conflict culminated in his resignation in 1951. He moved to Miami to become director of the Dade County Cancer Institute. He later went to New York City, and became president of the National Cancer Cytology Centre in Jericho, Long Island. Ayre did

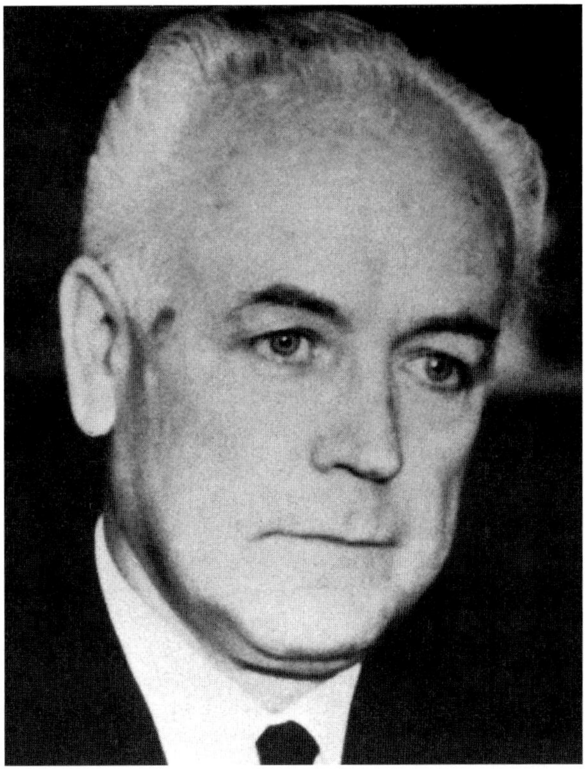

James Ernest Ayre

Ayre's spatula

not patent his spatula, which evolved from the wooden tongue depressors he used initially and with which millions of Pap smears have been and continue to be taken. In 1946 'Ayre's surface biopsy' scrapers were advertised for $2.00 per 100. He died in October 1974.

Selected Publications

Ayre JE. Selective cytology smear for diagnosis of cancer. *Am J Obstet Gynecol* 1947; 53: 609–17.

Bibliography References

91, 178, 383, 665, 1099, 1100, 1389.

B

Baer, Karl Ernst Ritter von (1792–1876)

Human Ovum/Germ Layer Theory

In early May 1827, while studying the embryology of the dog, Baer observed, as had others, the free blastocyst in the fallopian tube. He realised that such small cells could not be the whole Graafian follicle and undertook closer scrutiny. In so doing he discovered the mammalian ovum:

> *Examining the ovaries before making any incision I saw plainly in almost every follicle a yellowish-white point . . . Led by curiosity . . . I opened one of the follicles and took up the minute object on the point of my knife, finding that I could see it very distinctly and that it was surrounded by mucous. When I placed it under the microscope I was utterly astonished, for I saw an ovule just as I had already seen in the tubes, and so clearly that a blind man could hardly deny it.*

In his other classic work, *Entwicklungsgeschichte der Thiere* (*Developmental History of Animals*), Baer enunciated his 'germ layer theory'. He laid the foundation of modern embryology, proposing that the ovum forms four layers of tissue from which arise the organs and other structures of the adult. The two middle layers were later regarded as one, to establish the modern three germ layers of the embryo: ectoderm, mesoderm and endoderm.

> *Every animal which springs from the coition of male and female is developed from an ovum, and none from a simple, formative liquid. The male semen acts through the membrane of the ovum, which is not pervious by any foramen, and in the ovum it acts first on certain innate parts of the ovum. All development proceeds from the centre to the periphery. Therefore the central parts are formed before the peripheral. The same method of development occurs in all vertebrate animals beginning at the spine.*

Karl Ernst Ritter von Baer was born in Piep, Estonia, one of 10 children descended from German nobility. Initially trained for a military career, he switched to medicine and graduated from the University of Dorpat, Russia in 1814. He was not impressed with many of his professors, whom he said 'suffered from a surfeit of rather useless scholarship'. In 1812, while still a medical student, he volunteered for service in an army hospital when Napoleon invaded Russia. He continued his medical studies in Berlin and Vienna but forsook clinical medicine to pursue anatomy and embryology at Würzburg. He served successively as professor of zoology in Königsberg, where his work on the mammalian and human ovum was done, and at St Petersburg. Baer introduced the term 'spermatozoa', thinking the 'animalcules' in seminal fluid were parasites. Honoured during his lifetime, an island in the Russian north was named for him.

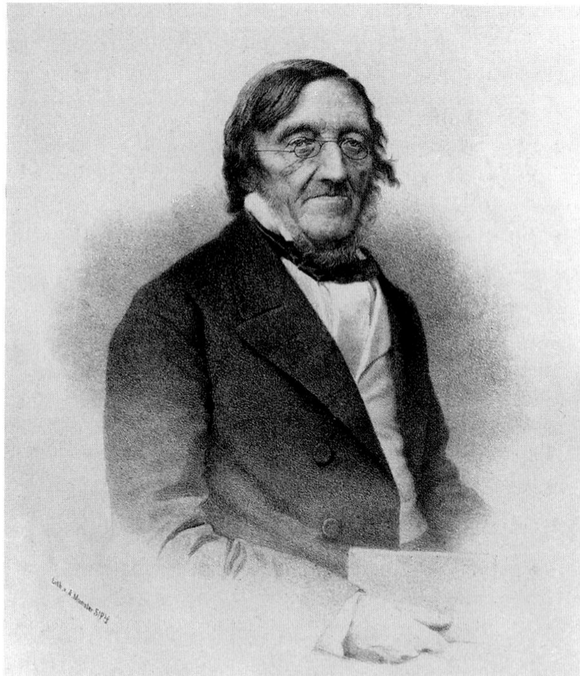

Karl Ernst Ritter von Baer

Selected Publications

Baer KE von. *De ovi mammalium et hominis genesi*. Leipzig: L. Voss, 1827.

Baer KE von. *Über Entwickelungsgeschichte der Thiere*. Königsberg: Gebrüder Bornträger, 1828.

Bibliography References

50, 286, 406, 615, 676, 873, 969, 1031, 1102, 1141, 1142, 1214, 1480, 1526.

Baillie, Matthew (1761–1823)

Ovarian Dermoid Cyst

Matthew Baillie, nephew of the famous Hunter brothers, William and John, was the first to give the definitive description of a dermoid cyst of the ovary. He described this in a paper to the Royal Society in 1789:

> *The fatty mass was of a yellowish white colour, in some places more yellow than others. It was very unctuous to the feeling . . . The hair with which the fatty substance was mixed grew out of the inner surface of the capsule containing it . . . They resembled much more the hairs of the head . . . There arose also from the inner surface of the capsule some vestiges of human teeth.*

Baillie dismissed the theory that such tumours were rudimentary ovarian pregnancies requiring intercourse and male semen to occur. As he was to write in his book, *Morbid Anatomy of Some of the Most Important Parts of the Human Body*, in 1793:

> *This change has been generally considered as the very imperfect rudiments of a fetus which had been formed in the ovarium. As, however, this change can take place in the ovarium before the uterus would appear capable of these functions which begin at the age of puberty and when the hymen in its entirety, it is highly probable that it is independent of impregnation.*

Matthew Baillie was born at the Manse of Shotts in Lanarkshire, Scotland on 27 October 1761. His father, Revd James Baillie, later became professor of divinity in the University of Glasgow. His mother, Dorothea, was the sister of William and John Hunter, the celebrated anatomists and surgeons. Matthew Baillie began his early education in the English and Latin schools at Hamilton and at the age of 13 went to the University of Glasgow, taking classics and philosophy. This was followed by a further two years of study at Balliol College, Oxford. Following the advice of his uncles he went to London in 1780 to live with his uncle, William Hunter, and attended his lectures in anatomy and dissection at the Great Windmill Street School. He quickly became an expert in anatomical dissection and also attended the surgical lectures of his other uncle, John Hunter, and lectures in medicine and in midwifery given by Thomas Denman.

Before William Hunter died in 1783, he arranged for Baillie to follow him as lecturer in anatomy at the Great Windmill Street School. He also left Baillie a legacy of £5,000 and a small estate at the Hunter birth place in Long Calderwood. Baillie felt that the estate should more properly belong to William Hunter's younger brother, John, and ceded Long Calderwood to him. Soon after this, Baillie received his BA and MD from Oxford University. He continued to lecture in anatomy at the Windmill Street school for 15 years. In 1787 he was appointed physician to St George's Hospital, London and in 1790 was awarded Fellowship of the Royal College of Physicians, London. In 1791 he made a career-enhancing move by marrying the youngest of twin daughters of Thomas Denman, whose lectures in obstetrics he had attended 10 years before. However, by this time his reputation was already growing and a large private practice began to consume most of his time. It is said that to meet the commitments of his practice he had to work from 6 a.m. until 11 p.m. each day.

In addition to his many papers, Baillie's *Morbid Anatomy* was extremely popular, running to eight editions in English as well as American, French, German and Italian editions. Using clinical, anatomical and pathological correlation he helped define the

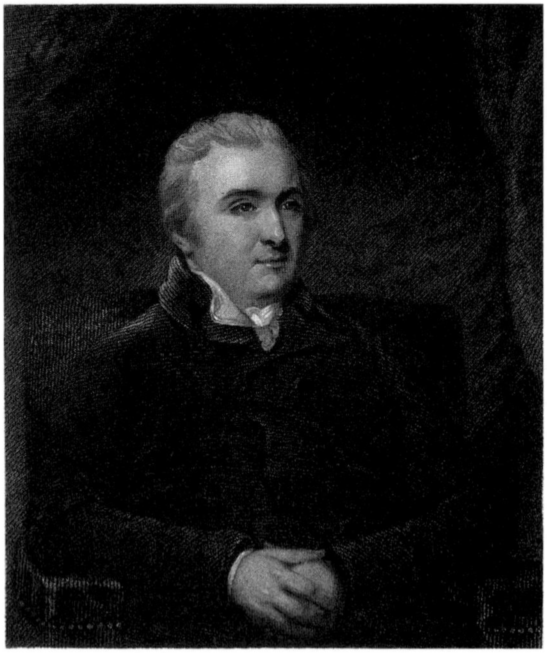

Matthew Baillie

diseases of cirrhosis and emphysema. In *Morbid Anatomy* he depicted the emphysematous lungs of Dr Samuel Johnson. He also made the link between cirrhosis and alcoholism: 'For this disease is most frequently found in hard drinkers'. Baillie also included an early description of hydrosalpinx or 'dropsy' of the fallopian tube. Over a period of 20 years, Matthew Baillie collected more than 1,200 anatomical and pathological museum specimens. In 1818 he presented this collection to the Royal College of Physicians of London, and in 1938 the specimens were transferred to the Royal College of Surgeons of England. Sadly, during the 1941 air raids in London the entire collection was destroyed, along with much of the Hunterian collection.

Baillie's reputation was such that he was appointed physician extraordinary to King George III. In the summer of 1823 he developed a severe and persistent cough and died on 23 September 1823. There are busts of Matthew Baillie in the Royal College of Surgeons of England, the Royal College of Physicians of London and in the Chapel of St Andrews, Westminster Abbey.

Selected Publications

Baillie M. An account of a particular change of structure in the human ovarium. *Phil Trans R Soc* 1789; 79: 71–8.

Baillie M. *The Morbid Anatomy of Some of the Most Important Parts of the Body*. London: J. Johnson & G. Nichol, 1793.

Bibliography References

108, 224, 322, 324, 577, 643, 753, 919, 1176, 1292, 1317, 1318, 1495, 1602, 1664, 1705.

Baird, Dugald (1900–1986)

Birth Control/Perinatal Epidemiology

In January 1941, Franklin Roosevelt delivered a speech in which he advocated a 'world founded upon four essential freedoms'. These were freedom of speech, freedom to worship, freedom from want and freedom from fear. In 1965 Sir Dugald Baird, Regius Professor of Midwifery at Aberdeen University wrote: 'I would suggest that it is time to consider a fifth freedom – freedom from the tyranny of excessive fertility'. No individual in Great Britain in the previous 30 years had done as much as Dugald Baird to make this fifth freedom a practical reality for women under his care.

Dugald Baird qualified in medicine in 1922 from the University of Glasgow. When he was a medical student and house officer the maternal mortality rate at the Glasgow Royal Maternity Hospital was approximately 25 per thousand, with an average of two maternal deaths in the hospital every week. His decision to practise obstetrics and gynaecology was partly influenced by his admiration for Munro Kerr, who appointed him resident registrar in his department at the Glasgow Royal Infirmary two years after his graduation. Dugald Baird was profoundly influenced by the squalid conditions in the slums of Glasgow when he was attending home confinements as a medical student:

> *The contrast between childbearing in the upper social classes and in the slum dwellers set me thinking about social class differences in the whole field of reproduction, so my lasting interest in social research in the field of obstetrics began.*

He once said, 'My maternal grandfather was a well-known breeder of Clydesdale horses. By the time I was 14 I was quite an expert on sex and reproduction. Mares received better attention in 1914 than some women today'.

In 1937 Baird was appointed Regius Professor of Midwifery at Aberdeen University and obstetrician-in-chief at the Aberdeen Maternity Hospital. On his arrival he set about improving the clinical services in obstetrics and gynaecology, resulting in an impressive fall in maternal and perinatal mortality. With the establishment of the National Health Service in 1948, Baird had an opportunity to do population-based research because of the city's centralised hospital service, and the additional responsibility for the whole northeastern region with a population of 500,000. During the 1940s and 1950s Baird published many papers on the different maternal and perinatal outcomes in pregnancy related to social class. He took the unprecedented step of appointing non-medical staff to his department, including dieticians, physiologists, social workers, health visitors, statisticians and psychologists. His research attracted the support of the Medical Research Council, which established an independent Obstetric Medicine Research Unit in Aberdeen with Baird as the honorary director. From 1948, all of the social and clinical data on pregnancies were recorded on cards, and this later formed the basis of the computerised Aberdeen Maternity and Neonatal Databank. Work from this unit highlighted the high perinatal mortality and maternal morbidity in women of lower social class, small stature and poor nutrition.

Baird did not neglect the gynaecological side of his professorial mandate. In 1960 he initiated one of the first cervical pap smear screening programmes. When the staff member responsible proudly informed him that she had screened 80 per cent of the women in the area, he acknowledged the achievement and asked, 'And when are you going to chase up the missing twenty?'

Early in his career at Aberdeen, Baird also turned his attention to the social welfare of women and, in particular, provided practical assistance for birth control. From the 1940s he provided termination of pregnancy and sterilisation services, when these were not generally available in Britain. He kept careful statistics on these patients and provided data in support of the Abortion Bill when it was put before the UK parliament in 1967. In both the fields of birth control and perinatal epidemiology he was a generation ahead of his time. He was knighted in 1959 and he and his wife, also a physician and chair of the Northeast Regional Hospital Board, were jointly given the freedom of the City of Aberdeen in 1966. He retired from the Regius chair in 1965 but continued his research, and by 1969 published results of a survey of the development of 16,000 seven-year-old children in Aberdeen. He and his wife, who died three years before him, had four

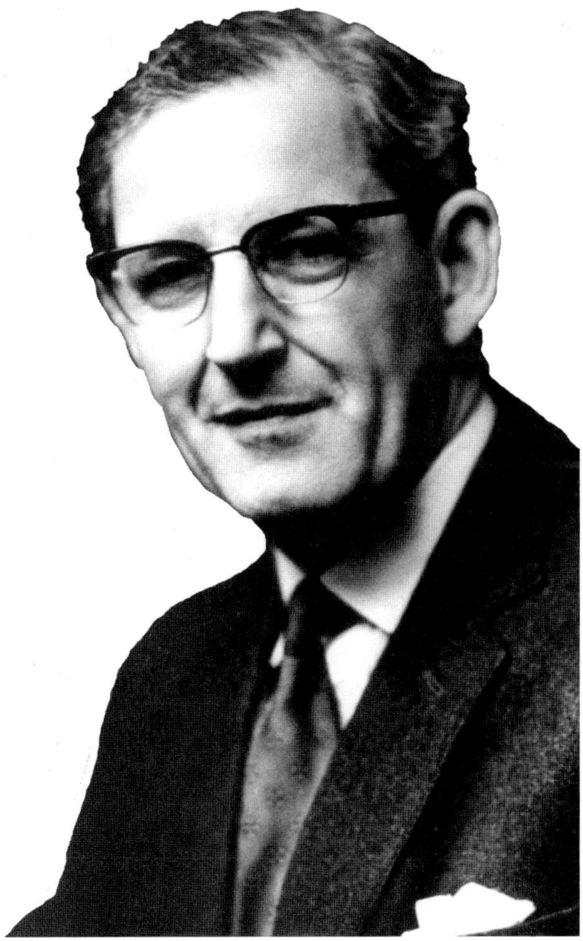

Dugald Baird

children, one of whom subsequently became professor of obstetrics and gynaecology at the University of Edinburgh. He was revered by staff and patients, one of the latter saying, 'He was a marvellous man, he would treat a tinker the same as a queen, making every one of his patients feel important'.

In his final publication, written when he was 85 years old, Baird reviewed the great improvements in maternal and perinatal mortality and discussed the social and emotional aspects of reproduction that faced women, particularly those with a career:

> *The number of people with the combination of intelligence, ability, personality, vigour, common sense and sense of humour necessary to 'get to the top' and make a success of it is limited. Society cannot therefore afford to neglect 50% of such people because they happen to be women. Nor indeed can it afford to do without the able children they might produce.*

During an interview in 1980 he said, 'Life's more interesting if you exert yourself, and do things, and you can hope that you're making the world, at the end of the day, a little more attractive for the people who are coming along'. Sir Dugald Baird died in Edinburgh in November 1986.

Selected Publications

Baird D. The influence of social and economic factors on stillbirths and neonatal deaths. *J Obstet Gynaecol Br Emp* 1945; 52: 339–66.

Baird D. Variation in reproduction patterns according to social class. *Lancet* 1946; 2: 41–4.

Baird D. Social class and fetal mortality. *Lancet* 1947; 2: 531–5.

Baird D. A fifth freedom? *BMJ* 1965; 2: 1141–8.

Baird D. Changing problems and priority in obstetrics. *Br J Obstet Gynaecol* 1985;92: 115–21.

Bibliography References

51–53, 263, 272, 288, 367, 936, 1019, 1124, 1186, 1587.

Baldy, John Montgomery (1860–1934) Webster, John Clarence (1863–1950)

Baldy–Webster Uterine Ventrosuspension

Webster, working in Chicago, and Baldy, from Philadelphia, independently developed a virtually identical surgical technique for uterine ventrosuspension. It came to be called the Baldy–Webster operation. In 1901 Webster published his half-page report of the operation he had carried out 'during the past year'. Baldy reported his technique in 1902 'after a few years' trial'. The essence of the procedure was described by Webster:

> *The fundus of the uterus is elevated and pushed forward. A small hole is then made through the broad ligament on one side under the utero-ovarian ligament near the uterus. Through it a pair of forceps is passed from behind in order to grasp the round ligament about an inch from its uterine end. The latter is then pulled through the broad ligament in a double fold. It is carried across the back of the uterus a short distance above the utero-sacral ligaments and is then stitched in this position with chromic catgut. A similar procedure is carried out on the other side, the second round ligament being stitched to the back of the uterus above or below the first one or crossing it. The amount of overlapping of the round ligaments depends upon their length and laxity.*

Baldy developed a sceptical attitude to the indications and benefits of ventrosuspension long before general medical opinion recognised the limitations and overuse of the operation. In his opening remarks to a symposium on the operative treatment of retroversion of the uterus, held at the Philadelphia Medical Society on 9 December 1914 he stated: 'In my opinion nine-tenths of the operations performed on women for retrodisplacements are uncalled for'. He went on to dismiss the need for the more than 50 variations of the operation for ventrosuspension and concluded with a cynical salvo:

> *I am sorry to say it, but it looks to me as though the possible number of retrodisplacement operations performed in this country is limited only by the number of females in existence.*

John Montgomery Baldy was born in Danville, Pennsylvania, and graduated from the University of Pennsylvania medical school in 1884. After general practice in the town of Scranton he returned to Philadelphia for postgraduate training in gynaecology. In 1891 he was appointed professor of gynaecology at the Philadelphia Polyclinic Hospital. He was president of the American Gynecological Society in 1908. Ten years after his retirement he died of a bullet wound by his own hand.

John Clarence Webster was born in Shediac, New Brunswick. His mother came from Yorkshire and his father was born at sea en route to Canada from Scotland. In 1882 he was about to embark for Edinburgh when he fell ill with typhoid fever. This was a fortuitous fever, as the boat on which he would have sailed was lost at sea with all hands. He took up his medical studies in Edinburgh the following year and excelled, graduating MB in 1888 and MD, with gold medal, in 1890. He spent time in the pathology laboratories of both Leipzig and Berlin. In 1890 he became first assistant to the professor of obstetrics and gynaecology in Edinburgh, Alexander Simpson (1835–1916). In the damp Scottish climate, he suffered badly from recurrent bronchitis and with reluctance, on medical advice, he returned to Canada in 1896. He spent two years as assistant gynaecologist at the Royal Victoria Hospital, Montreal. In 1899 he accepted the offer of the chair of obstetrics and gynaecology at Rush Medical College in the University of Chicago. He held this position until he retired in 1920, at the age of 57.

Returning to his hometown, Webster spent the last 30 years of his life in the research and restoration of Canadian historical sites and mementoes. During this time, he published more than 50 papers and several books on Canadian history. He served as chairman of the Historic Sites and Monuments Board of Canada from 1943 until his death. On 16 March 1950 he took his usual morning walk, returned home, sat down in his favourite chair and died.

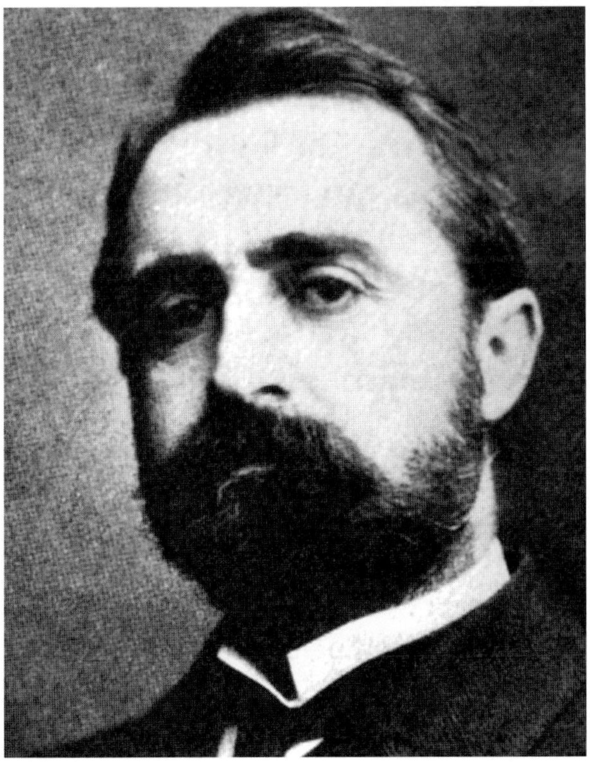

John Montgomery Baldy

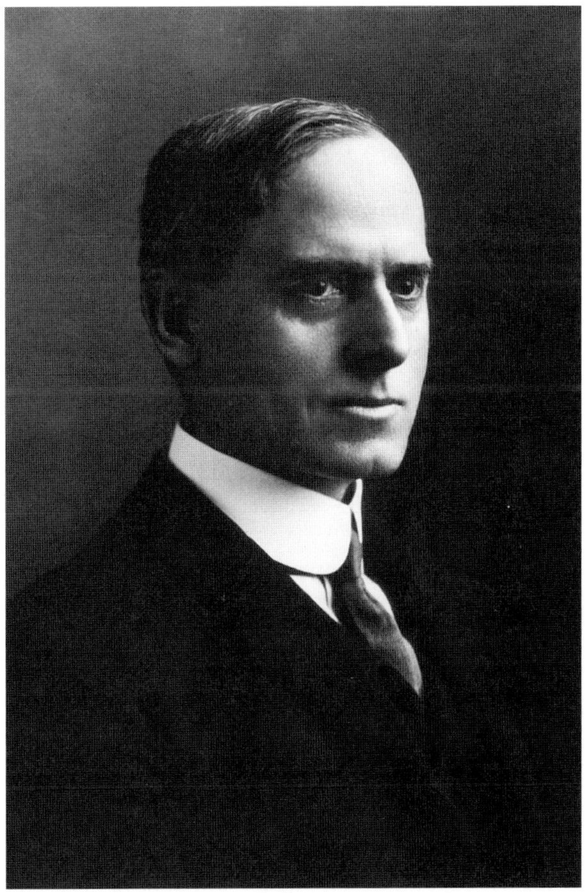

John Clarence Webster

Selected Publications

Baldy JM. A new operation for retrodisplacement. *Am J Obstet* 1902; 45: 650–4.

Baldy JM. The surgical treatment of retroversion of the uterus. *Surg Gynecol Obstet* 1915; 20: 614–5.

Webster JC. A satisfactory operation for certain cases of retroversion of the uterus. *JAMA* 1901; 37: 913.

Bibliography References

91, 163, 366, 648, 705, 801, 842, 1053, 1253, 1359, 1467, 1480, 1507.

Ballantyne, John William (1861–1923)

Antenatal Care

Until the early part of the twentieth century, there was virtually no antenatal care for pregnant women. Medical involvement was largely confined to antenatal catastrophes and the management of complicated labour. In 1901 John Ballantyne of Edinburgh requested, and was granted, one bed at the Royal Maternity Hospital for the care of unmarried mothers who became ill during pregnancy. Over the ensuing years he established the value of antenatal care and what he called 'pre-maternity hospital practice'. In recording the results in his report of 1909, he noted:

> *They prove completely that there exists a rapidly increasing demand among medical men for some place in which morbid pregnancies can be kept under observation and suitably treated. It needs no great powers of prevision to state that in fifteen or twenty years there will have arisen an important branch of obstetrics dealing with the management of abnormal pregnancy.*

Ballantyne was one of the first to recognise the hazards of prolonged pregnancy:

> *The post-mature infant has stayed too long in intrauterine surroundings: he has remained so long in utero that he has difficulty to be born with safety to himself and his mother.*

John William Ballantyne was born in Midlothian, Scotland, in 1861 and graduated in 1883 from Edinburgh, where he remained for the rest of his professional life. In 1885 he became assistant to Professor AR Simpson and by 1904 he was appointed chief physician to the Edinburgh Royal Infirmary. He was elected president of the Edinburgh Obstetrical Society in 1905.

His greatest work was the publication of *Antenatal Pathology and Hygiene: The Embryo and Foetus*, published in two volumes between 1902 and 1904. Many of his writings predicted the development of perinatal medicine:

> *. . . the varied and intricate relations which are or may be established between the maternal and foetal organisms through them and as a result of them: in no physiological or pathological laboratory could more elaborate or instructive experiments be devised and carried through than are to be witnessed in the uterus, when the mother is*

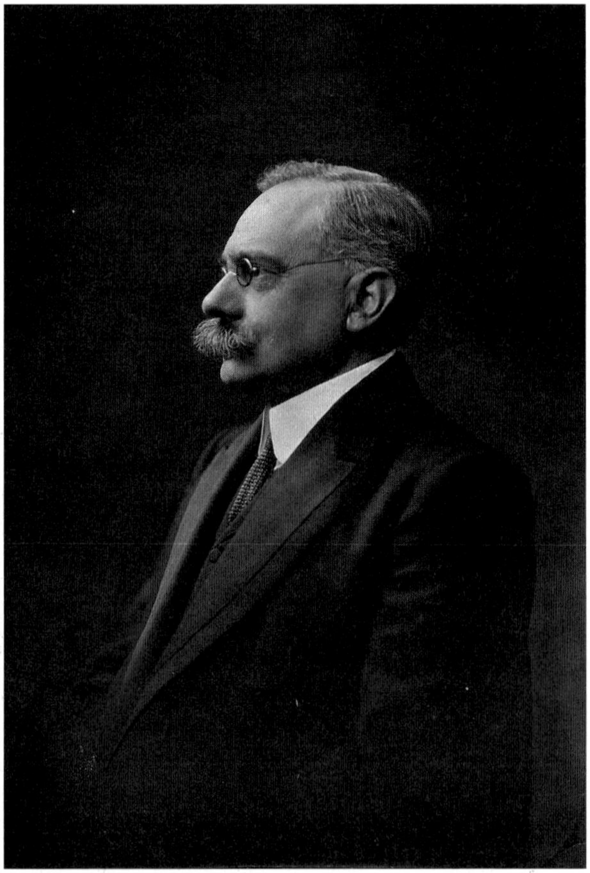

John William Ballantyne

> *the subject of a malady which is known to be transmissible . . . To some extent it may be said that the etiology of the transmitted foetal diseases is within our knowledge, and their diagnosis not altogether outside our grasp; with perseverance and skill their treatment will yet be hopefully undertaken by the well-informed physician.*

In his last publication Ballantyne foresaw the development of neonatology:

> *There is need for specialisation in neonatal medicine. This applies to doctors and nurses as well as teaching and construction of hospitals. The specialist in neonatal diseases and the nurse intensively trained and expert in the management of delicate newborns will be common place ere long.*

John Ballantyne died at the age of 61, shortly after the removal of a gangrenous appendix.

Selected Publications

Ballantyne JW. *Antenatal Pathology and Hygiene: The Embryo and The Foetus*. 2 vols. Edinburgh: William Green and Sons; 1902 and 1904.

Ballantyne JW. Pre-maternity hospital practice. *J Obstet Gynaecol Br Emp* 1909; 15: 93–107, 169–86.

Ballantyne JW. The new midwifery. *BMJ* 1923; 1: 617–21.

Bibliography References

37, 62, 72, 200, 305, 321, 464, 648, 777, 822, 956, 1181, 1202, 1279, 1435, 1558, 1665, 1690.

Bandl, Ludwig (1842–1892)

Bandl's Contraction Ring

Ludwig Bandl was professor of obstetrics and gynaecology at Vienna and Prague. He pointed out that the upper part of the uterus contracted to actively expel the fetus, while the lower part passively dilated. In cases of obstructed labour, rupture nearly always occurred in the lower uterine segment. One of the dramatic cases Bandl reviewed was of a despairing woman who drowned herself during labour in May 1870. Her body was recovered shortly thereafter and frozen. At longitudinal section Bandl noted a prominent muscular ring at the junction of the upper and lower uterine segments. Later this sign of advanced obstructed labour was to be called Bandl's contraction ring. In describing such a case Bandl wrote,

> *I found the internal os at the level of the umbilicus. The whole cervix was uniformly paper thin and enormously stretched out, so that it must surely have contained half the infant, while the body of the uterus and fundus sat on the infant like a cap . . . the conditions in this case were obviously most favourable for rupture of the uterus. It would have taken only one or two additional contractions of the uterus or the increased pressure of the physician's hand or an assistant to bring it about.*

Bandl was born on 1 November 1842 in Himberg, southern Austria. He studied medicine under Carl Braun in Vienna. In 1880 he was appointed professor of gynaecology at the University of Vienna. Bandl was

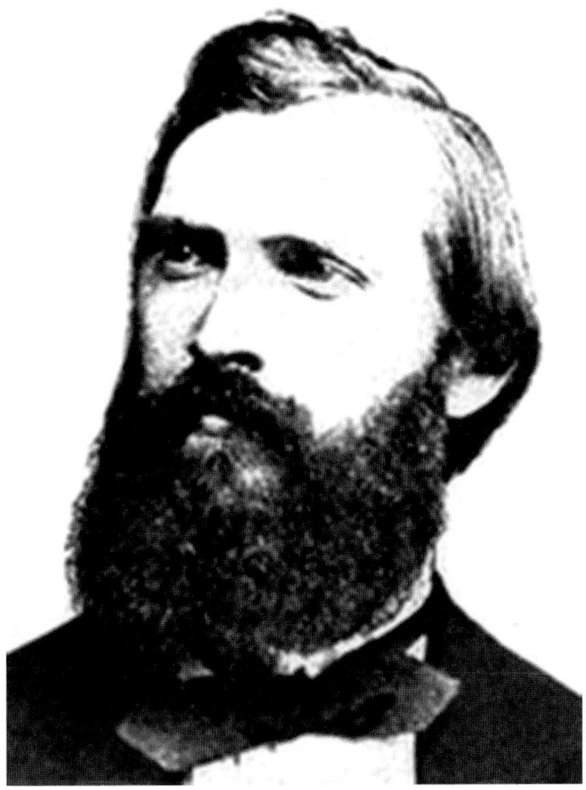

Ludwig Bandl

called to succeed August Breisky as professor of obstetrics and gynaecology at Prague in 1886. He suffered from depression and anxiety, feeling that he might not be up to the standards of his eminent predecessor. Indeed, he withdrew from his inaugural lecture. His obituary was prematurely published in the *American Journal of Obstetrics* in 1887, followed soon after by a retraction. Bandl's later years were plagued by melancholy and he was finally admitted to a psychiatric institution in Doebling, where he died on 26 August 1892.

Selected Publications

Bandl L. *Über Ruptur der Gebärmutter und ihre Mechanik.* Vienna: Czermak, 1875.

Bandl L. *Über das Verhalten des Uterus und Cervix in der Schwangerschaft und während der Geburt.* Stuttgart: F. Enke, 1876.

Bibliography References

648, 649, 987, 1480, 1486, 1595.

Barcroft, Joseph (1872–1947)

Fetal Physiology

Joseph Barcroft was born at the Glen, Newry, Northern Ireland on 26 July 1872. His parents were English Quakers and his father worked in the linen industry in Ulster. After schooling in England, Barcroft undertook his university studies in physiology at Cambridge, where he was to remain for the rest of his academic career. After obtaining a first-class honours degree at King's College, Cambridge, in 1896, he was made a fellow, later lecturer, at King's and was appointed professor of physiology in 1925. In his early years he worked on the circulation and respiratory function of blood. He was involved in high-altitude cardiopulmonary physiology and participated in three high-altitude expeditions to study the effects of hypoxaemia. Mount Barcroft in California was named for him.

In 1932, at the age of 60, Barcroft turned the focus of his scientific research to the physiology of the developing fetus. His studies included:

measurement of fetal blood volume and placental blood flow, the circulation through the chest and fetal heart, the passage of oxygen and carbon dioxide across the placental membrane, the differences between maternal and fetal haemoglobin at various stages, the nervous control of respiration and of growth rate of the fetus and a host of other cognate problems.

Barcroft found that the oxygen tension in fetal blood was low, being some 25 per cent of that in the adult. This is equivalent to the oxygen tension at 10,000 feet and led to the phrase 'Mount Everest in utero'. This term was attributed to Barcroft, although it does not appear in his classic text, *Researches on Pre-natal Life*. Barcroft found that the fetus maintained an adequate supply of oxygen because of a number of factors, including a higher haemoglobin concentration, and a greater oxygen-binding capacity of fetal haemoglobin – the so-called 'oxygen-dissociation curve'. In addition, Barcroft studied fetal circulation in sheep delivered prematurely by caesarean section but with intrauterine conditions preserved by leaving the umbilical cord attached to the placenta and covering the face of the fetus with a bag containing amniotic fluid to prevent respiration. These studies suggested that there was preferential blood flow to vital organs: 'the heart and brain are given preferential treatment with respect to the supply of oxygenated blood coming from the placenta'.

Barcroft summarised the work of himself and others on fetal physiology in his *Researches on Pre-natal Life* and outlined the rationale for his book as follows:

> *The general aim then, of this book is to trace the development of function in the mammalian foetus, never*

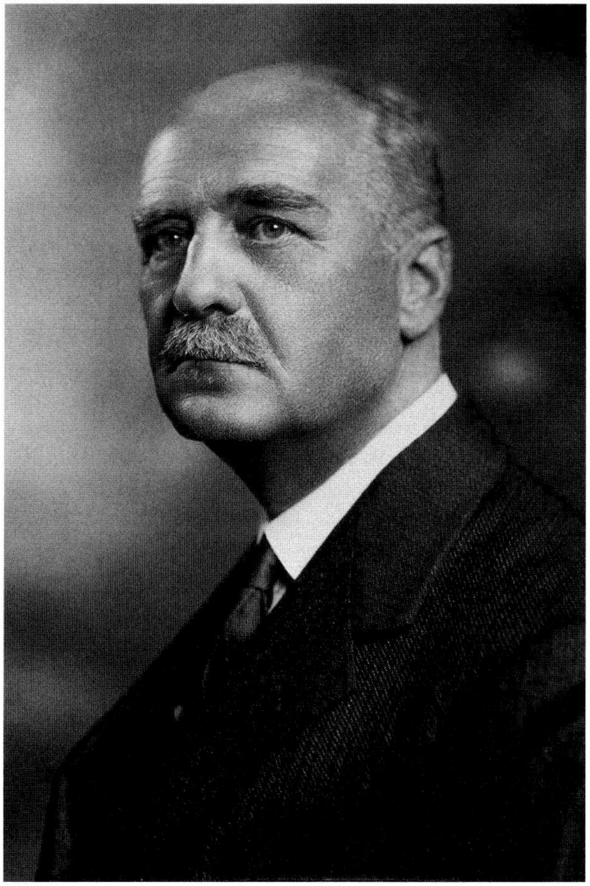

Joseph Barcroft

losing sight of the fact that one day the call will come and the foetus will be born. Not only has the foetus to develop a fundamental life which will suffice for intra-uterine conditions, but at the same time has to develop an economy which will withstand the birth and will suffice, nay more than suffice, for its new environment.

Many honours came to Barcroft in his time, including multiple honorary degrees and a knighthood in 1935. Sir Joseph Barcroft, Sir JB as he was known, was in his early seventies when, towards the end of the Second World War, he sat down to write *Researches on Pre-natal Life*. At the start of the preface he wrote,

> *This work partakes very much of the nature of a will – but I hope not my last. In the days of bombs it seemed to me only the due of the many who had given me encouragement and support, not least the Rockefeller Foundation, that I should sit down in some connected form such information as I had accumulated concerning pre-natal life; then, if the bomb came my way, the information, for what it was worth, would remain.*

Barcroft planned to write two volumes, the second of which was to deal largely with the nervous system and metabolic problems of prenatal life but died suddenly on 21 March 1947 of a myocardial infarction, soon after publication of the first volume. Sir Joseph Barcroft's work laid the scientific foundation for the next generation working in the field of fetal physiology, including Geoffrey Dawes. His research also paved the way for improved clinical perinatal and neonatal care, which was always the aim of his work.

Selected Publications

Barcroft J. *Researches on Pre-natal Life* (Vol. 1). Oxford: Blackwell; 1947.

Eastman NJ. Mount Everest in utero. *Am J Obstet Gynecol* 1954; 67: 701–11.

Bibliography References

474, 528, 873, 1202, 1215, 1267, 1737.

Bard, Samuel (1742–1821)

First American Obstetric Text

Samuel Bard, the son of a Philadelphia physician, was a second generation American descended from French Huguenots. He grew up in New York and at 19 years of age set out for his medical studies in Edinburgh. His ship was captured by French privateers and he spent five months as a prisoner in Bayonne Castle. Benjamin Franklin, a friend of his father's, negotiated his release. He received his MD from Edinburgh University and for his doctoral thesis, *De viribus opii,* reported the effects of one

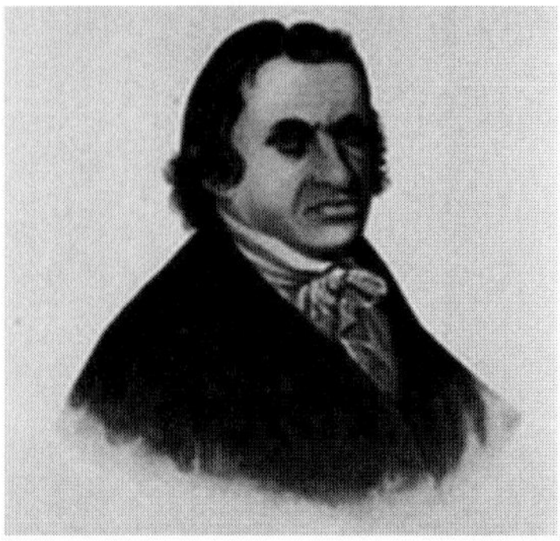
Samuel Bard

and a half grains of opium on the pulse rate. The ten subjects in his report included himself, three friends and six convalescent patients. Upon return to New York he established, along with five associates, the Medical School of King's College (now Columbia University) in 1768. He served as the first professor of physic and later dean of the medical school. Soon after the first presidential inauguration, on 17 June 1789, Bard operated on George Washington for an abscess of the left thigh. He was assisted by his father, John Bard (1716–1799).

After his retirement, Bard published the first American textbook on obstetrics in 1807, which was well received and went to five editions. He was an accomplished but conservative obstetrician, saying,

> *There is some reason to believe there is greater safety in this branch of medicine from modest unassuming ignorance, than from a meddling presumption which frequently accompanies a little learning . . . and I will venture to assert that the better the rules here laid down are understood, and the more steadily they are practised; the less frequently will the necessity of applying to instruments occur.*

In modern obstetrics the main reason for 'applying to instruments' is dystocia, necessitating caesarean section. More than 200 years ago Bard clearly identified the three maternal characteristics that predispose to dystocia, characteristics that represent an increasing proportion of the modern obstetric population:

> *First child . . . in some measure it may be said to be natural, and therefore necessary, for women with their first child . . . to have more tedious labours that with those which follow . . . The same delay happens more certainly, and in a greater degree, when women are advanced beyond thirty years of age before they have a child . . . Very fat women are observed to be subject to slow labours, from a remarkably feeble action of the womb.*

He remained active and interested after retirement to rural Hyde Park, New Jersey. Bard also served a term as president of the Agricultural Society of New York and later published a book, *The Shepherd's Guide*, on aspects of sheep rearing. He died within 24 hours of his wife of 56 years.

Selected Publications

Bard SA. *A Compendium of the Theory and Practice of Midwifery*. New York, NY: Collins and Perkins; 1807. Also published in The Classics of Obstetrics and Gynecology Library. Birmingham: Gryphon Editions; 1990 (facsimile).

Bibliography References

8, 61, 102, 444, 603, 648, 874, 967, 1156, 1325, 1480, 1586, 1597, 1629, 1702.

Barker, David James Purslove (1938–2013)

Barker Hypothesis

In the 1980s, David Barker and his colleagues at the Medical Research Council Environmental Epidemiology Unit at Southampton University published a series of studies showing that infants born of low birth weight were more prone to adult diseases including coronary heart disease, hypertension, stroke and diabetes mellitus. The hypothesis proposed, later called the Barker Hypothesis, was that fetal malnutrition at critical periods of intrauterine development led to reduced cell division and altered concentrations of growth factors and hormones, particularly insulin and growth hormone. This hypothesis has also been called the 'theory of fetal origins of adult disease'.

In 1986, Barker and his statistician colleague, Clive Osmond, reported in the *Lancet* that the distribution of coronary heart disease across England and Wales matched the distribution of infant mortality 50 and more years ago. It was more closely related to neonatal mortality, deaths in the first month after birth, than to post neonatal mortality, deaths from one month to one year. Their paper stated that:

The association of coronary heart disease with neonatal mortality suggests that the childhood influences predisposing to it are related to nutrition during prenatal and early postnatal life. The association with post neonatal mortality suggests a continued relation with nutrition throughout infancy.

They proposed that 'poor nutrition in early life increases susceptibility to the effects of an affluent diet'. This suggestion had been made before, but a possible link with poor nutrition in utero was a new hypothesis.

To pursue these ideas, it was necessary to identify people in later life whose size at birth and during infancy had been recorded at the time. After a three-year search Barker and his colleagues identified a large group of men in the county of Hertfordshire and found that death rates from coronary heart disease among 5,000 men born in the county during 1911–30 fell progressively across the normal range of birthweight and across the range of weight at one year of age. This was consistent with the geographical findings and suggested that what are regarded as normal variations in the supply of energy and nutrients from mothers to their infants have profound long-term effects on health.

Barker explained the vulnerability of the fetus to undernutrition as follows:

In the fetal period, from nine weeks after conception onwards, there begins the phase of rapid growth that continues until after birth. The main feature of fetal growth is cell division. Different tissues of the body grow during periods of rapid cell division, so-called 'critical' periods. The timing of these critical periods differs for different tissues. Growth depends on nutrients and oxygen, and the fetus's main adaptation to lack of these is to slow its rate of cell division, especially in those tissues that are undergoing critical periods at that time. Undernutrition slows cell division either as a direct effect or through altered concentrations of growth factors or hormones, of which insulin and growth hormone are particularly important. Disproportionate growth can occur because different tissues have different periods of growth at different times.

It was his sustained research, publications and presentations that eventually brought wide attention to the fact that fetal and infant development had long-term health consequences in adults. In his final paper, published in the month after his death, he wrote:

Many babies in the womb in the western world today are receiving unbalanced and inadequate diets. Many babies in the developing world are malnourished because their mothers are chronically malnourished. Protecting the nutrition and health of girls and young women should be the corner stone of public health. Not only will it prevent chronic disease but it will produce new generations who have better health and well-being through their lives.

David Barker was born on 29 June 1938 in London. He undertook his medical training at

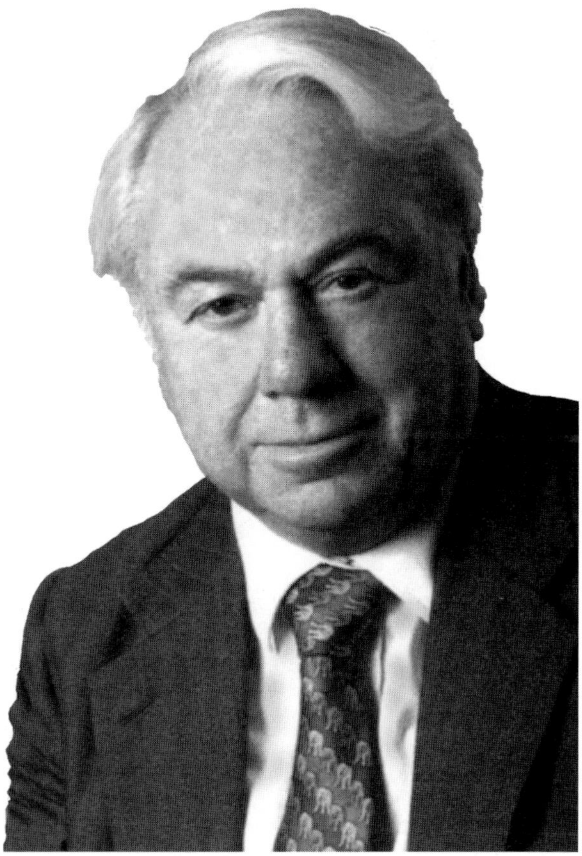

David James Purslove Barker

Guy's Hospital, London. His postgraduate training in internal medicine was done at Guy's Hospital and at the Queen Elizabeth Centre in Birmingham, where he was a lecturer in the department of medicine at the University of Birmingham. He then spent three years at Makere University in Uganda, supported by the Medical Research Council, to study the mode of transmission of *Mycobacterium ulcerans* and its relationship to epidemics of indolent skin ulceration. He moved to the University of Southampton in 1972 and subsequently became director of the Medical Research Council Environmental Epidemiology Unit, as well as consultant physician to the Southampton University Hospitals. He relinquished these posts in 2003 but continued his studies with a combined appointment as professor of clinical epidemiology at the University of Southampton and as professor of medicine in the Heart Research Center at the Oregon Health and Science University at Portland, Oregon. Barker's work was acknowledged by many awards, including an honorary DSc from the University of Birmingham, election to fellowship of the Royal Society of London in 1998 and the CBE in 2006. He was a gifted speaker with a wealth of whimsical anecdotes and jokes to help deliver his scientific message. David Barker died suddenly of a cerebral haemorrhage in Winchester, UK, on 21 August 2013.

Selected Publications

Barker DJ, Osmond C. Infant mortality, childhood nutrition and ischaemic heart disease in England and Wales. *Lancet* 1986; 1: 1077–81.

Barker DJP. Fetal origins of coronary heart disease. *BMJ* 1995; 311: 171–4.

Paneth N, Susser M. Early origin of coronary heart disease (the 'Barker Hypothesis'). *BMJ* 1995; 310: 1411–12.

Bibliography References

65, 66, 141, 263, 1208.

Barnes, Robert (1817–1907)
Neville, William Cox (1855–1904)

Barnes–Neville Forceps

Robert Barnes' long forceps were first displayed at a meeting of the Obstetrical Society of London in 1867. They were designed to grasp the moulded fetal head at or above the pelvic brim as an alternative to craniotomy or caesarean section. Barnes explained the principles involved in assisted forceps delivery from the level of the pelvic brim:

> *From this view it follows that, to extricate the head from the straitened brim, the traction must be made in the axis of the brim, or rather backwards in a curved line, taking the promontory as a centre. When this, the first curve, has been made, the traction must be directed in the axis of the outlet or in the curve of Carus. It is from want of attention to this law that I have known several practitioners fail to extract the head, although it came easily when the law was afterwards observed.*

In 1886 William Neville produced his axis-traction handle, which was a simple device that could be attached to most conventional forceps. He outlined the rationale and advantages as follows:

> *The general plan of the instrument will be understood by a reference to Fig. 4, which shows the forceps with its traction apparatus affixed. The forceps used may be a Barnes', Simpson's, or any other long double-curved forceps, according to individual fancy. I prefer the first-named because of its greater length, which allows the head to be easily seized, even when situated above the pelvic brim . . . When, with this forceps, traction is made through TH in the axis of the forceps – i.e., in the axis of the pelvic canal (approximately), as shown by the indicator (I), the force acts directly from J 1 . . . It is a much simpler instrument, and more easy to apply than Tarnier's or any of its modifications . . . It avoids the disadvantages of traction-rods, and the traction apparatus is entirely outside the vagina in sight . . . the traction apparatus described can be easily fitted to any ordinary double-curved forceps . . . the forceps can be used with or without the traction apparatus.*

Thus was born the Barnes–Neville forceps, which became one of the most popular instruments for axis

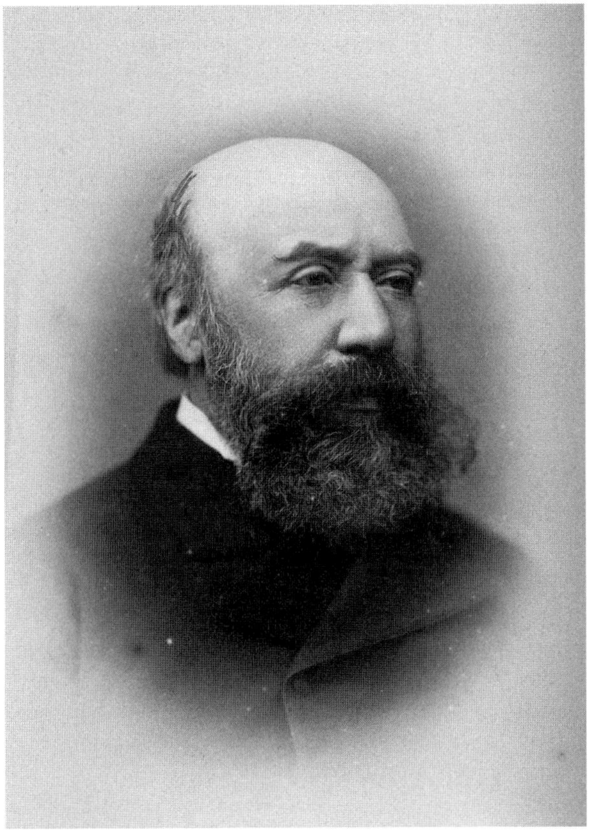

Robert Barnes

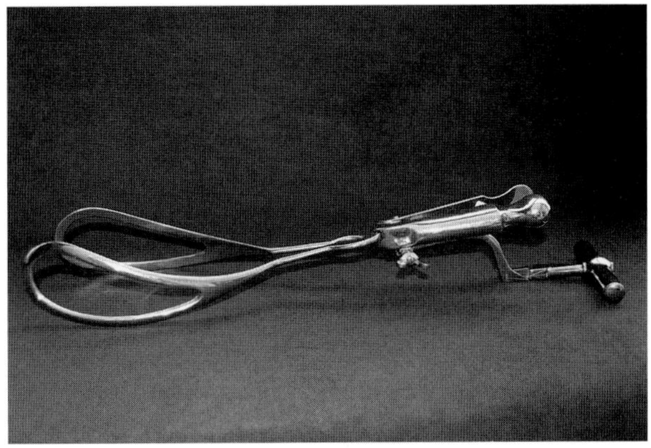

Barnes–Neville forceps

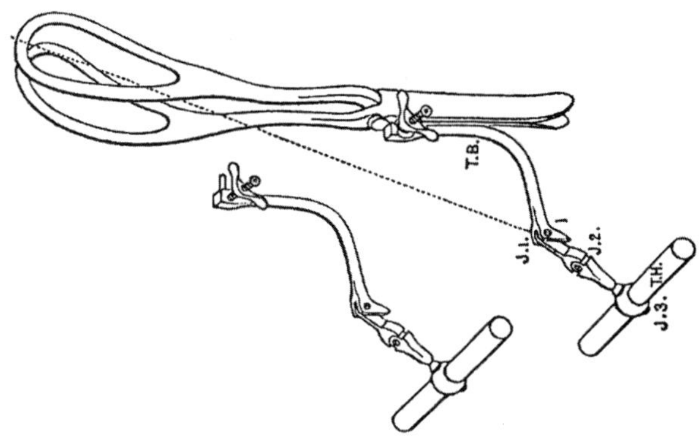

Figure 4 in Neville's paper explaining the rationale of the axis-traction handle

traction. Its main advantage was that the entire axis-traction component was outside the birth canal.

Robert Barnes was born in Norwich. His father was Philip Barnes, who founded the Royal Botanical Gardens in Regent's Park, London. He was initially apprenticed to a surgeon in Norwich and then studied medicine at University College London and St George's Hospital, qualifying in 1842. He spent a year studying in Paris, during which time he supported himself by writing and reputedly lived on one pound a week, no mean feat even then. He returned to London and general practice in Notting Hill. Barnes worked hard and was appointed obstetric physician successively to the London, St Thomas' and St George's hospitals. He became president of the Obstetrical Society of London and later a co-founder, with James Aveling, of the British Gynaecological Society. He also devised hydrostatic bags for dilatation of the cervix and induction of labour. This was placed through the cervix and distended with water from a syringe. 'Barnes' bag' was also used for tamponade in some cases of placenta praevia. Barnes was a large, self-confident and outspoken man. He died in Eastbourne.

William Neville (Sandy as he was known) was an obstetrician and assistant master at the Coombe Lying-in Hospital, Dublin when he designed his axis-traction apparatus. He was born in Louth, where his father was the county surveyor. He graduated first in his class at Trinity College Dublin. As a medical student he was captain of the Trinity rugby football team. From 1876 to 1880 he played rugby for Ireland. Neville studied both obstetrics and gynaecology as well as pathology in Berlin, Freiburg and Marburg. Ill health, probably tuberculosis, caused him to leave obstetrics and turn to pathology. He was appointed pathologist to the Rotunda Hospital, Dublin where he retained his interest in obstetrics and gynaecology. He died of pneumonia on 18 November 1904.

Selected Publications

Barnes R. On the indications and operations for the induction of premature labour and for the acceleration of labour. *Trans Obstet Soc Lond* 1861; 3: 132–9.

Barnes R. On the varieties of form imparted to the foetal head by the various modes of birth. *Trans Obstet Soc Lond* 1865; 7: 171–205.

Barnes R. *Lectures on Obstetrics Operations*. London: Churchill; 1869.

Neville WC. Axis traction in instrumental delivery, with description of a new and simple axis-traction forceps. *Dublin J Med Sci.* 1886; 81: 97–109, 295–8.

Bibliography References

32, 69, 88, 99, 201, 573, 643, 718, 721, 822, 983, 1108, 1224, 1338.

Barr, Murray Llewellyn (1908–1995)

Barr Body (Sex Chromatin)

In the course of studying the integration of nerve cell function and neuronal structure in the cat, Murray Barr and his graduate student Ewart Bertram discovered the sex chromatin. When they were working in the department of anatomy at the University of Western Ontario, Canada, their investigation involved the microscopic examination of Nissl stained sections of the hypoglossal nerve of the cat:

> *The difference in nuclear structure between neurones of adult male and female cats rests on the degree of development of a second body, which is much smaller than the nucleolus. The latter body is more or less intimately associated with the nucleolus and, like the latter stains well with basic dyes.*

This 'nucleolar satellite', as Barr called it, had been described by others, but the correlation of this chromatin mass with the sex of the animal had not. The relationship of the nucleolar satellite to the sex of the animal was a serendipitous finding, being absent in the only two male cats in the study. This was confirmed by studying additional cats of known sex. They extended their investigation to human tissue samples and found the same correlation:

> *A preliminary examination of sympathetic ganglia of human males and females indicates that a similar sex difference in nuclear morphology exists in the human.*

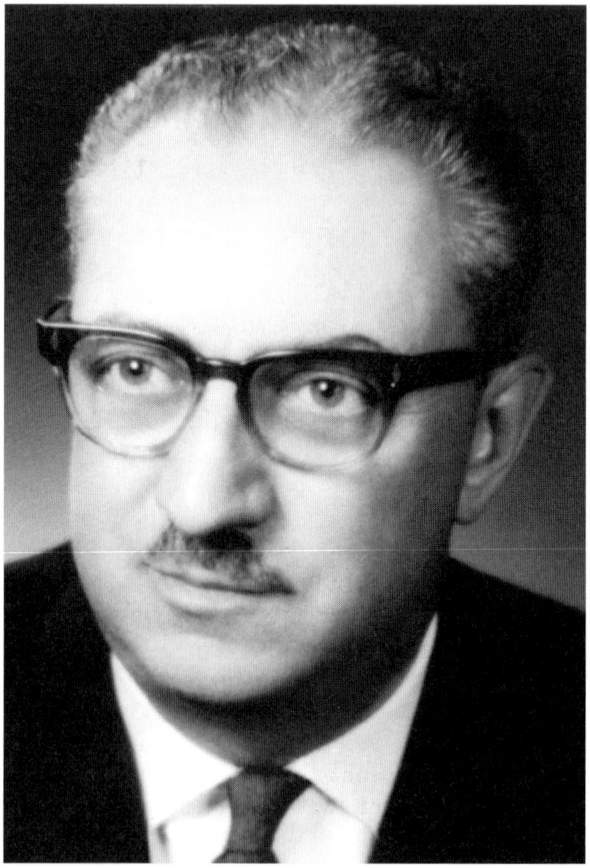

Murray Llewellyn Barr

Barr later called the nucleolar satellite the 'sex chromatin', but it also came into the eponymous lexicon as the 'Barr body'.

Later studies by Barr and another graduate student, Keith Moore, allowed identification of the sex chromatin in skin biopsies and buccal cytology smears. This brought the test into the realm of clinical utility until its replacement by chromosomal karyotyping.

Murray Llewellyn Barr was born, of Ulster extraction, on a farm near the small town of Belmont, Ontario. In 1933 he graduated in medicine from the University of Western Ontario. He initially worked in general practice in London, Ontario, as his wish to specialise in neurology was thwarted by the depression years. He joined the department of anatomy at the University of Western Ontario and did further study in Toronto and Minneapolis to enable him to develop research in neuroanatomy. During the Second World War he served as a medical officer in the Royal Canadian Air Force, achieving the rank of Wing Commander. He became professor of anatomy at the University of Western Ontario in 1949. Barr received many awards, including seven honorary degrees, and was inducted into the Order of Canada in 1968. Two of his sons became doctors. Murray Barr died in London, Ontario, on 4 May 1995.

Selected Publications

Barr ML, Bertram EG. A morphological distinction between neurones of the male and female, and the behaviour of the nucleolar satellite during accelerated nucleoprotein synthesis. *Nature* 1949; 163: 676–7.

Moore KL, Graham MA, Barr ML. The detection of chromosomal sex in hermaphrodites from a skin biopsy. *Surg Gynecol Obstet* 1953; 96: 641–8.

Moore KL, Barr ML. Smears from the oral mucosa in the detection of chromosomal sex. *Lancet* 1955; 2: 57–9.

Bibliography References

70, 71, 91, 303.

Bartholin, Caspar (1655–1738)

Bartholin's Glands

Caspar Bartholin and his eminent anatomy teacher, Guichard Duverney (1648–1730), described the vulvovaginal glands in cattle in 1676. The following year Bartholin outlined their presence and function in women. Both were apparently unaware of an earlier description some 50 years before by Francisco Plazzoni.

Caspar Bartholin the younger was born in Copenhagen into a distinguished family of scientists, physicians and authors. His grandfather, Caspar primus, was a physician, as was his father, Thomas primus. Caspar secundus was a precocious child and at the age of 13 is said to have edited and published his father's book on the anatomy of the swan. He became a medical student at the University of Copenhagen when he was 16 and, while still a student, was appointed professor of philosophy by King Christian V. For three years he visited universities in Holland, France, Germany and Italy. It was while in France that he worked with Duverney. Upon return to Copenhagen in 1677 he published his work and received his doctorate, from his father, the following year. In his middle years he largely forsook medicine for politics and rose to procurator-general in 1719 and deputy for finance in 1724. He was ennobled in 1731.

Selected Publications

Bartholin C. *De ovariis mulierum, et generationis historia.* Rome: Johann Zieger; 1677.

Bibliography References

406, 648, 968, 998, 1198, 1284, 1476, 1480.

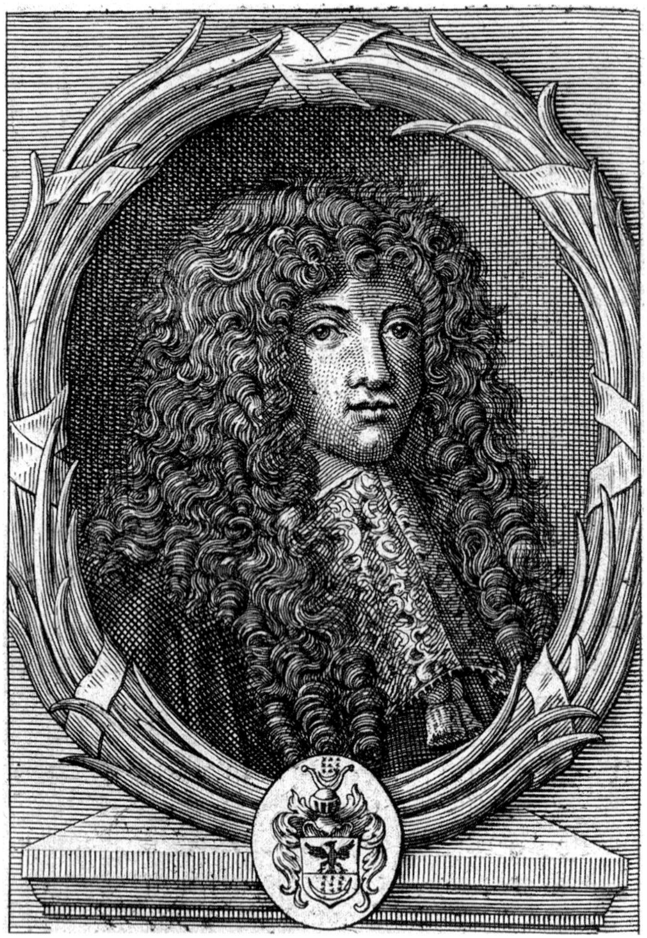

Caspar Bartholin

Barton, Lyman Guy (1866–1944)

Barton's Forceps

Lyman Barton conceived the idea of his forceps at a time when caesarean section still carried significant maternal risk. His forceps were specially designed for high application to the fetal head arrested in the transverse position at the pelvic brim. The anterior blade, which was hinged and flexible from 95–180 degrees, was applied into the hollow of the sacrum and wandered anteriorly under the symphysis. The hinge allowed application without displacement of the position or station of the head. The posterior blade was applied directly via the sacral bay. Axis traction was used to ensure descent via the pelvic curve from the upper pelvis.

Barton first presented his idea and design in 1907 to senior obstetricians, including Edwin Craigin, in Columbia University, New York, but they felt it was without merit and he dropped the proposal for several years. In early 1924 he showed his design to Archibald Campbell of McGill University, Montreal, who appreciated the features of the forceps and urged Barton to have them manufactured. He did, and again showed them to obstetrical colleagues

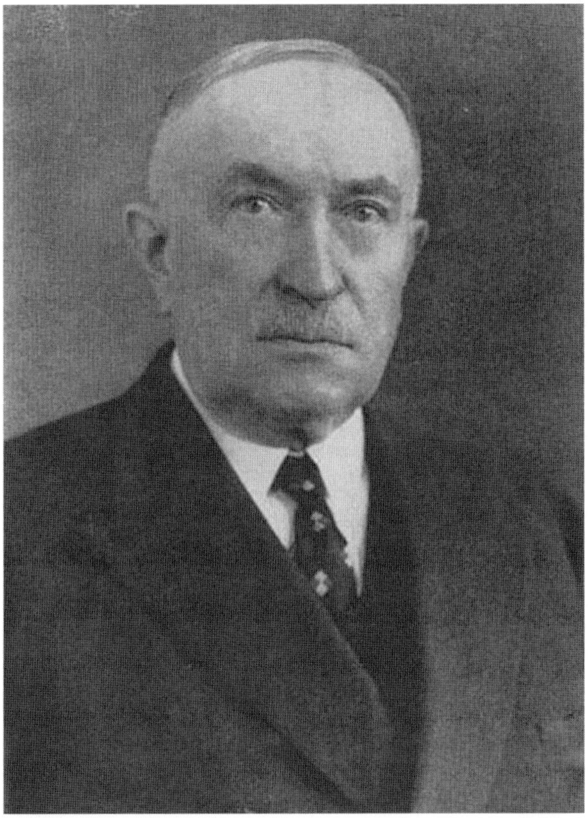

Lyman Guy Barton

in New York. Drs Caldwell and Studdiford (a classmate of Barton's from medical school) agreed to try them at the Sloane Maternity Hospital. Dr William Caldwell was the first to use them on 24 November 1924 and found them effective. His delivery record read in part:

> *Head resting at brim. Uterus becoming tonically contracted and at 7 am under ether anesthesia the Barton forceps were easily applied in a perfect cephalic application at the brim. The head coming down with very slight traction making an easy delivery. First use of Barton forceps.*

He then wrote to Barton:

> *The forceps work! After considerable practice on the mannikin we have had a case suitable for their use and found their application easy and most effective in the delivery of the child . . . I congratulate you on inventing a new and, I believe, a very serviceable forceps for use by expert hands . . .*

The forceps were presented at a meeting of the New York Obstetrical Society on 10 November 1925 and,

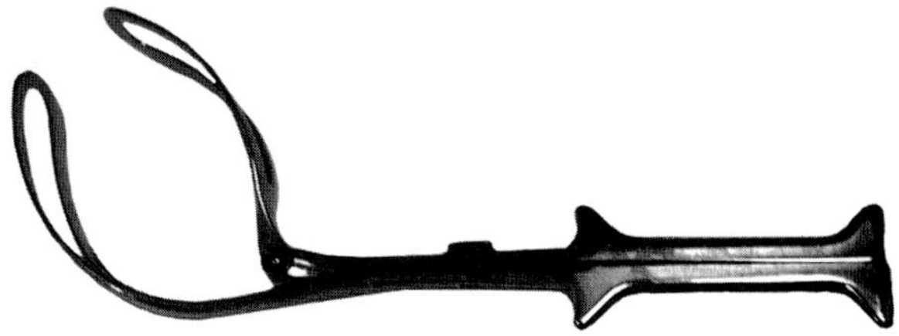

Barton's Forceps

after further experience, published in 1928 in a paper by Barton, Caldwell and Studdiford:

> *While at the present time, there are a number of different types of obstetric forceps which may be successfully employed in low forceps and midforceps operations, no one of them, however, in high forceps operations is equally efficient. This is due to the fact that the forms of the various forceps, as now constructed, render them not equally well adapted to both the head and the pelvic axis except in the low positions and necessitate, in the high forceps operation, the adoption of either the pelvic or cephalic methods of application. As a result of this lack of simultaneous adaptability in the pelvic method of application, the relation between the forceps and the head is faulty; in the cephalic application, the relation between the forceps and the pelvic axis is faulty.*

Lyman Guy Barton was born in Willsboro, Essex County, New York, on 1 July 1886. He initially studied mechanical engineering at Cornell University. However, as the only son of a doctor, he was persuaded to change to medicine and follow in his father's footsteps. He started in the Dartmouth Medical School and finished at Bellevue Hospital Medical School, New York, in 1891. He returned home to the family practice in Willsboro, at which point his 82-year-old father promptly retired. The younger Barton's first major operation in his new practice was a double leg amputation on a man in a railway accident: he survived. Barton moved to Plattsburg, New York in 1914. His engineering background was manifest in his invention or modification of many surgical instruments. He devised a collapsible and portable metal operating table for use in the patient's home, which was an advance on the proverbial kitchen table. Barton died in Plattsburg, New York on 21 November 1944, six weeks after the death of his wife, to whom he had been married for 59 years. Their two sons became doctors and their daughter was an artist.

Selected Publications

Barton LG, Caldwell WE, Studdiford WE. A new obstetric forceps. *Am J Obstet Gynecol* 1928; 15: 16–26.

Bibliography References

49, 361, 399, 555, 1032, 1132, 1169, 1170, 1229.

Basset, Antoine (1882–1951)

Radical Vulvectomy

In his postgraduate thesis, published in 1912, Antoine Basset was the first to describe the precise lymphatic drainage of the vulva. He pointed out that cancer of the vulva spread early to the regional nodes, and usually to both sides: 'It is thus a precocious adenopathy. It is furthermore usually, if not always, bilateral'.

Basset based his findings on a remarkable study of 147 cases of vulval cancer, which he called cancer of the clitoris. As a result, he advocated and performed 'extirpation of the tumour, the lymphatics and the nodes' – the first radical vulvectomy, which came to be called 'Basset's operation'. He wrote:

> *The evolution of the disease appears to be rather rapid without surgical treatment, at least after the tumour is ulcerated, and the prognosis is then always fatal. It is still very sombre after the mutilating operation, because of the great frequency of local, and above all nodal, recurrence. But this seems amenable to improvement by early and systematic extirpation including all the lymphatics and nodes that drain the clitoris.*

Antoine Basset was born and educated in Paris. He was a medical officer in the French army during the First World War. He was talented in many other branches of surgery, including gastrointestinal and orthopaedics. He died in Paris on 7 May 1951.

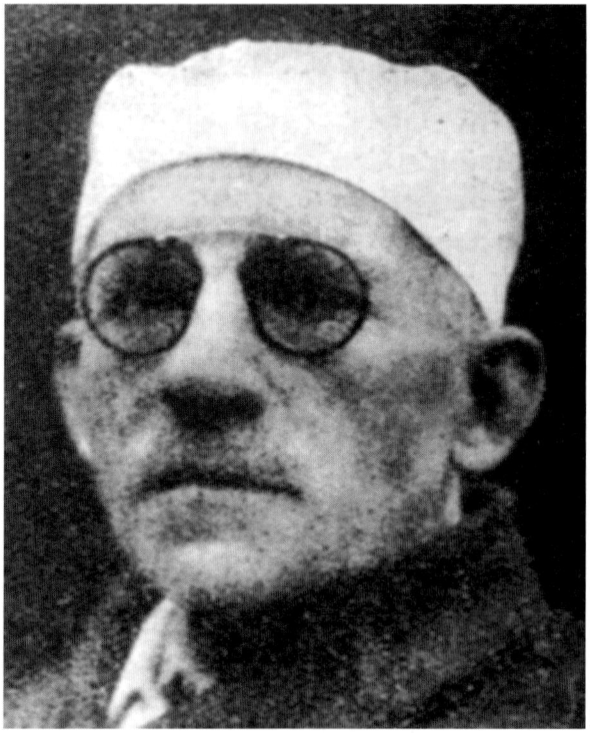

Antoine Basset

Selected Publications

Basset A. *L'épithélioma primitif du clitoris; son retentissement ganglionaire et son traitement opératoire.* Paris: G. Steinheil; 1912.

Basset A. Traitement chirurgical de l'épithélium primitif du clitoris. *Rev Chir* 1912; 46: 546.

Bibliography References

24, 648, 1460, 1480.

Battey, Robert (1825–1895)

Battey's Operation

Robert Battey was a thoughtful and skilful surgeon. Unfortunately, his well-intentioned promotion of bilateral oophorectomy, for some women with intractable symptoms associated with menstruation, ushered in one of the more shameful chapters in gynaecological surgery. Battey performed his first bilateral removal of normal ovaries on a young woman on 27 August 1872 in Rome, Georgia, because she 'was suffering serious detriment to her health and peril to her life by reason of an excessive menstrual flux'. Apparently she suffered convulsions during menstruation and after the operation showed 'all the evidence of perfect health'. Battey had performed this procedure only after considerable reflection. Believing that the artificial menopause induced by bilateral oophorectomy was the only way to relieve her debilitating symptoms, he consulted several senior colleagues before operating. Achieving good results in individual cases he continued to promote the procedure, although he emphasised that it should only be a last resort in carefully selected cases. Unfortunately, the procedure was taken up enthusiastically by the less thoughtful and the unscrupulous, so that 'Battey's operation' was widely used to relieve many physiological symptoms associated with menstruation and expanded to include other 'nervous disorders' in women.

Battey also described vaginal oophorectomy via an incision in the pouch of Douglas. In these cases he had an interesting approach to intra-operative bleeding: 'If any undue oozing of blood occurs, a small lump of ice slipped through the incision into the cul-de-sac quickly stops it, or it may be easily controlled by irrigating Douglas' space with hot water'.

Although ovarian function was not understood at this time, many in the profession spoke against this as unnecessary castration or 'spaying' of women. Battey was called to task and, in 1887, responded to the American Gynecological Society in these terms:

> *In my opinion the removal of the functionally active ovaries is indicated in the case of any grave disease which is either dangerous to life or destructive of health and happiness, which is incurable by other and less radical means, and which we may reasonably expect to remove by the arrest of ovulation or change of life. I do not propose it for any case which is curable by other means. If asked, 'do I operate for dysmenorrhea, for amenorrhea, for epilepsy, for mania?' I answer both no and yes: no, if the case be susceptible of other remedy; and yes, if the case be grave and otherwise without remedy. 'Do I operate for nymphomania?' No; never! There is no reason to expect its cure by the arrest of ovulation.*

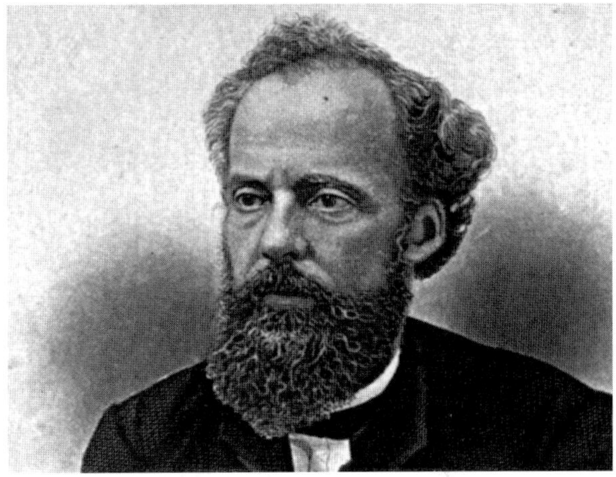

Robert Battey

Despite his defence of the procedure it was widely abused, mainly in the United States, and to a lesser extent in Europe where 'ovariomania' was less rampant.

Robert Battey was born in Augusta, Georgia on 26 November 1828. He was initially apprenticed to his physician brother but went on to graduate from Jefferson Medical College and settled in Rome, Georgia. During the American Civil War he gained considerable experience as a surgeon in the Confederate Army. After the war he returned to his original civilian surgical practice. He set up his own hospital and did the first oophorectomy in his own home. For two years he was professor of obstetrics and gynaecology at Atlanta Medical College before he returned to private practice.

Selected Publications

Battey R. Normal ovariotomy. *Atlanta Med Surg J* 1872; 10: 321–39.

Battey R. Battey's operation: its matured results. *Trans Am Gynecol Soc* 1887; 12: 153–74.

Battey R. Battey's operation In: Mann MD (ed.) *A System of Gynecology*. Vol. 2. Philadelphia, PA: Lea Brothers & Co; 1888, pp. 837–49.

Bibliography References

8, 104, 648, 924, 1018, 1480, 1728.

Baudelocque, Jean-Louis (1746–1810)

Baudelocque's Diameter

It was William Smellie who laid down the principles of clinical pelvimetry, including vaginal examination to estimate the internal or diagonal conjugate. The renowned French accoucheur, Jean-Louis Baudelocque, later emphasised the importance of pelvic mensuration and introduced his pelvimeter for external measurement of pelvic diameters. He wrote:

> *. . . one can determine, within one or two lines, to what degree the superior strait is abnormal in this regard, by measuring the thickness of the woman from the middle of*

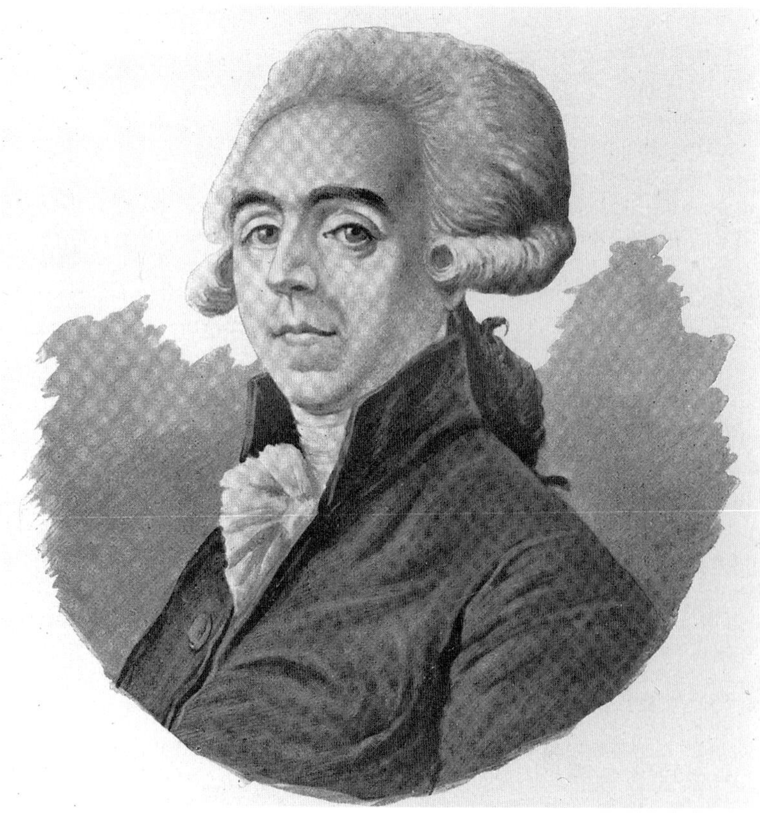

Jean-Louis Baudelocque

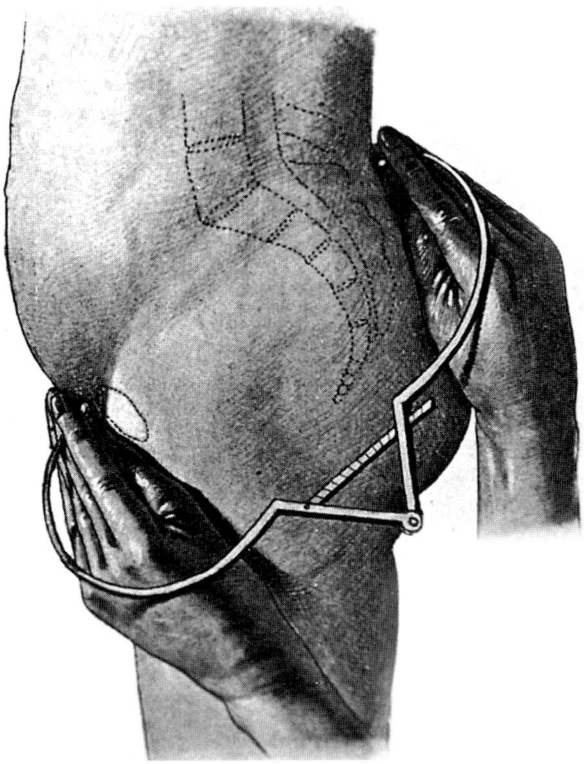

External pelvimeter measuring Baudelocque's diameter

the pubis to the tip of the spine of the last lumbar vertebra . . .

This measurement, the external conjugate of the pelvis, became known as Baudelocque's diameter, or line, and was used for over a century until radiology showed the poor correlation with internal pelvic diameters.

Jean-Louis Baudelocque was born in the village of Heilly in Picardie, France. His father was a surgeon and he followed his footsteps to Paris for medical training, concentrating upon anatomy, obstetrics and surgery. He quickly established himself in both the academic and private practice of obstetrics. After the French revolution he was appointed professor of obstetrics at the École de Santé and director of the Maternité in Paris, the latter being the main training centre for midwives in France. Baudelocque's reputation was such that he became known as *le grand Baudelocque* and attended Napoleon's wife, the Empress Marie Louise, in her first confinement. He spoke against symphysiotomy in the management of dystocia: 'a murderous and unphilosophical procedure'. Instead he advocated caesarean section for severe cases of pelvic contraction:

With respect to the child, it is the gentlest and most certain of all the methods we can employ for terminating labour.

Colleagues, jealous of his preeminence, criticised him and on one occasion he had to defend himself (successfully) in court when a contemporary called him an assassin for his views on caesarean section.

Selected Publications

Baudelocque JL. *L'Art des accouchements.* Vol. 1. Paris: Méquiqnon; 1781.

Bibliography References

38, 102, 347, 359, 419, 448, 482, 497, 648, 721, 1480, 1595, 1728, 1734.

Behçet, Hulusi (1889–1948)

Behçet's Syndrome

This uncommon syndrome of relapsing oral and genital ulcers associated with conjunctivitis and iridocyclitis was originally described by the Turkish dermatologist, Hulusi Behçet, in 1937. He observed this in both males and females, some recurring over a twenty-year span:

The cases which are considered here exhibit the following clinical picture: lesions in the mouth, on the genitalia, and

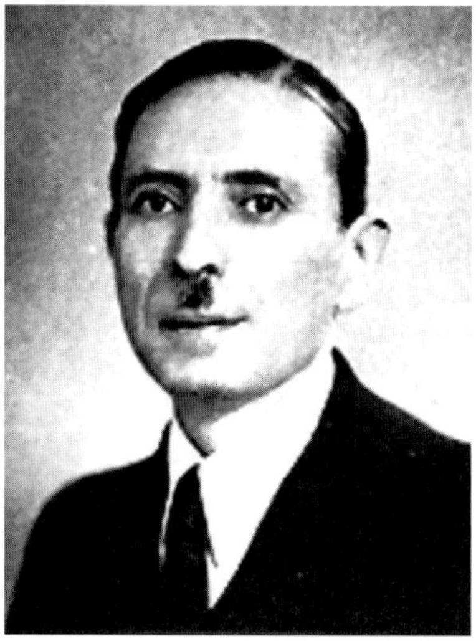

Hulusi Behçet

of the eyes . . . the lesions of the relapses which occurred several times a year appeared either simultaneously or successively in the mouth, on the genitalia, on the conjunctiva, and even as an inflammation of the iris . . .

This syndrome may be associated with other manifestations, such as arthralgia and thrombophlebitis, suggesting an underlying vasculitis or autoimmune disorder. Behçet recognised that the triad of local lesions may be part of a more systemic condition:

These facts, plus the observation that local therapy was of no help, and that internal therapy succeeded in lengthening the intervals between relapses, make it clear that we are dealing with a disease caused by a general infection, affecting the organism as a whole, and that the aphthous lesions have no relation to ordinary aphthae.

Hulusi Behçet was born in Istanbul, when it was still capital of the Ottoman empire. His father, a prominent businessman, was a friend of Mustafa Atatürk, the founder of the Turkish republic. Behçet's mother died when he was young, and he was raised by his grandmother; his childhood was said to be unhappy. He did receive a good education and graduated in 1910 at the age of 21 from the Gülhane Military Academy in Istanbul, there being no civil medical school at the time. Until the end of the First World War he served as a specialist in dermatology and venereal diseases at military hospitals in Istanbul. He then took postgraduate studies in Budapest and Berlin. He returned to Turkey in 1919 and worked in private practice and later in the university hospitals. In 1933 the University of Istanbul was established, and he became the first professor of dermatology and syphilology. In 1939 he was awarded the title 'Ordinarius', an acknowledgement of high academic achievement.

Behçet was a thin and abstemious man who tended to be gloomy and introverted. One colleague who admired him said 'the only thing he did was to read and work'. He married and had one daughter but separated from his wife seven years before his death. Ironically, Behçet was himself beset with a chronic triad of medical disorders through his adult life: insomnia, irritable bowel and angina. He was a heavy smoker and died on 8 March 1948 following a myocardial infarction. A commemorative stamp was issued by Turkey in his honour in 1980 and a silver coin in 1996.

Selected Publications

Behçet H. Über rezidivierende, aphthöse, durch ein Virul verursachte Geschwüre am Mund, am Auge und an den Genitalien. *Dermat Wochenschr* 1937; 105: 1152–7.

Behçet H. Considerations sur les lesions aphteuses de la bouche et des parties genitals, ainsi que sur les manifestations oculaires d'origine probablement virutique et observations concernant leur foyer d'infection. *Bull Soc Fr Dermatol Syph* 1938; 45: 420–33.

Behçet H. Some observations on the clinical picture of the so-called triple symptom complex. *Dermatologica* 1940; 81: 73–83.

Bibliography References

552, 864, 1094, 1350, 1640.

Bennewitz, Heinrich Gottleib (c.1824)

Diabetes in Pregnancy

The first case report of diabetes in pregnancy was published in Heinrich Bennewitz's thesis for the degree of doctor of medicine at the University of Berlin in 1824. In his thesis he reviewed the

DE

DIABETE MELLITO,
GRAVIDITATIS SYMPTOMATE.

DISSERTATIO
INAUGURALIS MEDICA
QUAM
GRATIOSI MEDICORUM ORDINIS
CONSENSU ATQUE AUCTORITATE
IN
UNIVERSITATE LITTERARIA BEROLINENSI
PRO SUMMIS
IN MEDICINA ET CHIRURGIA HONORIBUS
RITE OBTINENDIS
DIE XXIV. M. IUNII A. MDCCCXXIV
H. L. Q. S.
PALAM DEFENDET
AUCTOR
HENR. GOTTL. BENNEWITZ
BEROLINENSIS.

OPPONENTIBUS:
W. DE *MOELLER*, MED. ET CHIR. DDR.
A. TIETZEL, MED. ET CHIR. DDR.
O. ZIMMERMANN, MED. ET CHIR. DDR.

BEROLINI,
TYPIS IOANNIS FRIDERICI STARCKII.

Title page of Bennewitz's thesis on diabetes mellitus

knowledge of diabetes mellitus at that time and included a single case report of diabetes in the pregnancy of one Frederica Pape. She was 22 years old and in the seventh month of her fifth pregnancy when admitted to the Berlin Infirmary with polydypsia and polyuria. Her first three pregnancies had been normal, but in the fourth she had polyuria, which resolved after delivery. Bennewitz confirmed glycosuria by demonstrating 57 g of residual sugar crystals after boiling 7.25 kg of her urine. Her baby died during an obstructed labour, and Bennewitz gave a classic description of shoulder dystocia:

> *The child's head stuck out like a wedge and its shoulders stuck in the womb exit – moving neither up nor down. In the end he was born dead, but not without a great struggle.*

The infant weighed 5.4 kg and was of 'such robust and healthy character . . . whom you would have thought Hercules had begotten'.

Bennewitz observed that diabetes may be due to or worsened by pregnancy:

> *. . . the little fires which had hidden beneath the smouldering deceiving ashes broke forth and devoured again the women's condition in the most wretched manner.*

She recovered post-partum despite purges and the application of leeches: 'with nature to preserve and treat her, we dismissed our patient cured'.

The fact that this patient had at least partial resolution of her symptoms and glycosuria post partum raises the possibility of gestational diabetes, although the severity of her symptoms suggests insulin dependent diabetes worsened by pregnancy.

Bennewitz's thesis was rediscovered in the 1980s in the University of Munich library, and the translation of the Latin thesis into English was undertaken at the Queen's University of Belfast. No other details of his life are known.

Selected Publications

Bennewitz HG. *Diabetes mellitus: a symptom of pregnancy.* MD dissertation. Berlin: Johann Starck; 1824.

Hadden DR, Hillebrand B. The first recorded case of diabetic pregnancy (Bennewitz HG, 1824, University of Berlin). *Diabetologia* 1989; 32: 625.

Bibliography References

675.

Bevis, Douglas Charles Aitchison (1918–1994)

Amniocentesis in Rhesus Isoimmunisation

By the late 1940s the pathogenesis of rhesus isoimmunisation was well understood. However, although maternal anti-D antibody titres tended to reflect the severity of fetal disease, there were many exceptions and accurate prediction was not possible. In 1950 Bevis studied the amniotic fluid obtained at hind water rupture for induction of labour in 30 cases of rhesus isoimmunisation. He found the liquor contained increasing amounts of iron in relation to the severity of haemolytic disease in the newborn. He concluded this brief one-page report with the statement:

> *Possibly, if the test were applied to liquor obtained by paracentesis in the antenatal period, the induction of labour could be timed more accurately.*

He followed his own advice, and two years later reported his results on 158 specimens of amniotic fluid from 69 patients obtained at amniocentesis between 28 weeks gestation and term. He found no untoward side effects for mother or fetus and a clear relationship between amniotic fluid levels of non-haematin iron and urobilinogen and fetal outcome. Thus, his hopes of finding a reliable prognostic guide were realised:

> *An abnormal concentration, of either iron or urobilinogen at this time is therefore to be taken as a warning that the foetus is being affected by the haemolytic process, and appropriate decisions can then be made.*

It was several years before the safety and relevance of this seminal work was realised and incorporated into the management of isoimmunisation. In many ways this modestly presented work never received the recognition it deserved, as it undoubtedly led to a huge reduction in mortality and morbidity for thousands of infants worldwide.

Douglas Charles Aitchison Bevis was born in Ealing and educated in Manchester, qualifying as a doctor from the University of Manchester in 1943.

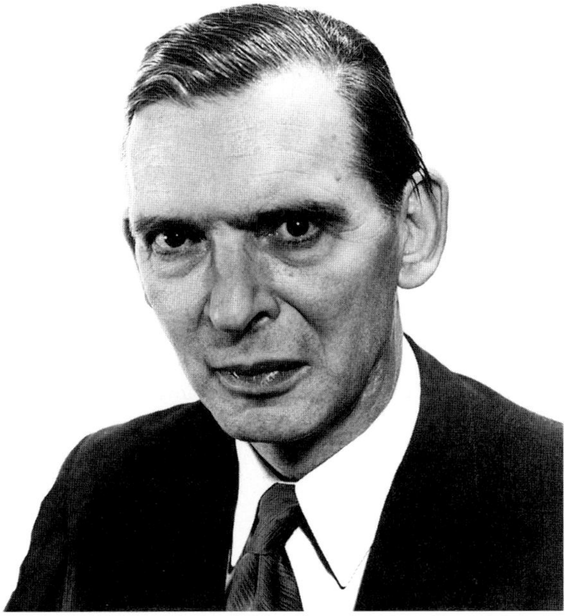

Douglas Charles Aitchison Bevis

He spent the last two years of the Second World War as a surgeon lieutenant in the Royal Navy. Following this he did postgraduate training in obstetrics and gynaecology at St Mary's Hospital, Manchester. It was as a senior registrar at this hospital that he did his work on amniotic fluid. He performed virtually all of the clinical and laboratory work on these cases himself. In 1952 he was appointed consultant at Park Hospital, Manchester. He became reader in the academic department of obstetrics and gynaecology at Sheffield University in 1967 and there changed the focus of his research endeavours to infertility. In 1973 he was appointed to a second chair of obstetrics and gynaecology at the St James Hospital, Leeds, where he remained until he retired in 1984. He provoked great controversy at the British Medical Association conference in 1974 when he announced that he had been involved with successful cases of in vitro fertilisation. He refused to divulge details and the ensuing pressure, both media and professional, led to his withdrawal from this area of research.

Bevis was a founder member of the Fothergill Club, a travelling gynaecological society. He was also a skilled silversmith and had his own hallmark. His nickname, 'Tiger' Bevis, bore no relation to his character, but was a hangover from his enthusiastic style of play when he represented his university at rugby football. He died in Sheffield on 25 June 1994.

Selected Publications

Bevis DCA. Composition of liquor amnii in haemolytic disease of newborn. *Lancet* 1950; 2: 443.

Bevis DCA. The antenatal prediction of haemolytic disease of the newborn. *Lancet* 1952; 1: 395–8.

Bibliography References

143, 144, 145, 388, 528, 1000, 1626, 1690, 1741, 1744.

Bird, Geoffrey Colin (1922–2001)

Vacuum Extraction

In the 1960s the vacuum extractor of Tage Malmström came into common use. Geoffrey Bird, a proponent of vacuum extraction working in Australia, felt there were weaknesses in the design of Malmström's cup, which had common traction and suction ports in the centre of the metal cup. Bird thought that this limited the ability to place the cup over the posterior fontanelle, particularly in deflexed occipito-transverse and occipito-posterior positions of the fetal head. In addition, he felt that oblique traction, sometimes necessary in these cases, commonly led to cup detachment. He therefore separated the traction and suction ports to reduce the leverage on the cup during traction and thereby diminish the risk of cup detachment. He later further modified the cup so that the suction port originated from the lateral margin. In correspondence with this author, Bird

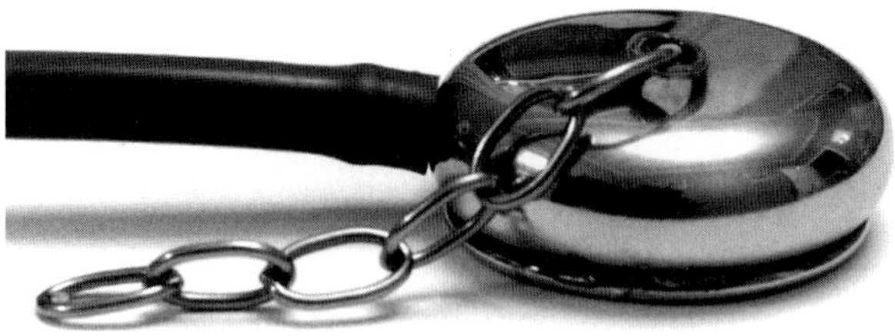

Geoffrey Bird's prototype OP cup

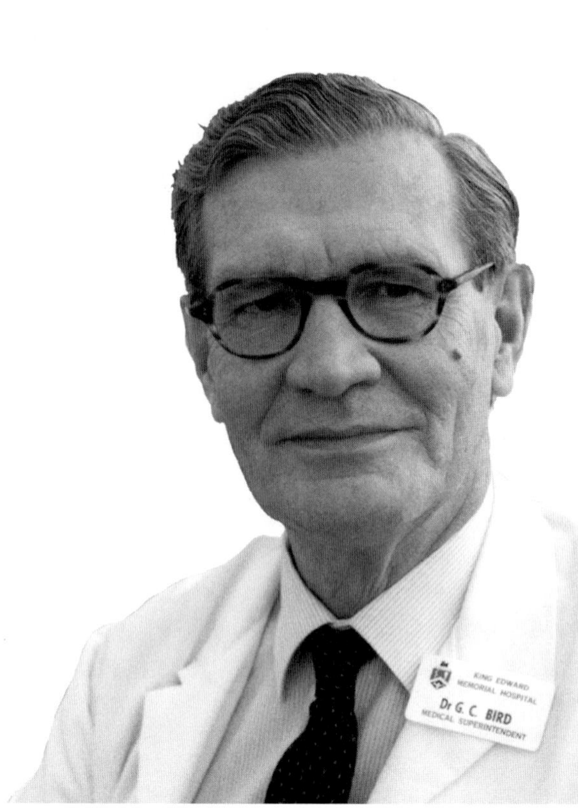

Geoffrey Colin Bird

gave one of his reasons for modifying the Malmström cup:

> *Examination of the position of the cup caput (chignon) on the infant's scalp after use of Malmström's vacuum extractor showed me that application of the cup was often far from ideal, particularly in posterior and lateral positions of the occiput. The ideal application site is over the posterior fontanelle with the sagittal suture pointing to the centre of the cup.*

Bird's modification, the so-called 'OP' cup, facilitated placement over the flexion point, 3 cm in front of the posterior fontanelle, thereby reducing the risk of deflexion with its larger diameter of the fetal head:

> *Cups with a dome attached suction tube are unsuitable for use in mid-cavity occipito-posterior positions because their limited manoeuverability results in a high incidence of deflexing applications . . . Deflexing applications can be largely avoided in mid-cavity occipito-posterior positions by using a cup that has the suction tube attached to the lateral wall. This 'OP' cup can be used whatever the position of the occiput . . . The use of cups that are more manoeuverable than Malmström's should, by permitting better applications, decrease failure rates, particularly when the occiput is obliquely posterior or lateral.*

Bird emphasised that:

> *Traction is a two-handed exercise. The thumb of the non-pulling hand, pressed firmly against the cup near the rim helps to prevent the cup from tilting off the scalp. The index finger of the non-pulling hand, resting on the shoulders of the cup with its tip touching the scalp, monitors descent.*

This latter point, the use of the index finger resting on the fetal scalp adjacent to the cup, was to detect scalp descent without descent of the bony skull, which Bird called 'negative traction'. The Bird cup, which was originally made in the hospital workshop, was used with good results at the King Edward Memorial Hospital for Women in Perth, Western Australia, where Bird worked at the time. He forwarded the prototype to the AB vacuum extractor manufacturers in Sweden and they later manufactured this along with the original Malmström cup. Recently a disposable vacuum extractor made of hard plastic has been designed. This uses the same principles of design as the Bird OP cup, which were put forward to the manufacturer by one of Bird's former students, Aldo Vacca, from Brisbane, Australia.

Geoffrey Bird was born on 24 March 1922 in Simla, India, where his father was an Anglican minister. He spent his early education in England, and when he left school in 1940 he immediately joined the British Army and served in the Royal Artillery in India and with the Infantry in Burma. After the war he returned to London, studied medicine and graduated from St Bartholomew's Hospital in 1953. He followed this with three years of postgraduate training in the London hospitals. In 1956 he went to Kenya, originally for one year to gain experience, but ended up staying until 1965.

He worked in the Kenya Government Service as a provincial maternal and child health specialist and gained huge clinical experience. In 1965 he immigrated to Australia and worked at the King Edward Memorial Hospital for Women in Perth, Western Australia, as senior lecturer in obstetrics and gynaecology at the University of Western Australia. He moved to the Port Moresby General Hospital in Papua New Guinea in 1972 as head of the department of obstetrics and gynaecology, remaining there until 1979. He then returned to the King Edward Memorial Hospital in Perth as deputy medical officer and later as medical superintendent. He retired in 1987. Geoffrey Bird died on 14 May 2001 of complications following hip replacement surgery.

Selected Publications

Bird GC. Modification of Malmström's vacuum extractor. *BMJ* 1969; 3: 526.

Bird GC. The importance of flexion in vacuum extractor delivery. *Br J Obstet Gynaecol* 1976; 83: 194–200.

Vacca A. Operative vaginal delivery: clinical appraisal of a new vacuum extraction device. *Aust NZ J Obstet Gynaecol* 2001; 41: 156–60.

Bibliography References

92, 99, 260, 532, 1133.

Bishop, Edward Harry (1913–1995)

Bishop Score

Since its introduction over 50 years ago, the Bishop score has become one of the most commonly used methods of clinical assessment in obstetrics. Edward Bishop developed his pelvic score in an attempt to reduce the chance of failed induction at a time when elective induction of labour was popular in the United States. Feeling that the methods of induction were well standardised he wrote:

> *... differences in results must ensue from variations in the method of selecting suitable candidates. Therefore, it would seem of benefit to develop some standardized, easily determined, and easily recorded plan for the selection of those patients most suitable for induction...*

Bishop felt that elective induction of labour should not be undertaken in the nulliparous woman:

> *Owing to the unpredictability of the duration of labor in the nullipara, even in the presence of apparently favorable circumstances, induction of labor brings little advantage for either obstetrician or patient.*

In correspondence with this author, Bishop wrote:

> *I decided to try to develop a set of standards or indications which would eliminate or at least minimize the risks of this elective procedure. About a thousand normal multiparous patients were examined pelvically at their final four prenatal visits. The pelvic findings were correlated with the time of onset of spontaneous labour – thus leading to the determination of a pelvic score which we hoped just preceded the onset of natural and normal labor. Incidentally, the graphic form of the scoring system*

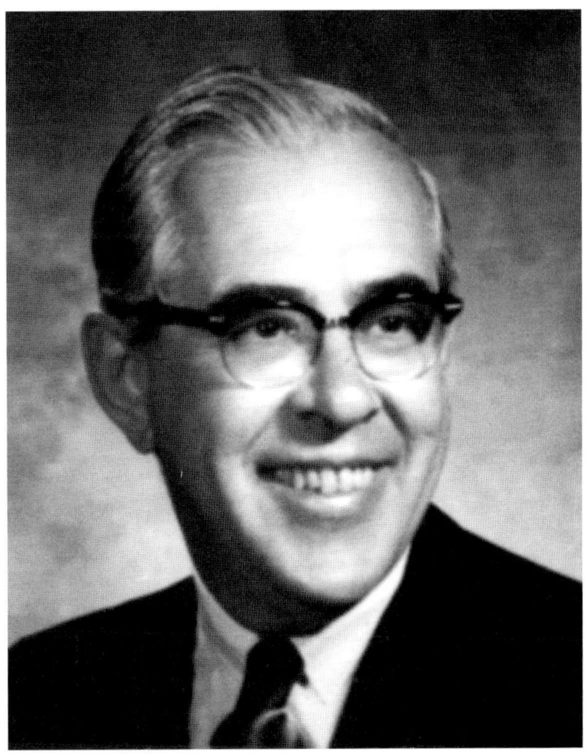

Edward Harry Bishop

was suggested by Virginia Apgar and uses the same graphic form and shape as the Apgar Score.

Bishop's pelvic score evaluates four cervical factors: position, consistency, effacement and dilatation, along with the station of the presenting part. The potential scores are 0–3 for all but station and cervical consistency, which range from 0–2. He correlated the total score with successful induction as well as the likelihood of spontaneous onset of labour. The Bishop score, or modification thereof, has been widely used in clinical practice and in trials involving different agents and methods for induction of labour. Bishop also carried out some of the early work with Doppler ultrasound monitoring of the fetal heart. He was one of the first to attempt uterine tocolysis with isoxuprine, reporting 156 cases of premature labour so treated between 1959 and 1961.

Edward Harry Bishop was born in Bethlehem, New Hampshire. He attended Dartmouth College and Medical School, graduating MD from the University of Pennsylvania in 1937. Most of his professional life was spent in Philadelphia at the Pennsylvania Hospital, rising to the rank of professor at the University of Pennsylvania. In 1972 he moved to Chapel Hill at the North Carolina Memorial Hospital and the University of North Carolina as professor of obstetrics and chief of perinatology. He retired in 1983 and died on 10 December 1995.

Selected Publications

Bishop EH, Woutersz TB. Isoxuprine, myometrial relaxant: a preliminary report. *Obstet Gynecol* 1961; 17: 442–6.

Bishop EH, Woutersz TB. Arrest of premature labor. *JAMA* 1961; 178: 812–14.

Bishop EH. Pelvic scoring for elective induction. *Obstet Gynecol* 1964; 24: 266–8.

Bishop EH. Instrument and method: the Doppler ultrasonic motion sensor. *Obstet Gynecol* 1966; 28: 712–3.

Bibliography References

126, 805, 1220, 1243.

Blair-Bell, William (1871–1936)

Posterior Pituitary Extract

William Blair-Bell, the son of a physician, was born in Wallasey, England. He received his medical education at King's College and King's College Hospital, London, graduating in 1896. As a student he was an accomplished cricketer, hurdler and table-tennis player. After hospital resident appointments he went into general practice in Wallasey. However, his main interest was obstetrics and gynaecology, and in 1905 he was appointed assistant consultant gynaecologist to the Liverpool Royal Infirmary. In addition to his clinical work he carried out laboratory-based research and published consistently. In 1921 he became professor of obstetrics and gynaecology at Liverpool University.

Blair-Bell was the first to use posterior pituitary extract in obstetrics, given to him by Henry Dale. He reported his preliminary clinical experience with the extract in 1909, being particularly impressed with its oxytocic property:

In two cases of caesarean section I have had the opportunity of observing the naked-eye effect of a single injection; it is immediate and convincing. The uterus contracts into a blanched 'ball', and only relaxes subsequently to a moderate degree . . . I am inclined to think, therefore, that in the future we shall rely on infundibular extract to produce contractions of the uterus in many serious obstetric complications and difficulties, although I should, perhaps, add that in my opinion it ought but rarely to be given before delivery. I have for some time carried it in my obstetric bag, and would not willingly be without it.

Blair-Bell is best remembered as one of the founders and the first president of the Royal College of Obstetricians and Gynaecologists. Before this, in 1911, he founded the Gynaecological Visiting Society of Great Britain and Ireland, which brought together the younger teachers and research-minded members of the specialty. From the membership of this society came much of the impetus to found the Royal

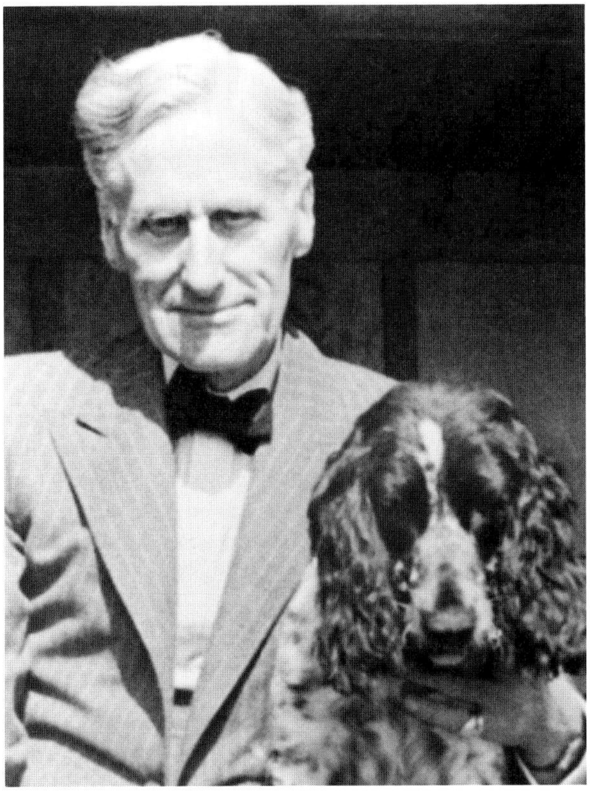

William Blair-Bell

College. Blair-Bell was obviously a man of enormous ability but with a ruthless, intolerant and autocratic side that often clouded his judgement. It also brought him many enemies, particularly in the London establishment of obstetrics and gynaecology. However, it was largely due to his tenacity and sustained strength of purpose that the college was established in the face of varying degrees of opposition, ranging from apathy to overt hostility.

Blair-Bell lost the second finger of his left hand after a surgical needle-stick injury with subsequent infection and gangrene. He was said to have been proud of this 'badge of war', and it can be seen in his portrait hanging in the Royal College. He married his first cousin Florence, who was chronically indisposed; they had no children and were never seen together outside their home. A certain streak of vanity was displayed when, in 1930, he changed his surname Bell to Blair-Bell, hyphenating his middle given name, Blair, to his original plain surname. Having no children of his own, he tried to persuade his nephew, Arthur Bell, to adopt the same hyphenated surname. Arthur Bell refused, although he later emulated his uncle by becoming president of the Royal College of Obstetricians and Gynaecologists.

Blair-Bell was a man of formality and tradition in college affairs. In large measure he designed the college coat of arms and gowns. He contributed the college motto *Super Ardua*, meaning 'over difficulties'. After one admission ceremony of new Fellows and Members in 1931 he felt that the proceedings ended rather abruptly. He therefore coined an appropriate phrase to conclude all formal college events: *Super Ardua Consurgamus Floreat Collegium* ('Together we shall rise above difficulties – may the College flourish'). This tradition continues.

William Blair-Bell died, age 64, following a coronary thrombosis suffered on a train journey as he returned home from a college meeting. At his request his original presidential gown, which he refused to give to his successor, was buried with him.

Selected Publications

Bell WB. The pituitary body and the therapeutic value of the infundibular extract in shock, uterine atony and intestinal paresis. *BMJ* 1909; 2: 1609–13.

Bibliography References

164, 263, 564, 720, 753, 822, 1159, 1183–1186, 1392, 1394, 1395, 1605, 1661.

Blond, Kasper (1889–1964) Heidler, Hans (1889–1955)

Blond–Heidler Saw

In the early part of the twentieth century, a neglected shoulder presentation with a dead fetus posed a formidable dilemma. Caesarean section, with its significant maternal mortality, was not appropriate for a dead fetus. Internal version with a retracted and thinned lower uterine segment held considerable risk of uterine rupture. One common solution was fetal decapitation using the Braun hook. This instrument took time and carried some risk of trauma to adjacent maternal tissues.

In this clinical context Kasper Blond, working in the University Clinic at Vienna, devised a thimble attachment to a thin chain saw or decapitation wire. Later that same year Hans Heidler, working in the same clinic, modified the thimble device. The thimble allowed easy, atraumatic passage of the chain saw around the fetal neck. Handles were then attached to each end of the wire which, when pulled to and fro, achieved rapid fetal decapitation without maternal trauma. In its time this instrument represented a considerable advance in the rather barbarous management of a dangerous clinical conundrum. It still has occasional use in low-resource settings.

Kasper Blond's medical studies were interrupted by the First World War, during which he served in the Austrian army. He was taken by the Russians and imprisoned in Siberia. He escaped via Persia and Turkey back to Vienna, where he completed his MD in 1917. Blond worked as a surgeon in the Allgemeines Krankenhaus in Vienna. In 1938 he left Vienna for London and became senior surgeon to the Ministry of Health. His main research interest was liver disease, upon which subject he wrote a book. He died in London.

Hans Heidler was born in Gmunden, Austria and took his MD at the University of Vienna in 1912. From 1913 to 1918 he worked as an assistant in the first department of surgery in Vienna, gaining considerable experience in military surgery. In 1918 he

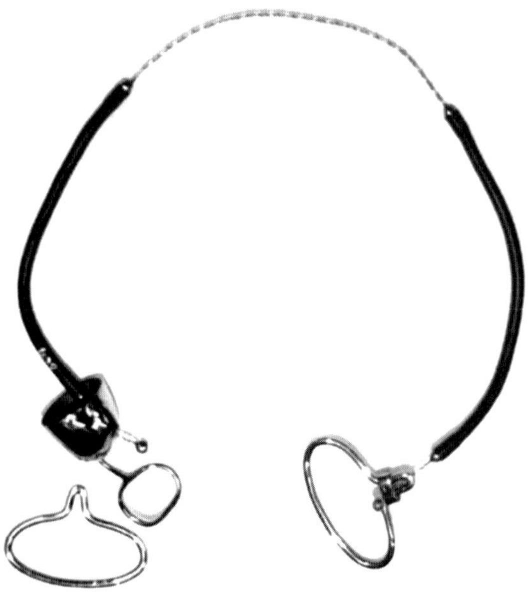

Blond–Heidler saw

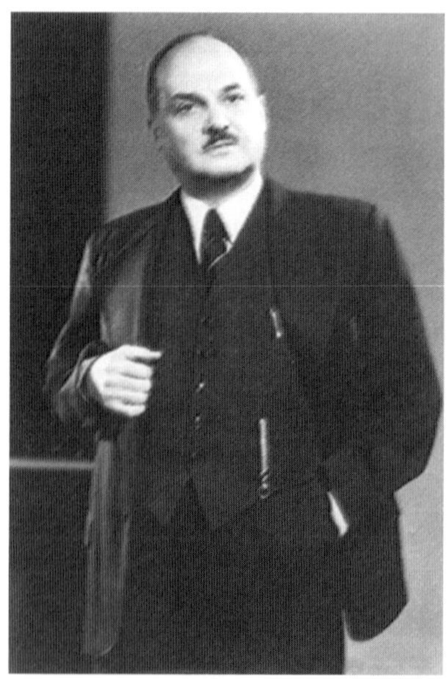

Hans Heidler

transferred to the second university department of obstetrics and gynaecology and worked under Ernst Wertheim. In 1945 he became head of the Semmelweis Frauenklinik and extraordinary professor at the University of Vienna. He died in Vienna.

Selected Publications

Blond K. Der Dekapitationsfingerhut. *Zentralbl Gynäkol* 1923; 47: 1097–100.

Heidler H. Zum Dekapitationsfingerhut von Kasper Blond. *Zentralbl Gynäkol* 1923; 48: 1815–17.

Bibliography References

105, 648, 986, 1118, 1189.

Blundell, James (1790–1878)

Blood Transfusion

James Blundell, obstetrician and physiologist, was born in London and initially studied under Sir Astley Cooper. He continued his medical training in Edinburgh and graduated MD from that university in 1813. He returned to London and became lecturer in midwifery and physiology at St Thomas' and Guy's hospitals. A careful and honest investigator, he carried out extensive experiments with transfusion in animals. He was the first to carry out transfusion of human blood and point out the dangers of heterologous blood transfusion. In 1825 his first case of successful human blood transfusion was reported by Dr Waller in a woman with post-partum haemorrhage:

> *The vein in the bend of the arm was laid bare, and an incision of sufficient extent to admit the pipe of the syringe was made into it . . . the syringe used by Dr B. was similar to the common injecting syringe, and contained two ounces . . . The blood was drawn from the patient's husband into a tumbler, and Dr B. stood ready with his syringe to absorb it instantly, in fact, while it was flowing: it was then immediately introduced into the orifice in the vein, and cautiously injected. No effect appeared to be produced by the first injection of two ounces, but towards the end of the second there was an approach to syncope; the pulse fell a little; there was sighing . . .*

Blundell foresaw the potential opposition to this treatment, saying, 'The operation will after the usual ordeal of neglect, opposition and ridicule, hereafter be admitted into general practice'. He also acknowledged the potentially serious risks:

> *. . . therefore seems right, as the operation now stands, to confine transfusion to the first class of cases only, namely, those in which there seems to be no hope for the patient, unless blood can be thrown in the veins.*

Blundell's ideas and writings predicted tubal ligation, hysterectomy, caesarean section and other

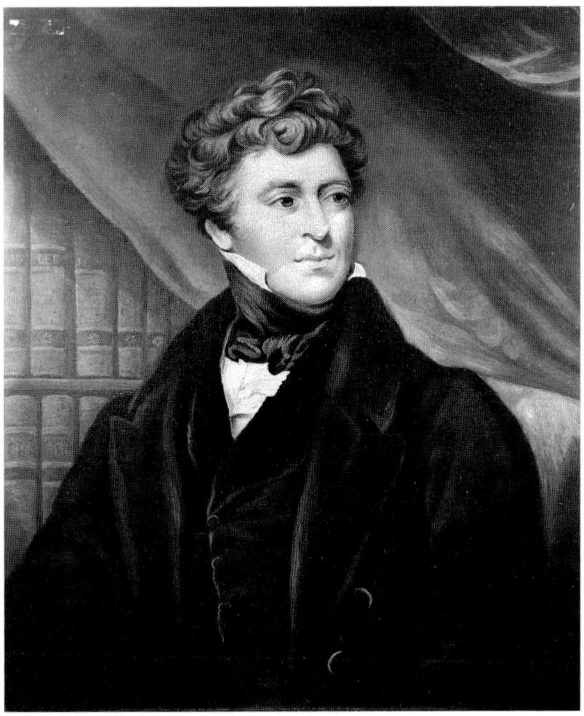

James Blundell

surgical developments in obstetrics and gynaecology. He was criticised for his experiments on abdominal surgery with living animals. He responded to his critics, saying: 'Strike gentlemen, but hear! . . . which will you sacrifice, your women or your cats?'

Although he felt that puerperal sepsis was due to vapours, his prescient observations led him to suspect the correct vector when he wrote in his lectures reported in the *Lancet* of 1827–9:

> *That its infectious nature may be plausibly disputed, I do not deny; but I add, considerately, that in my own family I had rather that those I esteemed the most should be delivered unaided, in a stable, by the mangerside, than that they should receive the best help, in the fairest apartment, but exposed to the vapours of this pitiless disease. Gossiping friends, wet-nurses, monthly nurses, the practitioner himself, these are the channels by which, I suspect, the infection is principally conveyed.*

Blundell published a comprehensive text on obstetrics, including clear instructions for endotracheal intubation of asphyxiated infants with his silver 'tracheal pipe':

> *Never hastily despair of the means of resuscitation. Many a foetus is laid aside as dead which, by a diligent use of resuscitants, might have been saved . . . the bud of life may appear withering, dying, nay dead – when unexpectedly, nature, from her deep and hidden recess, comes forth and raises the sinking embryo to vigorous life.*

In 1836 a dispute with the administration of Guy's Hospital led to his resignation. He continued with an extensive private practice and often made his calls late in the evening. His carriage was distinguishable by its illumination, allowing him to read as he travelled between houses. He died at his home in Piccadilly on 15 January 1878.

Selected Publications

Waller C. Case of uterine haemorrhage, in which the operation of transfusion was successfully performed. *Med Phys J* 1825; 54: 273–7.

Blundell J. Experiments on the transfusion of blood by the syringe. *Medico Chir Trans* 1818; 9: 56–92.

Blundell J. Successful case of transfusion. *Lancet* 1828; 1: 431.

Blundell J. *Principles and Practice of Obstetricy.* London: E Cox, 1834.

Bibliography References

34, 42, 57, 89, 102, 160, 161, 168, 171, 459, 648, 721, 758, 787, 826, 891, 976, 1057, 1130, 1205, 1509, 1736, 1745.

Boivin, Marie Anne Victoire (1773–1841)

Bivalve Vaginal Speculum

Madame Boivin was one of the most famous and well-educated Paris midwives, having studied at the Hospice de la Maternité in Paris, where she worked from 1797 to 1811. She wrote widely on midwifery, devised the first bivalve vaginal speculum in 1825 and was one of the first to advocate amputation of the cervix for cancer. She also wrote one of the early classic descriptions of hydatidiform mole, pointing out that it was of chorionic origin.

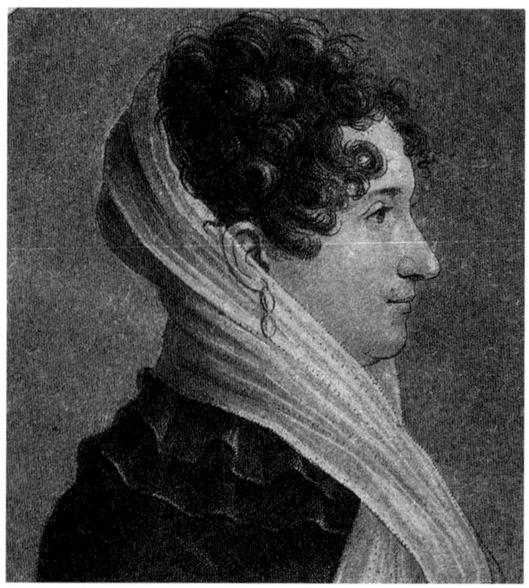

Marie Anne Victoire Boivin

Her maiden name was Gillian, and her husband died when she was in her thirties. Her first publication in 1812 was as the Widow Boivin. For her extensive and respected publications, she was awarded an honorary MD degree by the University of Marburg.

Near retirement, she was persuaded by Dupuytren to deliver his daughter, her last professional act. Dupuytren's opinion of her skill was summed up in his statement: 'She has an eye on the tip of her finger'.

Selected Publications

Boivin M A V. *Mémorial de l'art des accouchements.* Paris: Méquignon Père; 1812.

Boivin MAV. *Nouvelles recherches de la mole vesiculaire ou grossesse hydatique.* Paris, 1827.

Boivin MAV, Duges A. *Traité pratique des maladies de l'utérus et de ses annexes.* Two vols and atlas. Paris: JB Bailliere; 1833. (English Translation by GO Heming. London: Sherwood, Gilbert & Piper; 1834)

Bibliography References

63, 347, 419, 534, 648, 676, 982, 1278, 1303, 1595.

Bonney, William Francis Victor (1872–1953)

Bonney's Test/Myomectomy

Victor Bonney was a master pelvic surgeon with an international reputation as a surgical teacher. Along with Sir Comyns Berkeley, he modified and perfected Wertheim's radical hysterectomy for cancer of the cervix in the era before radiotherapy. He developed techniques for myomectomy and ovarian resection that ensured maximum conservation of healthy tissue, at a time when uterine fibroids and benign ovarian cysts tended to be treated by removal of the whole uterus or ovary. His technique using a flap to cover the bare area of myometrium left by removal of fibroids is called the 'Bonney hood'. The greatest number of fibroids he removed in one patient was 225 and the heaviest combined weight was 9.5 kg. In promoting conservation of the uterus and ovaries Bonney stated in his book, *The Technical Minutiae of Extended Myomectomy and Ovarian Cystectomy*:

> *As I have personally performed myomectomy rather over 800 times and ovarian cystectomy just over 300 times, more often, I believe, than anyone else in this country, and being able to draw, I thought it would be well to set down and illustrate, in more detail than has hitherto appeared, the technical minutiae of these two operations as I perform them, in the hope of being of assistance to those whose gynaecological work is already imbued with the spirit of conservatism, and a stimulus to those who have not yet appreciated the scope of reparative surgery as applied to the uterus and ovaries.*

He designed a number of surgical instruments, including dissecting forceps and a myomectomy corkscrew. 'Bonney's blue' solution, a mixture of crystal violet 0.5%, brilliant green 0.5 %, rectified spirit 50% and distilled water 49%, is still used by many as an antiseptic and marker in the vaginal fornices before abdominal hysterectomy.

Bonney also described a test to predict the likelihood of successfully curing stress incontinence with an anterior repair:

> *Before deciding upon it the following test should be applied. The patient, whose bladder should not recently have been emptied, is told to cough violently and the escape of urine noted. The index and middle finger of the examiner's hand should now be inserted into the vagina and the anterior vaginal wall pressed against the subpubic angle, but without pressing on the urethra. The patient is now told to cough again. If the pressure of the fingers prevents the leak, the operation if properly carried out will cure her.*

This became known as 'Bonney's test'. A more elaborate form of this test was later described by Marshall.

William Francis Victor Bonney was born in Chelsea, London, the son of a general practitioner. He studied medicine at the Middlesex Hospital and graduated in 1896. He initially intended to be a physician but, failing to get a training appointment at the Brompton Hospital, he chose surgery. After postgraduate training in London and a research fellowship in the Cancer investigation laboratories of the Middlesex Hospital, he was appointed obstetric tutor in 1905 and assistant gynaecological surgeon in 1908. He succeeded Berkeley as the senior gynaecological surgeon at the Middlesex Hospital in 1930. He also had a long association with the Chelsea Hospital for Women. Although he did little obstetrics, he helped promote the development and acceptance of the

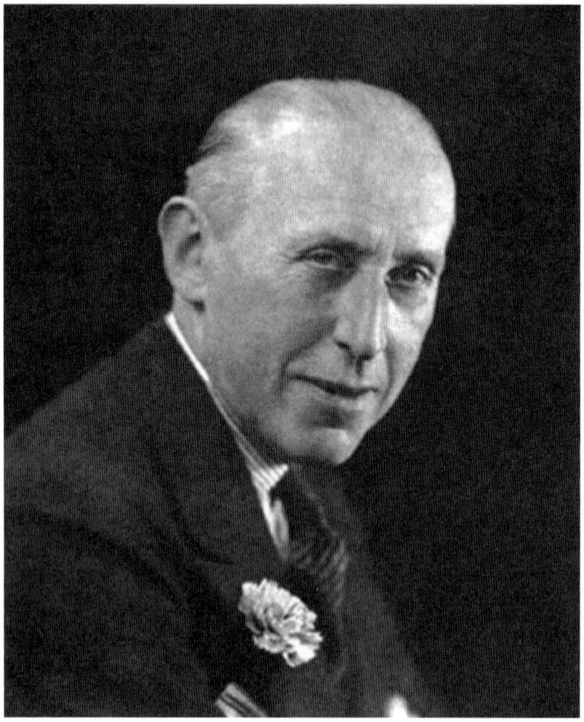

William Francis Victor Bonney

lower-segment caesarean operation in Britain. He regarded pregnancy as a 'surgical tumour'.

Bonney was a strong supporter and vice-president of the Royal College of Surgeons. He opposed the formation of the new British College of Obstetricians and Gynaecologists, feeling it did not adequately emphasise the surgical side of training. He influenced other London colleagues against the new college, creating a rift between him and those who supported it. Having helped elevate gynaecology to an accepted surgical specialty, he did not want it to descend again to the 'pill and pessary' era. He later changed his views and in 1946 accepted an honorary fellowship from the college in recognition of his enormous contribution to gynaecological surgery. Bonney's *Textbook of Operative Gynaecology,* originally co-authored with Berkeley, went through six editions in his lifetime and has continued in the hands of junior colleagues. A talented artist, Bonney went to art school and illustrated his book with line drawings, 611 of them in the sixth edition. He was a knowledgeable admirer of Rudyard Kipling's work and a vice-president of the Kipling Society. As an expert fly-fisherman, Bonney once played a foul-hooked salmon for six hours before landing it successfully. A small, dapper man who wore a monocle and a home-grown carnation in his button hole, Bonney died in the Middlesex Hospital from the sequelae of myocardial infarction on 4 July 1953.

Selected Publications

Berkeley C, Bonney V. *A Textbook of Gynaecological Surgery.* 4th edn. London: Cassell; 1942, pp. 537–8.

Bonney V. *The Technical Minutiae of Extended Myomectomy and Ovarian Cystectomy.* New York, NY: Paul B Hoeber Inc; 1946. Also published in The Classics of Obstetrics and Gynecology Library. New York: Gryphon Editions; 1992 (facsimile).

Bibliography References

165–167, 261, 262, 822, 965, 1056, 1183, 1505.

Bourgeois, Louyse (1563–1636)

Haemolytic Disease of the Newborn

It is possible that Louyse Bourgeois gave the earliest description of haemolytic disease of the newborn in her 1609 midwifery text. This was the first book on obstetrics published by a midwife. She reports a case of twins in a multiparous woman: one was born hydropic and soon died, while the other later developed jaundice and died on the fourth day.

Most of the obstetric advice in her book was based on the teachings of Guillemeau and Paré. She did, however, have her own quaint remedies, including one for arm presentation. In such cases she advised placing the infant's hand in a pan of cold water to stimulate its withdrawal back into the uterus. She acknowledged that, if the child was too feeble,

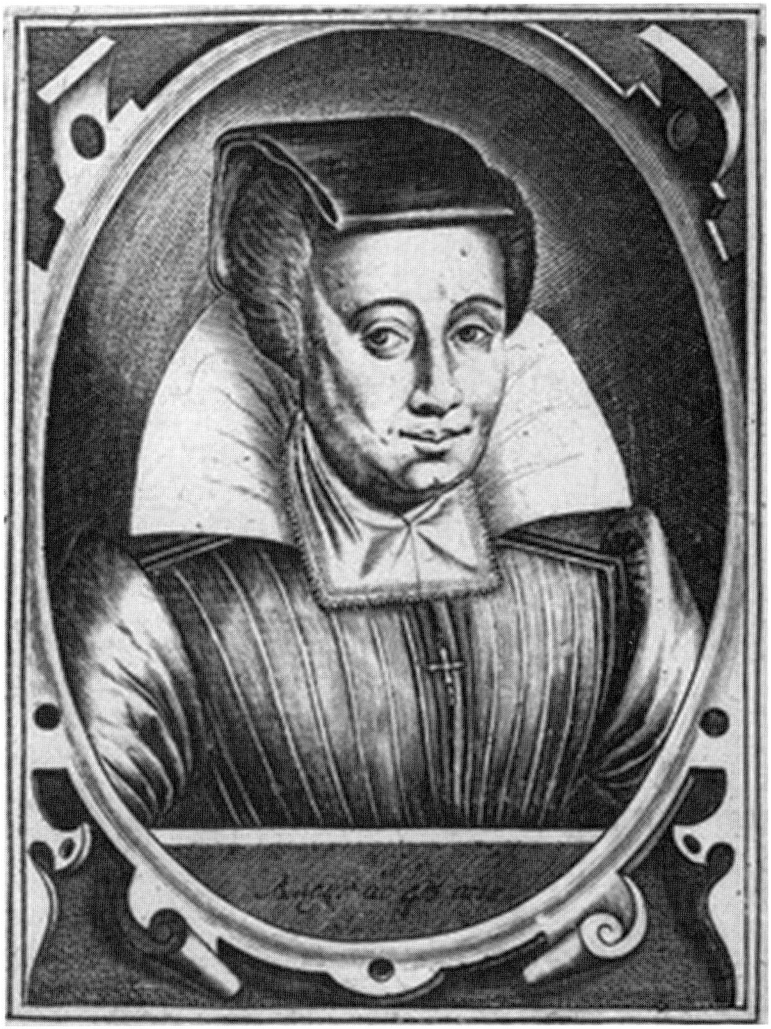

Louyse Bourgeois

the accoucheur might have to replace the arm and do an internal version and breech extraction.

Louyse Bourgeois was born in the Faubourg Saint-Germain, near Paris. She married Martin Boursier, a surgeon and pupil of Ambroise Paré. After the birth of her first child she received instruction from her husband and Paré and began acting as midwife to the poor of her own neighbourhood. In 1598 she passed the examination of the Municipal Authority of Paris and received her licence to practice as a midwife. Her reputation spread, and in 1601 she was called to attend Marie de Medici, the wife of Henry IV, at the birth of the future Louis XIII. She became midwife to the court and royal family of France for the next 26 years. Her book, *Observations diverses*, was published in 1609 at the height of her career as the royal midwife. However, in 1627, Marie de Bourbon-Montpensier, sister-in-law of Louis XIII, died under her care with puerperal sepsis. Although the review report of her death by a number of physicians was left 'open' and did not accuse her of incompetence, she felt it implied criticism and attacked the report in her *Apologie*. Effectively, this ended her career as a midwife and she spent her remaining years writing.

In the introduction to *Observations diverses*, she said she was 'the first woman practising my art to take up the pen'. The text went through four editions between 1609 and 1634 and was translated into Dutch, English and German. She was against intervention unless absolutely necessary: 'You should wait for the time which God has ordained, and especially in normal births where there is no accident'.

She died in December 1636, three years after her husband. They had three children: her daughter became a midwife and the two sons did medicine. One of her sons became physician to Louis XIII, whom she had delivered when first appointed royal midwife.

Selected Publications

Bourgeois L. *Observations diverses, sur la stérilité, perte de fruict, foecondité, accouchements, et maladie des femmes, et enfants nouveaux-naiz.* Paris: Saugrain; 1609.

Bourgeois L. *Apologie contre le rapport des médecins.* Paris, 1627.

Bibliography References

23, 347, 480, 632, 633, 648, 795, 912, 983, 1131, 1193, 1194, 1302, 1417, 1690.

Bourne, Aleck William (1886–1974)

Therapeutic Abortion

At 10 a.m. on 14 June 1938, Aleck Bourne, a respected consultant gynaecologist at St Mary's Hospital, London, terminated the early pregnancy of a 14-year-old girl by dilatation and curettage. He informed the police, and that evening he was arrested and later released on £200 bail.

The young girl in question had been raped in the Whitehall Barracks by three Horse Guardsmen, who were later found guilty and received jail sentences. She was referred to Bourne by a sympathetic general practitioner, who had diagnosed her pregnancy with an Aschheim–Zondek test. Bourne had her admitted to his ward at St Mary's Hospital 'to be sure of the type of girl I was dealing with'. When he examined her to take a swab for infection, 'She had a complete breakdown of her morale ... and wept beyond control ... This decided me that she had to be relieved of her pregnancy'.

The relevant law under which Bourne was charged in 1938 was the Offences Against the Person Act of 1861. The act stated that 'therapeutic' abortion was only justified if the woman's life was in danger. Bourne had performed therapeutic abortion in the past but felt that the definition, 'life was in danger', was too narrow and precluded even serious risks to the woman's health – in particular, her psychological or mental health. He decided this case was ideal to test the system and see if aspects of the woman's physical and mental health could be interpreted as 'a danger to life'. Thus, he informed the police so that the case would come before the court. Bourne did not seek to have the law changed, but he sought clarification vis-à-vis serious physical and mental health risks as valid reasons for therapeutic abortion, rather than the current absolute life-threatening indications, such as severe tuberculosis or cardiac disease.

The case went to trial on 18 July 1938 at the Old Bailey criminal court before Justice Macnaghten and a jury. Bourne was charged as follows: 'That on June 14th, 1938, he used an instrument with intent to procure the miscarriage of a girl'. At the outset, the defence lawyer asked that the word 'unlawful' be added to the indictment to acknowledge that there were occasions when the operation was lawful. This was granted. Supporting medical opinions were called by the defence. In Bourne's own testimony he explained that his rationale for termination was based on risks to the girl's physical and mental health:

> *I could not draw a line between danger to life and danger to health, if one waited for danger to life the woman would be past assistance. He would terminate pregnancy if he believed there was serious danger to health.*

On the second day of the trial, on hearing all the evidence, Justice Macnaghten instructed the jury:

> *If the doctor is of opinion on reasonable grounds and on adequate knowledge that the continuance of pregnancy would probably make the woman a physical or mental wreck, the act is lawful ... Life depends on health and it may be that health is so gravely impaired that death results.*

He also pointed out that if the prosecution had proved, beyond a reasonable doubt, that Bourne had not acted, 'in good faith for the purpose only of preserving the life of the girl', then the verdict must be guilty.

The jury retired for 40 minutes and returned a verdict of not guilty.

This established case law that made it feasible for physicians to provide therapeutic abortion for risk to the woman's health and not only for the risk of death if the pregnancy continued. It was, however, largely provided in the private sector, and the carnage of illegal backstreet abortion continued. Septic abortion remained a major cause of maternal death. It was not until 1967 that new statute law, in the form of the Abortion Act, made therapeutic abortion legal in government hospitals and licensed private clinics throughout Britain. Similar laws followed in Canada (1969) and the United States (1973).

Aleck Bourne was born in 4 June 1886 in the small town of Totteridge, England. His father was a Wesleyan minister of modest means. Young Bourne won a scholarship to Cambridge University and began his medical studies there, completing his clinical work at St Mary's Hospital, London. At the outbreak of the First World War he volunteered and served as a medical officer in Egypt and France. In 1918 he was appointed to the consulting staff of St Mary's and began a private practice of obstetrics and gynaecology, with rooms in Harley Street, London.

Ironically, Aleck Bourne was opposed to the Abortion Act, which was passed some 15 years after he retired. He was a founding member of the Society for the Protection of Unborn Children, which was set up in opposition to the Act. He felt there was enough flexibility with the case law of Rex v Bourne to allow a reputable doctor to provide therapeutic abortion in the rare cases it was necessary.

Selected Publications

A charge of illegal abortion. Rex v Bourne. *Lancet* 1938; 232: 220–6.

Bourne A. Correspondence: Rex v Bourne. *Lancet* 1938; 232: 280.

Bourne A. *A Doctor's Creed: The Memoirs of a Gynaecologist*. London: Victor Gollancz Ltd; 1962.

Bibliography References

172, 173, 263, 375, 1129.

Bovie, William T (1882–1958)

Electrosurgery

The application of heat via cautery was used to stop bleeding in Egyptian medicine circa 2000 BC. In the Smith papyrus, the use of incisional cautery by a hot scalpel was described: 'The knife should be heated in the fire; the bleeding is not great'. There was no mention, however, of how the surgeon would hold the hot knife.

Electrosurgery was a descendant of cautery, and the first practical application came with the development of high frequency electrical current. By the late nineteenth and early twentieth centuries there was sporadic application for haemostasis and cautery-excision of superficial tumours.

By 1926, William Bovie, working in Boston at the Huntington Hospital of the Harvard Cancer Commission, had developed a practical electrosurgical unit and was exploring its use in excising tumours in his laboratory. Just up the street, in the Peter Bent Brigham Hospital, the neurosurgeon, Harvey Cushing, struggled and failed to remove a patient's vascular brain tumour. Cushing heard of Bovie's work and asked for his assistance. Bovie brought his unit, the size of a small desk, down the street on a handcart. Thus, on 1 October 1926, Cushing reoperated on the same patient and, using Bovie's 'electrified loop', successfully removed the tumour:

> *I had persuaded Dr Bovie to bring his electrosurgery unit over here to let me see what I could do with his cutting loop. This had necessitated re-electrifying the operating room . . . So far as I am aware, the principles of electrosurgery have heretofore not been utilised in cranio-cerebral operations . . . Not until the autumn of 1926 when, in the Huntington Hospital nearby, I happened to see Dr Bovie's electrified loop being used for the purpose of bloodlessly scooping out bits of malignant tissue for examination, did I realise that here was a new tool which might possibly be utilised for the piecemeal removal of*

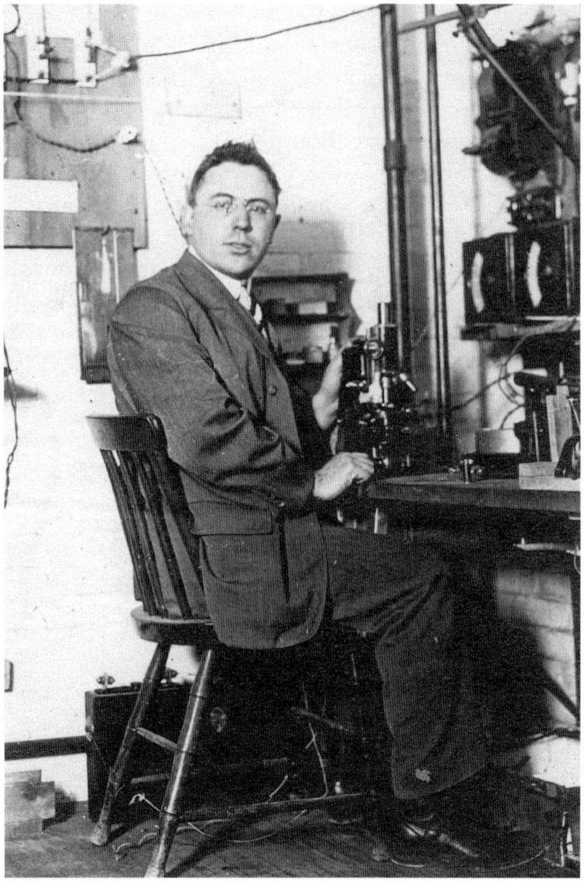

William T Bovie

some of the more inaccessible intracranial tumours. The results have exceeded all expectations.

With Bovie's help, Cushing operated with success on many more cases of vascular brain tumours, previously thought to be inoperable.

William Bovie was born in Augusta, Michigan on 11 September 1882. He grew up in the small town, where his father was the local general practitioner and also managed the family farm. His father died in 1901 and William had limited finances to pursue higher education. He obtained his bachelor's degree from the University of Michigan and his master's from the University of Missouri. In between he worked as a college instructor; it took him three years to pay off his debts sufficient to allow receipt of his bachelor's degree. In 1911 he went to Harvard University and received his PhD in plant physiology in 1914.

Bovie felt that the subjects of physics and biology overlapped: 'I have an idea that there is a field between physics and biology – a field that should be known as biophysics'. Harvard University agreed and he was appointed assistant professor of biophysics from 1920 to 1927. His research was based at the Cancer Commission and, in addition to his development of the electrosurgical unit, he carried out studies with radium. Suitable precautions for handling radium were not used and he later suffered chronic radiation damage to his hands.

In 1927, Bovie was appointed chairman of the new biophysics department at Northwestern University in Chicago. Two years later he moved to Bar Harbor, Maine, at the behest of a friend who had started the Jackson cancer research laboratory. In 1939 he moved to the small, liberal arts, Colby College in Waterville, Maine, as lecturer in social technology. Here he saw out the final 10 years of his professional career.

Bovie's inventive mind and wide range of interests meant that he started but did not complete many projects. His hero was Leonardo da Vinci. He was said to be irascible and, on occasions, pompous. Although he felt his work was under appreciated, he was awarded the prestigious John Scott Medal from the city of Philadelphia in 1928.

In retirement Bovie suffered from obesity, arthritis and diabetes, which caused him to become housebound. When he patented his electrosurgical unit in 1931 he signed over the patent rights to the manufacturing company for one dollar, feeling he should not benefit from his invention. Unfortunately, his final years were plagued by poverty. He died on New Year's Day 1958 after a stroke and was buried in Fairfield, Maine.

Selected Publications

Cushing H, Bovie WT. Electrosurgery as an aid to the removal of intracranial tumours with a preliminary note on a new surgical-current generator by WT Bovie. *Surg Gynecol Obstet* 1928; 47: 751–84.

Bibliography References

247, 812, 863, 973, 990, 1127, 1268.

Bowen, John Templeton (1857–1940)

Bowen's Disease of the Vulva

In 1912 John Bowen drew attention to what he termed a pre-cancerous dermatosis in two patients with chronic skin lesions recurring after local destructive treatment over ten and 20 years respectively:

> *They appeared as papular and tubercular lesions, only slightly elevated above the normal skin, of a moderately firm consistency, and dull red in color. The surface was in some places slightly crusted; in other places it had a papillomatous character.*

While Bowen felt these cases had some features in common with extramammary Paget's disease, there were differences:

> *With regard to the clinical appearances, the cases I am reporting resembled Paget's disease in very few respects . . . At no time was there any oozing, exposed or weeping surface. The lesions were more organised and solid, the only symptoms of exudation being expressed by the rather moist crusts and scales that covered the surface.*

He predicted the ultimate development of malignancy in these cases:

> *As yet no signs of malignancy have appeared in these cases. It can hardly be doubted that such a sequel is imminent.*

Bowen's original cases were described in two males, one on the buttock and one on the lower leg. The same lesions are seen on the vulva and are usually classified as carcinoma in situ.

John Templeton Bowen was born in Boston and graduated MD from Harvard in 1884. He spent two years in Berlin, Munich and Vienna, returning to Boston as an assistant physician at the Massachusetts General Hospital in 1889. He became professor of dermatology at Harvard in 1907. A shy bachelor, he was a reluctant lecturer.

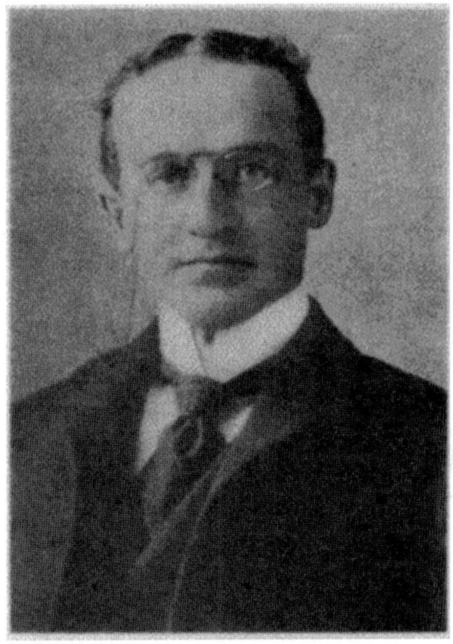

John Templeton Bowen

Bowen retired in 1927 and became quite reclusive. He spent his summers in Europe, usually in France. His final years were beset by vertigo and ill health. He died in Boston on 3 December 1940.

Selected Publications

Bowen JT. Precancerous dermatoses: a study of two cases of chronic atypical epithelial proliferation. *J Cutan Dis* 1912; 30: 241–55.

Bibliography References

174, 801, 1398, 1480.

Bozzini, Philipp (1773–1809)

Endoscopy

The beginnings of endoscopy lie in the development of the *Lichtleiter* (light conductor) by Philipp Bozzini in 1805. This consisted of a light source, 'a good wax candle', and a mirror system with conducting tubes, 'made of brass or silver which are modified according to the opening they are meant for'. He reported his work in 1806 and advocated physiological and pathological studies of all 'interior cavities . . . by looking through natural openings or at least small wounds'.

In support of the efficiency of his *Lichtleiter* Bozzini wrote:

> *To give an idea how distinctly the light transmitter reflects the rays, I would like to cite just one example: if, observing proper cleanliness, one places a piece of writing in the fundus of the uterus of a woman who died during delivery, it can be read through the vagina with the help of the light transmitter containing an ordinary wax candle as clearly as by the light of a candle standing at the same distance on a table.*

He also anticipated the development of endoscopically guided surgery:

> *Surgery will not only develop new and previously impossible procedures, but all uncertain operations which depended on luck and approximation will become safe under the influence of direct vision, since the surgeon's hand will now be guided by his eyes.*

One year before he published his work, Bozzini sent the text of his paper along with a letter dated 8 June 1805 to the Archduke Karl of Austria, in which he wrote:

> *I feel that it is the holiest duty of my most humble thankfulness to most humbly submit my invention by which a clear and easy view is given into all the inner cavities and spaces of the living body, either through the normal or through artificial openings . . . the latter have convinced me that by the use of the device (a description of which I am adding) among other things all surgical operations in cavities of the living body will gain an ease and safety, since the use of the sense of sight for knowledge of the state of illness and for guiding instruments will be more effectively facilitated.*

Bozzini was subsequently reprimanded by the medical faculty of Vienna for 'undue curiosity', after he had inspected the interior of the urethra in a living patient. Later his *Lichtleiter* was dismissed as a 'mere toy' by the same group, led and dominated by a jealous colleague. However, other physicians embraced his invention and ideas, which he shared freely.

Bozzini also invented a repositor to replace a prolapsed umbilical cord in labour. In response to a negative report by a physician who had never tried it, Bozzini said, 'It means nothing for an invention when somebody gives a judgement, based only on his own authority and not on his own experiments and clinical experience'.

Philipp Bozzini was born in Mainz, Germany. His father was Italian but had to leave his homeland after a fatal duel. Bozzini studied medicine at Jena and Mainz graduating in 1796. He started practice in Mainz but left when it was conquered by the French in 1797. He served as a military physician in the Austrian army during the War of the Coalition from 1799 to 1802. In 1803 he settled in Frankfurt am Main

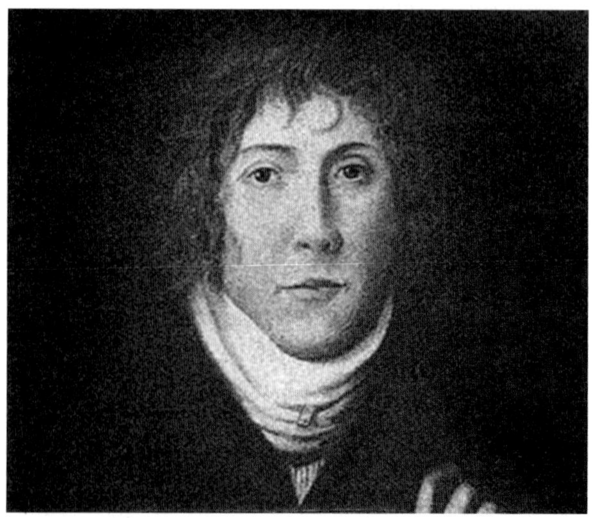

Philipp Bozzini

and became 'physicus extraordinarius' in 1808. In the course of his duties he contracted and died from typhoid fever on April 4 1809, at the age of 35. He left a wife and three young children.

Selected Publications

Bozzini P. Lichtleiter, eine Erfindung zur Anschauung innerer Theile und Krankheiten nebst der Abbildung. In: Hufeland CW (ed.) *Journal der Practischen Arzneykunde und Wundarzneykunst (Berlin)* 1806; 24: 107–24.

Bush RB, Leonhardt H, Bush IM, Landes RR. Nr Bozzini's lichtleiter: a translation of his original article (1806). *Urology* 1974; 3: 119–23.

Bibliography References

127, 128, 544, 612, 670, 895, 1084, 1096, 1111, 1178, 1271, 1315, 1361, 1364, 1449.

Bracht, Erich Franz (1882–1969)

Bracht's Manoeuvre

The safe conduct of a breech vaginal delivery requires a fine balance between the spontaneous forces of labour and guided assistance by the accoucheur. Erich Bracht felt that too much interference during the process was unnecessary and harmful. His manoeuvre involved allowing spontaneous delivery of the breech to the umbilicus and trunk. The body and extended legs are then grasped in both hands with the fingers around the lower back and the thumbs around the posterior aspect of the thighs. While an assistant applies suprapubic pressure, the body is drawn up towards the maternal abdomen. The symphysis acts as a fulcrum around which the occiput rotates as the head delivers.

Bracht first described his manoeuvre to the Berlin Obstetrical and Gynaecological Society on 4 October 1935. This was outlined in his first publication in 1936. In May 1938 he presented a motion-picture of the manoeuvre to the International Congress of Obstetrics and Gynaecology in Amsterdam. He also reported his experience of 206 cases without death. The Bracht manoeuvre was adopted in Europe but never much used in North America or the United Kingdom.

Erich Franz Bracht, the son of a doctor, was born in Berlin. He studied medicine in Freiburg, Kiel and Berlin, qualifying in 1906. His postgraduate studies were taken in Freiburg, Heidelberg and Kiel, where he was a pupil of Herman Pfannenstiel and Walter Stoeckel.

He settled back in Berlin and became extraordinary professor there in 1922. From 1945 to 1955 he was head of the department of obstetrics and gynaecology at the provincial Frauenklinik at Berlin-Neukölln. He is also known eponymously for Bracht–Wächter bodies, which are perivascular microabscesses seen in the myocardium in acute bacterial endocarditis. He carried out this work during his first postgraduate job working in the pathology laboratory of Ludwig Aschoff (1866–1942) in Freiburg.

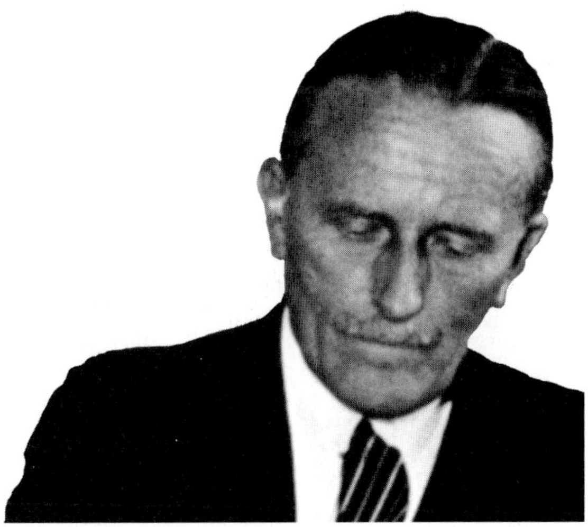

Erich Franz Bracht

Selected Publications

Bracht E. Zur Manualhilfe dei Beckenendlage. *Ztschr Geburtshilfe Gynäkol* 1936; 271: 6–10.

Bibliography References

790, 1225, 1480.

Brandt, Murray Lampel (b. 1892) Andrews, Charles James (1876–1950)

Brandt–Andrews Method of Placental Delivery

Over the centuries various methods of placental delivery have been advocated, from immediate manual removal to observation with no intervention. In 1933, the New York obstetrician, Murray Brandt, helped clarify the clinical distinction between separation and expulsion of the placenta in the third stage of labour. In a series of 30 cases he injected sodium iodide into the umbilical vein of the placenta immediately after delivery and took an X-ray within three minutes. He found 'the placenta detached and folded on itself in every case lying in the lower segment of the uterus'. He therefore advised waiting 5–10 minutes after delivery of the infant and proceeding as follows:

> *An artery clamp is placed on the umbilical cord close to the vulva and held in one hand while the other hand is placed on the abdomen of the mother, in such a manner that the thumb lies parallel to the symphysis and palm and fingers approximate the surface of the uterine body. Holding the umbilical cord taut, a gentle upward push is made on the lower segment by the hand on the abdomen, without attempting to grasp the uterus. If the placenta lies in the dilated cervical canal or upper vagina, the uterus will rise upward and there will be but slight tension on the cord held in the artery clamp. If it rises, a further series of gentle pushes causes the uterus to ascend towards the diaphragm while the placenta remains in the vagina. It is usually sufficient to raise the uterus to a level where the umbilicus is about at the middle of the uterine body. Frequently in performing this maneuver, one feels the membranes peeling off the lower uterine segment.*

He emphasised that 'although the cord must be held taut, traction must be avoided'.

In 1940, Charles Andrews of Norfolk, Virginia advocated a similar approach. Initially he was unaware of Brandt's publication but he did acknowledge it in his own report. He described his technique thus:

> *The cord is then clamped about two to three inches from the vulva. The palmar surfaces of the fingers of the left hand are placed on the abdomen over the anterior surface of the uterus at the junction of the body and lower relaxed portion of the cervix. By gentle pressure backward and upward the fundus is carried out of the pelvis into the abdomen. If the placenta is separated the cord does not rise. If separation has occurred downward pressure above the pubis, below the fundus will cause the placenta to appear at the vulva. If the placenta has not been separated the cord will be drawn upward. In such case the left hand is placed with the fingers over the fundus and the thumb below, and very slight stimulation by massage will give a contraction which may bring the placenta down to be expelled as previously described.*

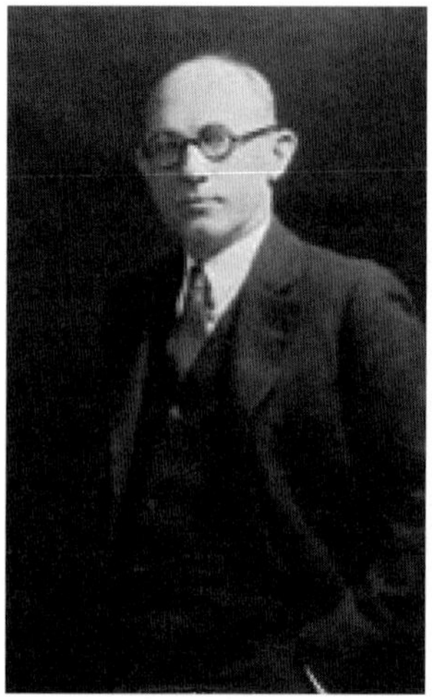

Charles James Andrews

The English obstetricians FCR Picton and Norman Kimball later emphasised the use of this technique in association with ergometrine at the time of delivery. Thus began the modern principle of active management of the third stage of labour with an oxytocic drug and controlled cord traction.

Murray Brandt was born in 1892 and received his MD from Bellevue Hospital Medical School, New York in 1914. He was assistant obstetrician to the Fordham Hospital and assistant gynaecologist at the Mount Sinai Hospital, New York.

Charles Andrews graduated MD from the Medical College of Virginia in 1902, followed by an internship at the New York Lying-in Hospital. He returned to Norfolk, Virginia in 1904 and later became director of the department of obstetrics and gynaecology at the Norfolk General Hospital. His son, Mason (1919–2006), became a prominent obstetrician in Norfolk and Mason's younger brother, William (1924–2008), was president of the American College of Obstetricians and Gynecologists in 1994.

Selected Publications

Andrews CJ. The third stage of labour with an evaluation of the Brandt method of expression of the placenta. *J South Med Surg* 1940; 102: 605–8.

Brandt ML. The mechanism and management of the third stage of labor. *Am J Obstet Gynecol* 1933; 25: 662–7.

Kimball N. Brandt–Andrews technique of delivery of the placenta. *BMJ* 1958; 1: 203–4.

Picton FCR. Use and abuse of the umbilical cord in the third stage of labour. *J Obstet Gynaecol Br Emp* 1951; 58: 764–73.

Bibliography References

27, 85, 94.

Braun, Carl Rudolph (1823–1891)

Braun's Decapitation Hook

In neglected cases of shoulder presentation, before the era of safe caesarean section, fetal decapitation was the treatment of choice. Carl Braun devised a decapitation hook which was widely used until the advent of the Blond–Heidler saw. This consisted of a long stem with a blunt hook at one end and a transverse handle at the other. The hook was guided over the fetal neck and, by a twisting motion with the handle, the vertebral column was dislocated and severed. Other decapitation hooks used in that era were designed by Bernhard Schultze, Robert Jardine (1862–1932) and Paul Zweifel (1848–1927).

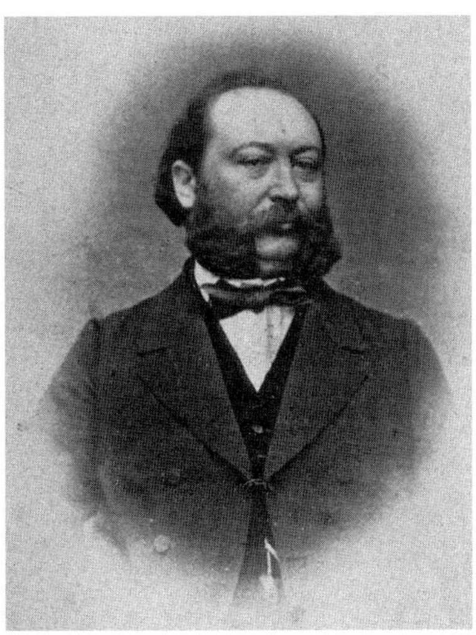

Carl Rudolph Braun

Carl Rudolph Braum was born in Zistersdorf, Austria. He followed Ignac Semmelweis as assistant to Johann Klein at the Vienna Maternity Clinic in 1847 and became head of the clinic in 1856. He added a gynaecological section in 1858, being convinced that

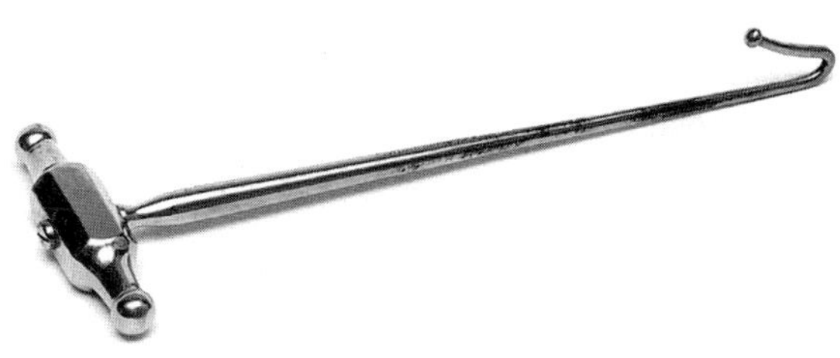

Braun hook

obstetrics and gynaecology belonged together. In 1867 he was appointed dean of the medical faculty at the University of Vienna. He was knighted in 1872 and thus entitled to the name Carl Ritter von Fernwald Braun. His younger brother, Gustav August Braun (1829–1911), followed in his footsteps, and it was he who published the paper drawing attention to the value of his older brother's invention. For the highly skilled bimanual examiner, his name is also associated with the asymmetrical enlargement and softening of the uterine fundus at 4–6 weeks gestation: the Braun-Fernwald sign.

Selected Publications

Braun GA. Über das technische Verfahren bei vernachlässigten Querlagen und über Decapitationsinstrumente. *Wien Med Wochenschr* 1861; 11: 713–6.

Bibliography References

542, 648, 1291, 1480.

Breisky, August (1832–1889)

Kraurosis Vulvae

In 1885, August Breisky published his classic description of kraurosis vulvae:

> *On the external genitalia of adult females I have observed in a few cases – 12 in all – peculiar alterations, an atrophic shrivelling of the skin . . . The generalised effect of this extensive shrivelling is a striking smallness and inflexibility of the vestibular portion of the vulva . . .*

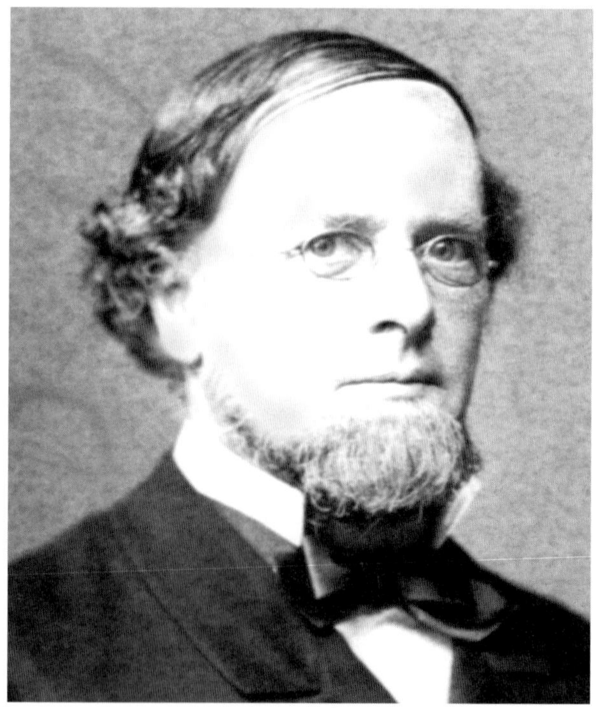

August Breisky

August Breisky was born in Klattau, Bohemia, and took his medical degree in Prague, qualifying in 1855. He did postgraduate training in both pathology and obstetrics and gynaecology. He was appointed professor successively at Salzburg, Berne, Prague and Vienna. Breisky made many contributions to gynaecological surgery, and his name is linked with Ernst Navratil in the Breisky–Navratil vaginal retractor. He was said to be a genial and kindly man.

Selected Publications

Breisky A. Über Kraurosis vulvae, eine wenig beachtete Form von Hautatrophie am pudendum muliebre. *Zeitschr für Heilk* 1885; 6: 69–80.

Bibliography References

187, 543, 765, 1123, 1398, 1441, 1443.

Brenner, Fritz (1877–1969)

Brenner's Tumour

Fritz Brenner was born in Osthofen, Germany in 1877. He received his medical degree from Heidelberg in 1904.

During his studies at the Senckenbergsche Pathology Institute in Frankfurt he published his work on the ovarian tumour that was later designated the 'Brenner tumour' by Robert Meyer. In his report of three cases Brenner thought the tumour was related to abnormal follicular growth and suggested the name 'oophoroma folliculare'.

Brenner left Germany in 1910 for Southwest Africa, then a German colony, moving into general practice in Johannesburg in 1935. It was not until the 1950s, when Harold Speert tracked him down, that Brenner was informed of his eponymous fame. He died on 26 December 1969.

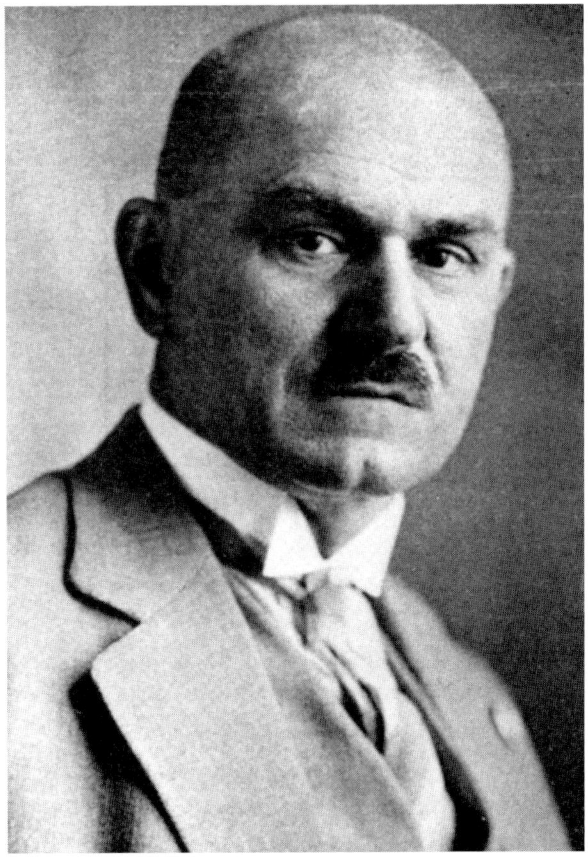

Fritz Brenner

Selected Publications

Brenner F. Das Oophoroma folliculare. *Ztschr Path Frankfurt.* 1907; 1: 150–71.

Bibliography References

968, 1244, 1465, 1480.

Browne, Thomas (1605–1682)

Teratology

In 1919, when Sir William Osler's body lay in the chapel of Christ Church College, Oxford, placed upon the coffin was his personal copy of a small book he cherished: *Religio medici.* Written almost three centuries before by another famous medical scholar, Thomas Browne, it embodied his observations and philosophy of life, pleading for religious tolerance in an intolerant era. The book became and remains a bestseller, even though it was placed on the *Index expurgatorius* by the Vatican, as forbidden reading for Catholics. One of the most famous quotations could be said to predict the essence of teratology:

> *And surely we are all out of the computation of our age, and every man is some months elder than he bethinks him; for we live, move, have a being, and are subject to the actions of the elements, and the malice of diseases, in that world, the truest microcosm, the womb of our mother . . .*

Thomas Browne was born in London. He received a classical education and graduated MA from Oxford in 1629. He embarked upon his medical training by visiting Montpellier, Padua and Leyden, obtaining his medical degree from the latter university in 1633. He returned to England, entered practice in Shipden Dale near Halifax and there wrote *Religio Medici* before his thirtieth birthday. It was originally written in 1635 as

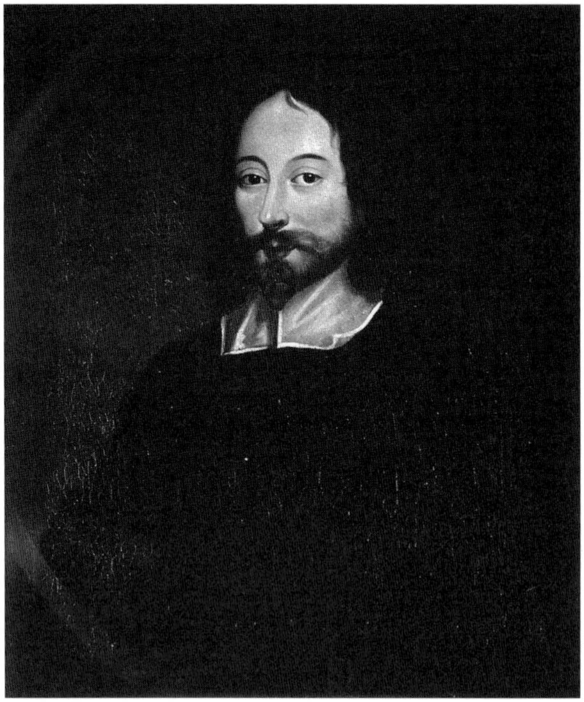

Thomas Browne

a personal memoir for private circulation. However, the response was such that it was published in 1642. Browne moved to Norwich in 1636, where he remained and practised medicine until his death. He became Sir Thomas Browne in 1671 when he was knighted by Charles II. When he wrote *Religio Medici* Browne was unmarried and had a rather jaundiced view of the act of procreation:

> *I could be content that we might procreate like trees without conjunction, or that there were any way to perpetuate the world without this trivial and vulgar act of coition: it is the foolishest act a wise man commits in all his life nor is there any thing that will more deject his cooled imagination, when he shall consider what an odd and unworthy piece of folly he hath committed.*

Most of his other observations of the human condition were more optimistic and uplifting. Moreover, six years later he married and managed to overcome his inhibitions sufficiently to father 12 children. In his tract, *Urn Burial*, a meditation on mortality, he wrote movingly:

> *Time which antiquates Antiquities, hath an art to make dust of all things . . . the iniquity of oblivion blindly scattereth her poppy, and deals with the memory of men without distinction to merit of perpetuity.*

This sentiment, despite the passage of four centuries, has not applied to him. Sir Thomas Browne died on his birthday in 1682. He is buried at the church of St Peter Mancroft in Norwich, marked by a memorial and a statue.

Selected Publications

Browne T. *Religio Medici*. London: William Pickering; 1845. The Classics of Medicine Library. Birmingham: Gryphon Editions; 1981 (facsimile).

Bibliography References

185, 466, 546, 571, 750, 755, 867, 1148, 1149, 1251, 1387, 1388, 1657, 1674, 1688, 1715.

Burch, John Christopher (1900–1977)

Burch Colposuspension

Surgical innovation is often required during an operation when the planned or standard technique proves impossible. Such were the circumstances that led John Burch to develop his technique of colposuspension, now accepted as one of the simplest and most effective methods of elevating the urethrovesical junction in cases of urinary stress incontinence. As he was to write in his 1961 publication on the procedure:

> *One day while we were doing a Marshall–Marchetti–Krantz operation, the sutures in the periosteum continued to pull out and it was necessary to look for another point of attachment. An examination of the field revealed that the intravaginal finger was pushing the anterior vaginal wall*

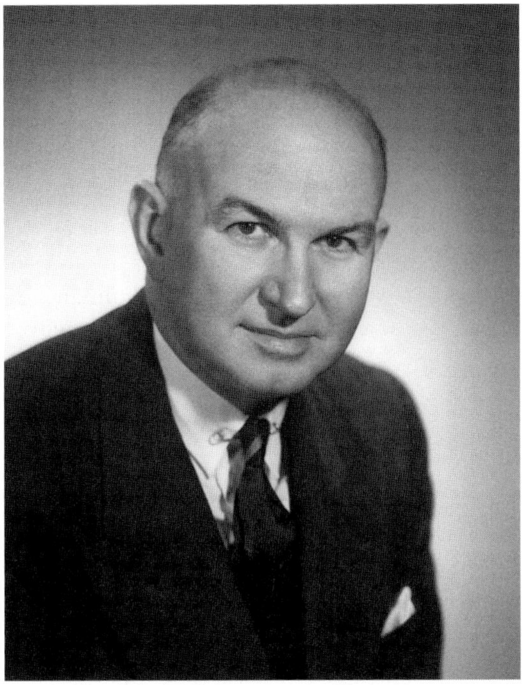

John Christopher Burch

up to a level as high as the origin of the levator muscle from the white line of the pelvis. Since the white line is the usually accepted origin of the so-called fascia surrounding the vagina it seemed reasonable and anatomically correct to suture this perivaginal fascia to the white line and the underlying levator muscle with three interrupted sutures on each side. This maneuver produced a most satisfactory restoration of the normal anatomy of the bladder neck and, in addition, a surprising correction of most of the cystocele involving the base of the bladder ... The white line, however, had the same disadvantage as the symphysis. It holds the sutures poorly. The final step in the development of the operation to be described was the utilization of Cooper's ligament as a point of fixation. This strong thick band of fibrous tissue runs along the superior surface of the superior ramus of the pubic bone and is ideal from the standpoint of both passing and holding a suture.

John Christopher Burch was born in Nashville, Tennessee. His father, Lucius Burch, was head of the department of obstetrics and gynaecology and later dean of the medical school at Vanderbilt University. John Burch graduated in medicine from Vanderbilt University in 1923. After resident training in Boston and New York he visited Edinburgh and Vienna as a Rockefeller Foundation fellow. He returned to Nashville in 1926 and joined his father's private practice in the Burch Clinic. During the Second World War he served in the US army as colonel and chief of the surgical service at Brooke General Hospital in Fort Sam Houston, Texas. Upon return to Nashville he was appointed professor and head of the department of obstetrics and gynaecology. In addition to gynaecology at the university hospital he practised general surgery at St Thomas' Hospital, Nashville. He was elected president of the Southern Surgical Association in 1953, as was his father before him in 1929. He was also a long-serving vestryman in the local Episcopal church. In 1965 he received the Distinguished Service Award from the American College of Surgeons. He continued in private practice until his death, in 1977.

Selected Publications

Burch JC. Urethrovaginal fixation to Cooper's ligament for correction of stress incontinence, cystocele, and prolapse. *Am J Obstet Gynecol* 1961; 81: 281–90.

Burch JC, Cooper's ligament urethrovesical suspension for stress incontinence. Nine years' experience – results, complications, technique. *Am J Obstet Gynecol* 1968; 100: 764–74.

Bibliography References

103, 390, 442, 443, 1236, 1455.

Burnham, Walter (1808–1883)

Subtotal Abdominal Hysterectomy

Walter Burnham performed the first – albeit unplanned – abdominal subtotal hysterectomy in which the patient survived. The patient, a 42-year-old woman, was known to have a slowly growing tumour arising from her pelvis for the previous six years. Initially the tumour was symptom-free, but by

1853 persistent pain made her seek consultation with Dr Walter Burnham of Lowell, Massachusetts. After examining the woman, Burnham diagnosed a large ovarian cyst and informed the woman 'that she could not be cured by any remedial plan of treatment, and that nothing short of the removal of the tumour could in any way be expected to benefit her, and even this course could not be adopted without placing her life in imminent danger'. He advised her to seek a second opinion and 'also to consult her friends as to the propriety of running so great a risk'. She elected to proceed with the operation, which was performed on 25 June 1853. Burnham made a midline incision and found to his surprise that the tumour was not an ovarian cyst but a large pedunculated fibroid which, once it pushed out through the abdominal incision could not be replaced:

> *I was now enabled to determine the nature and extent of the tumour and found that its principle portion was attached by a small neck – about one inch in diameter – to the fundus of the uterus, instead of being an enlargement of the ovarium as I had supposed; and also that the uterus itself was implicated in the disease occupying and filling the pelvis literally full. I also ascertained that the left ovarium was enlarged to the size of a man's fist, and of the same fibrous structure. To the right ovarium was attached a cyst containing about six ounces of dark sero sanguinous fluid.*

The operation was carried out under chloroform anaesthesia, with two surgical assistants and in the presence of a 'large number of medical gentlemen'. His description of the operation included ligation of the uterine arteries:

> *... with great caution, I had at length removed all the attachments down to the cervix uteria, this part not appearing to be implicated in the disease was divided at the point where the vagina is reflected upon it. Two arteries – the uterine – only required ligatures.*

The patient recovered fully with the aid, among other things, of brandy and opium and, ultimately, she outlived her surgeon. Although the operation concluded successfully, Burnham was honest enough to emphasise the difficulty he encountered:

> *Although this case terminated favourably, I would not easily be induced to make another attempt to extirpate the uterus and ovaries, or even remove the uterus under almost any condition ...*

Water Burnham, the son of a doctor, was born in Brookfield, Vermont, on 12 January 1808. He studied medicine with his father and graduated in medicine from the University of Vermont in 1829. He practised in Vermont until moving to Lowell, Massachusetts in 1846. He carried out general surgery and was one of the early advocates of ovariotomy at which he became expert, performing some 300 such procedures in 30 years with a 75 per cent survival rate – a good showing at the time. He ultimately performed 15 hysterectomies with only three survivors, including the first case described above.

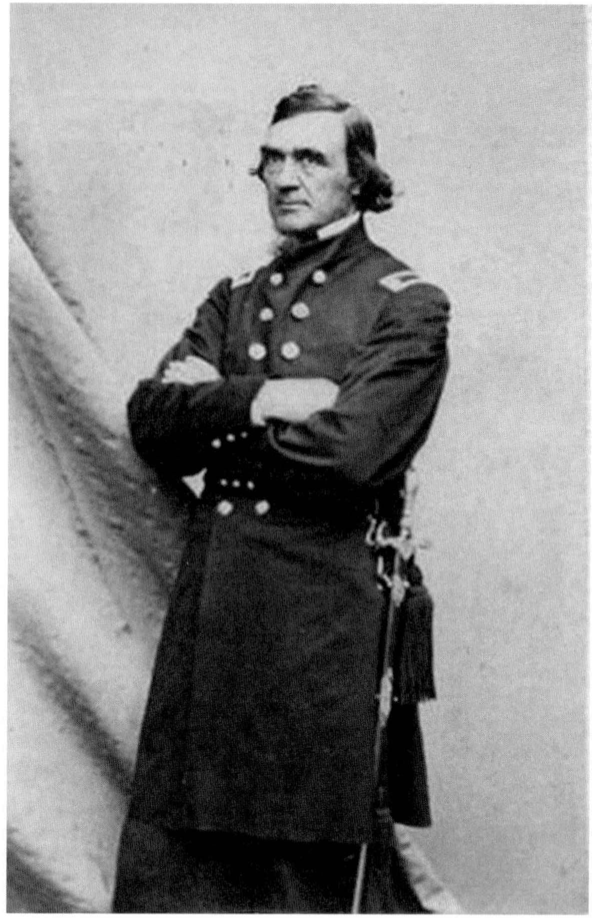

Walter Burnham

Dr Burnham was surgeon of the Sixth Massachusetts Regiment of Volunteers in the Civil War from 1862 to 1870. He was a member of the Massachusetts House of Representatives and was instrumental in securing passage of the Anatomy Act in 1855, which authorised the medical profession to obtain bodies of dead paupers for dissection and anatomical instruction. He died at his home in Lowell on 16 January 1883.

Selected Publications

Burnham W. Extirpation of the uterus and ovaries for sarcomatous disease. *American Lancet* 1854; 8: 147–51.

Bibliography References

97, 125, 215, 345, 678, 690, 691, 810, 1001, 1291, 1292.

Burns, John William (1884–1950) Marshall, Charles McIntosh (1901–1954)

Burns–Marshall Manoeuvre for Breech Delivery

Working in Liverpool, Burns and Marshall developed a technique for controlled delivery of the aftercoming head of the breech. They reported this at the North of England Obstetrical and Gynaecological Society meeting in Liverpool on 6 April 1934 and later in the *Journal of Obstetrics and Gynaecology of the British Empire*. Burns wrote:

> *To effect delivery various two-handed grips have been devised; grips which, in my opinion, induce the operator to use more force than is necessary. Unfortunately, these two factors, haste and force, are the Scylla and Charybdis between which the accoucheur is wrecked and the passenger lost.*

The manoeuvre involved allowing the body to hang after delivery of the arms to facilitate flexion of the fetal head, and then sweeping the legs down, out and up in an arc with one hand as the other controlled the release of the head over the perineum. In so doing, 'the fetal head is forced to rotate about the point of contact between the sub-occipital area and ischiopubic rami'.

John William Burns received his medical degree from Trinity College Dublin in 1905 and, after early training at the Rotunda Hospital, moved to Liverpool. He became consultant to the Liverpool Women's and Maternity hospitals and lecturer in the department of obstetrics and gynaecology at Liverpool University.

Charles McIntosh Marshall was born at Invercargill, New Zealand and educated at Otago University. He held resident posts in New Zealand and later, with

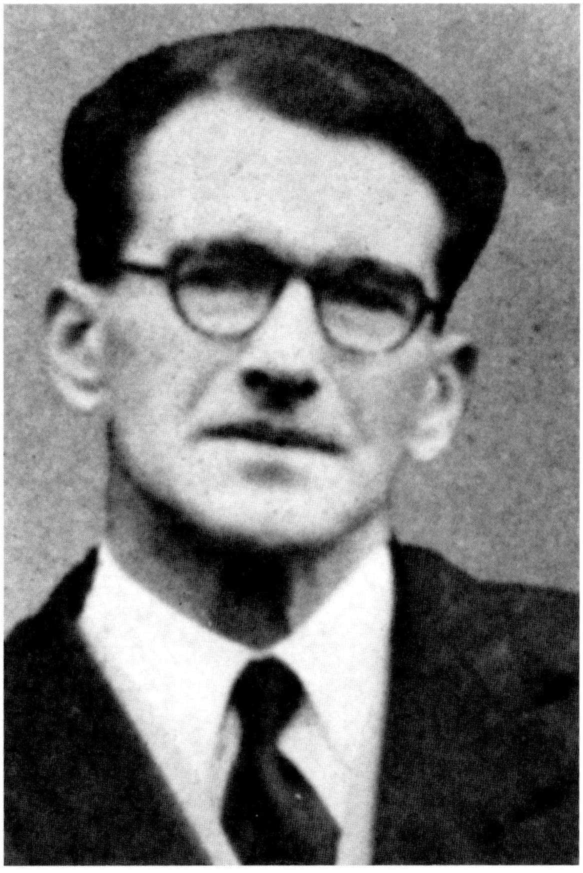

Charles McIntosh Marshall

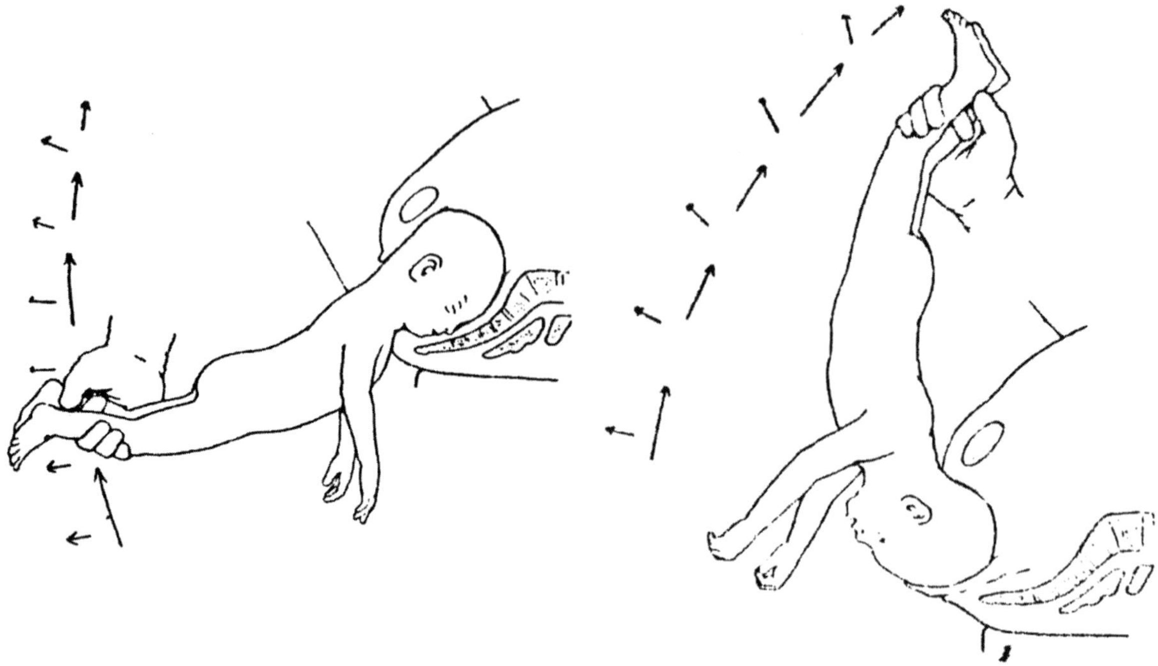

Diagram illustrating the Burns–Marshall manoeuvre for breech delivery

a Dominion scholarship, studied in London. In 1932 he moved to Liverpool and remained at the Liverpool Maternity and Women's hospitals for the rest of his life. He wrote extensively on caesarean section and did much to popularise the lower-segment operation.

Selected Publications

Burns JW. Breech: a method of dealing with the aftercoming head. *Br J Obstet Gynaecol Br Emp* 1934; 41: 923–9.

Marshall CM. A technique for delivery of the breech with extended legs in primiparae. *Br J Obstet Gynaecol Br Emp* 1934; 41: 930–5.

Bibliography References

102, 263, 822, 987–989.

C

Caldeyro-Barcia, Roberto (1921–1996)

Uterine Contractility/Electronic Fetal Heart Rate Monitoring

The first attempt to record uterine contractions was by Shatz in Germany in 1872. He used a fluid-filled bag passed through the cervix, attached by fluid-filled tubes to a smoked drum and a mercury manometer. In the modern era it was Caldeyro-Barcia and his colleague Hermógenes Álvarez in Montevideo who first used transabdominal fluid-filled catheters to record intrauterine pressure in labour. They started this work in 1947 and reported it in the Uruguayan and English literature in 1948 and 1950 respectively. Two years later, transcervical intrauterine pressure catheters were developed by Williams and Stallworthy in England.

Continued systematic research by Caldeyro-Barcia and Álvarez resulted in their formula for quantification of uterine activity known as the 'Montevideo unit', which they reported in 1957:

> *The intensity (amplitude) of each contraction is measured by the rise in pressure (mm Hg) it produces in the amniotic fluid. The frequency of the contractions is expressed by the number of contractions per 10 minutes. The product (intensity × frequency) of the contractions is called 'uterine activity' and is expressed in Montevideo Units.*

In the late 1950s Caldeyro-Barcia began to study the response of the fetal heart rate to uterine contractions using a fetal scalp electrode. He classified type I dips in the fetal heart rate as due to fetal head compression, equivalent to the 'early' deceleration of Edward Hon. His type II dips were indicative of potential fetal hypoxia and equivalent to the 'late' deceleration of Hon and the 'alarm' dip of Erich Saling's classification. This work was reported in the Spanish and English literature in 1962 and 1963 respectively. Thus, Caldeyro-Barcia was instrumental in developing two of the components for monitoring the fetus during labour: continuous intrauterine pressure and fetal heart rate recording.

Roberto Caldeyro-Barcia was born in Montevideo, Uruguay on 26 September 1921. He took his MD at the University of Uruguay School of Medicine in 1947. As a student he was already carrying out research in the medical school's institute of physiology. Indeed, his initial work on uterine contractility was started in the same year as he qualified in medicine. He carried on a remarkable career of teaching and research in the physiology of parturition from the late 1940s. Recognising his contribution, the University of Uruguay created the service of obstetrical physiology in 1959, with Caldeyro-Barcia as chairman. In 1970 the Pan-American Health Organisation asked him to direct the Latin American Centre of Perinatology and Human Development, which was established to facilitate the work of his group. From these two posts Caldeyro-Barcia trained more than 300 fellows in perinatal medicine from all over the world. There are few countries that do not have former fellows of Caldeyro-Barcia in

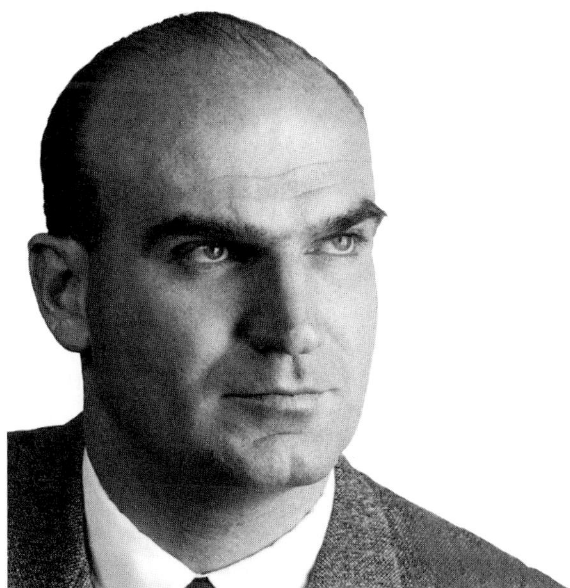

Roberto Caldeyro-Barcia

senior positions. Through them his high standards of basic and clinical perinatal research have been disseminated worldwide.

Appropriately, Caldeyro-Barcia lectured and was honoured around the world. He received honorary degrees from 16 universities. He remained active in university education and perinatal research in Montevideo for over half a century, until his death following cardiac surgery on 2 November 1996.

Selected Publications

Álvarez H, Caldeyro R. Estudios sobre las fisiologia de la actividad contractil del utero humano. *Arch Giniecol Obstet Urug* 1948; 7: 7.

Álvarez H. Caldeyro-Barcia R. Contractility of the human uterus recorded by new methods. *Surg Gynecol Obstet* 1950; 91: 1–13.

Caldeyro-Barcia R, Sica-Blanco Y, Poseiro JJ et al. A quantitative study of the action of synthetic oxytocin on the pregnant human uterus. *J Pharmacol Exp Ther* 1957; 121: 18–31.

Caldeyro-Barcia R, Poseiro JJ. Efecto de las contracciones uterinas sobre el feto humano. *Pediatra* 1962; 29: 91–120.

Mendez-Bauer C, Poseiro JJ, Arellano-Harnandez G, Zambrana MA. Caldeyro-Barcia R, Effects of atropine on heart rate of the human fetus during labour *Am J Obstet Gynecol* 1963; 85: 1033–53.

Shatz F. Beiträge zur physiologischen Geburtskunde. *Arch Gynäkol* 1872; 5: 58.

Williams EA, Stallworthy JA. A simple method of internal tocography. *Lancet* 1952; 1: 330–2.

Bibliography References

277, 635, 819, 1341, 1536, 1537, 1731.

Caldwell, William Edgar (1880–1943) Moloy, Howard Carman (1903–1953)

Radiological Classification of the Female Pelvis

Based on work involving dried bony pelves in the museums of Washington DC, Cleveland and New York, along with their own radiological studies, Caldwell and Moloy produced a classification of the female pelvis. They reasoned:

> *A classification of pelves which will prove of maximum clinical value and lead to a better understanding of the mechanism of labour is based necessarily upon morphology.*

They concluded that there were four bony pelves of distinct morphology:

> *1) The so-called normal female pelvis or Gynaecoid; 2) Female pelvis with masculine characters or Android; 3) Transversely contracted or 'assimilation pelvis' or Anthropoid; 4) The simple flat type or Platypelloid.*

Through the 1940s and 1950s in many affluent societies, radiological pelvimetry became very common. By the late 1950s Stewart pointed out the possible relationship between childhood malignancy and irradiation in utero. By the 1960s the clinical uselessness of radiological pelvimetry became evident.

William Edgar Caldwell was born in Northfield, Ohio. He graduated in medicine from New York University in 1904. By 1927 he rose to the rank of professor of clinical obstetrics and gynaecology at

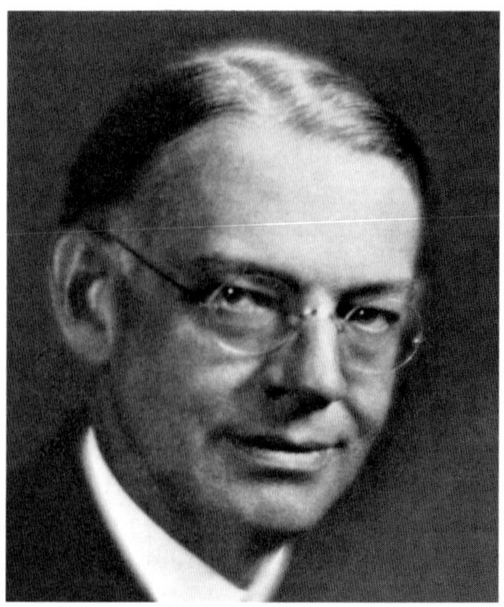

William Edgar Caldwell

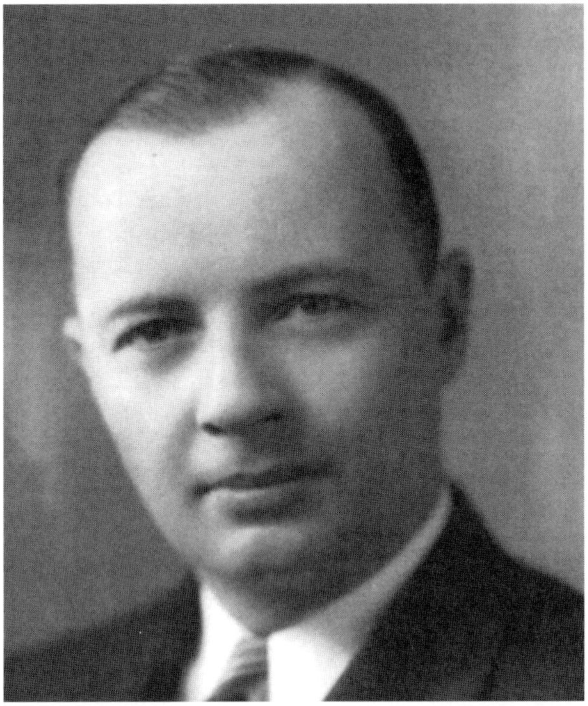

Howard Carman Moloy

Columbia University, New York. He worked in the Sloane Hospital for Women as director of the obstetric division. There he was the first to use the forceps designed by Lyman Barton.

Howard Carman Moloy was born in Thedford, Ontario and received his medical training at the University of Western Ontario, graduating in 1927. He moved to the United States and served his residency in obstetrics and gynaecology at Long Branch, New Jersey and at the Sloane Hospital for Women. On completion of his training he was appointed to the staff of the Sloane Hospital and began his productive partnership with Caldwell. He devoted the major part of his professional career to the study of the female pelvis. He was awarded the gold medal of the American Roentgenological Association for his design of a stereoscope used in pelvimetry. Moloy died in the Sloane Hospital in his fiftieth year on 13 March 1953, shortly after performing a caesarean section on a private patient.

Selected Publications

Caldwell WE, Moloy HC. Anatomical variations in the female pelvis and their effects in labour with a suggested classification. *Am J Obstet Gynecol* 1933; 26: 479–505.

Stewart A, Webb J, Giles D, Hewitt D. Malignant disease in childhood and diagnostic irradiation in utero. *Lancet* 1956; 2: 447.

Bibliography References

536, 607, 648, 721, 801, 1480, 1484, 1532, 1563.

Call, Emma Louise (1847–1937)
Exner, Siegmund (1846–1926)

Call–Exner Bodies

In 1875, Emma Call, working in Vienna as a postgraduate student under the guidance of the distinguished physiologist, Siegmund Exner, reported their studies on the rabbit ovary. They noted tiny cells among the ovarian granulosa cells which resembled ova and suggested that ova may arise from the epithelium of the Graafian follicle as well as from the germinal epithelium. These tiny vacuolar areas of cystic degeneration surrounded by granulosa cells are indicative of granulosa growth. Their presence is an aid to the diagnosis of granulosa cell tumours, which can have a variable microscopic pattern. In the classic variety, the granulosa cells are arranged in clusters around the cystic cavity: Call–Exner bodies or rosettes.

Emma Louise Call was born in Newburyport, Massachusetts and, upon receiving her medical degree with honours from the University of Michigan in 1873, became one of the first female physicians in the United States. After graduation she studied in

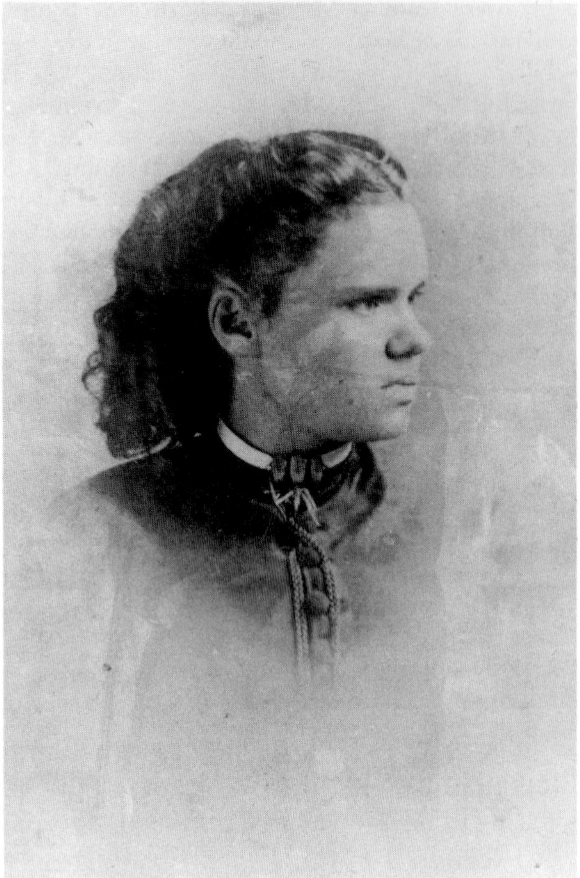

Emma Louise Call

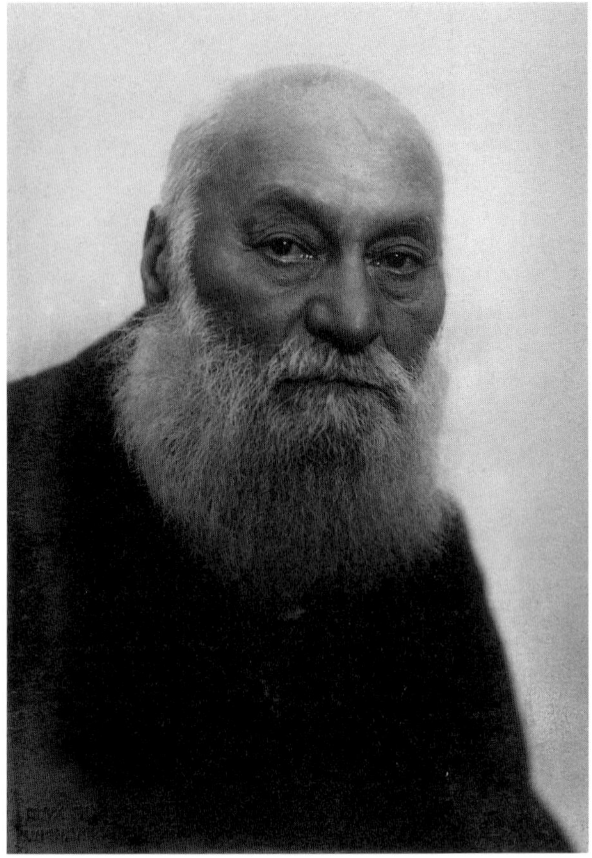

Siegmund Exner

Vienna with Exner. She returned to Boston in 1875 and worked as a consultant in obstetrics at the New England Hospital for Women and Children for 40 years. She also served as physician to the Massachusetts Infant Asylum. Call was the first woman member of the Massachusetts State Medical Society. Her single contribution to the medical literature secured her eponymous fame. She died in her ninetieth year on 3 May 1937 at the hospital she had served for so long.

Siegmund Exner was born in Vienna into a distinguished academic family. His medical studies were undertaken in Vienna and Heidelberg. He became professor at the Physiological Institute in Vienna and made many significant contributions to the understanding of neurophysiology.

Selected Publications

Call LE, Exner S. Zur Kenntnis des Graafschen Follikels und des Corpus luteum beim Kaninchen. *Sber Akad Wiss Wien. Math-naturw.* 1875; 71: 321–8.

Bibliography References

227, 228, 968, 1480, 1557.

Campbell, Kate Isabel (1899–1986)

Retrolental Fibroplasia

In the 1940s oxygen therapy was enthusiastically used to improve survival of premature infants. In 1942 the first case of retrolental fibroplasia causing blindness in a six-month-old infant was described by Terry in Boston. The pathogenesis of the condition involves retinal vessel spasm, proliferation, haemorrhage and fibrosis. In 1951 Kate Campbell, working at the Royal Women's Hospital in Melbourne, established the clinical link between intensive oxygen therapy and retrolental fibroplasia. She was stimulated to study the condition by reports suggesting a link between oxygen therapy and retrolental fibroplasia:

> *I heard, from colleagues returning from overseas, the suggestion that oxygen might be responsible for producing retrolental fibroplasia. The idea arose apparently from a comparison of the treatment of premature infants in America, where retrolental fibroplasia is a problem and where oxygen was used freely, with the treatment in England, where retrolental fibroplasia is seen rarely, and where oxygen was used sparingly . . . As I had under my care at the same time three series of premature infants, whose management was identical except for the amount of oxygen used, I was able to compare the incidence of retrolental fibroplasia in the three groups.*

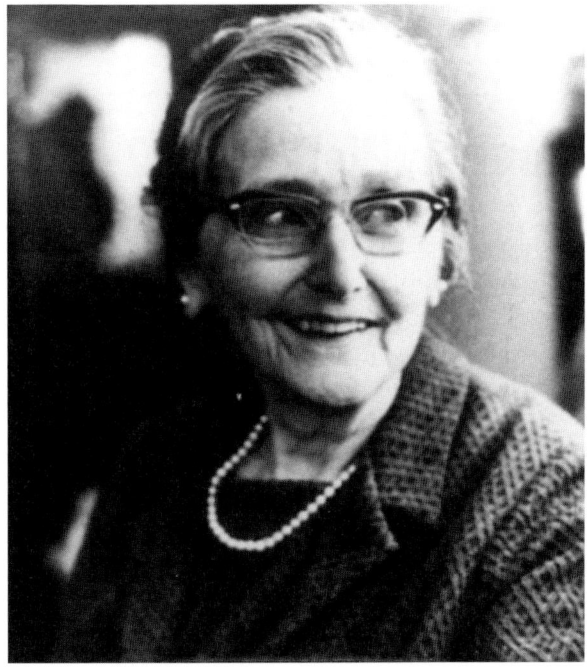

Kate Isabel Campbell

From her clinical study she concluded:

1. *The normal oxygen environment of the newborn full-term infant is abnormal for the premature infant.*
2. *This is particularly so for infants of thirty-two weeks gestation or less.*
3. *The potential toxic effect of oxygen on premature infants can be enhanced, i) by administration of a high concentration of oxygen therapeutically, ii) by pyrexia, iii) by toxaemia.*
4. *The generalised vascular spoiling and oedema so produced affect the eye and are the starting points of retrolental fibroplasia.*

This was later confirmed by others in animal and clinical studies.

Kate Isabel Campbell was born in Hawthorn, Australia to parents of Scottish descent. She was a home delivery, weighing 11 pounds. She graduated in medicine in 1922 from the University of Melbourne. Over the next two years she held resident posts in paediatrics and obstetrics.

She spent 10 years in general paediatric practice with a particular emphasis on infant welfare services. In 1929 she was appointed the first lecturer in neonatal paediatrics in the University of Melbourne. She was amused to learn that her constant questioning of obstetricians at perinatal mortality rounds earned her the title of 'paediatric policeman'. She was president of the Australian Paediatric Association in 1965–6. Among the many honours she received were the Doctorate of Laws from the University of Melbourne, Fellowship ad eundem of the Royal College of Obstetricians and Gynaecologists and Dame Commander of the Order of the British Empire. Dame Kate Campbell died on 12 July 1986.

Selected Publications

Campbell K. Intensive oxygen therapy as a possible cause of retrolental fibroplasia: a clinical approach. *Med J Aust* 1951; 2: 48–50.

Terry TL. Extreme prematurity and fibroblastic overgrowth of persistent vascular sheath behind each crystalline lens: a preliminary report. *Am J Ophthalmol.* 1942; 25: 203–4.

Bibliography References

237, 238, 572, 1202, 1265.

Camper, Pieter (1722–1789)

Camper's Fascia

Pieter Camper was born in Leyden, the son of a clergyman and grandson of a physician. An exceptional scholar, he entered university at the age of 12. He held degrees in philosophy and medicine as well as being multilingual and a capable artist. He practised midwifery in Leyden. In 1748 Camper went to England, studied with William Smellie in London, and took lessons at the Painters' Academy. He recorded that on 5 January 1749, 'I subscribed on Dr Smellie's course of midwifery for three guineas'. Camper returned to London in 1752 and assisted with dissections and drawings for Smellie's anatomical atlas. He ultimately contributed 11 illustrations from which plates were made. The original drawings are now in the library of the Royal College of Physicians of Edinburgh. He became professor of anatomy, medicine and surgery at Amsterdam and Groningen, also holding chairs in philosophy and botany. He spoke against caesarean section and in favour of symphysiotomy, although he had only performed the latter on pigs. Camper described the superficial layer of abdominal fascia with which his name is linked. After his wife died from breast cancer in 1776, he retired from medicine and spent the final years of his life as a politician. In his time, he discovered that the bones of birds contained air and dissected an elephant, rhinoceros and orangutan. He died at The Hague.

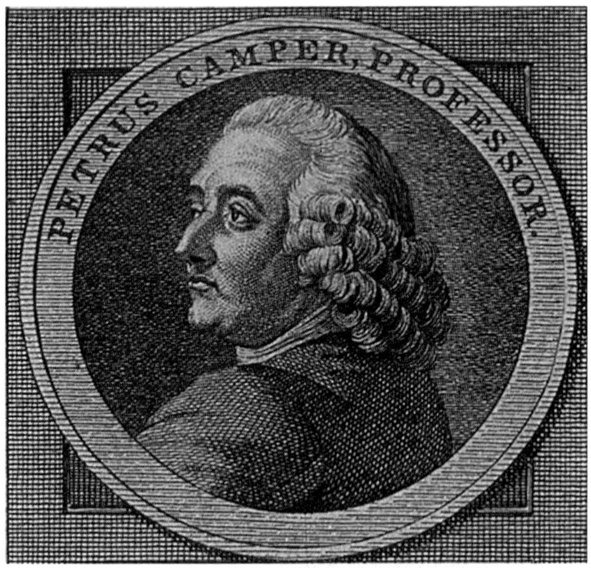

Pieter Camper

Selected Publications

Camper P. *Oeuvres de Pierre Camper qui ont pour objet l'histoire naturelle, la physiologie et l'anatomie compareé.* Paris; 1803.

Bibliography References

8, 239, 271, 406, 648, 774, 906, 907, 1261.

Carus, Carl Gustav (1789–1869)

Curve of Carus

Defining the axis of parturition occupied many prominent obstetricians of the eighteenth century, as they attempted to better understand the mechanisms of labour and assist accurate forceps delivery. Most involved intricate descriptions of various pelvic axes and geometric formulae. In reviewing the work of others Carus said:

> *It was therefore found necessary to abandon entirely the idea of one or several pelvic axes and to adopt a curved line instead ... One takes the middle of the pubic symphysis, where the conjugate of the pelvic cavity begins, and using a radius of 2 1/4 inches, describes a circle around the synchondrosis, whereupon it will then be seen that the arc of this circle falling inside the pelvic cavity transects the middle of the inlet as well as the outlet. Coursing in general through the middle of the pelvic cavity, it indicates the true axis of the pelvis in the most precise way.*

Franz Naegele later pointed out that the axis was straight in the upper half and curved from the mid-pelvis to the outlet. However, the elegant simplicity of Carus' description became rapidly accepted in obstetric teaching as the 'curve of Carus'.

Carl Gustav Carus was born in Leipzig, Germany. He gained both philosophy and medical degrees from the University of Leipzig. In 1814 he became professor of obstetrics and director of the lying-in hospital at Dresden. In 1827 he was appointed royal physician. He published widely on a range of subjects outside medicine, including, art, anthropology, philosophy and zoology.

Selected Publications

Carus CG. Lehrbuck der Gynäkologie. (Vol. 1.) Leipzig: G.Fleischer; 1820, pp. 32–3.

Bibliography References

406, 648, 721, 968, 1261, 1480.

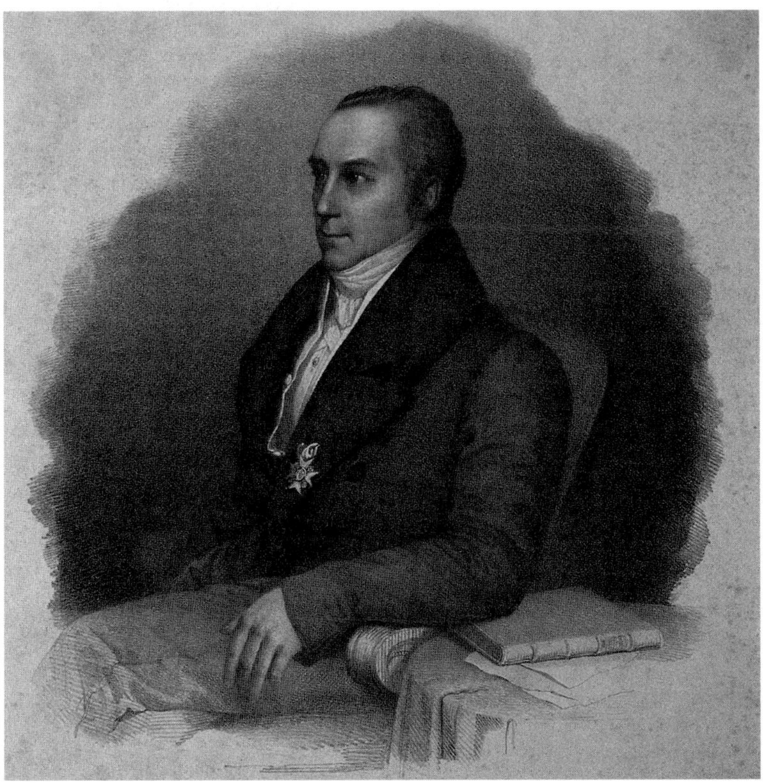

Carl Gustav Carus

Cary, William Hollenback (b. 1883)

Salpingography

One of the major advances in the investigation of infertility was presented by William Cary to the Brooklyn Gynecological Society in February 1914. He reported the injection of the radiopaque silver colloid solution, collargol, through the cervix followed by X-ray. He performed the first test just before a laparotomy, and the operative findings of one patent and one blocked tube were confirmed on the radiographic salpingogram. Cary outlined the potential of this investigation:

> *In taking up the question of sterility in the individual case we can seldom feel that our diagnosis is accurate or any prognosis warranted because of our inability to determine if the tubes are unobstructed . . . frank lesions may be present which prevent fertility. More frequently, however, we are consulted by the patient who had no reason to suspect pelvic disease and in whom we find no gross lesion . . . If in this large group of causes of sterility we can now bring to bear definite knowledge regarding the patency of the tubes, the most important single factor is determinable so far as the woman is concerned. An intelligent prognosis may be given.*

He added a cautionary note: 'This procedure will not be safe if infection in any form exists'.

Independently in the same year, Isidor Rubin reported a similar technique. A preface to these efforts occurred in 1910 when Rindfleisch injected a watery paste of bismuth into the uterine cavity of a woman with suspected ectopic pregnancy and outlined the uterus and left fallopian tube.

William Hollenback Cary was born in Barton, New York on 13 August 1883. He obtained his MD from Syracuse University, New York in 1905. He was an attending obstetrician and gynaecologist at the Brooklyn Hospital and at St Marks Hospital, New York.

Selected Publications

Cary WH. Note on determination of patency of Fallopian tubes by the use of collargol and X-ray shadow. *Am J Obstet Dis Women Child* 1914; 69: 462–4.

Rindfleisch W. Darstellung des Cavum uteri. *Klin Wschr* 1910; 47: 780–1.

Rubin IC. Röntgendiagnostik der Uterustumaren mit Hilfe von intrauterin Collargolinjektionen. *Zentralbl Gynäkol* 1914; 38: 658–60.

Rubin IC. X-ray diagnosis in gynecology with the aid of intra-uterine collargol injection. *Surg Gynecol Obstet* 1915; 20: 435–43.

Bibliography References

1409.

Chadwick, James Read (1844–1905)

Chadwick's Sign

James Chadwick was one of the founders of the American Gynecological Society and served as its president in 1897. Indeed, it was Chadwick who conceived and organised the first meeting of the society, held at the Academy of Medicine in New York on 3 June 1876. He presented his paper, describing the sign of early pregnancy, before that society in 1886. Chadwick's sign refers to the blue-violet colour of the vagina in early pregnancy. He described this as follows:

> *The color begins as a pale violet in the early months, becomes more bluish as pregnancy advances, until it often assumes finally a dusky, almost black tint; the last is familiar to every obstetrician.*

This sign had been clearly described 50 years earlier by Étienne Jacquemin, a fact that Chadwick acknowledged. Chadwick spent 10 years in a study of more than 6,000 women to confirm the value of the sign and also to show that non-pregnant causes of pelvic congestion did not produce the same discolouration. He later noted that the sign was manifest at the introitus and particularly prominent on the anterior vaginal wall just below the urethral orifice. He cautioned that the absence of this sign, especially in the first three months, did not rule out pregnancy. The clinical value of this observation was considerable in the days before pregnancy tests based on the detection of human chorionic gonadotrophin.

James Read Chadwick was born in Boston and graduated from Harvard Medical School in 1871. After qualification he spent two years studying gynaecology in the centres of Berlin, Vienna, Paris and London. He returned to practice in Boston and in 1875 was appointed to the gynaecological department of the Boston City Hospital. A great bibliophile, Chadwick was instrumental in founding and sustaining the Boston Medical Library. He also organised the Harvard Medical Alumni Association in 1890 and served as its first president. As a strong proponent of cremation, he became the clerk of the Massachusetts Cremation Society. On September 23 1905, Chadwick was found dead at his summer residence in Chocorua, New Hampshire, apparently due to an accidental fall from the second-floor balcony.

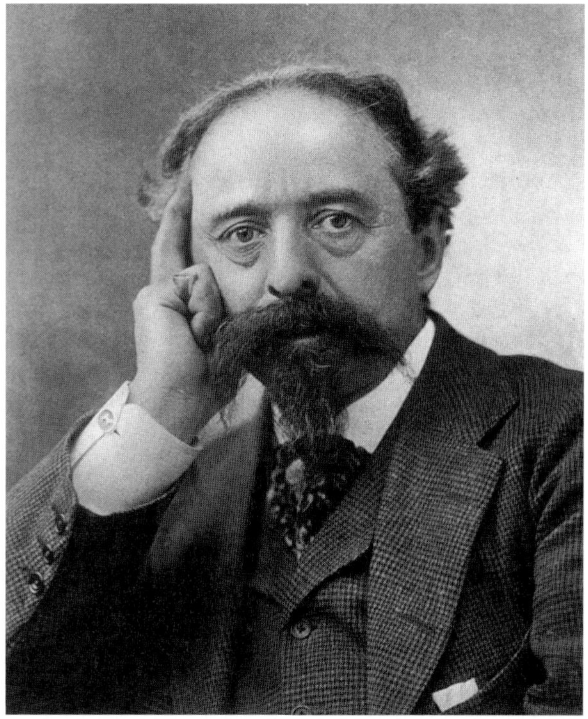

James Read Chadwick

Selected Publications

Chadwick JR. The value of the bluish coloration of the vaginal entrance as a sign of pregnancy. *Trans Am Gynecol Soc* 1887; 11: 399–418.

Bibliography References

111, 216, 257, 625, 801, 1480, 1713.

Chamberlen, Peter (1601–1683)

Obstetric Forceps

The forerunner of modern obstetric forceps was devised by the Chamberlens and kept secret within the family for about a century. Much has been written about the Chamberlen family and only a brief outline will be given here.

William Chamberlen (d. 1596) was a Huguenot surgeon in Paris who, facing religious persecution, fled to England in 1569. He had two sons named Peter who became barber-surgeons in London: Peter the Elder (d. 1631) and Peter the Younger (1572–1626). The son of Peter the Younger was also named Peter (1601–1683). He studied at Cambridge, Padua and Heidelberg universities and received medical degrees from Padua, Oxford and Cambridge. Thus, in the confusing trio of Peters, he is known as Dr Peter. He had a son, Hugh Senior, who in turn had a son, Hugh Junior. Both Hughs were qualified doctors and practised obstetrics. Just to complete the confusion and sharpen up the historians, Dr Peter had another son, Paul, who practised obstetrics and often signed himself PC.

It is likely that Peter the Elder devised the forceps and, along with his younger brother, established the family's reputation with the secret instrument. In his privately published, largely autobiographical booklet in 1647, *A Voice in Rhama, or the Crie of Women and Children,* Dr Peter wrote,

> *Fame begot me envie and secret enemies which mightily increased when my father added to me the knowledge of deliveries.*

As had his uncle before him, Dr Peter became physician to the Royal Court in London. In 1670, Hugh Senior went to Paris to sell the family secret to the physicians of the French court. As a suitable test of the secret instrument's ability, François Mauriceau presented Chamberlen with a rachitic dwarf who had been in labour for eight days, with such a small deformed pelvis that all attempts to deliver her vaginally had failed. One can imagine Mauriceau retiring from the room with a quiet Gallic chuckle as he left the confident Chamberlen to his impossible task.

After an unsuccessful struggle, Hugh Chamberlen had to admit defeat and leave Paris without selling his forceps. He did, however, bring back a copy of Mauriceau's *Treatise*, and translated it into English for considerable personal profit. In the preface to this book Hugh Senior explained why this secret was kept within the family for four generations, throughout the seventeenth century:

> *My Father, Brothers, and my self (tho' none else in Europe as I know) have, by God's Blessing, and our Industry, attain'd to, and long practis'd a Way to deliver Women in this Case, without any prejudice to them or their Infants; tho all others (being oblig'd for want of such an Expedient, to use the common Way) do, and must endanger, if not destroy one or both with Hooks . . . I will now take leave to offer an Apology for not publishing the Secret I mention we have to extract Children without Hooks, where other Artists use them, viz., there being my Father and two Brothers living, that practise this Art, I cannot esteem it my own to dispose of, nor publish it without Injury to them.*

Dr Peter moved to Woodham Mortimer Hall near Malden, Essex. He was survived by his wife, who preserved the forceps along with 'my husband's last tooth' and other family mementoes in a box under a trap door in the attic. These were discovered in 1813, and the four pairs of Chamberlen forceps are now in the museum of the Royal College of Obstetricians and Gynaecologists.

Selected Publications

Chamberlen P. *A Voice in Rhama or, The Crie of Women and Children.* London: Printed by William Bentley for John Marshall; 1647.

Bibliography References

32, 45, 249, 361, 373, 399, 473, 657, 718, 719, 1131, 1230, 1257, 1260, 1261, 1495, 1516.

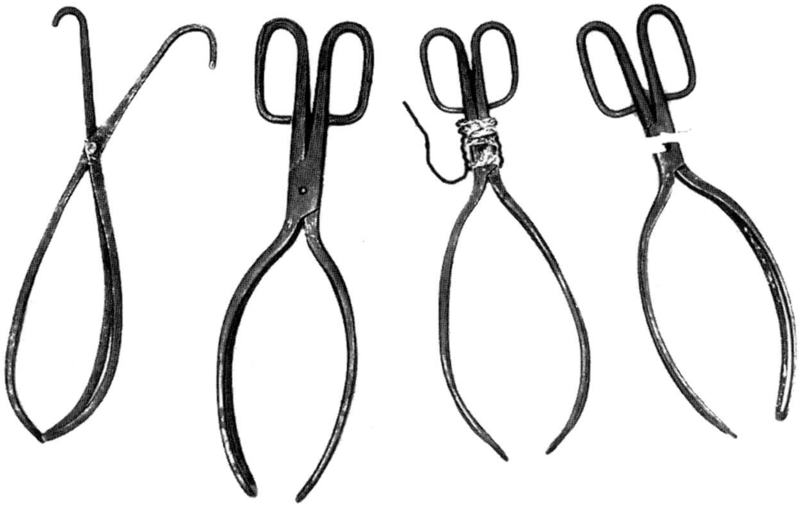

The original Chamberlen forceps

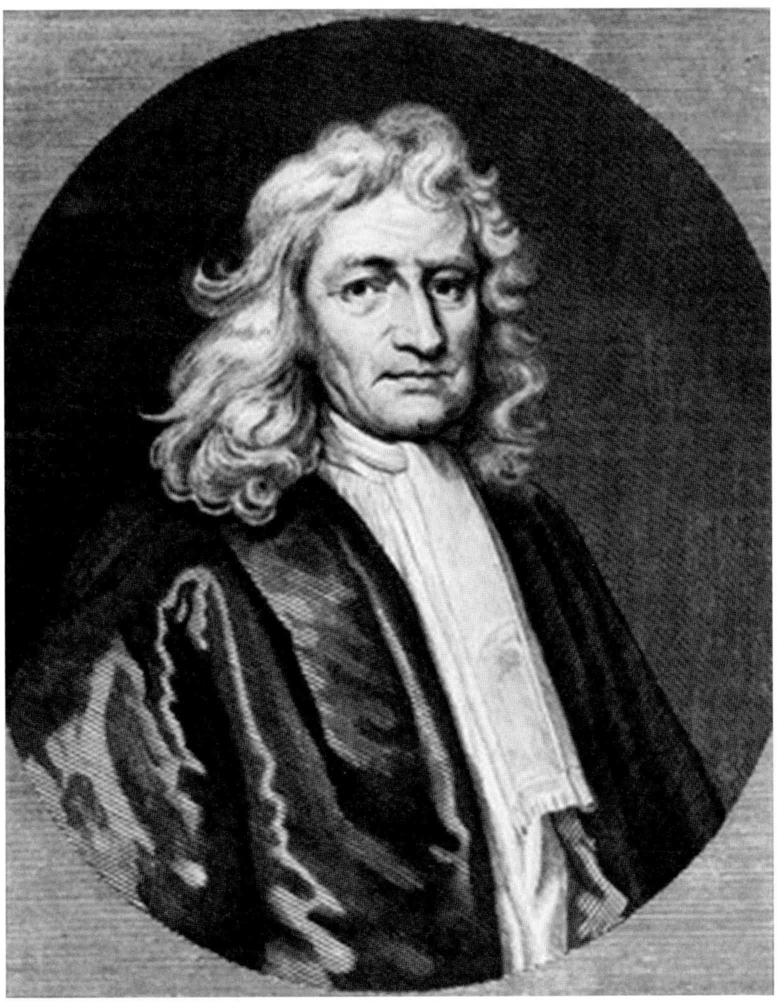

Peter Chamberlen

Champetier de Ribes, Camille Louis Antoine (1848–1935)

De Ribes' Balloon

Since the early nineteenth century a variety of balloon-like objects (metreurynters) have been inserted into the uterus, usually in an attempt to induce labour or arrest haemorrhage from placenta praevia. Champetier de Ribes was first introduced to the principle when he worked as an intern for Étienne Tarnier in the Maternité of Paris in 1878. He felt that the existing models were too small and, after much experimentation, eventually designed a silk balloon, covered in rubber, of conical shape and 21 cm in circumference. His main indication for its use was induction of labour in cases of contracted pelvis:

> *I have sought a method to induce labour surely and rapidly, and at the same time to dilate the whole birth canal in order to remove the obstacles presented by the soft parts at the time of delivery, whether left to nature or terminated by operation. I believe I have attained this objective by a simple, harmless procedure, easy to use. In order to accomplish this result I insert an impermeable empty balloon, made of nondistensible material, above the internal os; I inject it with fluid: then its largest circumference becomes equal to or a little larger than that of the fetal head; then I let the maternal organism expel the foreign body spontaneously.*

Champetier de Ribes was born in Draveil, France. He took his medical degree in Paris and became a pupil of Tarnier's at the Maternité. His balloon was used widely in the late nineteenth and early twentieth century for induction of labour and to provide tamponade and arrest of haemorrhage in placenta praevia.

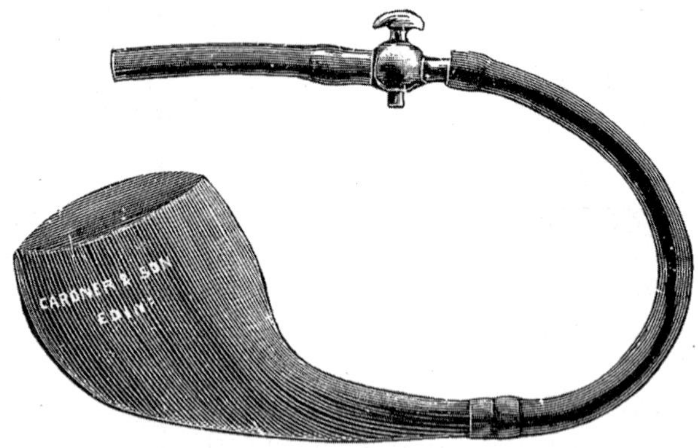

Champetier de Ribes' balloon expanded

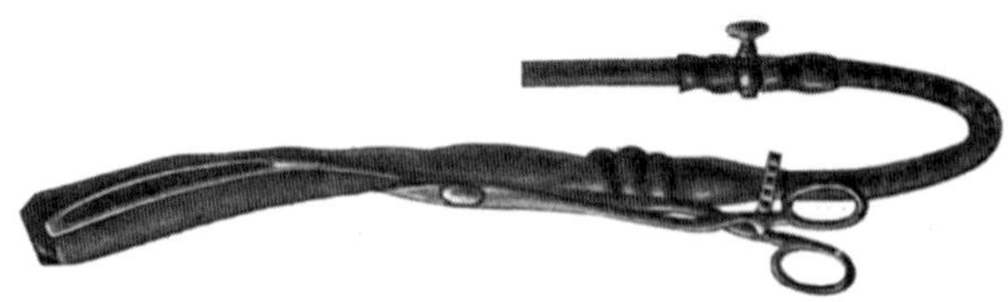

Champetier de Ribes' balloon collapsed, with forceps for its introduction

Selected Publications

Champetier de Ribes CLA. De l'accouchement provoqué. Dilatation du canal genital (col de l'uterus, vagin et vulve) a l'aide de ballons introduit dans la cavité uterine pendant la grossesse. *Ann Gynéc* 1888; 30: 401–38.

Bibliography References

99, 542, 648, 721, 983, 1462, 1480.

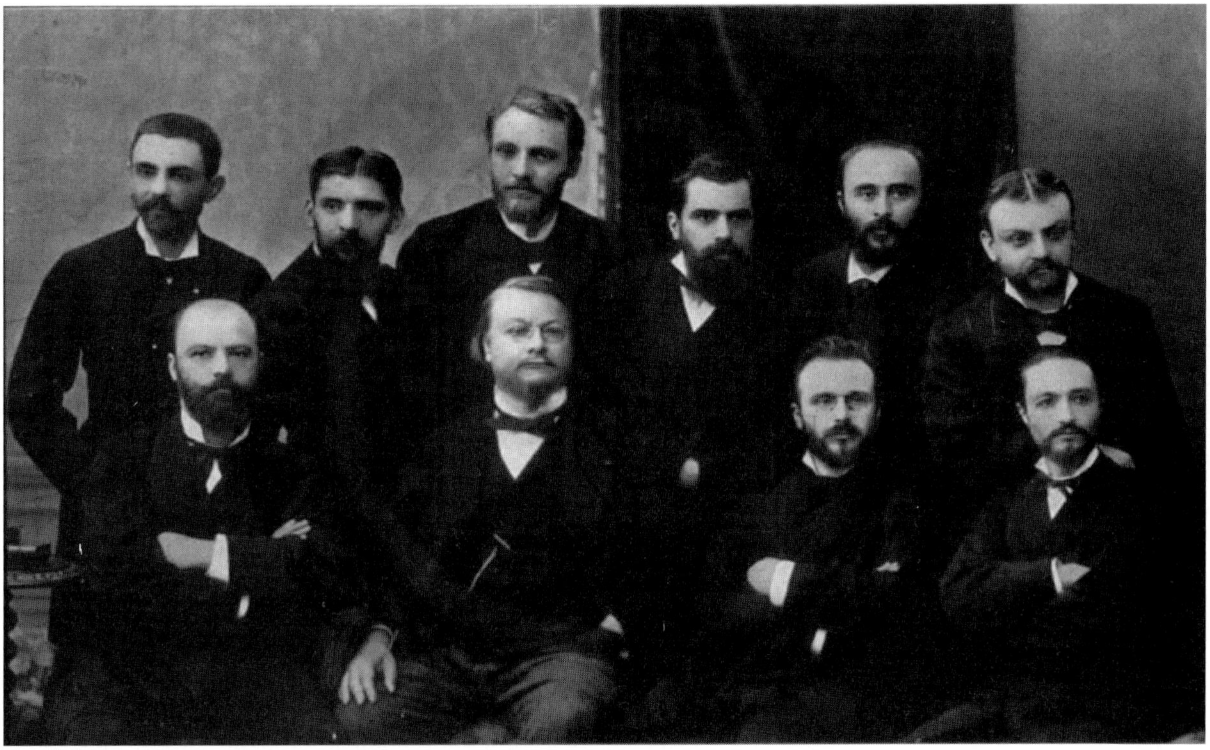

Camille Louis Antoine Champetier de Ribes (back row, far left)

Channing, Walter (1786–1876)

Ether Anaesthesia in Obstetrics

Through the pioneering efforts of two men, James Young Simpson of Edinburgh and Walter Channing of Boston, chloroform and ether inhalation analgesia and anaesthesia became widely available in obstetrics. Channing was on the staff of the Boston Lying-in Hospital and the Massachusetts General Hospital. Through his association with the latter institution, he was aware of the first operations performed under ether anaesthesia in 1846.

The first case of ether inhalation in labour in the United States was administered by Nathan Cooley Keep on 7 April 1847 in Boston. This and a few other cases under his own guidance were reported by Channing in a pamphlet published in May 1847, with an enlarged version produced in July the same year. Channing then set about analysing the results of his own experience and, through a questionnaire and interviews, the results of other physician's cases. Just over a year after the first use of ether in labour Channing published *A Treatise on Etherization in Childbirth*, with details of 581 cases.

Like Simpson, Channing came under critical fire from segments of the lay and medical public on both the morality and safety of the practice. He dismissed those who quoted the book of Genesis in the Bible, 'in sorrow thou shalt bring forth children', with the argument that those who relieved pain with ether were using their God-given powers to apply God-given means. To Channing, he wrote,

> *The whole question resolves into safety alone. It has nothing to do with man's notion of the value or the pleasure of pain . . . Let the reader, then, look at the true point at issue; and, above all, let him not be misled in his*

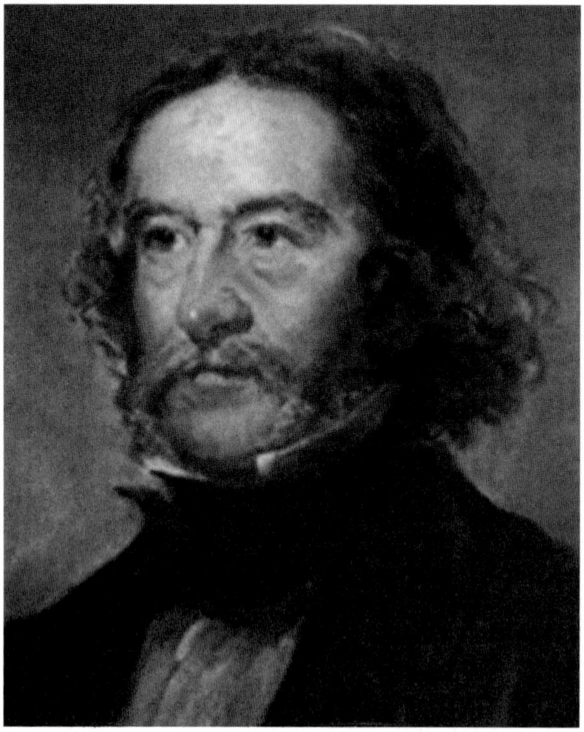

Walter Channing

judgements by ignorance, by prejudice, or more especially by a priori reasoning.

Channing thought that ether was safer than chloroform, as the progression from light to deep anaesthesia was slower. With his analysis of the cases in his treatise, Channing felt the question of safety was answered, and largely through his efforts, the acceptance and availability of ether anaesthesia in obstetrics in the United States was established.

Walter Channing was born on 15 April 1786 in Newport, Rhode Island, to a prominent family. His maternal grandfather signed the Declaration of Independence. He entered Harvard University in 1804, but because of his participation in a student rebellion in 1807 he did not graduate. He left and studied medicine in London, Edinburgh and Philadelphia and was granted his MD from the University of Pennsylvania in 1809. In 1812 he returned to Boston, was granted his MD *ad eundem* from Harvard Medical School and in 1818 became the first professor of obstetrics and medical jurisprudence there. He served as dean from 1819 to 1847. Channing's brother, William Ellery Channing, was a distinguished Unitarian minister. On one occasion, when he was mistaken for his clergyman brother, he replied, 'My brother preaches, while I practise'. Channing had a profound knowledge of the Bible and Shakespeare and published a volume of poetry. His son, William Ellery II, became a well-known poet. Channing stayed at Simpson's house in Queen Street when he visited Edinburgh. Of his treatise Channing said, 'It treats of a noble subject – the remedy of pain'. Walter Channing died peacefully at his home in Brookline, Massachusetts on 27 July 1876.

Selected Publications

Channing W. *A Treatise on Etherization in Childbirth.* Boston, MA: William D Ticknor and Company; 1848. Also published in: The Classics of Obstetrics and Gynecology Library. Birmingham: Gryphon Editions; 1991 (facsimile).

Bibliography References

111, 216, 252, 253, 265, 287, 457, 578, 709, 710, 765, 796–799, 1120, 1217, 1336, 1397, 1592, 1648, 1682.

Chapman, Edmund (c.1680–1756)

Obstetric Forceps

The Chamberlen-type obstetric forceps slowly came into limited use in Britain in the 1720s. Edmund Chapman was the first to describe the forceps in print in his *Essay on the Improvement of Midwifery*, published in 1733. He expanded this into a treatise in 1735 and included an illustration with enough details of the dimensions of the forceps to allow their construction by others. Chapman spoke against the use of destructive instruments to deal with the obstructed head when the fetus was alive:

> *The use of hooks and some other instruments, by which living children, presenting with the head, are destroyed, when they might very easily have been extracted in a few minutes by the fillet or forceps, is, in my opinion, a most cruel and unwarrantable practice. But yet, however inhuman, it is, to my certain knowledge, by some kept up to this day.*

Chapman was clearly enamoured of the forceps, as his writings attest:

> *I can, from my own experience, affirm it to be a most excellent instrument, and so far from hurting or destroying, that it frequently saves the mother's life, and that of the child, as will appear in the course of this treatise . . . All I can say in praise of this noble instrument, must necessarily fall short of what it justly demands.*

Both William Smellie and Jean-Louis Baudelocque acknowledged Chapman's role in communicating the existence of forceps to the profession.

Edmund Chapman was a surgeon and man-midwife in South Halstead, Essex, for many years. He moved to London just before the publication of his treatise. Chapman was one of the earliest teachers of midwifery in London. How he acquired his forceps is unknown, but he did live close to the Chamberlen home in Essex.

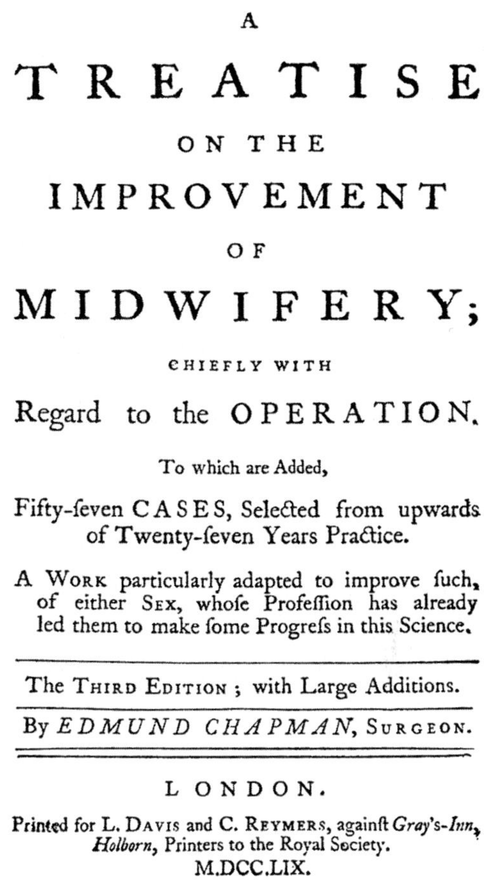
A

TREATISE

ON THE

IMPROVEMENT

OF

MIDWIFERY;

CHIEFLY WITH

Regard to the OPERATION.

To which are Added,

Fifty-ſeven CASES, Selected from upwards of Twenty-ſeven Years Practice.

A WORK particularly adapted to improve ſuch, of either SEX, whoſe Profeſſion has already led them to make ſome Progreſs in this Science.

The THIRD EDITION; with Large Additions.

By *EDMUND CHAPMAN*, SURGEON.

LONDON.

Printed for L. DAVIS and C. REYMERS, againſt *Gray's-Inn*, *Holborn*, Printers to the Royal Society.
M.DCC.LIX.

Title page of Edmund Chapman's *Treatise on the Improvement of Midwifery*

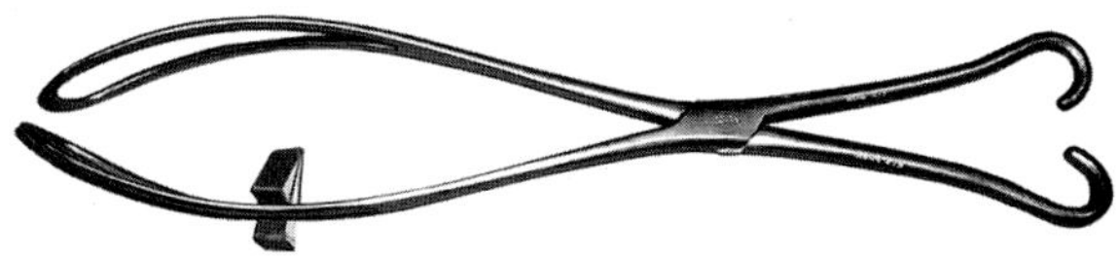

Chapman's forceps

Selected Publications

Chapman E. *A Treatise on the Improvement of Midwifery. Chiefly with Regard to the Operation.* London: Brindley, Clarke and Corbett; 2nd edn 1735, 3rd edn 1759. Also published in: The Classics of Obstetrics and Gynecology Library. Birmingham: Gryphons Editions; 1991 (facsimile).

Bibliography References

99, 361, 373, 418, 423, 503, 721, 1260, 1261, 1285, 1286, 1495, 1710.

Chaussier, François (1746–1828)

Chaussier's Sign/Neonatal Resuscitation

The association of epigastric pain as a prodrome of eclampsia is attributed to François Chaussier of Dijon and Paris and is known as Chaussier's sign.

Chaussier was born on 2 July 1746 and grew up in Dijon but studied medicine in Besançon. He returned to Dijon and was appointed physician to the hospital and to the prison. He was an accomplished anatomist and surgeon-accoucher, who carried out research in forensic medicine and was a pioneer in neonatal resuscitation.

Chaussier was the first to administer oxygen to the newborn in 1781 and devised a laryngeal tube for neonatal resuscitation in 1806. This was a curved metal tube that was guided to the infant's larynx along the accoucheur's little finger, which was placed behind the base of the tongue. Artificial respiration was then given, either mouth-to-tube or via small bellows applied to the tube.

After the French revolution the royal colleges and societies of medicine and surgery were abolished and replaced with Écoles de Santé. In 1794 Chaussier was summoned to Paris to advise on medical education in the new order. He submitted his report in late 1794 and, among other recommendations, advised that all medical students be taught both medicine and surgery, these having previously been regarded as separate professions. Chaussier remained in Paris and was appointed professor in the École d'Accouchement and chief physician at the Hospice de la Maternité, in which role he was a close colleague of Jean-Louis Baudelocque. Among his pupils was the midwife Marie Boivin. He died in Paris on 19 June 1828 at the age of 81.

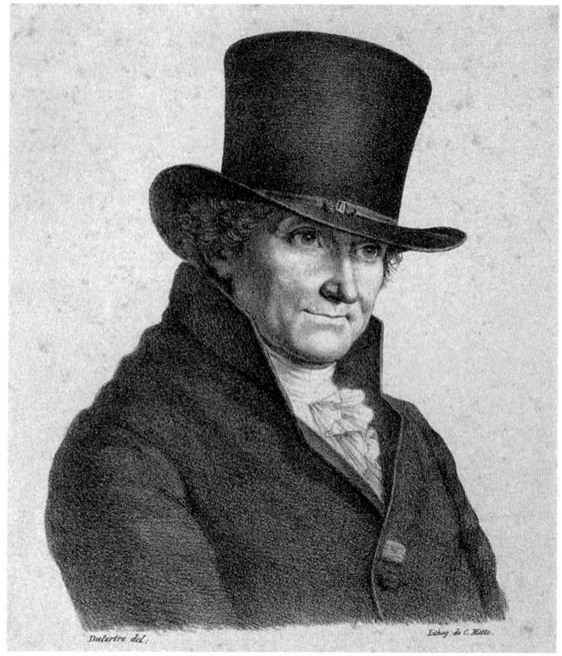

François Chaussier

Selected Publications

Chaussier, F. *Mémoire médico-legal sur la viabilitié de l'enfant naissant.* Paris; 1826.

Bibliography References

347, 1265, 1291, 1523, 1719.

Cherney, Leonid Sergius (1907–1963)

Cherney Incision

The advantages of the transverse lower abdominal incision, originated by Hermann Pfannenstiel, were manifest, with reduced incisional hernia and improved cosmetic results. However, Pfannenstiel's incision provided limited access for complex pelvic surgery. Alfred Maylard had improved the exposure by cutting both rectus muscles transversely. However, many surgeons were reluctant to cut through the rectus muscles.

Leonid Cherney suggested a modification that avoided cutting through the body of the muscle. The start of the incision is the same as that of Pfannenstiel, until just before entry to the peritoneum:

> *Near their attachment to the pubis, the recti are fibrous, frequently entirely tendinous. They are cut at their very insertion into the pubis. Even in the rare cases in which the muscle fibers are abundant, bleeding is negligible. The muscles are then reflected upward . . . In the closure of the incision, the peritoneum is sutured in the customary manner. The pyramidalis muscles are allowed to fall on top of the peritoneum without any sutures. The ends of the rectus tendons are securely united with mattress sutures to the under surface of the rectus sheath.*

Cherney's incision is less bloody and quicker than the Maylard incision. The exposure is superior to the Pfannenstiel incision, especially for work in the space of Retzius.

Leonid Sergius Cherney was born in Siberia. His family moved to the United States and he attended the University of California San Francisco Medical School at Berkeley. He graduated MD in 1934, doing his residency in surgery at San Francisco, New York and Cincinnati. He returned to practice surgery in San Francisco in 1937. Here he served his alma mater as an instructor in anatomy and assistant clinical professor of surgery.

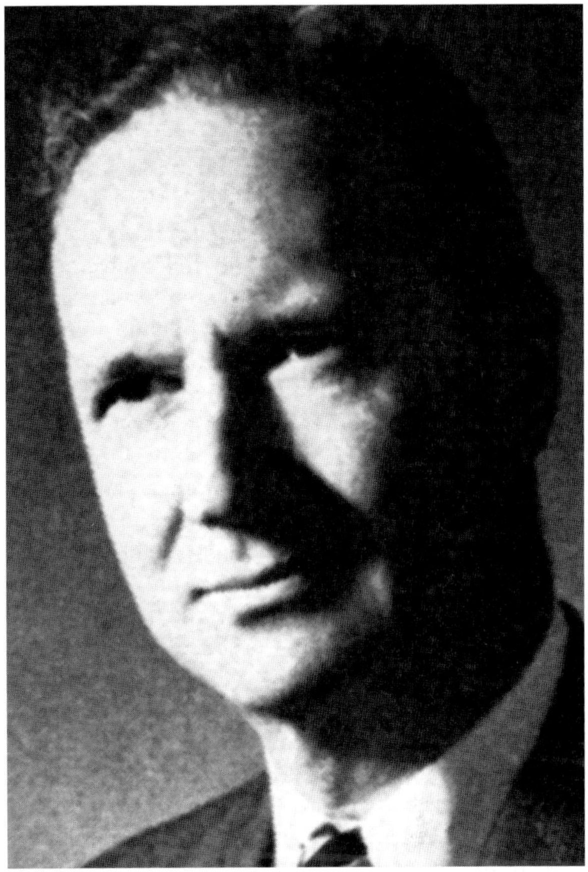

Leonid Sergius Cherney

Selected Publications

Cherney LS. A modified transverse incision for low abdominal operations. *Surg Gynecol Obstet* 1941; 72: 92–5.

Bibliography References

274.

Clarke, Cyril Astley (1907–2000)

Prevention of Rhesus Haemolytic Disease

It was the swallowtail butterfly that led Cyril Clarke to an interest in rhesus blood groups and ultimately to the method of preventing Rh immunisation in pregnancy. Clarke had been an avid butterfly collector since childhood. After his appointment as consultant physician in Liverpool he renewed his work with butterflies and devised a technique of 'hand-mating'. From this evolved his interest in hybridisation and genetics. With his colleagues he studied, and refuted, the apparent relationship between blood group type and duodenal ulcer. He was also struck by the similarities of the inheritance pathways of mimetic butterfly wing patterns and the rhesus blood groups.

In the late 1950s it had been shown that ABO incompatibility between the mother and fetus afforded a degree of protection against Rh immunisation. This was assumed to be due to the naturally occurring anti-A or anti-B eliminating Rh-positive paternal fetal cells before they could stimulate the mother's immune system to produce Rh antibodies. In 1959 Zipursky and the Winnipeg group first used the Kleihauer–Betke test to detect fetal red cells in maternal blood after delivery. Using this test, Dr Ronald Finn, working on his MD thesis under Clarke's guidance, demonstrated that ABO incompatibility did give a high degree of protection against Rh immunisation. As Clarke later wrote:

> *... it occurred to us that it might be possible to mimic the protection afforded by ABO incompatibility by giving the mother anti-D after delivery, thereby destroying any Rh-incompatible foetal cells (which we assumed had at some time crossed the placental barrier) before they had time to sensitize her.*

This suggestion was first put forward by Finn at a symposium on 'The Role of Inheritance in Common Diseases', held in Liverpool on 18 February 1960. They had begun the year before by injecting 40 Rh-negative male volunteers (Liverpool policemen) with chromium-tagged Rh-positive cells. This was followed by anti-D serum with saline (complete) antibody. To their disappointment, this did not prevent the development of immunisation. Based on work from the United States by Stern and Berger, they changed to albumin (incomplete) antibody and found it gave significant protection. In the United States the New York group of Freda, Gorman and Pollack independently carried out a similar study using gammaglobulin on volunteers from the local Sing Sing Prison. It was later confirmed that the use of gammaglobulin with incomplete anti-D was effective, without the risk of hepatitis carried by serum.

The Liverpool clinical trial in high-risk primiparous women was started in 1964. Anti-D gammaglobulin was given within 48 hours of delivery to alternate women with Kleihauer–Betke test evidence of a fetomaternal bleed. None of those treated with anti-D became immunised, as opposed to 24 per cent of those not treated. Similar trials in the United States, Canada and Germany confirmed these findings. Later studies would refine the dose and define the additional role of antenatal administration. The development of this safe and effective method of preventing the potentially lethal effects of a common disease is one of the major landmarks in preventive medicine. Since its introduction, tens of thousands of infants have been saved.

Cyril Astley Clarke was born in Leicester, England. He received his undergraduate education at Caius College, Cambridge and his medical degree from Guy's Hospital medical school in 1932. His postgraduate medical training in London and Birmingham was interrupted by service in the Royal Navy during the Second World War as a medical

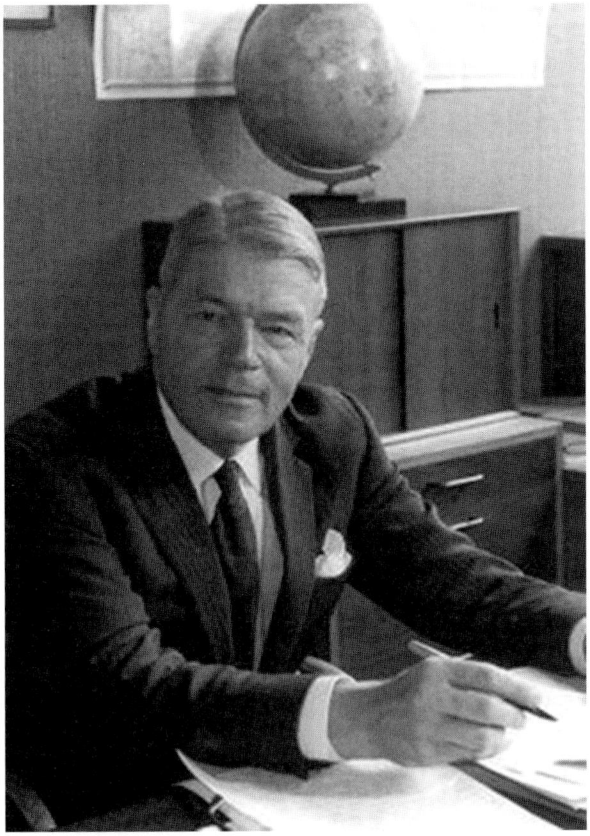

Cyril Astley Clarke

officer on the hospital ship *Amarapoora* and later at the Royal Naval Hospital in Sydney, Australia.

In 1946 he was appointed consultant physician to the United Liverpool Hospitals and professor of medicine at the University of Liverpool in 1965. From 1963 to 1972 he was director of the Nuffield Unit of Medical Genetics. For his services to medicine, Clarke was knighted in 1974. His contributions have been recognised by honorary fellowships in many colleges, including the Royal College of Obstetricians and Gynaecologists, and the granting of honorary degrees from 10 universities. He was president of the Royal College of Physicians from 1972–7. In 1990 he was awarded the Buchanan Medal from the Royal Society for his work on the prevention of rhesus immunisation. Living in retirement in Merseyside, Professor Sir Cyril Clarke continued his life-long interests in writing and small-boat sailing, having taken part in the 1948 Olympic sailing Firefly trials. He continued to breed and study the swallowtail butterfly, which is where it all started 50 years before. Sir Cyril Clarke died on 21 November 2000.

Selected Publications

Clarke CA, Donohoe WTA, McConnell RB et al. Further experimental studies on the prevention of Rh haemolytic disease. *BMJ* 1963; 1: 979–84.

Clarke CA. Prevention of Rh-haemolytic disease *BMJ*. 1967; 4: 7–12.

Finn R. Erythroblastosis. *Lancet* 1960; 1: 526.

Finn R, Clarke CA, Donohoe WTA et al. Experimental studies on the prevention of Rh haemolytic disease. *BMJ* 1961; 1: 1486–90.

Freda VJ, Gorman JG, Pollack W. Successful prevention of experimental Rh sensitization in man with anti-Rh gammaglobulin antibody preparation: a preliminary report. *Transfusion* 1964; 4: 26–32.

Zipursky A, Hull A, White FD, Israels LG. Foetal erythrocytes in the maternal circulation. *Lancet* 1959; 1: 451–2.

Bibliography References

82, 175, 279–284, 550, 551, 921, 1624–1626, 1677, 1690, 1741, 1744, 1748.

Clay, Charles (1801–1893)

Abdominal Hysterectomy/Ovariotomy

Charles Clay of Manchester, England had performed four ovariotomy operations in the preceding year when he confidently approached his fifth on 17 November 1843. He opened the abdomen but encountered a huge fibroid uterus rather than the ovarian cyst he had expected. He therefore carried out the first abdominal hysterectomy in the midst of 'great haemorrhage'. The patient died shortly after the operation. Four days later, AM Heath, another surgeon from Manchester, performed the same operation under the same circumstances with the same outcome. Clay did have a short-term success a year later with a total abdominal hysterectomy and bilateral salpingo-oophorectomy for uterine fibroids weighing 9 kg, but the patient died 15 days after the operation. The exact cause of her death was unclear, but it may have been related to her being dropped while the bed linen was being changed.

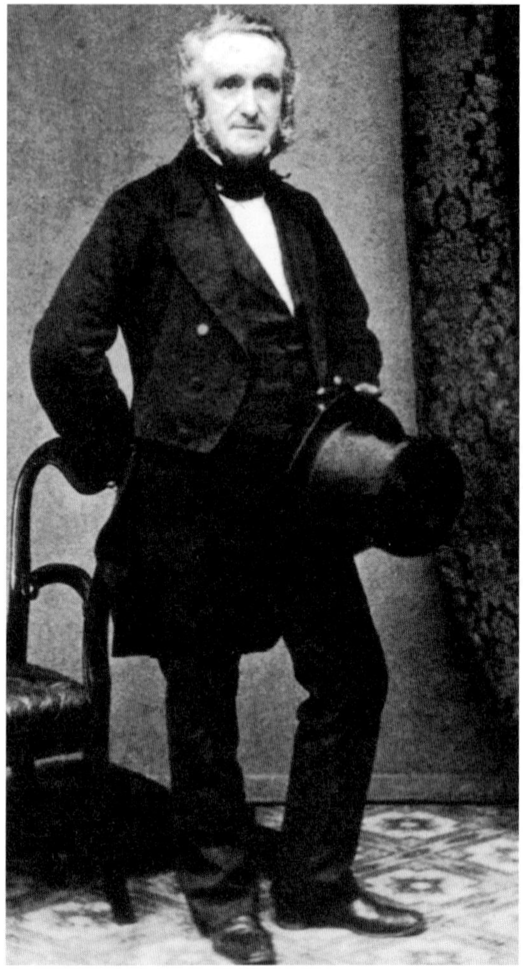

Charles Clay

The first successful abdominal hysterectomy was performed 10 years later in June 1853. Again, the circumstances leading to the procedure were dictated to the surgeon, Walter Burnham of Lowell, Massachusetts. Rather than finding the ovarian cyst he expected, he was faced with large uterine fibroids. Under chloroform anaesthesia and in the presence of 'a large number of medical gentlemen', he removed the uterus and ovaries. The first successful, planned subtotal abdominal hysterectomy for fibroids was carried out under chloroform anaesthesia on 1 September 1853 by Gilman Kimball, also of Lowell, Massachusetts.

The achievements of these pioneer surgeons should be placed in the context of the time, with limited or no anaesthesia and no knowledge of asepsis. Only a few years before, the editor of the London *Medico-Chirurgical Review* summed up the prevailing opinion on the possibility of abdominal hysterectomy:

We consider extirpation of the uterus, not previously protruded or inverted, one of the most cruel and unfeasible operations that ever was projected or executed by the head or hand of man.

Clay performed his early operations without anaesthesia and later, when it became available, with chloroform. However, he disliked this anaesthetic:

I should infinitely prefer to operate without it, as the patient would bring to bear on her case a nerve and determination to meet so great a trial, which would assist beyond all value the after-treatment; it would also relieve the case from that most distressing retching, and vomiting, so common after all abdominal operations where it is used . . .

Charles Clay was born in Bredbury, England. He was apprenticed to Kinder Wood (1785–1830) in Manchester, who did one of the first caesarean sections in Britain. After this he spent four years studying in Edinburgh and then worked as a general practitioner in Ashton-under-Lyne from 1823–39, when he moved to establish his practice in Manchester. He carried out the first successful ovariotomy in England on 12 September 1842 in the pre-anaesthetic era. The patient was 45 years old with eight children, and repeated tapping of the huge ovarian cyst failed to control her pain and disability. Clay explained the risks of surgery quite frankly, but he was emboldened to operate by the women's character:

Still she was determined I should operate, and the calm deliberate manner in which she weighed the matter convinced me I had a woman of no ordinary nerve to deal with – and that, in itself, was a point of considerable promise towards ultimate success.

Clay performed several hundred ovariotomies in his time and is said to have measured his results in the weight of tumours removed rather than the number of patients. His mortality rate was one of the lowest on record. He demonstrated his technique to Spencer Wells, who was later to belittle Clay's role as a pioneer of ovariotomy. The two men became, and remained, bitter antagonists.

Clay was to wait 19 years before he again attempted a hysterectomy. On 2 January 1863 he performed a planned abdominal subtotal hysterectomy and salpingo-oophorectomy for uterine fibroids. This was the first successful hysterectomy in Europe. By this time anaesthesia, antisepsis and asepsis were beginning to make the operation safer.

His efforts received approval from Sir James Young Simpson, who fortuitously arrived in Manchester just after the operation. He took the specimen back to Edinburgh and later wrote to Clay:

Your case may turn out as a precedent for operative interference in some exceptional cases of large fibroids of the uterus, and I congratulate you most sincerely on the happy recovery of your patient.

In 1848 he became editor of the *British Record of Obstetrics and Surgery*, the first English language journal devoted to obstetrics and gynaecology. In his time, he also designed a pair of short obstetric forceps.

Selected Publications

Burnham W. Extirpation of the uterus and ovaries for sarcomatous disease. *Nelson's Amer Lancet* 1853; 7: 147–51.

Clay C. Observations on ovariotomy statistical and practical. Also, a successful case of entire removal of the uterus, and its appendages. *Trans Obstet Soc Lond* 1863; 5: 58–74.

Kimball G. Successful case of extirpation of the uterus. *Boston Med Surg J* 1855; 52: 249–55.

Bibliography References

97, 125, 1001, 1393, 1538, 1539.

Cloquet, Jules Germain (1790–1883)

Cloquet's Node

Cloquet's node, a landmark in the operation of radical vulvectomy, was first described in Cloquet's monograph on the surgical anatomy of inguinal and femoral herniae based on 340 dissected cases:

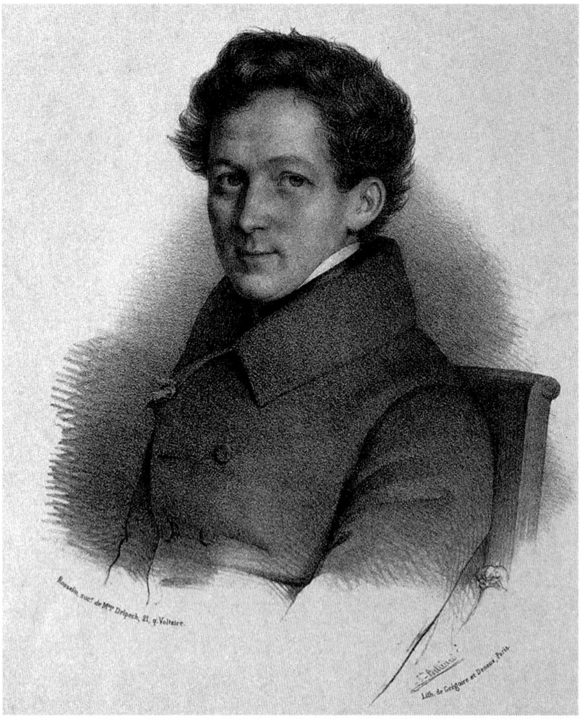

Jules Germain Cloquet

> *The upper surface of the septum crurale is towards the abdominal cavity . . . This septum is always perforated by small apertures for the passage of lymphatics, and which are sometimes so numerous, that the superior part of the canal appears to be closed simply by a fibro-cellular network. One of these apertures, more considerable than the others, is central, and is sometimes occupied by an elongated absorbent gland.*

Cloquet was born in Paris, the son of an art teacher. He was such a brilliant student that in 1812 the University of Paris sought, and obtained, a special decree from Napoleon exempting him from military service. An accomplished anatomist and surgeon, he held the chair of surgical pathology at the University of Paris for 27 years. In 1852 he was appointed surgeon to the Emperor Napoleon III and was created a Baron. He received international acclaim and, although he was always worried about his frail constitution, Baron Cloquet lived to the age of 93.

Selected Publications

Cloquet JG. *Recherches anatomiques sur les hernies de l'abdomen*. Paris; 1817.

Bibliography References

406, 968, 1288, 1290–1292, 1460.

Clover, Joseph Thomas (1825–1882)

Clover's Crutch

Joseph Clover designed this cunning device to allow a single practitioner to work with a patient in the lithotomy position when there was limited assistance and no operating table with leg supports. It also served to immobilise the patient. It was originally used for lithotomy operations, but later adopted for domiciliary obstetric practice and was carried by general practitioners and obstetric flying squads in Britain well into the twentieth century.

Clover's crutch consists of two firm leather braces encircling the legs just below the knees and separated by a metal bar. A long leather strap attached to the outer aspect of each knee brace was looped over one shoulder, behind the neck and below the other shoulder. Thus, the patient was firmly held in the lithotomy position.

Joseph Thomas Clover was born in Aylesham, Norfolk. He was initially apprenticed to a surgeon in Norwich and for two years acted as surgical dresser in the Norfolk and Norwich Hospital. At the age of 19 he became a medical student at University College Hospital, London, and he became a Fellow of the Royal College of Surgeons in 1850. He was involved with lithotomy operations and invented a bladder aspirator to remove

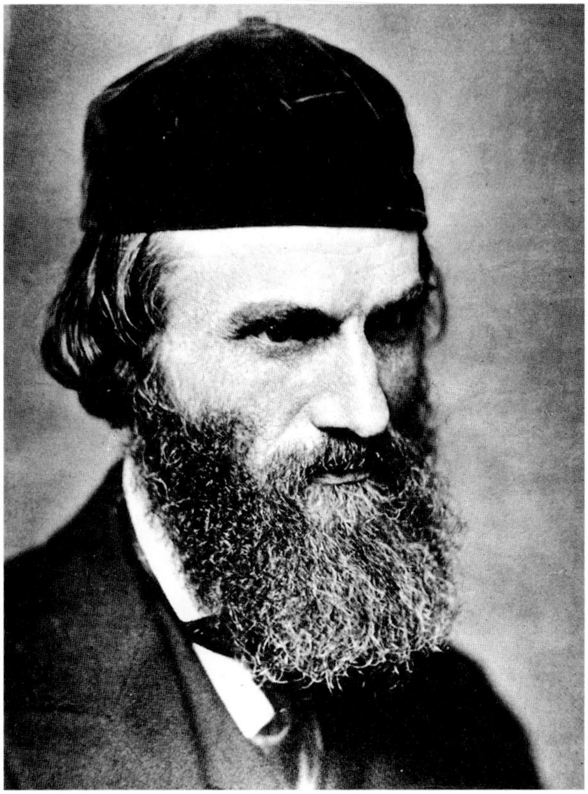

Joseph Thomas Clover

stone fragments. However, chronic pulmonary disease, probably tuberculosis, forced him to relinquish his surgical career for the less arduous life

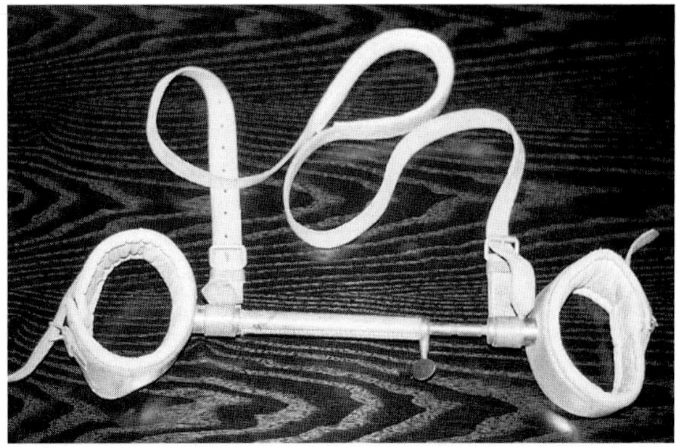

Clover's crutch

of anaesthesia. He worked at the Westminster and University College hospitals, becoming one of the leading anaesthetists in London. He devised several pieces of anaesthetic apparatus. In his time, he anaesthetised the Princess of Wales and Florence Nightingale. Along with John Snow, he is regarded as the founder of anaesthesia in Britain. The figures of Snow and Clover support the armorial crest of the Royal College of Anaesthetists.

Joseph Thomas Clover is buried in Brompton cemetery, London, as is John Snow.

Bibliography References

14, 14, 290–292, 457, 832, 881, 958, 991, 992, 1336, 1438, 1530, 1579, 1582, 1584, 1722.

Cochrane, Archibald Leman (1909–1988)

Cochrane Collaboration

Over the past 40 years much of obstetric practice has changed from an often-technical specialty, and to some extent *secundum artem*, to a more logical science. A major factor in this change was the development of evidence-based medicine, of whom one of the earliest and most ardent proponents was Archie Cochrane, a Scot imbued with a sharp mind and a caustic wit.

In 1972 Cochrane published *Effectiveness and Efficiency: Random Reflections on Health Services*. In this book he lamented the dearth of evidence-based medicine and the paucity of randomised controlled trials (RCTs) in the allocation of health resources in the National Health Service (NHS) in the United Kingdom. In a later essay in 1979 he reiterated the importance of RCTs to guide the effectiveness of medical treatment. In this context he rated the various medical specialties and awarded the 'wooden spoon' to obstetrics and gynaecology as the specialty making the least use of evidence-based medicine. He wrote, 'G and

O stands for gynaecologists and obstetricians, but it could also stand for GO ahead without evaluation'.

At this time Cochrane was director of the epidemiology unit at the Medical Research Council in Cardiff. Also working in Cardiff was another Scot, the obstetrician Ian Chalmers, who was profoundly influenced by Cochrane and in 1974 established a registry in Cardiff to identify and collate RCTs in perinatal medicine. In 1978 Chalmers and others set up the Oxford Database of Perinatal Trials at the National Perinatal Epidemiology Unit in Oxford, funded in part by the World Health Organization. Chalmers was appointed director and, as well as the classification and appraisal of previous studies, established a clinical trials unit to advise clinicians undertaking clinical trials. The culmination of this work was the publication in 1989 of *Effective Care in Pregnancy and Childbirth*. The rate of progress in obstetrics was such that, in a foreword to this book, Cochrane graciously withdrew his condemnation and wrote:

> *In 1979 I finally chose obstetrics as the specialty most deserving of the 'wooden spoon'. I think that I made a reasonable defence of my choice. That, however, was nearly a decade ago and a great deal has happened since. There has been a marked increase in the use of randomized trials in the world of obstetrics. Moreover, the systematic review of randomized trials of obstetric practice that is presented in this book is a new achievement. It represents a real milestone in the history of randomized trials and in the evaluation of care, and I hope that it will be widely copied by other medical specialities. I now have no hesitation whatsoever in withdrawing the slur of the wooden spoon from obstetrics ...*

There is no doubt that the publication of *Effective Care in Pregnancy and Childbirth* – ECPC as it came to be known – was a major landmark in obstetric care. In 1992 Chalmers was able to establish, with funding from the research and development branch of the NHS, the UK Cochrane Centre with a mandate to organise structured reviews of evidence from RCTs in all areas of health care following the ECPC model. Indeed, the forest plot of the original systematic review, showing that corticosteroids given to women in preterm labour had the beneficial effect of reducing neonatal respiratory distress syndrome, was adopted as the logo for the Cochrane Collaboration. There are now more than 10,000 volunteers in 90 countries who systemically review trials for the Cochrane Collaboration.

Archie Cochrane was born on 12 January 1909 at Galashiels, Scotland. He played rugby for his school and won a scholarship to King's College, Cambridge, where he completed his preliminary medical studies. He took a year off to be a research student in the Strangeways Laboratory, Cambridge, which taught him that basic science research was not his métier. For the next three years he combined informal medical studies in Vienna and Leiden with psychoanalysis, which he found unhelpful. In 1934 he returned to London and started his clinical studies at University College Hospital. He took another year away from his formal medical studies in 1936 to serve with a Field Ambulance Unit in the Spanish Civil War. He returned to London in 1937 and finally qualified in medicine in 1938. With the outbreak of war in 1939 he served as a Captain in the Royal Army Medical Corps. He was taken prisoner of war in Crete in June 1941 and spent the rest of the war as a medical officer in a number of prisoner of war camps in Egypt and Germany, for which service he was awarded the MBE. After the war he completed his diploma in public health in London and was subsequently awarded a Rockefeller fellowship to study in Philadelphia.

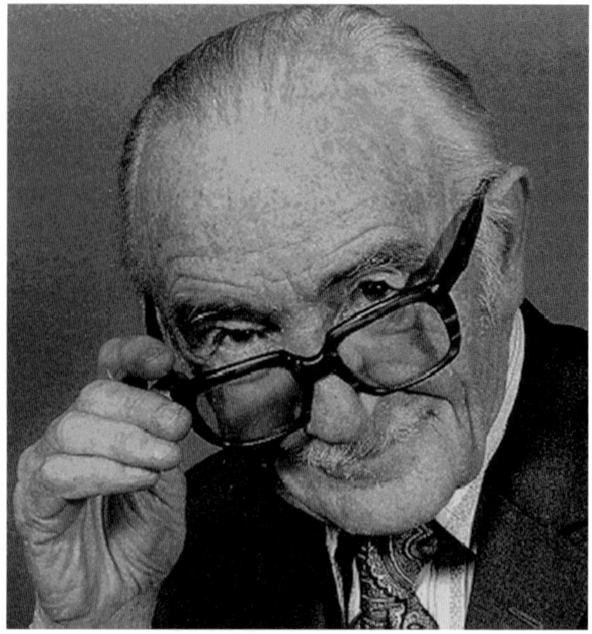
Archibald Leman Cochrane

He developed his research interest in the radiological study of pulmonary tuberculosis and observer error in the interpretation of X-ray films. He returned to the Medical Research Council Pneumoconiosis Research Unit in Cardiff, South Wales. Here began his life-long interest in the study of pulmonary fibrosis among coal miners, culminating in the 1980s in a 30-year follow-up. Although his work as an epidemiologist was admired, it was his critique of the National Health Service efficiency in 1971 that brought him international recognition. In the 1960s and 1970s he was the David Davies Professor at the Welsh National School of Medicine in Cardiff and director of the Medical Research Council Epidemiology Unit. He died on 18 June 1988 at Rhoose, Wales. He had previously written his own obituary which concluded, 'He was a man with severe porphyria who smoked too much and was without consolation of a wife, a religious belief, or a merit award – but he didn't do so badly'.

Selected Publications

Cochrane AL. *Effectiveness and Efficiency: Random Reflections on Health Services*. London: Nuffield Provincial Hospital's Trust; 1972.

Cochrane AL. 1931–1971: A critical review with particular reference to the medical profession. In: *Medicine for the Year 2000*. London: Office of Health Economics, 1979; pp. 1–11.

Cochrane AL. Foreword: In: Chalmers I, Enkin M, Keirse MJNC (eds) *Effective Care in Pregnancy and Childbirth*. Oxford: Oxford University Press; 1989.

Bibliography References

258, 295, 296, 392, 757, 838, 1007.

Colebrook, Leonard (1883–1967)

Chemotherapy for Puerperal Sepsis

In 1928, when Leonard Colebrook was appointed bacteriologist to the British Minister of Health's Committee on Maternal Mortality, some 2,000 women died each year from puerperal sepsis in England and Wales; this figure had not changed since records began in 1880.

From an earlier era, Jacques François Hervieux (1818–1895), the medical director of the Maternité Hospital in Paris, had compared the scourge of puerperal sepsis in women to the carnage of war in men:

> *Epidemics of puerperal fever are to women what war is to men. Like war they carry off the healthiest, the most courageous and the most useful part of the population; like war, they strike the victims in the prime of their life, spreading terror, sorrow and devastation in communities.*

The work of Alexander Gordon, Oliver Wendell Holmes and Ignac Semmelweis had established the contagious nature of outbreaks of puerperal sepsis and Louis Pasteur (1822–1895) had isolated the infecting agent, later identified by Rebecca Lancefield (1895–1981) and others as haemolytic streptococci.

Colebrook worked with Maeve Kenny, the resident medical officer of the isolation ward established in Queen Charlotte's Hospital, London to study and treat cases of puerperal fever. Improvements were made in prevention of the disease using better hygiene with asepsis, antisepsis, face masks and rubber gloves. However, their attempts to treat the disease, once it occurred, with arsenicals, blood transfusions and antistreptococcal sera made no impression on the case mortality rate of about 25 per cent, unchanged throughout the 1920s and early 1930s.

It was the work of Gerhard Domagk (1895–1964) that provided Colebrook and Kenny with the drug that would dramatically improve the outlook for women with puerperal sepsis. Domagk was a medical graduate of Kiel University and the director of research at the bacteriology laboratory of IG Farben Industries in Wuppertal, Germany. In 1935 he reported the use of a red dye, which he subsequently named prontosil, in the treatment of peritonitis in mice infected with streptococci. The untreated mice all died, whereas those given prontosil all survived.

After Colebrook repeated the work in mice and confirmed Domagk's findings, he and Kenny turned their attention to the more severe cases of puerperal infection with haemolytic streptococci. In two papers, published in June and December 1936, they reported the first clinical study with a mortality of 4.7% in 64 cases treated with prontosil. In the previous year, without prontosil, one in four mothers with puerperal haemolytic streptococcal infection had died. At that time these results were almost magical and provided the first real breakthrough in the treatment of this devasting disease:

> *Almost at once, with the new drug there was a surprising and most gratifying change. Signs of incipient peritonitis*

did not develop as we expected; positive blood cultures changed quickly to negative . . . This was something we had never seen before in ten years experience of the disease . . . It seemed clear to most of us that in red prontosil we had at last got a drug which could change the course of a haemolytic streptococcal infection in human beings as well as in mice.

In the Pasteur Institute in Paris a group led by Jacques Tréfouel (1897–1977) showed that the red dye was broken down in the body to a simpler compound, p-aminobenzine sulphonamide, and that this was the active ingredient against streptococci. This simpler and cheaper drug, the first of the sulphas, was named sulphanilamide. Colebrook later confirmed that sulphanilamide was as effective as prontosil and helped usher in the antibiotic era that came with the availability of penicillin towards the end of the Second World War.

Leonard Colebrook, the son of a farmer, was born in Guildford, England on 2 March 1883. He was brought up in an abstemious, teetotal environment with an emphasis on work and education. He took his medical degree at St Mary's Hospital, London, along with fellow classmate, Alexander Fleming (1881–1955); the two men were destined to play major roles in the development of the chemotherapeutic conquest of infections with sulpha drugs and penicillin.

After a year as a ship's doctor, Colebrook decided not to follow his original intention to become a missionary and instead took an appointment as a research bacteriologist in the pathology department of Sir Almroth Wright (1861–1947) at St Mary's Hospital. Both before and after his research on puerperal sepsis he worked on the treatment of wound infections in both World Wars. Later in his career he modernised the prevention and treatment of infection at the Medical Research Council Burns Unit in the Accident Hospital in Birmingham.

In retirement he and his second wife campaigned vigorously for the prevention of burn injuries. They were instrumental in the passage of the Fireguards Act of 1952, which made it illegal to sell a gas or electric heater without an effective guard and legislation to ensure the flame-proofing of children's clothes.

Leonard Colebrook, 'Coli' as he was known to his friends, died on 24 September 1967.

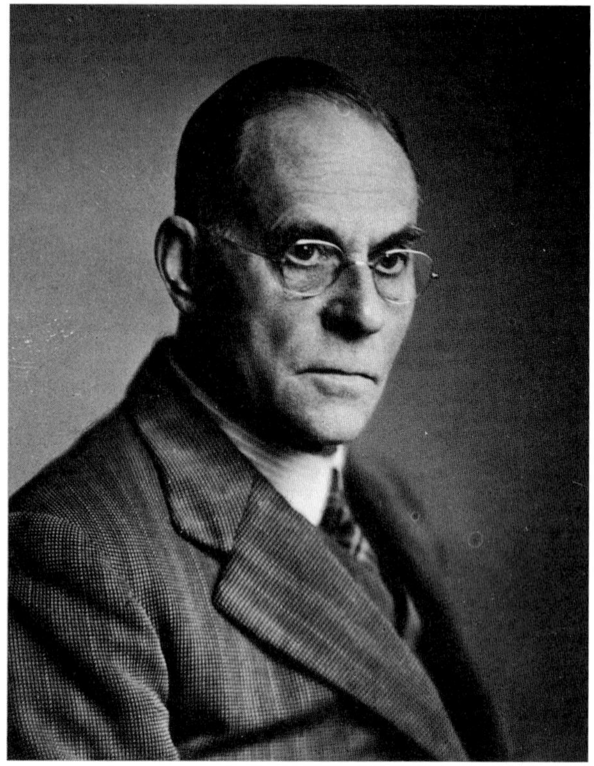

Leonard Colebrook

Selected Publications

Colebrook L, Kenny M. Treatment of human puerperal infections and of experimental infection in mice with prontosil. *Lancet* 1936; 1: 1279–86.

Colebrook L, Kenny M. Treatment with prontosil of puerperal infections due to haemolytic streptococci. *Lancet* 1936; 1: 1319–22.

Domagk G. Ein Beitrag zur Chemotheropie der bakterillen Infektionen. *Dtsch Med Wochensch* 1935; 61: 250–3.

Hervieux JFE. *Traité clinique et practique des maladies puerpérales.* Paris; 1870.

Pasteur L. Septicémie puerpérale. *Bull Acad Méd (Paris)* 1879; 8: 271–4.

Bibliography References

301, 489, 939, 940, 944, 1635.

Collip, James Bertram (1892–1965)

Oestrogen Hormone Replacement

James Bertram Collip was born in the town of Belleville, Ontario, on 20 November 1892. At the age of 15 he left the one-room school in Belleville and started his studies in physiology and biochemistry at Trinity College in the University of Toronto, receiving his PhD in 1916. He was appointed lecturer in physiology at the University of Alberta in Edmonton, where his research focus was on blood chemistry. In late 1921, while on sabbatical in Toronto, he was assigned to work with Frederick Banting and Charles Best as they attempted to treat diabetes with pancreatic extract. It was Collip's skill at chemistry that helped produce the pure injectable form of insulin in early 1922.

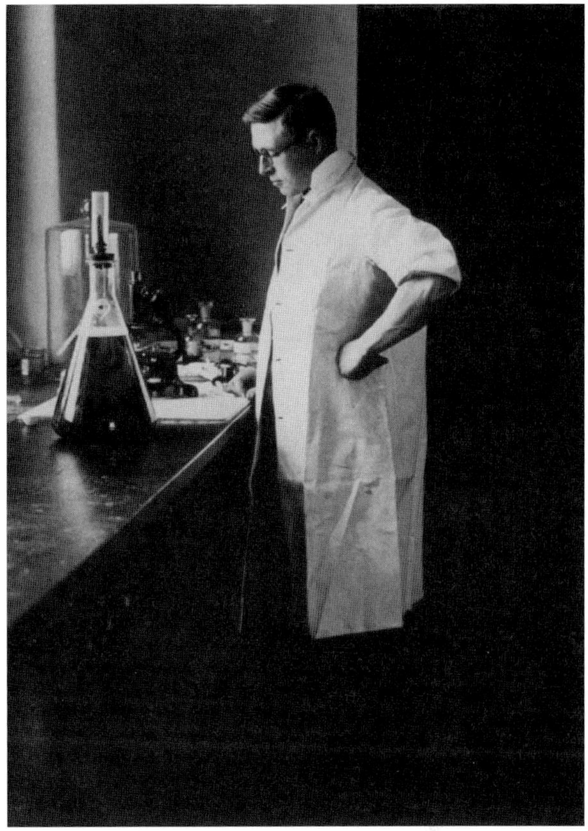

James Bertram Collip

Collip returned to Edmonton in 1922 as professor and head of biochemistry and, pari passu, he completed his medical degree in 1926. In the same year he isolated the parathyroid hormone. In 1928 he was recruited to become head of the department of biochemistry at McGill University in Montreal.

In 1929, Collip 'became interested in the problem of the isolation of the oestrogen hormone from the placenta'. He always regarded himself as a 'boiling biochemist' and, following a series of intricate distillations of human placental tissue, he produced an orally active substance that he called emmenin. Dr Archie Campbell (1887–1961), a gynaecologist at the Montreal General Hospital, first used emmenin in women with oestrogen deficiency in 1930. They were heartened by the response:

> *It is too early to make a definite pronouncement on the value of this treatment ... It may be said, however, that definite results of a most encouraging character have been obtained in five cases of oligo-menorrhoea, in two cases of distressing menopause symptoms ...*

A small local pharmaceutical company, Ayerst, McKenna and Harrison (later to become Wyeth-Ayerst), had backed some of Collip's research and continued to work with Collip's group to develop emmenin for clinical use. As the market for oestrogen replacement grew, it became clear that the placenta was an inadequate source, so they used the urine of humans in late pregnancy. This also proved to be too high-cost and low-yield. Ultimately the most productive and cost-effective source came from the urine of pregnant mares and, to meet the demand, Ayerst set up farms in Brandon, Manitoba and the Eastern Townships in Quebec.

The name emmenin was later dropped and replaced with premarine (PRegnant MAre uRINE), shortened to premarin. The pharmaceutical product, premarin, was introduced to the Canadian market in 1941, and received United States FDA approval in May 1942. It became the most widely prescribed oestrogen for replacement therapy.

During the Second World War, Collip oversaw the medical military research of the National Research Council, which involved liaison with his counterparts in the United Kingdom and the United States. For this work he received the CBE from King George VI and the United States Medal of Freedom. He was also the recipient of 12 honorary degrees.

After the war, he was appointed dean of medicine at the University of Western Ontario from 1947 to 1961. He had an aversion to flying and undertook all of his many trips in North America by train and car.

James Collip died following a stroke on 19 June 1965.

Selected Publications

Collip JB. The ovary stimulating hormone of the placenta: preliminary paper. *Can Med Assoc J* 1930; 22: 215–19.

Campbell AD, Collip JB. On the clinical use of the ovary-stimulating hormone of the placenta. *Can Med Assoc J* 1930; 22: 219–20.

Collip JB. Further observations on an ovary stimulating hormone of the placenta. *Can Med Assoc J* 1930; 22: 761–4.

Bibliography References

587, 837, 1031, 1113, 1114.

Coombs, Robert Royston Amos (1921–2006)

Coombs' Test

Coombs and his colleagues devised a test for detecting red cell antibodies on the red cell (direct Coombs) or in the serum (indirect Coombs), using antihuman immunoglobulin serum, an antiglobulin prepared by animal injection. This test is used on cord blood and, if positive, shows that antibody has coated the fetal erythrocytes, confirming the presence of erythroblastosis fetalis. The preliminary communication of this work covered half a page in the *Lancet* in July 1945: 'In our hands the test has proved most specific and reliable, showing up weak Rh sensitisation and sensitisation with "incomplete" antibody'.

His co-worker Mourant later wrote of Coombs' inspiration for the test:

> *He states that he was travelling on an ill-lit wartime train from London to Cambridge . . . when he visualized the cells, already coated with molecules of incomplete antibody, which of course was a globulin, but still floating free, becoming linked together by molecules of another antibody, an antiglobulin antibody.*
>
> *He realised that this idea could be the basis of a practical test, and he formulated in some detail its possible applications – essentially as the direct and indirect antiglobulin test.*

Coombs later said, 'In a flash I could see the globulin antibody on the red cells, and these red cells should be agglutinated with an antibody to serum globulin, i.e., an antiglobulin'.

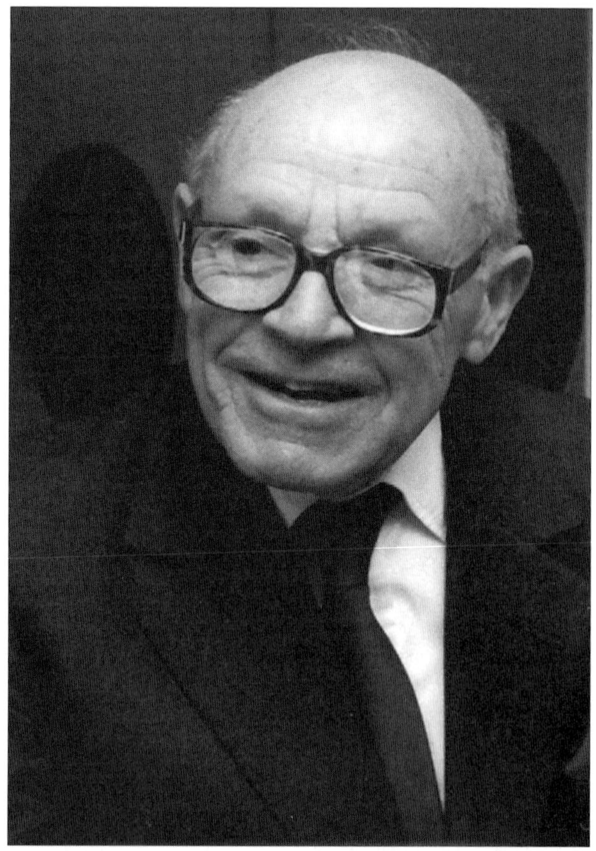

Robert Royston Amos Coombs

The general principles of this test had been elucidated before by the Italian, Carlo Moreschi, in 1908. This work was unknown by Coombs at the time of his own studies, but later came to his notice, as he acknowledged in his subsequent publications.

Robert Royston Amos Coombs, known to his friends as Robin, was born in London and grew up in South Africa. He returned to Britain and graduated in veterinary medicine from Edinburgh University in 1943. He became Quick Professor of Biology and head of the division of immunology, department of pathology at Cambridge University from 1966 to 1988. He is said to have stated, 'erythrocytes were primarily designed by God as tools for the immunologist and only secondarily as carriers of haemoglobin'. He was a fellow of both the Royal Society and Corpus Christi College, Cambridge. He retired to Cambridge and died on 25 January 2006.

Selected Publications

Coombs RRA, Mourant AE, Race RR. Detection of weak and 'incomplete' Rh agglutinins: a new test. *Lancet* 1945; 2: 15.

Coombs RRA, Mourant AE, Race RR. A new test for the detection of weak and 'incomplete' Rh agglutinins. *Br J Exp Path* 1946; 26: 255.

Moreschi C. Nune tatsachen über die blutkörperchen agglutination. *Zentralbl Bakt* 1908; 46: 49–51.

Mourant AE. The discovery of the anti-globulin test. *Vox Sang* 1983; 45: 180–3.

Bibliography References

248, 307, 308, 899, 1626, 1690, 1746, 1748.

Cooper, Astley Paston (1768–1841)

Cooper's Ligament

Sir Astley Paston Cooper described the ligament on the upper posterior aspect of the pubic bone that is used as a point for suture and elevation of the urethrovesical junction in operations for stress incontinence:

> *The pubis is covered by a ligamentous substance, which forms a particularly strong production above the linea ileo-pectinea, extending from the tuberosity of the pubis outwards and projecting beyond the bone above that line.*

Cooper also described the contracture of the palmar fascia 10 years before Guillaume Dupuytren. He was born at Brooke Hall near Norwich, where his father was a minister and his mother an author. At the age of 15 he became an apprentice to his uncle, William Cooper, surgeon to Guy's Hospital. He attended the lectures of John Hunter. After an additional year in Edinburgh he returned to London and became an accomplished anatomist, surgeon and teacher. He was appointed demonstrator in anatomy at St Thomas' Hospital in 1789. His lectures were attended by up to 400 students, and he reputedly gave his customary lecture on the evening of his wedding day. In 1800 he succeeded his uncle as surgeon to Guy's Hospital and became a contemporary of Thomas Addison, Richard Bright and Thomas Hodgkin. He was knighted by George IV, following the successful removal of a sebaceous cyst from the royal scalp in 1821. In the era of fatal post-operative sepsis, this was not a trivial procedure. Indeed, Cooper later wrote, 'I was very averse from doing it . . . I saw that the operation, if it were followed by erysipelas, would destroy all of my happiness, and blast my reputation'.

One student at Guy's Hospital during Cooper's tenure was the poet John Keats (1795–1821), who was licensed as an apothecary in 1816. Keats initially served as a surgical dresser under Cooper, but his later apprenticeship with a notoriously unsuccessful surgeon may have influenced him to give up medicine for poetry. Cooper died in 1841 and was attended in his final illness by Bright. Two days before his death, increasingly ill and short of breath, he responded to his doctors' suggestion that they change his treatment with a terminally courteous statement: 'My dear sirs, I am fully convinced of your excellent judgement and of your devotion to me, but your good wishes will not be fulfilled in my case, and you must excuse me, for I will take no more medicine'. Two days later his last words to assembled family and friends were, 'Good-bye, God bless you'. The post-mortem findings showed healed tuberculosis of the lungs and the small granular kidneys of chronic glomerulonephritis (Bright's disease).

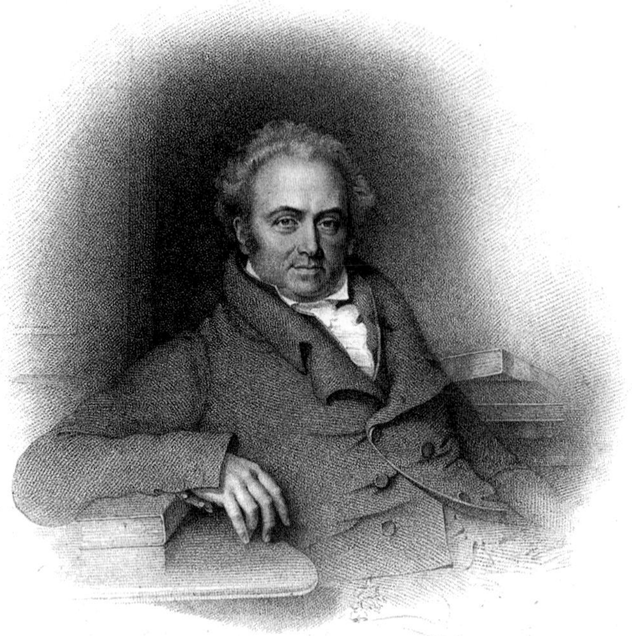

Astley Paston Cooper

Selected Publications

Cooper AP. *Anatomy and Surgical Treatment of Hernia.* London; 1804.

Bibliography References

149, 196, 210, 406, 519, 626, 648, 1588, 1679.

Corner, George Washington (1889–1981) Allen, Willard Myron (1904–1993)

Progesterone

Although George Corner was professor and head of anatomy at the Medical School of Rochester, New York, he had physiological research tendencies towards reproductive endocrinology. In the 1920s the existence of ovarian and pituitary hormones and the timing and stimulation of ovulation were a matter of speculation. Edgar Allen and Edward Doisy had isolated the ovarian hormone oestrogen in the early 1920s. In 1927 Corner had the good sense to enlist the assistance of Willard Allen, at that time a first-year medical student in Rochester, who had earlier training in organic chemistry. In this era the classic research approach was to remove organs and then see if various extracts from those organs could replace their function. In 1928 Corner had shown that ovariectomy in rabbits blocked progestational changes and embryo implantation, but that this could be restored by injecting a 'mash' of corpus luteum tissue. By 1929 they had enough evidence to declare that the corpus luteum produced a hormone that caused progestational proliferation of the endometrium and that this allowed for implantation of the blastocyst:

The experiment described . . . shows that alcoholic extracts of the corpus luteum, freed from phospholipids, contain a substance which when injected into castrated adult female rabbits induces a characteristic alteration of the endometrium identical with the progestational proliferation previously shown to be due to the presence of corpora lutea in the ovaries . . .

It appears therefore, that extracts of the corpus luteum contain a special hormone which has for one of its functions the preparation of the uterus for reception of the embryos by inducing progestational proliferation of the endometrium . . .

The evidence is now complete that, in the rabbit, the corpus luteum is an organ of internal secretion which has for one of its functions the production of a special state of the uterine mucosa (progestational proliferation) and that in turn the function of the proliferated endometrium is to nourish or protect the free blastocysts and to make possible their implantation.

The isolation of the pure crystalline hormone was a laborious business and was achieved in 1934 by Allen and Wintersteiner, and simultaneously by four other groups in Europe, including Adolf Butenandt (1903–1995). Allen and Corner named the hormone progestin, but a year later an international conference, including Allen, agreed to the name progesterone.

George Washington Corner was born in Baltimore on 12 December 1889. He enrolled in Johns Hopkins University as a classics student but later switched to biology and ultimately gained his MD in 1913. He chose a career in anatomy and did his early training at the Carnegie Institute in Washington, DC, Berkeley, California, and Johns Hopkins University. In 1923 he was appointed the first professor and head of anatomy at the new medical school in Rochester, New York. In addition, he was a noted medical historian. He died on 21 September 1981.

Willard Myron Allen was born in Macedon, New York, on 5 November 1904. His first degree was in organic chemistry from Hobart College, New York. In 1926 he started his medical training at Rochester, New York, where he did his work with Corner on the isolation of progesterone. After this he did his residency training in obstetrics and gynaecology at Rochester's Strong Memorial Hospital. He remained on staff there until 1940, when he was appointed head of the department of obstetrics and gynaecology at the Washington University School of Medicine in St Louis. Here he collaborated with William Masters (1915–2001), a local gynaecologist who would later achieve fame for his research on the human sexual response. They described laceration of the base of the broad and Mackenrodt ligaments, secondary to obstetric or gynaecological surgical trauma. This is known as the Allen–Masters syndrome and is familiar to laparoscopists as the 'window' seen at the base of the broad ligament. It leads to increased mobility of the uterine cervix, but its relationship to gynaecological symptoms is moot.

In 1971 Allen retired from his position in St Louis but worked for another 10 years at the University of Maryland School of Medicine. He received an honorary DSc from his alma mater, Hobart College, in 1940. Willard Allen died in an automobile accident in August 1993.

Selected Publications

Corner GW, Allen WM. Physiology of the corpus luteum II. Production of a special uterine reaction (progestational proliferation) by extracts of the corpus luteum. *Am J Physiol* 1929; 88: 326–39.

Allen WM, Corner GW. Physiology of the corpus luteum III. Normal growth and implantation of embryos after very early ablation of the ovaries, under the influence of extracts of the corpus luteum. *Am J Physiol* 1929; 88: 340–6.

Allen WM, Wintersteiner O. Crystalline progestin. *Science* 1934; 80: 190–1.

Allen WM, Masters WH. Traumatic laceration of uterine support. The clinical syndrome and operative treatment. *Am J Obstet Gynecol* 1955; 70: 500–13.

Bibliography References

22, 315, 316, 642, 1031, 1166, 1480, 1485, 1486, 1491.

Cotte, Gaston (1879–1951)

Cotte's Operation

The operation of presacral neurectomy was first described by Mathieu Jaboulay (1860–1913) of Lyon, France and, in the same year (1899), by the Italian, Guiseppe Ruggi (1844–1925). However, it was Gaston Cotte of Lyon who reported, in 1925, an unusually high success rate for cure of severe dysmenorrhoea in 300 patients. Thus, it is often known as Cotte's operation. In his publication of 1937 Cotte wrote:

> *After an experience of twelve years with the operation, I may say that I am more and more convinced of the value of resection of the presacral nerve in every syndrome associated with an anatomic or functional disturbance of the hypogastric plexus, and that I know of no other therapeutic method that may be substituted for it . . . In the absence of precise and certain physiologic data concerning the nature and origin of the constituents of the presacral nerve, it is difficult to explain the successful results of presacral sympathectomy. Is it due to the suppression and interruption of abnormal sensory-motor reflexes or modification of the pelvic circulatory system? . . . Resection of the presacral nerve is effective because it suppresses the connections of the genital organs with the nervous centres . . . Accordingly, when all of the known therapeutic measures have been ineffective, it seems wisest to advise early operation.*

The level of acceptable operative mortality in that era is shown by his statement:

> *The mortality rate is that of all simple abdominal operations, about 1 per 100. In more than 300 operations I lost only two patients who died from acute pulmonary complications.*

Gaston Cotte was a well-known professor of gynaecology at the Hôtel Dieu in Lyon, and was noted for his conservative surgical approach. In the First World War he served in the French Ambulance Corps in Paris and Salonika. He received both British and French honours for his service (the DSO and Légion d'Honneur, respectively). A street in Lyon was named for him.

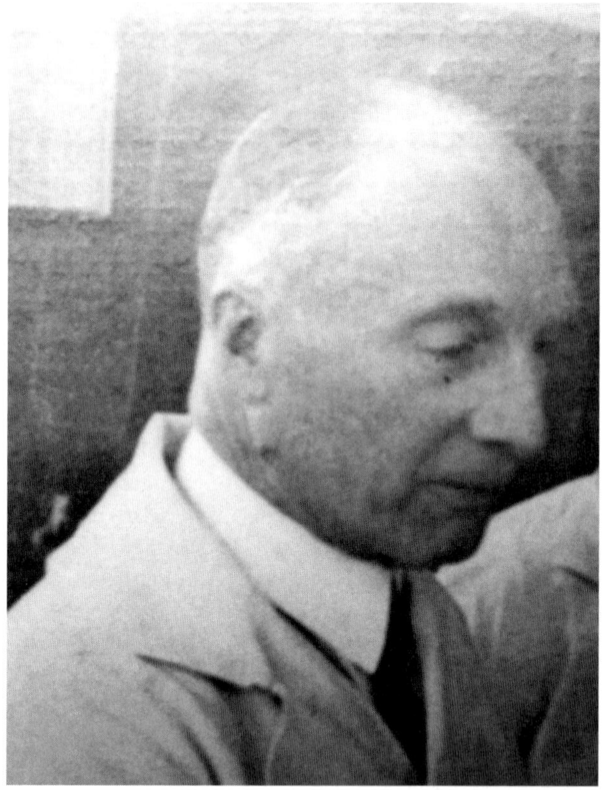

Gaston Cotte

Selected Publications

Cotte G. La sympathectomie hypogastrique, sa place dans la thérapeutique gynécologique. *Presse Med* 1925; 33: 98.

Cotte G. Resection of the presacral nerve in the treatment of obstinate dysmenorrhea. *Am J Obstet Gynecol* 1937; 33: 1034–40.

Jaboulay M. Le traitment de la neuralgie pelviènne par la paralysie du sympathique sacre. *Lyon Med* 1899; 90: 102.

Ruggi G. *La simpathectomia abdominale utero-ovarica come mezzo di cura di alcune lesioni interne degli organi genitali della donna.* Bologna: Zanichelli;1899.

Bibliography References

318, 448, 1480.

Coudray, Angelique Marguerite Le Boursier du (1715–1794)

Obstetric Mannequin

In February 1740, Marguerite Le Boursier, 'mature maiden', was officially registered as 'mistress matron midwife' of Paris. She was 25 years old and had just completed a three-year apprenticeship with senior midwives and passed an examination at the College of Surgery. After gaining experience as a midwife in Paris, she took on and trained apprentice midwives. By 1751 she moved to the provinces, practising and training midwives in Auvergne and Clermont. She began to teach increasing numbers of women the elements of midwifery. She found that the limited education of the women was a barrier. As she wrote, 'The only obstacle I found to my project was the difficulty of making myself understood by minds unaccustomed to grasping things except through the senses'. It was this barrier that led her to design and build her obstetrical mannequin.

I took the task of making my lessons palpable by having them manoeuvre in front of me on a machine I constructed for this purpose, and which represented the pelvis of a woman, the womb, its openings, its ligaments, the conduit called the vagina, the bladder and rectum intestines. I added a model of a child of natural size, whose joints I made flexible enough to be able to put it in different positions; a placenta with its membranes, the demonstration of waters that they contain; the umbilical cord composed of its two arteries and of the vein, leaving one half withered up, the other inflated, to imitate somewhat the cord of a dead child and that of a live child in which one feels the beating of the vessels that compose. I added the model of the head of the child separated from the trunk, in which the cranial bones are caved in on each other. I thought that with a demonstration this tangible, if I could not make these women very skilled, I would at least make them feel the necessity of asking for

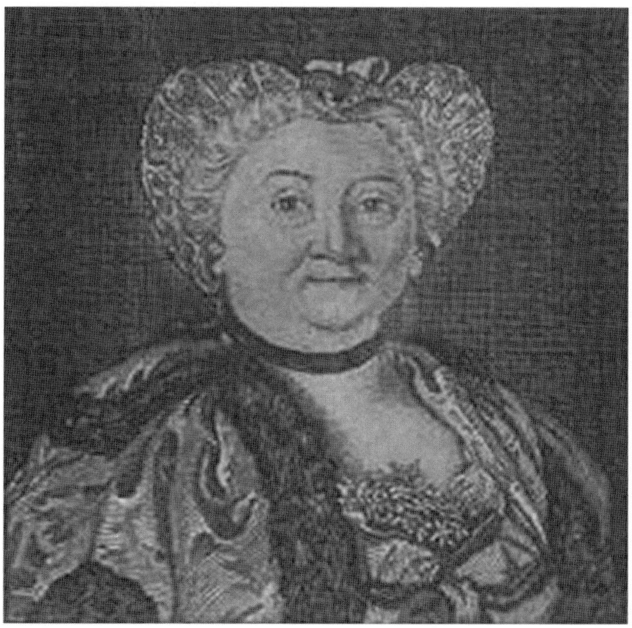

Angelique Marguerite le Boursier du Coudray

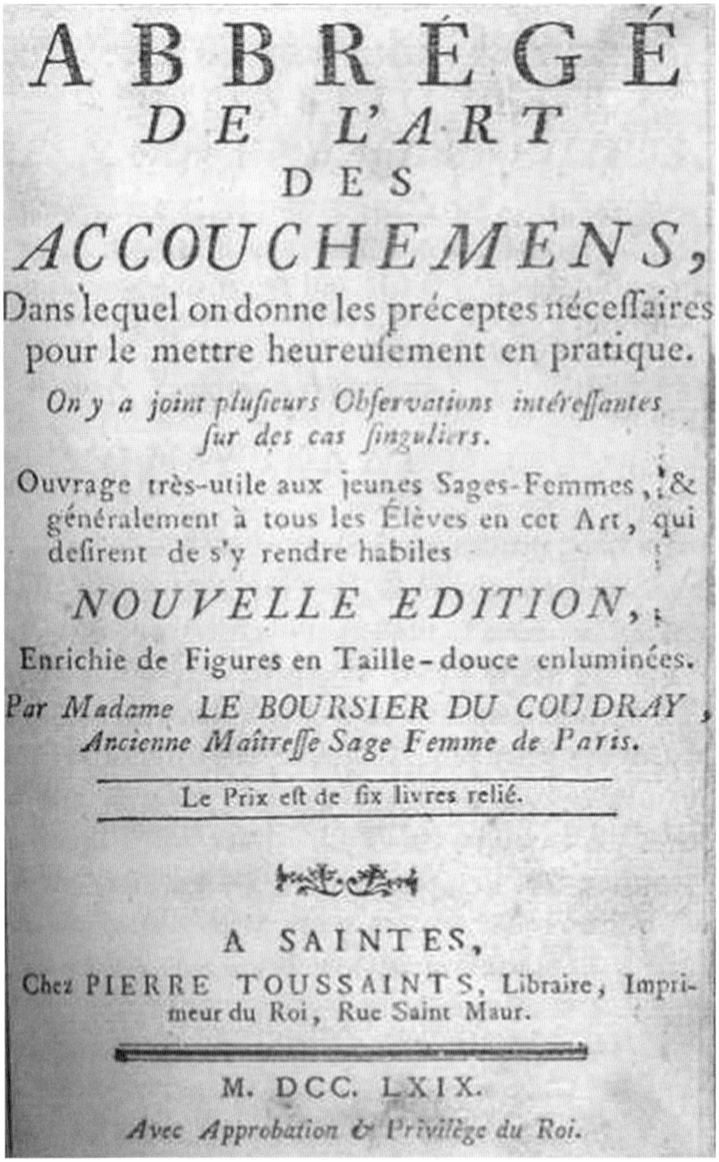

ABBRÉGÉ
DE L'ART
DES
ACCOUCHEMENS,

Dans lequel on donne les préceptes néceſſaires pour le mettre heureuſement en pratique.

On y a joint pluſieurs Obſervations intéreſſantes ſur des cas ſinguliers.

Ouvrage très-utile aux jeunes Sages-Femmes, & généralement à tous les Élèves en cet Art, qui deſirent de s'y rendre habiles.

NOUVELLE EDITION,

Enrichie de Figures en Taille-douce enluminées.

Par Madame LE BOURSIER DU COUDRAY,
Ancienne Maîtreſſe Sage Femme de Paris.

Le Prix eſt de ſix livres relié.

A SAINTES,
Chez PIERRE TOUSSAINTS, Libraire, Imprimeur du Roi, Rue Saint Maur.

M. DCC. LXIX.

Avec Approbation & Privilège du Roi.

Title page of Madame du Coudray's book *Abrégé de L'art des Accouchemens*

help soon enough to save the mother and child . . . where the skill of a surgeon called too late is often useless . . . Thus my project was to have these women recognize the diverse dangers to which the incapacity exposes the mother and child.

In this context she was the midwifery counterpart of William Smellie, who in the same era devised similar machines for the instruction of both male and female midwives in London. The only one of her models that remains intact is in the Musée Flaubert in Rouen. At the Royal Academy of Surgery in Paris, her 'machine' was approved and endorsed by the eminent obstetrician André Levret. She followed this with a publication of the first edition of her book *Abrégé de l'art des accouchemens.*

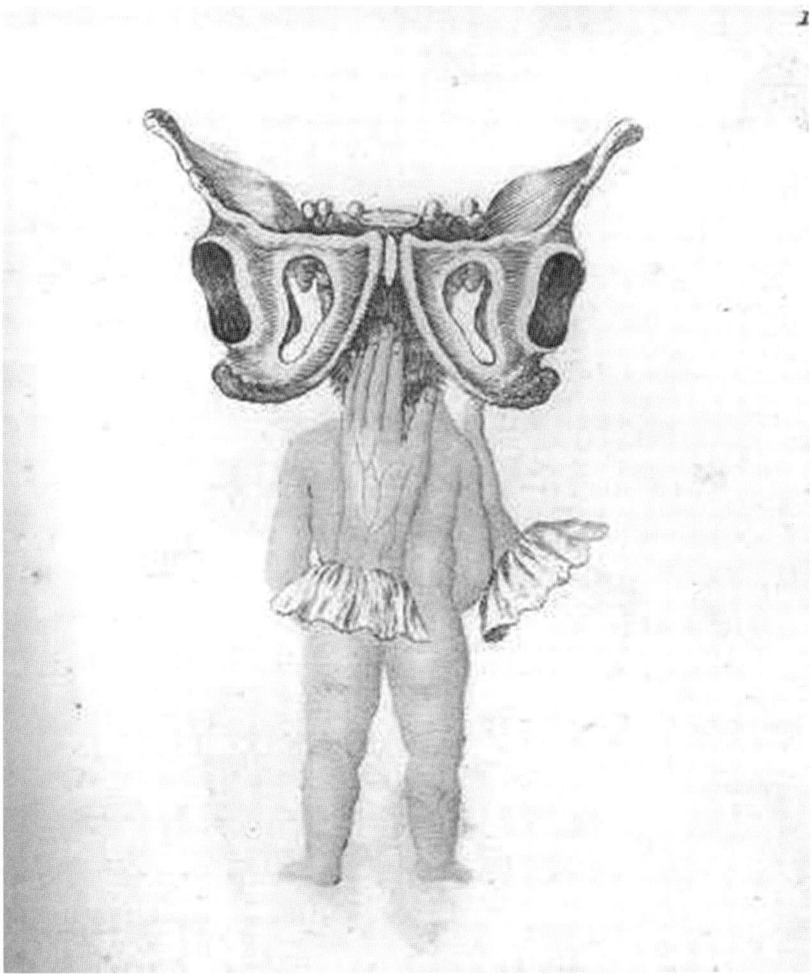

Illustration from du Coudray's book showing assistance to the aftercoming head in breech delivery

At this time the Government of France, in order to increase the population, set about raising the standards of midwives practice through training and licensing programmes. Under the authority of Louis XV and the authorities at Versailles, Madam Le Boursier du Coudray, as she now called herself, embarked upon a life of roving instruction in midwifery between 1759 and 1783. She visited 40 cities in France and by her own reckoning instructed 10,000 pupils. She managed to avoid confrontation with authority and particularly with the medical profession, saying, 'I asked the Grace that I not be accused of passing myself off as a doctor. I speak here from only a pure zeal for unfortunates deprived of all aid, because the distance of the villages does not permit doctor or able surgeon getting there in time, or because the poverty of these women prevents them from paying the suitable fees'.

Little is known about the private life of Madam Le Boursier du Coudray. Neither her birthplace or grave site is known. It seems she never married or had children. She lived the final 10 years of her life with her niece, Mme Coutanceau, a midwife whom she had trained, in Bordeaux. She died there in April 1794.

Selected Publications

Le Boursier du Coudray AM. *Abrégé de L'art des Accouchemens*. Paris: Delaguette; 1959.

Bibliography References

162, 298, 347, 419, 609, 610.

Couvelaire, Alexandre (1873–1948)

Couvelaire Uterus

Extensive haemorrhage into the myometrium associated with abruptio placentae was first described in detail in a case report by Alexandre Couvelaire in 1911. The patient had severe abruptio placentae, causing death of the fetus. Despite amniotomy she did not progress in labour and, with her condition deteriorating, Couvelaire did a caesarean section to control the bleeding. The placenta had completely separated and the myometrium, broad ligament and adnexa were infiltrated with blood. The surface of the uterus was striking in the extent of subserosal haemorrhages. Couvelaire performed a hysterectomy and bilateral salpingo-oophorectomy. The patient survived. He described the condition as one of utero-placental apoplexy:

> *The lesions observed during the course of the operation and later on histological examination could not be exactly characterised by the classic term retroplacental haematoma . . . The whole utero-ovarian apparatus seemed covered with blackish splotches. The uterine wall, in the zone of membranous insertion as well as the zone of placental insertion, was the site of a tremendous bloody infiltration separating the muscle bundles . . . The ovaries were peppered with a punctiform bloody suffusion. The broad ligaments were infiltrated with blood. This was indeed a true case of uteroplacental apoplexy . . . These lesions made it extremely unwise to conserve the uterus and sufficed in themselves to justify hysterectomy.*

In the early part of the twentieth century, with a lack of oxytocic drugs, blood transfusion or knowledge of coagulopathy, this early surgical approach in selected severe cases made some sense.

Alexandre Couvelaire was born in Bourg, France. He trained as an assistant with Adolphe Pinard. He worked at the Baudelocque Clinic in Paris and was made chief in 1901. In 1914 he was appointed professor in the University of Paris. Couvelaire was an early proponent of caesarean section in selected cases of placenta praevia.

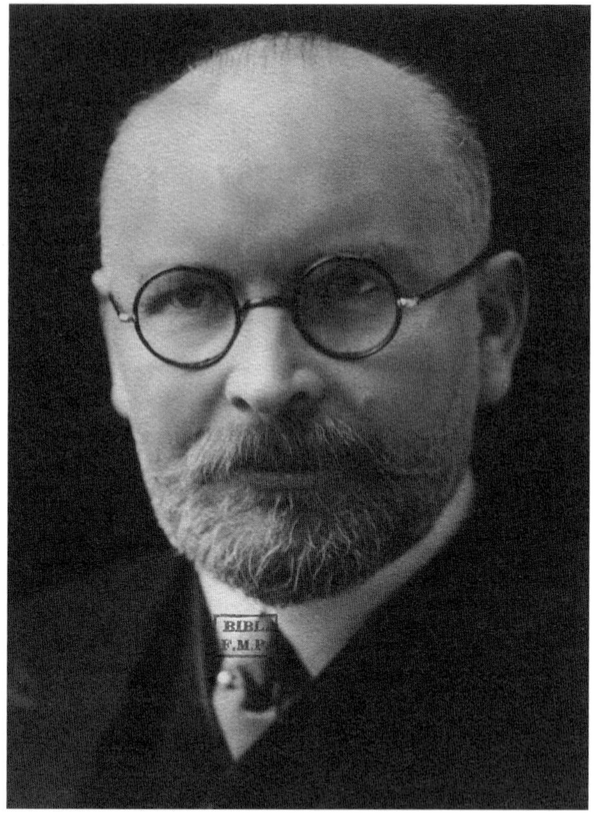

Alexandre Couvelaire

Selected Publications

Couvelaire A. Traitement chirurgical des hémorrhagies utéro-placentaires avec décollement du placenta normalement inséré. *Ann Gynéc* 1911; 8: 591–608.

Bibliography References

648, 865, 893, 902, 1231, 1477, 1480, 1486.

Craigin, Edwin Bradford (1859–1918)

Once a Caesarean . . .

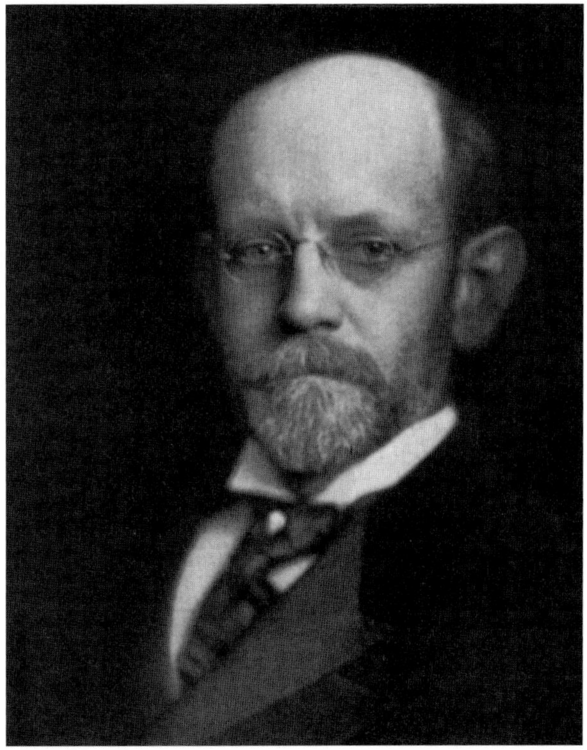
Edwin Bradford Craigin

Edwin Craigin was responsible for one of the most widely quoted and influential obstetric dictums in the United States: 'Once a caesarean, always a caesarean'. At the time Craigin made this statement, caesarean sections were uncommon, usually done for a contracted pelvis, and of the classical, upper uterine segment variety with a significant risk of rupture in a subsequent pregnancy. Thus, at this time, his pronouncement made good obstetric sense. This warning note was part of a lecture entitled 'Conservatism in Obstetrics', read before the Eastern Medical Society of the City of New York on 12 May 1916:

> *One thing must always be borne in mind, viz., that no matter how carefully a uterine incision is sutured, we can never be certain that the cicatrized uterine wall will stand a subsequent pregnancy and labor without rupture. This means that the usual rule is, once a Caesarean always a Caesarean. Many exceptions occur . . . The general rule holds, however, that we cannot depend on a sutured uterine wall, whether it is done in a Caesarean section or a myomectomy, hence I believe that the extension of Caesarean section to conditions other than dystocia from contracted pelvis or tumors should be exceptional and infrequent.*

With the advent of the lower uterine segment incision and clear evidence of its low risk of subsequent scar rupture, the change to allow labour after previous caesarean section became widespread. This did not apply often in the United States, however, where Craigin's dictum held sway until overwhelming data forced a slow change in the 1980s. Until then, this represented one of the main differences in common obstetric practice between North America and the rest of the world.

Edwin Bradford Craigin was born in Colchester, Connecticut, a descendant of one of the Mayflower settlers and governor of the Plymouth Colony. His undergraduate studies were taken at Yale and his medical degree in 1886 at the College of Physicians and Surgeons of Columbia University in New York. In 1899 he became professor of obstetrics and gynaecology at his alma mater and worked at the Sloane Hospital for Women and the City Maternity Hospital in New York. Craigin's early training was mainly gynaecological and, indeed, he was once gently upbraided at a meeting by Montgomery Baldy for having performed two hundred uterine ventrosuspensions in one year. In 1898 Craigin was appointed director of the Sloane Maternity Hospital, which at that time had no gynaecology unit. Craigin convinced the trustees to build an adjacent gynaecological pavilion, and in 1910 the institution's name was changed to the Sloane Hospital for Women. However, the obstetric and gynaecological units were staffed separately.

Before Craigin's appointment, there had not been a single caesarean delivery at the hospital. By 1913 Craigin was able to report a series of 122 caesarean sections, of which he performed 112. He was a swift operator, and the average time to delivery of the infant was recorded as 38 and 1/7 seconds.

Craigin was a small dapper man and, in keeping with his upbringing, of puritan character with a strong Presbyterian outlook. Reputedly, when he arrived at the hospital, the doorkeeper sounded three long whistles 'to alert the staff to proper obeisance to the chief'. He established and funded a medical mission in China and always gave 10 per cent of his income to charity. In 1905 he endowed a library in his hometown of Colchester, now the Craigin Memorial Library. He was awarded an honorary MA by Yale in 1907. Craigin died on 21 October 1918.

Selected Publications

Craigin EB. Cesarean section. *Sloane Hosp Women Obstet Gynecol Rep* 1913; 1: 13–19

Craigin EB. Conservatism in obstetrics. *NY Med J* 1916; 104: 1–3.

Bibliography References

99, 102, 348, 350, 351, 436, 648, 987, 1484, 1485, 1734.

Credé, Carl Siegmund Franz (1819–1892)

Credé's Method of Placental Delivery/Credé's Prophylaxis of Ophthalmia Neonatorum

Carl Credé was born in Berlin of French parents. He received his medical training in Berlin and at Heidelberg when Franz Naegele was the professor of obstetrics.

In 1852 he was made director of the Berlin School of Midwives and physician-in-chief of the lying-in division of the Charité hospital. It was here that he described his method of placental delivery. In 1856 Credé was appointed professor of obstetrics at Leipzig, which position he held for 32 years. As an author and teacher, he influenced many, including his pupils Christian Leopold and Max Sänger. He was the founder and editor of *Archive für Gynäkologie.* Prostate cancer caused his death on 14 March 1892.

Credé's method of placental delivery was first described in 1854 in *Klinische Vortrage über Geburtshülfe.* This involved massage of the uterine fundus if the placenta was not delivered within 15 minutes. The massage was gradually increased until, when the uterus was strongly contracted, manual compression was used to expel the placenta. In 1861 he advocated a more rapid method, using strong massage and compression to force expulsion of the placenta within five minutes of delivery. This method was soon condemned as a cause of haemorrhage, and Credé himself abandoned it and returned to his gentler original approach. Credé did not claim to be the first to advocate uterine massage to encourage placental delivery; François Mauriceau and John Harvie, among others, also used this technique.

Credé's greatest contribution was in the prevention of gonococcal ophthalmia neonatorum. In confronting this condition, he came to the conclusion that:

> *almost without exception, the affected infants in my institution became infected only through direct transfer of the vaginal discharge into their eyes during the act of birth.*

Efforts to cleanse the vagina during pregnancy and labour failed. In October 1879 he began experiments to disinfect the infant's eyes at birth, first with a solution of borax and then with silver nitrate.

In 1881, two years after Albert Neisser identified the bacterium gonococcus as the responsible organism for ophthalmia neonatorum, Credé published his results of prophylaxis of this condition. Within minutes of birth a few drops of 2% silver nitrate solution were placed in each eye. Using this method, he observed only two cases of ophthalmia

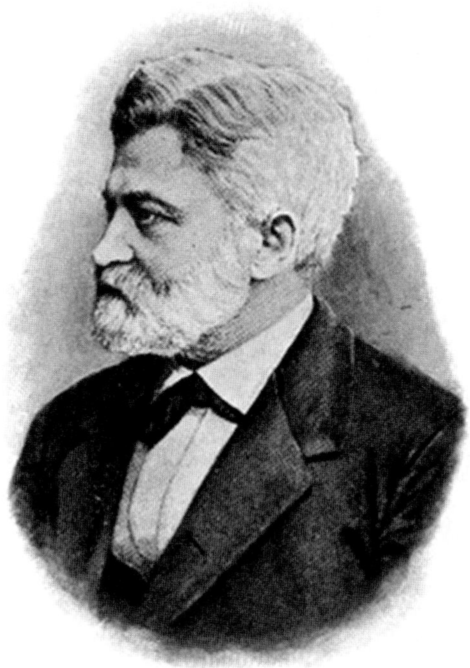

Carl Siegmund Franz Credé

neonatorum in 1,160 infants. At that time this condition occurred in almost 10 per cent of infants and was responsible for 25–50 per cent of all cases of blindness. Credé wrote:

> *A goal long striven for has been attained. Now all infants born in lying-in hospitals are sure to be protected . . . this prophylactic measure cannot fail to blaze a trail for itself in private practice.*

How right he was: the introduction and acceptance of Credé's prophylaxis remains one of the greatest triumphs of preventive medicine.

Selected Publications

Credé CSF. Handgriff zur Entfernung der Placenta. *Klin Vortr Geburtshülfe* 1854; 599–603.

Credé CSF. *Monatschr Geburtshülfe* 1861; 17: 274.

Credé CSF. Die Verhürtung der Augenentzündung der Neugeborenen. *Arch Gynäkol* 1881; 17: 50–3.

Bibliography References

476, 542, 648, 1145, 1146, 1328, 1408, 1478, 1480, 1595.

Cullen, Thomas Stephen (1868–1953)

Cullen's Sign

Thomas Cullen first noted the sign that was to bear his name in the spring of 1918. He reported it briefly in the *American Journal of Obstetrics and Diseases of Woman and Children* and later expanded this report in *Contributions to Medical and Biological Research,* which was dedicated to Sir William Osler on the occasion of his seventieth birthday on 12 July 1919. The report began in graphic terms:

> *On March 21 1918, there entered the Church Home and Infirmary a thin, wiry woman (CHI. No. 18744) who looked to be nearly sixty years of age, but who was actually only thirty-eight. She was the mother of seven children. For three weeks she had pain in the right lower abdomen with intermittent attacks of abdominal distension. One week after the onset of the trouble the umbilical region suddenly became bluish black (Plate), although there had been no injury whatever in this region.*

Cullen's extensive knowledge of the literature recalled a case report by Joseph Ransohoff of Cincinnati in which there was jaundice of the umbilicus associated

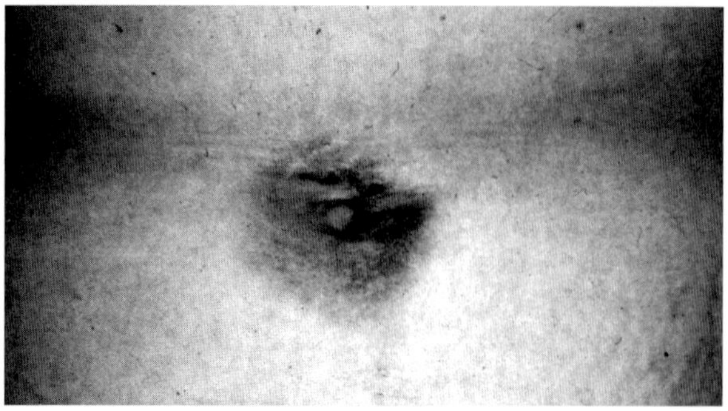

Cullen's sign: the umbilical 'black eye'

with a ruptured common bile duct with free bile in the peritoneal cavity. Cullen therefore reasoned:

> *The bluish black appearance of the navel unassociated with any history of injury, together with the mass to the right of the uterus, makes the diagnosis of extrauterine pregnancy relatively certain, although the patient has not missed any period and although there has been no uterine bleeding.*

These findings were confirmed at laparotomy with a right tubal pregnancy and extensive haemoperitoneum. The paper was accompanied by a watercolour plate of the umbilicus by Max Brödel (1870–1941), the famous medical artist, whom Cullen was responsible for bringing to Johns Hopkins to establish the first department of medical illustration.

Cullen noted a diminution in the discolouration after operation and its disappearance within a few days. The sign is sometimes referred to as the 'umbilical black eye' as depicted by Cullen:

> *The gradual change in color that took place in the umbilical region reminded one strikingly of the changes in color that occur in a black eye resulting from a blow.*

Thomas Stephen Cullen was born in Bridgewater, Ontario, the son of a Methodist minister. His grandparents on his mother's side came from Cornwall and on his father's side were of Ulster-Scots descent from County Fermanagh, Northern Ireland. He graduated in medicine from the University of Toronto in 1890. After his internship at the Toronto General Hospital, he moved to Baltimore and Johns Hopkins Hospital. For the first four years he worked with William Welch (1850–1934) and helped establish the discipline of gynaecological pathology. He spent 1893 visiting the major pathology centres in Europe.

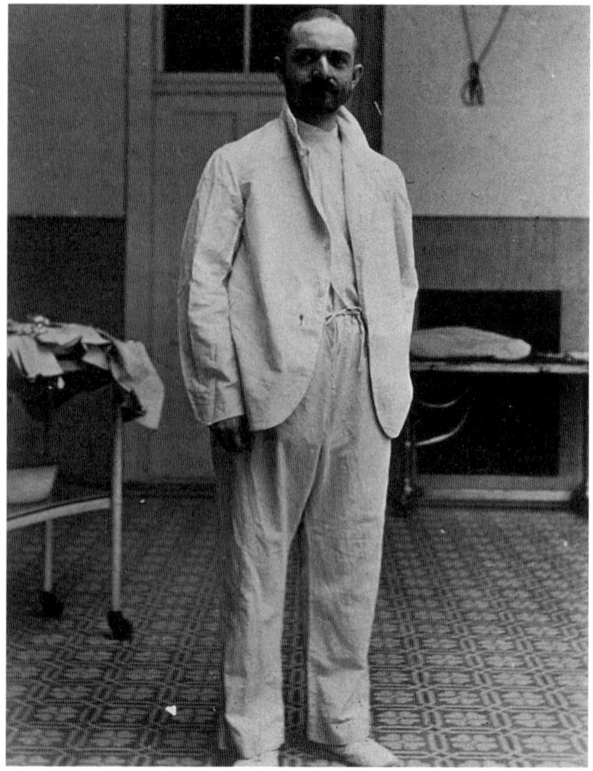

Thomas Stephen Cullen

He then worked as a resident in gynaecology with Howard Kelly and remained as his assistant. Cullen was a prodigious investigator and writer. His first book, *Cancer of the Uterus,* was published in 1900 and included the first description of endometrial hyperplasia. He also wrote a 680-page treatise on *The Embryology, Anatomy and Diseases of the Umbilicus.* It is ironic that the paper describing the sign for which his name is remembered was one and a half pages long.

In 1919 Cullen followed Kelly as professor of clinical gynaecology at Johns Hopkins. At that time gynaecology and obstetrics were separate departments. In 1932 he was appointed professor of gynaecology and held this position until he retired in 1939 at the age of 70. He married twice; his first wife died 18 years after marriage. There were no children. He died at the age of 85 on 4 March 1953, four days after a stroke.

Selected Publications

Cullen TS. A new sign in ruptured extra-uterine pregnancy. *Am J Obstet Dis Women Child* 1918; 78: 457.

Cullen TS. Bluish discolouration of the umbilicus as a diagnostic sign when ruptured extrauterine pregnancy exists. In: *Contributions to Medical and Biological Research*. New York, NY: Hoeber; 1919.

Ransohoff J. Gangrene of the gall bladder: Rupture of the common bile duct with new sign. *JAMA* 1906; 46: 395–7.

Bibliography References

77, 91, 121, 198, 269, 552, 648, 695, 780, 1040, 1311, 1314, 1480, 1485, 1488, 1568, 1569, 1738.

Culpeper, Nicholas (1616–1654)

English Midwifery Text

In the first half of the seventeenth century most of the medical texts in Britain were published in Latin. In his short life of 37 years, Nicholas Culpeper wrote or translated 79 books, several of which were published after his death. As a result, he made available a broad medical literature for the apothecaries, barber-surgeons and physicians in England who did not have a classical education. In addition, Culpeper wrote books aimed at the lay public. His unauthorised translation, in 1651, of the Latin *Pharmacopoeia Londinensis* to the *London Dispensator* in English earned him the strong disapproval of the College of Physicians in London. He responded in kind, 'They cry out against me for writing in my mother tongue, they bring, no other arguments than what the papists bring for themselves. One holds the word of God, the other physick to be a mystery, and the vulgar must be ignorant in both'. His most famous work was his herbal, *The English Physitian*, first published in 1652 and produced in more than 100 editions in several countries before and after his death.

In 1651 he published *A Directory for Midwives: or A Guide for Women* which was one of the earliest books on obstetrics in the English language. Culpeper's experience as an accoucher was limited, and he concentrated on anatomy, physiology and preventive medicine in this text rather than the manual skills required in abnormal labour and delivery: 'I have not meddled with your callings nor manual operations, lest I should discover my ignorance'. He was one of the first to postulate that the ovaries produced an egg that combined with the male seed to form the embryo. At this time the general belief was that the woman's contribution was more passive and that the embryo was formed entirely from the male seed. The book finished with a section 'Of Nursing Children', which at the time exhibited an advanced level of common sense:

> *No part of medicine is of more general importance than that which relates to nursing and management of children. Yet few parents pay proper attention to it. They leave their tender offspring in the sole care of nurses, who are either too negligent to do their duty or too ignorant to know it. I venture to affirm that more human lives are lost by the carelessness and inattention of parents and nurses than are saved by physicians. A sensible lady therefore should read a medical treatise which will instruct her in the management of her children. A little medical knowledge about cleanliness and care can do more good than many costly potions from the apothecary.*

Nicholas Culpeper, Gent, as he signed himself, was born on 18 October 1616 to an upper-class family in London. His father, who died before he was born, was a clergyman and his grandfather a knight and baronet, Sir Thomas Culpeper. He was brought up by his widowed mother with the help of her clergyman father. He received a good education in the classics and attended Cambridge University for some time but did not graduate. Against his family's wishes, he did not study for the Church

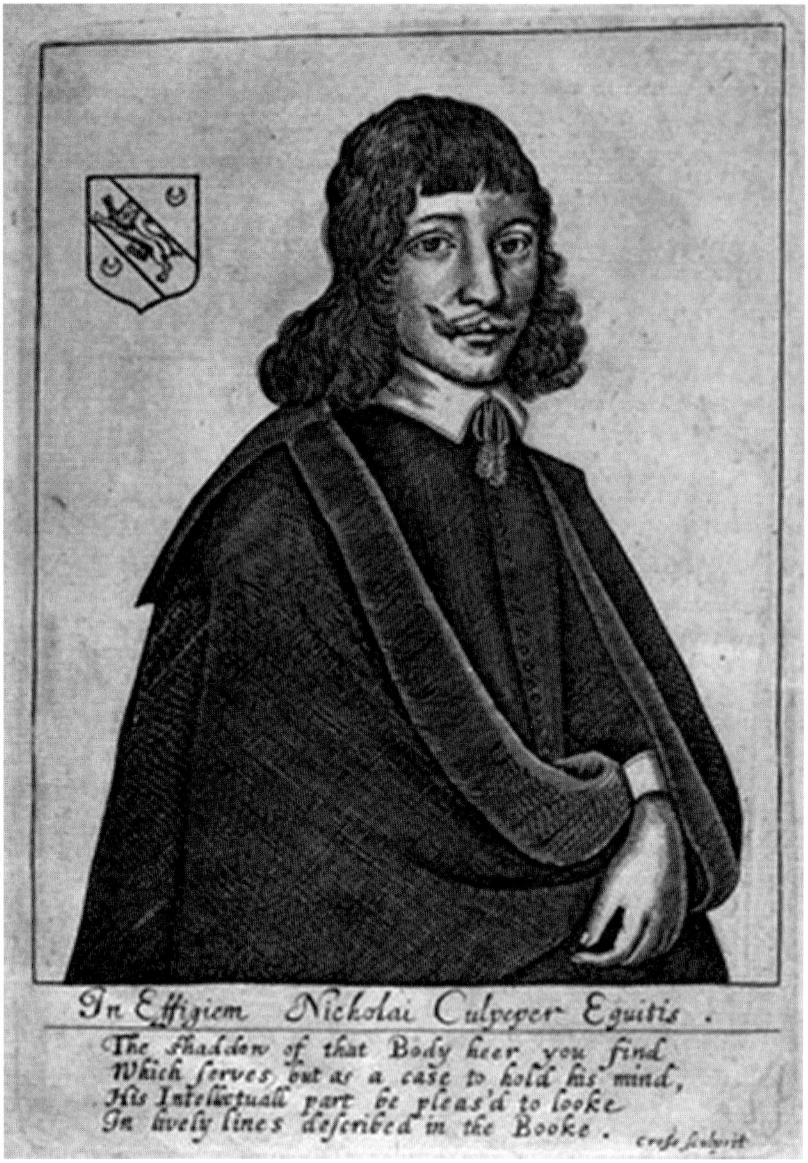
In Effigiem Nicholai Culpeper Equitis.
The shaddow of that Body heer you find
Which serves but as a case to hold his mind,
His Intellectuall part be pleas'd to looke
In lively lines describ'd in the Booke.

Nicholas Culpeper

of England ministry and at the age of 18 was apprenticed to a London apothecary. He ultimately served apprenticeships with two other London apothecaries but never achieved membership in the Society of Apothecaries. At odds with both physicians and apothecaries, Culpeper developed a thriving practice and provided herbal cures for conditions he diagnosed mainly by astrological means. On the title page of his book he described himself as 'Student in Physick and Astrologie'.

Despite his often sensible advice for pregnancy and child rearing, he and his wife, whom he married when she was 15, had seven children with only one surviving to adulthood. Culpeper's views on fertility

Title page of Culpeper's *A Directory for Midwives*

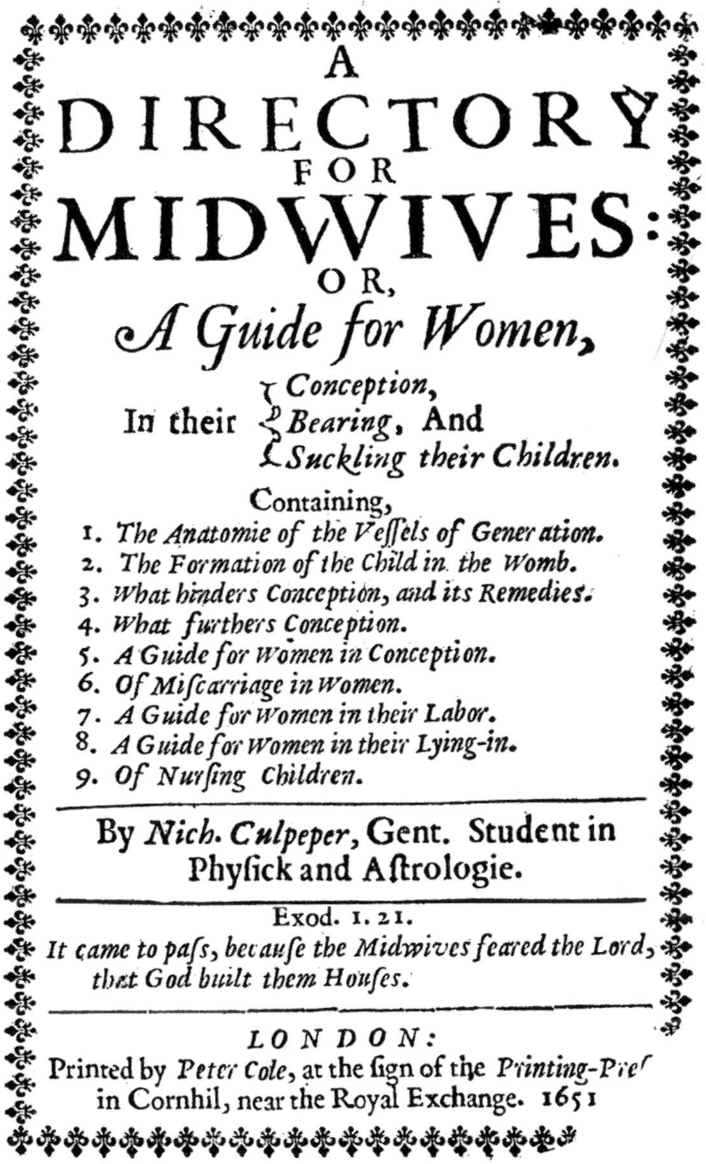

A
DIRECTORY
FOR
MIDWIVES:
OR,
A Guide for Women,
In their { *Conception,* *Bearing,* And *Suckling their Children.*
Containing,
1. *The Anatomie of the Veſſels of Generation.*
2. *The Formation of the Child in the Womb.*
3. *What hinders Conception, and its Remedies.*
4. *What furthers Conception.*
5. *A Guide for Women in Conception.*
6. *Of Miſcarriage in Women.*
7. *A Guide for Women in their Labor.*
8. *A Guide for Women in their Lying-in.*
9. *Of Nurſing Children.*

By *Nich. Culpeper*, Gent. Student in Phyſick and Aſtrologie.

Exod. 1. 21.
It came to paſs, becauſe the Midwives feared the Lord, that God built them Houſes.

LONDON:
Printed by *Peter Cole*, at the ſign of the *Printing-Preſ* in Cornhil, near the Royal Exchange. 1651

were at odds with the ecclesiastical approach: 'Lust is the cause of begetting more children than the desire of the blessings of God'. His prolific publication rate secured him a comfortable living. However, over the last 10 years of his life, his health deteriorated, probably due to tuberculosis that was not helped by his tobacco-smoking habit. He died on 10 January 1654 and was buried in the new church yard of Bethlehem in London, an annex to the cemetery of Bedlam Mental Hospital.

The true character of Culpeper is hard to determine some three and a half centuries distant. He is regarded by some historians as a charlatan and 'quacksalver' and by others as an enlightened anti-establishment figure who, through his translation of the European medical authors of the day, brought this valuable medical literature to English doctors and patients in their own language.

Selected Publications

Culpeper N. *Directory for Midwives: or A Guide for Women in their Conception, Bearing, and Suckling their Children.* London: Peter Cole; 1651.

Culpeper N. *The English Physitian: or An Astrologo-Physical Discourse of the Vulgar Herbs of this Nation.* London: Peter Cole; 1652.

Bibliography References

158, 1010, 1249, 1612, 1613, 1617, 1655, 1723.

Curtis, Arthur Hale (1881–1955) Fitz-Hugh, Thomas (1894–1963)

Curtis–Fitz-Hugh Syndrome

In 1930 Arthur Curtis reported the 'not uncommon' finding at laparotomy of 'violin-string adhesions between the anterior surface of the liver and the anterior abdominal wall'. He noted:

> *I wish particularly to emphasise the location and the character of these adhesions . . . anterior liver surface to anterior abdominal wall adhesions usually occupy an area several inches in diameter, are ordinarily numerous, and are usually of sufficient length to allow considerable play between the liver and the parietal peritoneum. I have been impressed with the frequency with which we encounter evidence of gonorrheal disease of the tubes in patients with adhesions of this character; salpingitis is so frequently coexistent that we anticipate tubal disease as soon as the palpating hand reveals characteristic bands on exploration of the anterior surface of the liver.*

Curtis finished his paper with the statement, 'The female patients with symptoms suggestive of gallbladder disease or pleurisy may be suffering liver-abdominal wall adhesions complicating a pelvic gonorrhoeal infection'. Four years later, Thomas Fitz-Hugh described three cases presenting with pain in the right hypochondrium, which he attributed to acute gonococcal peritonitis and postulated this as the forerunner of the violin-string adhesions previously described by Curtis:

> *The following three cases, encountered within the past six months in the practice of an internist would seem to represent incidences of the hitherto undescribed acute and early manifestations of gonococcal peritonitis of the right upper quadrant. They would seem to complete the picture of the condition previously described in the end stage by Curtis.*

Fitz-Hugh described one of the physical signs thus: 'a crunching to and fro type of friction rub may be readily heard just over this area of the abdominal wall, at least during the subsiding stage of the acute process'. In one case he likened this friction rub to 'the crunching of new snow'.

In fact, the condition had previously been described in the Spanish literature by Carlos Stajano (1891–1976), professor of surgery in Montevideo.

Arthur Hale Curtis was born in Portage, Wisconsin and took his undergraduate science degree from the University of Wisconsin in 1902. He was a good athlete and captained both the university football and baseball teams. He later acted as head football coach at both the Universities of Kansas and Wisconsin. He graduated MD in 1905 from Rush Medical College, Chicago. Curtis served overseas as a medical officer in the US army during the First World War. He took his post graduate training in obstetrics and gynaecology at Cook County Hospital, Chicago and in Berlin and Vienna. He then entered private practice in Chicago with Thomas Watkins. He rose through the academic ranks of the department of obstetrics and gynaecology at Northwestern University Medical School and became professor and chairman in 1929. He was president of the American Gynecological Society in 1927. Arthur Hale Curtis died after a sudden heart attack on 13 November 1955.

Thomas Fitz-Hugh was born in Baltimore but grew up in Charlottesville, Virginia, where his father was professor of Latin. He enlisted as a private in the US army during the First World War and served at the base hospital at Saint Denis, France. He returned to the study of medicine and graduated MD from the University of Pennsylvania in 1921. He became chief of the haematology section there in 1929 and retired in 1955. Thomas Fitz-Hugh died of lung cancer on 26 September 1963.

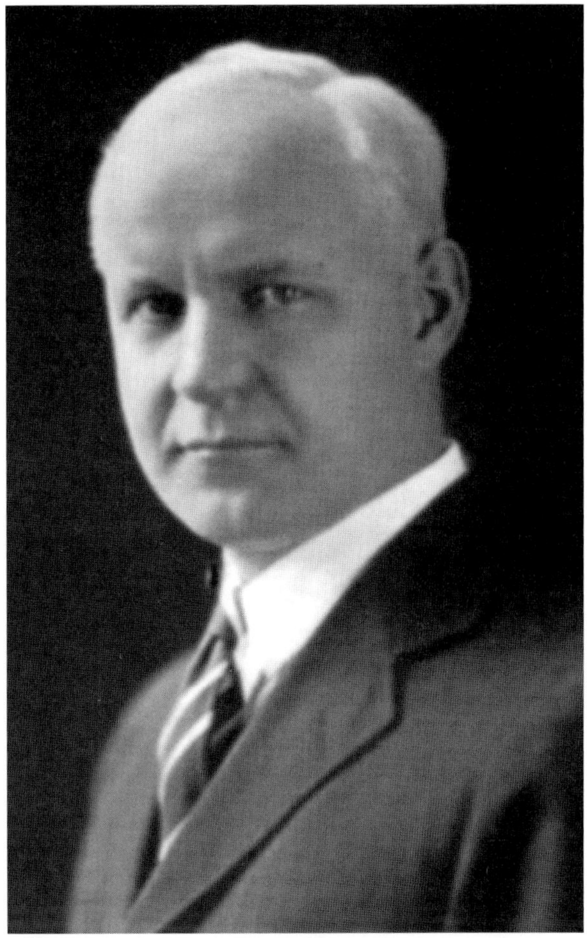

Arthur Hale Curtis

Selected Publications

Curtis AH. A cause of adhesions in the right upper quadrant. *JAMA* 1930; 94: 1221–2.

Curtis AH. Adhesions of the anterior surface of the liver. *JAMA* 1932; 99: 2010–12.

Fitz-Hugh T. Acute gonococcic peritonitis of the right upper quadrant. *JAMA* 1934; 102: 2094–6.

Stanjano C. La reaction frenica en ginecologia. *Sem Med Buenos Aires* 1920; 27: 243–8.

Bibliography References

342, 343, 646, 801, 1326, 1480, 1485.

Cyprianus, Abraham (1655/1660–1718)

Abdominal Pregnancy

Abraham Cyprianus, a surgeon in Amsterdam, was sent for consultation in nearby Leeuwarden where a 32-year-old woman was suffering abdominal pain in the twentieth month of her third pregnancy: 'When the time of parturition had come, she suffered severe pain, while other signs of childbirth were lacking . . . At last all hope for a normal delivery vanished when the movements of the foetus ceased . . .'. A month after term the woman developed abdominal pain and started to menstruate. Cyprianus was consulted 11 months after term. By this stage the patient had continuous abdominal pain and had developed a 'fungeus ulcer' near her umbilicus. Cyprianus summarised the case:

> *After I had examined the patient and all other circumstances . . . I didn't doubt to declare that the child was dead . . . when I pushed the abdomen with both hands I discovered a large solid tumour . . . This solid tumour was also felt near the fungeus ulcer, in which easily a stiletto was introduced besides I bumped on something hard. After I had widened the ulcer so far that I could introduce my little finger, I had no further doubt that I could feel and reach the parietal bone of the fetus. Based on these findings, I became less fearless and declared, that the foetus was in the right fallopian tube, and I pointed out to the woman, that the only hope of a good outcome was to perform a caesarean section, and if she would consent to such a procedure, otherwise, a miserable death would become her part.*

The woman, who was not eating and in constant pain, readily agreed. Cyprianus made his incision with the umbilical ulcer as the starting point and 'extended the incision on both sides to the length of a foot and after I had shoved away the intestines with my left hand . . . I extracted the child without any difficulty'. The placenta was 'thin and mostly decomposed and was attached to the fallopian tube, as I discovered later when I prized it off with my finger'. Cyprianus demonstrated an otherwise normal uterus,

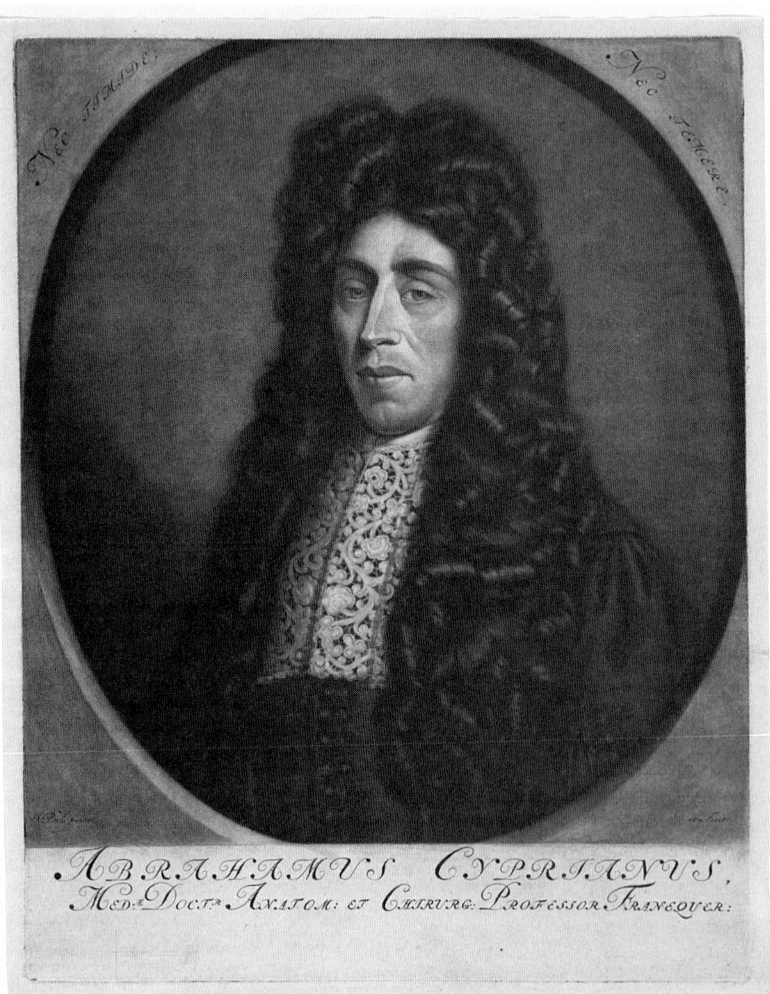
Nec TIMIDE,
Nec TEMERE.
ABRAHAMVS CYPRIANVS,
MED: DOCT.R ANATOM: ET CHIRURG: PROFESSOR FRANEQUER:

Abraham Cyprianus

left ovary and left fallopian tube to the spectators. The infant he extracted was preserved in 'liquor balsamicus' and was apparently 'a girl of normal length . . . without any putrefaction'. He used four sutures to close the abdomen taking the 'skin, muscles and peritoneum at the same time'. The patient's recovery was satisfactory, in part, in Cyprianus' opinion, because 'the patient had gone along with everything and was very obedient'. So swift was her recovery that 'in the third month after the operation, on 17 March 1695 she was able to come out of her bed'. She was to have two subsequent pregnancies, both born normally, one of which was a twin pregnancy.

Abraham Cyprianus was born between 1655 and 1660 in Amsterdam. His father was a surgeon in Leeuwarden. Abraham obtained his surgical qualification at the Surgeon's Guild of Amsterdam in July 1680. He also studied medicine and obtained his MD from the University of Utrecht in the same year. His surgical practice in Amsterdam mainly consisted of the treatment of bladder stones, and he was such an expert that he was known as 'lithotomus expertissimus'. In 1693 he was appointed professor of medicine at the University of Fraenker. He died on 16 April 1718 in Amsterdam.

Selected Publications

Cyprianus A. *Epistola historiam exhibiens foetus humani post XXI, menses ex uteri tuba, matre salva ac superstiete excisi.* Lugduni Batavorum: Jordanum Luchtmans; 1700.

Bibliography References

727, 851, 1097.

D

Dale, Henry Hallett (1875–1968)

Posterior Pituitary Extract

Henry Dale was, along with Joseph Barcroft, the pre-eminent British research worker in physiology during the first half of the twentieth century. He is known mainly for his physiological studies that led to advances in clinical medicine. In 1938 he was awarded, with Otto Loewi, the Nobel Prize for developing the theory of combined electrical and chemical transmission of nerve impulses.

In obstetrics his legacy is in the application of posterior pituitary extract and ergot to clinical practice. He was the first to describe the oxytocic effect of posterior pituitary extract in animals in 1906. Following this observation, he gave some of the extract to William Blair-Bell, who reported similar effects in the human. The initial work of Dale would lead to subsequent investigators discovering oxytocin, its structure and its synthesis. It was in Dale's laboratory that Harold Dudley, working in conjunction with Chassar Moir, discovered the active oxytocic alkaloid in ergot: ergometrine. Dale gave much guidance in the laboratory aspect of this work and suggested the name ergometrine. He also decided, in view of the life-saving potential of ergometrine, that no proprietary interest should be sought, and its chemical structure and method of preparation was made immediately available.

Henry Dale was educated at Trinity College, Cambridge and qualified in medicine at St Bartholomew's Hospital, London in 1903. He immediately embarked upon his life-long career of research in physiology. He served as director of the Wellcome Physiological Research Laboratories at Herne Hill for 10 years and was then appointed the first director of the National Institute for Medical Research. He was one of the most distinguished and best loved men of science and received multiple honours, including a knighthood and that most exclusive of British honours, the Order of Merit. He died on 23 July 1968 at the age of 93, 'both venerated and venerable'.

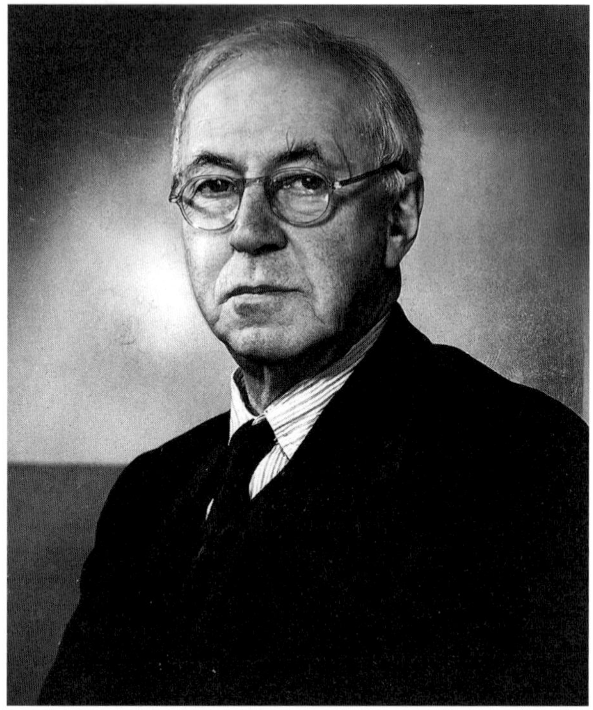

Henry Hallett Dale

Selected Publications

Dale HH. On some physiological actions of ergot. *J Physiol* 1906; 34: 163–97.

Dale HH. The action of extracts of the pituitary body. *Biochem J* 1909; 4: 427–47.

Bibliography References

94, 354, 355, 363, 528, 590, 703, 955, 1031, 1129, 1130, 1338, 1417, 1556, 1644.

Dawes, Geoffrey Sharman (1918–1996)

Fetal Physiology

Geoffrey Dawes was born in Mackworth, Derbyshire, a son of the manse, on 21 January 1918. He attended Oxford University and qualified in medicine in 1943. He immediately began a life of research, starting in the Department of Physiology at Oxford. This was followed with a Rockefeller Traveling Fellowship to the United States in 1946. He returned to Oxford in 1947 as a demonstrator in pharmacology and was also awarded a Foulerton Research Fellowship of the Royal Society.

At the age of 30, Dawes was appointed director of the Nuffield Institute for Medical Research in Oxford. Originally the Institute was situated in the old astronomical observatory designed by Christopher Wren in the seventeenth century. Later the Institute moved to the outskirts of Oxford, alongside the obstetrical and neonatal units of the Radcliffe Hospital. Dawes developed a first-rate laboratory of experimental physiology and, following along the work of Joseph Barcroft, studied the fetal and neonatal mammal, mostly with sheep, concentrating on the preparation of mechanisms for adaptation to extrauterine life. In 1967, during a sabbatical in San Francisco he wrote his classic text, *Foetal and Neonatal Physiology*, published in 1968. He wrote in the preface:

> *The main theme of this book is the development in the foetus and newborn of the integrated responses which are needed to conserve their energy supply for maintenance of their internal environment, growth and development.*

Dawes attracted many visiting fellows from all over the world who spent one to two years in his laboratory. Many of these were clinical perinatologists and neonatologists who later established significant research careers. Dawes also had a whimsical turn of phrase and once described the foetus in the following manner:

> *The human foetus has been likened to a spaceman; passive, insulated and preserved from stimuli, which is only half the truth. On the contrary one could think of the mammalian embryo as a hitch-hiker with a large pack on his back getting into a rather small car; he is a friendly fellow who chatters away all the time and is prepared to do some driving if given half a chance – he takes you off your route and tells when and where he would like to get out.*

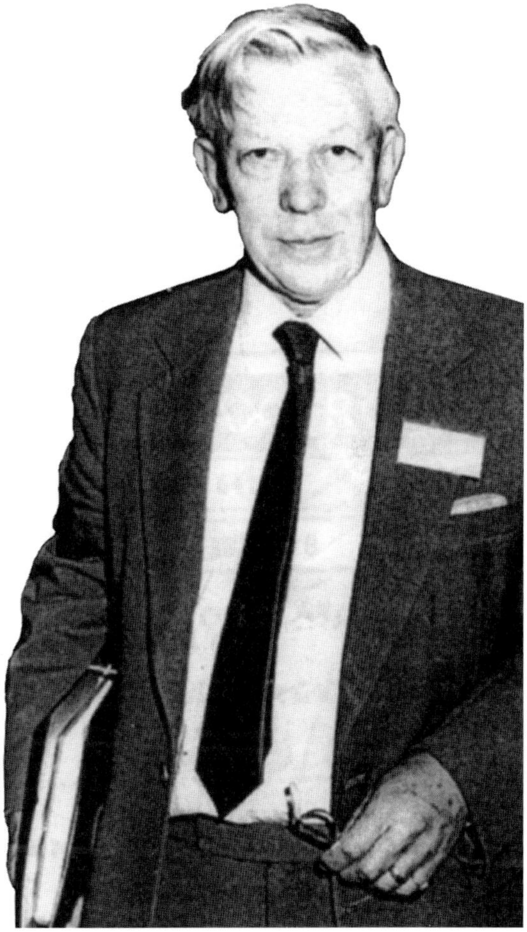

Geoffrey Sharman Dawes

Dawes retired from the Nuffield Institute in 1985 but remained active and was soon appointed director of the Sunley Research Centre at Charing Cross Hospital. He directed much attention in his later years to the analysis of human fetal heart rate patterns. He helped develop systems to apply computer technology to this analysis. As well as his research work, in his retirement he enjoyed his lifelong pursuits of gardening and fly-fishing. He suffered from asthma his whole life but was active until his death on 6 May 1996.

Selected Publications

Dawes GS. *Foetal and Neonatal Physiology*. Chicago, IL: Yearbook Medical Publishers Inc; 1968.

Dawes GS. Foetal autonomy. In: Wolstenholme GE, O'Connor M (eds) *Ciba Foundation Symposium*. London: J&A Churchill Limited; 1969, p. 316.

Bibliography References

370, 371, 688, 903, 1202, 1215.

DeLee, Joseph Bolivar (1869–1942)

Prophylactic Forceps Delivery

In his famous paper on the prophylactic forceps operation, first read before the American Gynecological Society in Chicago on 24 May 1920, DeLee advocated elective low forceps delivery in all labours. His routine included morphine, scopolamine and other sedatives in the first stage of labour, and ether anaesthesia and forceps delivery in the second stage, combined with a wide medio-lateral episiotomy and manual removal of the placenta. He justified this approach by claiming that childbirth was a pathological rather than a physiological process. He stated, 'I have often wondered whether nature did not deliberately intend women should be used up in the process of reproduction, in a manner analogous to that of the salmon, which dies after spawning'.

He defended the early use of forceps as follows:

> *One may well ask himself whether the short, and moderate in amount, compression of the head in a skilfully performed forceps operation is not less dangerous to the integrity of the brain than the prolonged pounding and congestion it suffers from a hard spontaneous delivery.*

DeLee correctly anticipated criticism for his recommendations and in his paper made the rather contradictory statement:

> *It is not a complete reversal of watchful expectancy that is universally taught but I cannot deny that it interferes with nature's process. Were not the results I have achieved so gratifying, I myself would call it meddlesome midwifery. For unskilled hands it is unjustifiable.*

DeLee believed that compression of the fetal head on the perineum in normal labour could cause brain damage and rationalised this by claiming, 'not the firstborn, but the children of subsequent labours, were the people who moved the world'.

DeLee was one of the first to report a fatal case of haemorrhage associated with abruptio placentae and postulate the association with a haemorrhagic diathesis, later known as disseminated intravascular coagulation:

> *Is there such a disease as acquired haemophilia? . . . I believe there is such an affliction as a temporary haemophilia, but the demonstration of the same, I admit, presents no little difficulty.*

Perhaps the first such observation was in 1771, when William Hewson of the British Lying-in Hospital in London observed a woman with bleeding that failed to clot. He concluded that the patient's blood was probably 'without the coagulable lymph'.

In the 1920s the early use of posterior pituitary extract – the forerunner of oxytocin, but of variable purity and potency – was associated with fatal cases of uterine rupture. DeLee addressed the American Gynecological Society with a scathing condemnation of its use before delivery. With his usual dramatic flair, he held a ruptured uterus in one hand and a dead fetus in the other, declaring, 'It biteth like the adder, it stingeth like the asp'. This quote, Proverbs 23:32 was, in the Bible, a cautionary note about alcohol which, ironically, would later be used in attempts to inhibit uterine contractions.

Joseph Bolivar DeLee was the ninth of 10 children born in New York's Lower East Side to a Polish-Jewish immigrant family of modest means. His grandfather was a surgeon in Napoleon's army. At six years of age he was rescued by his oldest brother when their house was destroyed by fire. His father hoped he would become a rabbi, but his dominant mother supported his quest to study medicine. He enrolled in the Chicago Medical College, forerunner of Northwestern University Medical School, graduating in 1891.

He financed his studies by installing door bells and working in a drugstore. As a student he also worked as a medical attendant at a home for illegitimate and unwanted infants. Many of these died, and DeLee performed the autopsies. He was struck by the frequent finding of cerebral haemorrhage, which led him to regard labour and delivery as pathological. In retrospect, in such an environment, it is possible that the haemorrhage was incurred post-partum rather than intra-partum.

His postgraduate education included hospital work at Cook County Hospital, Chicago and a study tour of centres in Berlin, Vienna and Paris, after which DeLee returned to Chicago and the practice of obstetrics. He was moved by the plight of the poor, and after persistently seeking philanthropic aid, he founded the Chicago Lying-in Dispensary in 1895. Under his supervision this institution provided obstetric care for the poor and clinical instruction for students. It later evolved into the Chicago Lying-in Hospital. DeLee became professor of obstetrics at Northwestern University and was one of the most influential of American obstetricians. He designed many instruments, including the widely used DeLee obstetric forceps. His popular text, *The Principles and Practice of Obstetrics,* went through seven editions in his lifetime. He appeared on the cover of *Time* magazine in 1936.

DeLee was obsessional, arrogant and autocratic. On his ward rounds he would scrutinise the charts of other physician's patients and write 'RO' (rotten obstetrics) when he disagreed with their management. He never married and had few friends, devoting himself totally to his work and his personal mission against maternal mortality and infant brain damage. He was vehemently opposed to midwives. DeLee kept a daily diary for 46 years, from which emerges an inherently insecure and unhappy man, plagued by recurrent depression and minor illness. Once asked to give his advice to young doctors, he said, 'If he selects obstetrics as his field of work, he must be prepared to sacrifice time, comfort, convenience and sometimes health for his ideal'. To a large extent DeLee himself lived this ideal, albeit in a rigid, and on occasions, misguided way. Perhaps he suffered for it. On his study wall hung a sign: 'In case of fire, save my books'.

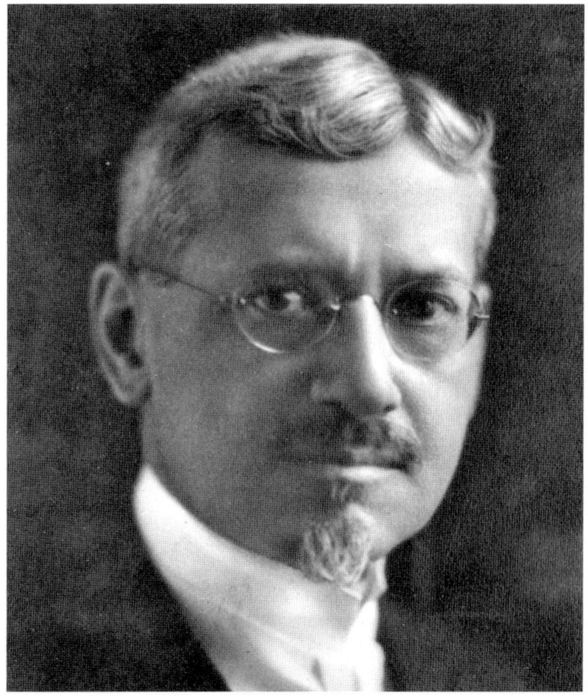

Joseph Bolivar DeLee

Selected Publications

Hewson W. *An Experimental Inquiry into the Properties of the Blood, with Remarks on Some of Its Morbid Appearances*. London: Cadell;1771. (In: Gulliver G., ed., The Works of William Hewson, FRCS. Sydenham Society, London: 1846).

DeLee JB. A case of fatal haemorrhagic diathesis, with premature detachment of the placenta. *Am J Obstet Dis Women Child* 1901; 44: 785–92.

DeLee JB. The prophylactic forceps operation. *Trans Am Gynecol Soc* 1920; 45: 72–6.

DeLee JB. The prophylactic forceps operation. *Am J Obstet Gynecol* 1921;1: 34–44.

Bibliography References

32, 99, 102, 358, 379, 380, 556, 637, 648, 721, 777, 793, 879, 880, 987, 1059, 1205, 1333, 1734.

Denman, Thomas (1733–1815)

Denman's Aphorisms/Denman's Law/Spontaneous Evolution

There are four possible outcomes with a shoulder presentation in labour: 1) spontaneous version to a longitudinal lie if the membranes are intact, 2) total obstruction with uterine exhaustion or rupture, 3) vaginal delivery of a small fetus with the body doubled up *partus conduplicato corpore*, or 4) spontaneous evolution, in which the shoulder becomes impacted behind the symphysis and the trunk, breech and limbs are driven past, followed by the shoulders and head.

The first to describe spontaneous evolution was Thomas Denman. Between 1772 and 1774 he observed three cases in term infants of 'usual size'. He reported these in 1784. In all three cases attempts at internal version had failed:

> *In the year 1772, I was called to a poor woman in Oxford-street . . . I found the arm much swelled and pushed through the external parts in such a manner, that the shoulder nearly reached the perinaeum. The women struggled vehemently with her pains, and during their continuance, I perceived the shoulder of the child to descend . . . I remained at the bed-side till the child was expelled, and I was very much surprised to find, that the*

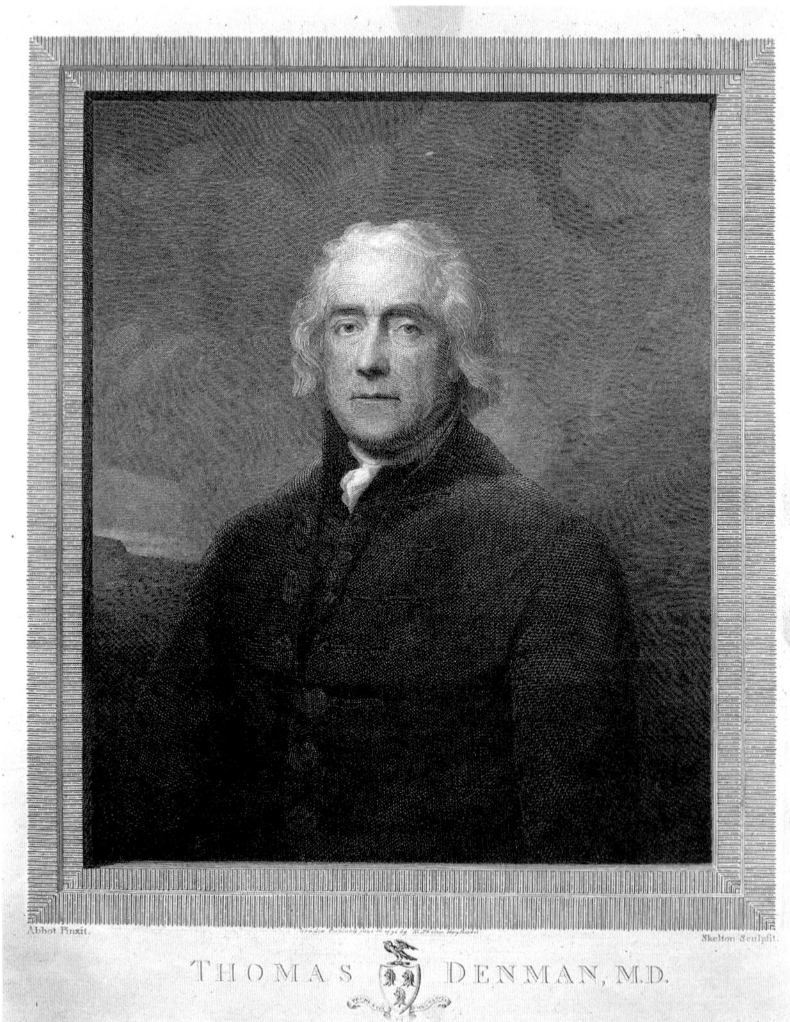

Thomas Denman

> *breech and inferior extremities were expelled before the head, as if the case had originally been a presentation of the inferior extremities ...*

Thomas Denman, the son of an apothecary, was born in the village of Bakewell, England. He began the study of medicine at St George's Hospital, London. However, running out of money, he joined the navy as a ship's mate and surgeon. He spent nine years at sea, much of it on fighting ships. He returned to England in 1763 and, after attending further lectures, obtained his medical degree from Aberdeen University. He set up practice in Haymarket Square, London and concentrated on the study of midwifery. In 1769 he was appointed physician man-midwife to the Middlesex Hospital. His stature increased as he lectured on midwifery, and after the death of William Hunter, he became the leading obstetric teacher in London. Denman was a very conservative practitioner of the art of obstetrics, as summed up in his philosophy: 'The abuse of art produces more and greater evil than are occasioned by all the imperfections of Nature'. In particular he was against the excessive use of forceps. He developed a guiding rule that came to be known as 'Denman's Law':

> *A practical rule has been formed, that the head of the child shall have rested for six hours, as low as the perineum, that is, in a situation which would allow of their application, before the forceps are applied, though the pains should have altogether ceased during that time.*

However, Denham also advised against excessive conservatism:

> *Care is also to be taken that we do not, through an aversion to the use of instruments, too long delay that assistance we have the power of affording them.*

Denham developed a number of aphorisms which he published as an appendix to his text. These were brief, single sentence instructions, and 50 of them, including the above, applied to the use of forceps. Among these was the following:

> *The lower the head of the child has descended and the longer the use of the forceps is deferred, the easier will in general their application be, the success of the operation more certain, and the hazard of doing mischief less.*

Another of his aphorisms regarding forceps delivery still resonates:

> *In some cases, the mere excitement occasioned by the application of the forceps, or the very expectation of their being applied, will bring on a return or an increase of the pains sufficient to expel the child without their assistance.*

Denman's conservative obstetrics was passed down to his son-in-law Richard Croft, who joined him in practice. Later, Croft's very conservative management of Princess Charlotte's labour, in which he did not use forceps despite a low head many hours in the second stage, was criticised as contributing to both her and her infant's death in childbirth. Sir Richard Croft later shot himself.

Thomas Denman died on 25 November 1815.

Selected Publications

Denman T. Observations to prove that in cases where the upper extremities present, at the time of birth, the delivery may be effected by the spontaneous evolution of the child. *London Med J* 1784; 5: 64–70.

Denman T. *An Introduction to the Practice of Midwifery.* London: J. Johnson; 1795.

Denham T. *Aphorisms on the Application and Use of the Forceps and Vectis.* 2nd US edn. Newburyport, MA: Isiah Thomas; 1806.

Bibliography References

99, 263, 298, 463, 648, 676, 736, 980, 1407, 1495, 1714, 1728.

Denonvilliers, Charles Pierre (1808–1872)

Denonvilliers' Fascia

The rectovesical fascia in the male was described by Denonvilliers in 1836: he called it the 'rectovesical septum'. It was previously recorded by the British anatomist and surgeon, Frederick Tyrrell (1797–1843), working in St Thomas' Hospital, London and is also known as 'Tyrrell's fascia'. Tyrrell was a nephew of Astley Cooper and, as a student, shared lodgings with the poet John Keats at Guy's Hospital in 1815.

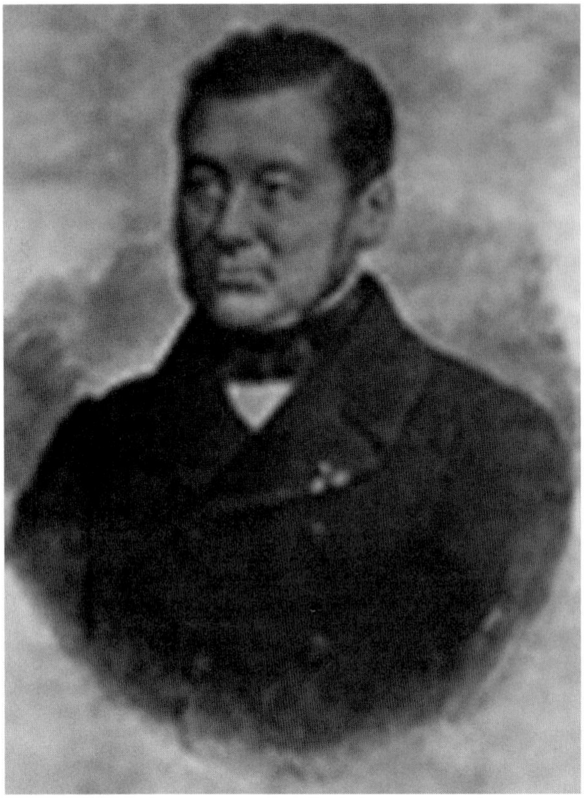

Charles Pierre Denonvilliers

The counterpart in the female is the rectovaginal septum, which represents the fusion of the walls of the fetal peritoneal pouch and extends from the pouch of Douglas to the perineal body. It is adherent to the posterior vaginal wall and not easily demonstrated as a separate layer. Indeed, some dispute its existence as an anatomical entity.

Charles Pierre Denonvilliers was born in Paris and graduated in medicine from the University of Paris in 1837. In 1842 he became chief of the school of practical anatomy and surgeon at the Hôtel Dieu. He had a special skill in plastic surgery and was appointed professor of surgery in 1856.

He was greatly saddened by his only son's death in 1864 and stopped all his public activities. He died following a stroke in 1872. At his memorial service, a close friend said Denonvilliers 'was dying for eight years'.

Selected Publications

Denonvilliers CP. Anatomie du perinée. *Bull Soc Anat* (Paris) 1836; 11: 105–7.

Tyrrell F. In: Cooper A. (ed.) *Lectures on Surgery with Additional Notes and Cases by F. Tyrrell.* (Vol. 1). London; 1824–27, p. 311.

Bibliography References

397, 406, 1294, 1616.

Deventer, Hendrik van (1651–1724)

Anatomy of the Pelvis

The belief that the symphysis pubis separated during labour to allow passage of the infant held sway from the time of Hippocrates. Although Vesalius had discounted the theory some 150 years before in his anatomical studies, this was not applied to clinical practice. Hendrik van Deventer was one of the first obstetricians to refute this dogma in his publication of 1701:

> *It does not seem to happen too often, and it is not a necessity: we cannot expect too much from it, and therefore we should not rely on too much help from that side.*

Deventer was the first to make a serious study of the pelvis and spinal deformities. As justification for his work and its publication, he noted:

> *It is absolutely necessary to have thorough knowledge of the pelvis; without this we would just be messing around, either with our brains or with our hands. The final result would be disastrous, and we would be unable to perform our duties properly.*

Hendrik van Deventer was born on 16 March 1651 in The Hague. He was initially an apprentice goldsmith but abandoned this for the study of medicine in Groningen, whence he received his MD in 1694. He returned to The Hague to practice obstetrics. His wife had 10 children and became a midwife. His work was published in Latin and later translated into French and English. He died in Voorburg on 12 December 1724.

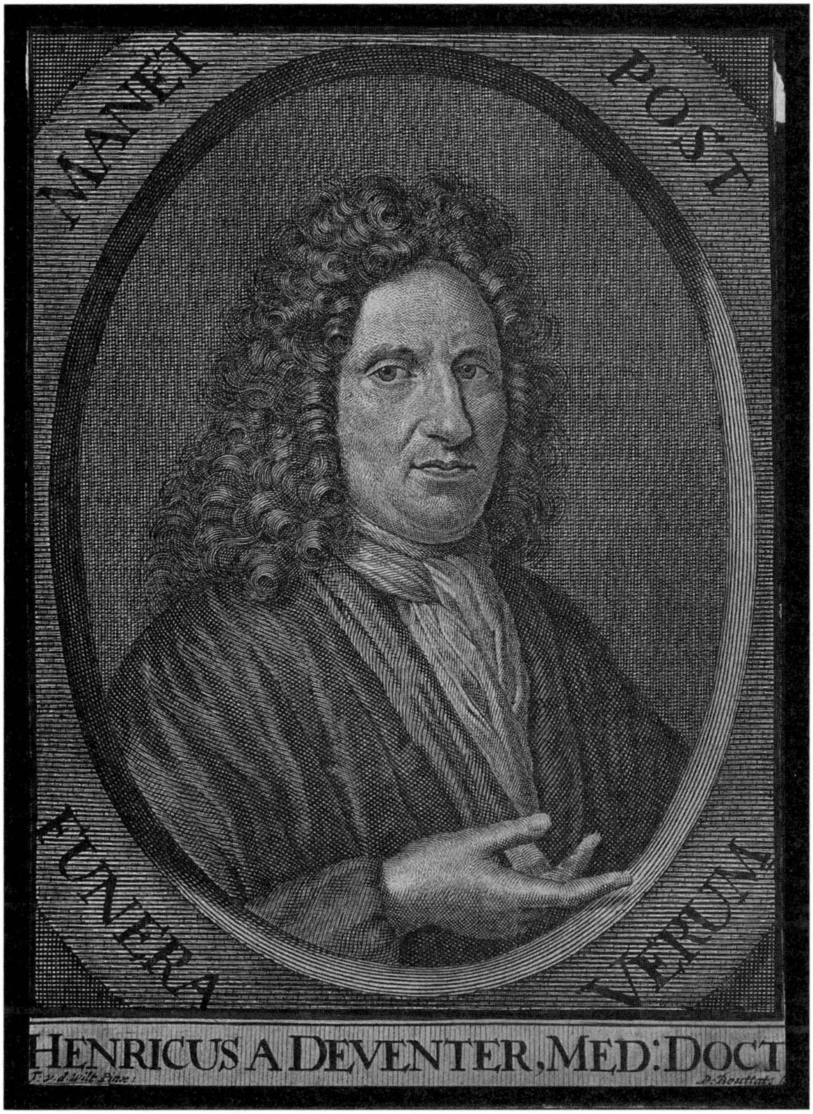

Hendrik van Deventer

Selected Publications

Deventer H von. *Operationes chirugicae novum lumen exhibentes obstetricantibus.* Lugduni Batavorum: Andream Dyckhuisen; 1701.

Deventer H von. *The Art of Midwifery Improved (English Translation)* London: Bettesworth; 1716. Also published in: The Classics of Obstetrics and Gynecology Library. New York, NY: Gryphon Editions; 1993 (facsimile).

Bibliography References

648, 721, 741, 1131, 1261, 1373, 1480, 1678, 1711.

Dickinson, Robert Latou (1861–1950)

Birth Control/Sex Education

Robert Latou Dickinson was born in Jersey City, New Jersey on 21 February 1861, the son of a hat manufacturer. His early education was at Brooklyn Polytechnic Institute followed by four years in Germany and Switzerland. He returned to the United States and graduated MD, first in his class, from Long Island College Hospital in 1882. There he studied under Alexander Skene. For almost 40 years he practised obstetrics and gynaecology in three Brooklyn hospitals: Long Island College Hospital, King's County Hospital and the Brooklyn Hospital. He served in the medical corps of the United States Army in 1919.

After the war he did little clinical practice and devoted himself to the physiological and social aspects of reproduction. Before it was fashionable, he supported a number of feminist causes, including sex education and birth control. The medical establishment did little to oppose the Comstock Law of 1873, which classified birth control information and contraceptive material as obscene and prohibited. Dickinson was one of the first to openly challenge and defy this law. He chastised those who maintained the 'hush and pretend' secret dogmas of sex as both 'non-compos mentis' and 'non-compos testis'. He organised and chaired the first report of the Committee on Maternal Health of New York which reviewed the state of contraception in 1924:

> *The data concerning contraception which can be brought together at this time are only sufficient to indicate on what lines research, clinical tests and records of effects should be undertaken. There is general recognition of the necessity of an inquiry – one that will be exempt from inclination to prove or disapprove any particular theory. The subject should be capable of handling as clean science, with dignity, decency and directness, but with due consideration of the danger that certain forms of publication may pander to pruriency and give safety to license. The medical profession is not yet cognizant of any guaranteed contraceptive. In the very large number of cases where contraception works securely as well as harmlessly and happily, we shall expect to find a choice rightly adapted to the particular couple, often with two measures combined or in sequence, and above all with attention to detail. It is our business to discover and define such conditions.*

In 1924 Dickinson published in the *American Journal of Obstetrics and Gynecology* a summary of the committee's findings and added detailed illustrations of the various contraceptive methods. In direct defiance of the Comstock Law, he mailed 3000 copies of this article to doctors across the country. It was in 1908, while Dickinson was still carrying on a busy clinical practice, that he began to promote his ideas of birth control and sex education within the medical profession:

> *In all marriages whatever, except a marriage where both partners are ascetic, sterile or impotent, birth control and the mechanism of love loom large as techniques of happiness. Honoring all honorable acts of love means teaching them. Herein nature is no better guide than other works of art. No act of life is without a technique of*

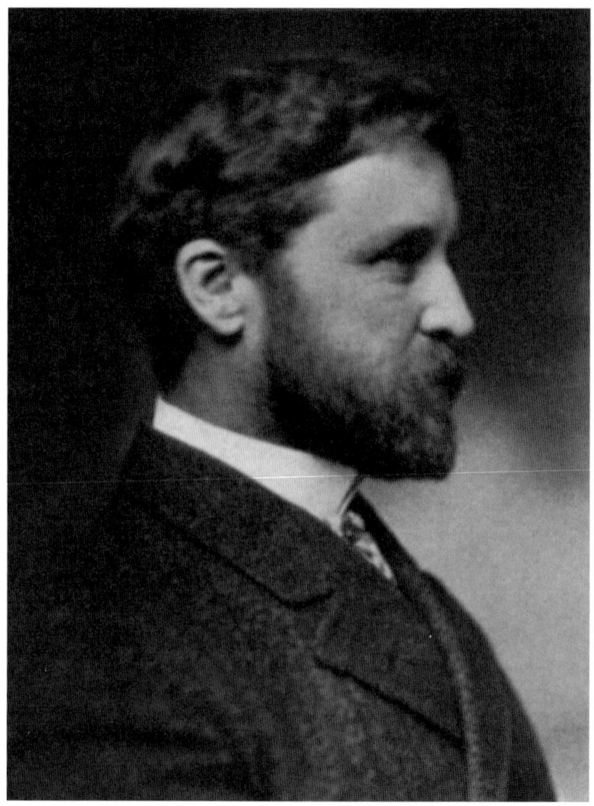

Robert Latou Dickinson

training ... No single cause of mental strain in married women is as widespread as sex fears and maladjustments.

Dickinson was President of the American Gynecological Society in 1920 and as such carried a certain amount of clout in medical circles, despite his progressive and strongly stated views on contraception and sex education. In 1935 a committee of the American Medical Association released a report condemning lay organisations that promoted and provided birth control information, and particularly the involvement of the medical profession with these organisations. Dickinson met with the committee and systematically dismantled their report to such good effect that the following year the same committee released a second report which endorsed birth control and recommended its teaching in medical school. Dickinson was the most prominent physician in the United States to be associated with the early birth control movement. He worked closely with a number of the pioneers, including Margaret Sanger. Dickinson's education, erudition, eloquence and energy allied to his logic and humanity helped change the medical profession's attitudes towards sex and reproduction. In his later years as he coped with the effects of prostate cancer, he wrote to a younger colleague, 'I have argued that instruction in sex behaviour and all its phases should be subject to the same processes and principles as other preparation for living and vocation. You recall my outcry that for every life work there was examination for fitness save for the most important of all, marriage'.

Robert Dickinson died on 29 November 1950.

Selected Publications

Dickinson RL. Contraception: a medical review of the situation. *Am J Obstet Gynecol* 1924; 8: 583–604.

Dickinson RL. *Human Sex Anatomy: A Topicographical Atlas.* Baltimore, MD: Williams and Wilkins; 1930.

Bibliography References

193, 288, 393, 394, 536, 596, 726, 801, 1026, 1274, 1485, 1562.

Döderlein, Albert Siegmund Gustav (1860–1941)

Döderlein's Bacillus/Döderlein–Kronig Hysterectomy

As part of his study of puerperal sepsis, Albert Döderlein investigated the bacteriology of the vagina in pregnancy. In his report of the vaginal secretions of 195 healthy pregnant women he noted:

The reaction of this normal secretion is always intensely acid on blue litmus paper. In this easily demonstrable characteristic lies one of the principle features of the normal secretion. Bacteriological examination of it reveals the almost exclusive presence of a special kind of bacillus, whose biological characteristics are to be seen in the vagina as well as in the culture tube.

Through later efforts he cultured the organism: the gram-positive, acid-producing *Lactobacillus acidophilus* or Döderlein's bacillus. He subsequently delineated its appearance at the time of puberty and its acid-producing, antibacterial action.

Albert Döderlein was born in Augsberg, Germany and qualified in medicine from the University of Erlangen in 1879. He first worked in Leipzig, where he carried out his studies on the lactobacillus. He subsequently occupied the chair of obstetrics and gynaecology in Tübingen for 10 years and in 1907 moved to a similar post in Munich. Döderlein was a renowned clinician and gynaecological surgeon. In conjunction with Bernard Kronig (1863–1918), he wrote a text on operative gynaecology and developed a vaginal hysterectomy technique via an anterior colpotomy incision: the Döderlein–Kronig hysterectomy. There is renewed interest in this technique, as it can be modified to allow subtotal vaginal hysterectomy.

Selected Publications

Döderlein A. *Das Scheidensekret und seine Bedeutung für das Puerperalfieber.* Leipzig: O. Durr; 1892.

Döderlein A. *Die Scheidensekretuntersuchungen Zentbl Gynäk* 1894; 18: 10–14.

Döderlein A, Kronig S. *Die technik der Vaginaden bauchohlen-operationen.* Leipzig: Verlag von Hirzel; 1906.

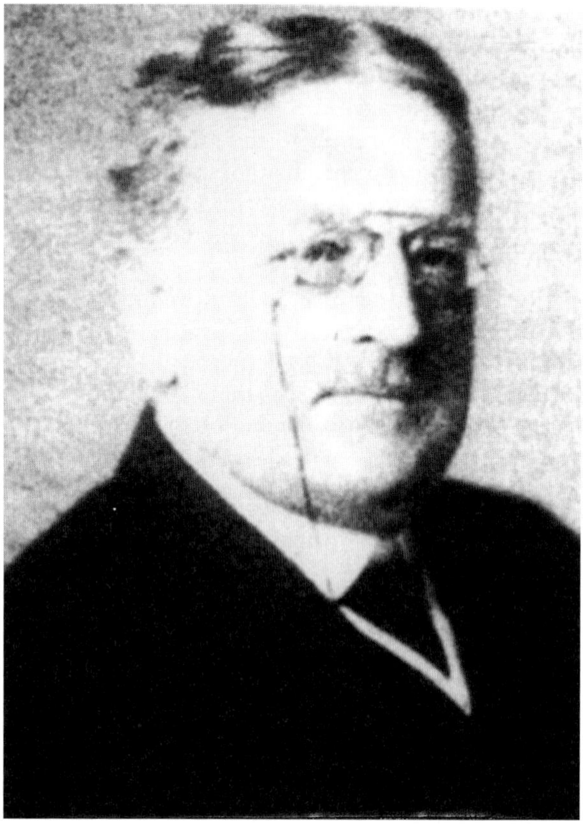

Albert Siegmund Gustav Döderlein

Bibliography References

501, 548, 553, 648, 968, 1123, 1145, 1291.

Donald, Archibald (1860–1937)

Manchester Repair Operation

Born in Edinburgh and educated at Edinburgh University, Archibald Donald later worked at St Mary's Hospital, Manchester and the Manchester Royal Infirmary. He was appointed professor of obstetrics and gynaecology at Manchester University in 1912 but resigned in 1920 to become clinical professor and allow more time for clinical work. Donald developed a vaginal repair for uterine prolapse, which was common among the women who worked in the local mills. As he later wrote,

> *When I was resident surgical officer at St Mary's Hospital during the years 1884–87, I was struck by the numbers of women who came to the outpatients department suffering from the more serious degree of prolapse . . . the condition seemed to me to be one in which operative treatment on lines similar to what was employed in cases of hernia ought to be possible and successful.*

He performed the first of these operations, an anterior and posterior colporrhaphy combined with amputation of the cervix at the Manchester Royal Infirmary on 30 July 1888. He used silver wire in the first two cases and catgut thereafter. Before this development, the main operation for prolapse was to tighten up the perineum so that a pessary could be retained. Renowned for his small hands and dexterous surgical technique, he wrote little but taught many

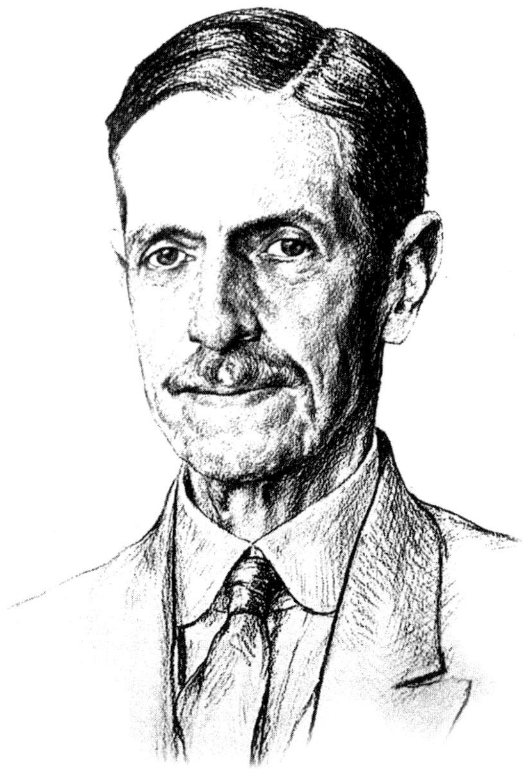
Archibald Donald

others. William Fothergill later made minor modifications to Donald's operation and published his technique. Thus, for a time it became known as Fothergill's operation. However, it later came to be called the Manchester operation, acknowledging both Donald's and Fothergill's contributions

Selected Publications

Donald A. Operation in cases of complete prolapse. *J Obstet Gynaecol Br Emp* 1908; 13: 195–6.

Bibliography References

412–414, 501, 822, 1086, 1390, 1391.

Donald, Ian (1910–1987)

Obstetric Ultrasound

Ian Donald was born in Liskeard, Cornwall, the son of a Scottish general practitioner father and a concert pianist mother. His father later practised in Paisley, Scotland, and young Donald's early education was at Fettes College, Edinburgh (which he did not enjoy). When he was 14 his family moved to Cape Town, South Africa. Donald graduated BA from the University of Cape Town and returned to Britain to gain his medical degree from the University of London in 1937. He served in the Royal Air Force as a medical officer from 1942–1946. He was awarded the MBE and mentioned in dispatches for his role in saving several airmen from a crashed, burning aircraft. Following the war, he pursued training in obstetrics and gynaecology at St Thomas' and Hammersmith hospitals in London, where he did some of the earliest research on neonatal resuscitation and infant respirators.

Appointed to the Regius chair of midwifery at Glasgow in 1954, Donald soon turned his attention to the potential use of ultrasound in obstetrics. In the two World Wars a joint committee of the French and British Admiralties had formed the anti-submarine detection and investigation committee (ASDIC) that developed echo sounding for U-boat detection. Shortly after his arrival in Glasgow, Donald, who had seen ASDIC in action during his RAF service, remarked to his consultant colleague, Wallace Barr (1920–2015), 'I think the ASDIC technique could be applied to medicine'. He was aware of an engineering firm in Renfrew that used ultrasound to detect flaws in boilers. He made contact with this firm and, after initial discussion, he and Barr put specimens of fibroids and ovarian tumours in their car, drove to Renfrew and to their delight saw different echo patterns between cystic and solid tumours using the ultrasound scanner.

Shortly thereafter the brilliant young engineer, Tom Brown (b. 1933), started work with Donald and together they produced the first contact compound sector scanner, described in the *Lancet* in 1958. The early images were poor, but Donald's obsessive drive ensured the practical development and application of ultrasound to diagnosis in obstetrics and gynaecology. The initial work was done at the Royal Maternity Hospital in Glasgow and later at the Queen Mother's Hospital, opened in 1964. Later one of his co-workers, John MacVicar (1927–2011), then a registrar in Donalds' department, wrote,

> *All that was available then was a crude machine, which used ultrasound to detect flaws in metals and with it we were attempting to detect flaws in women. Hours of continuous work often late at night became usual. Examination of countless patients and experiments with mechanical developments and picture display took up much of our time. Feelings of fatigue and frustration, despair and delusion, excitement and elation became well known to us. Recognition of the birth of a new science was slow. Personally, I might have given up the whole idea in the face of the current carping criticism but that was not for Ian Donald. He proved himself a man of vision who could see, despite all the criticism, the amazing potential which the new technique had. He pioneered something which as it developed was used worldwide, and on which much of modern obstetric practice depends.*

Donald was an enthusiastic and didactic teacher, and his book, *Practical Obstetric Problems*, first published in 1955, became a standard and went through five editions in his lifetime. He had cardiac surgery for rheumatic heart disease on three occasions, and the patient's perspective is reflected in his book. Some idea of his entertaining style of writing is shown in his cautionary words about the third stage of labour:

> *This is indeed the unforgiving stage of labour, and in it there lurks more unheralded treachery than in both the other stages of labour combined. The normal case can, within a minute, become abnormal and successful delivery can turn swiftly to disaster. The obstetrician's judgement must be sure and swift, and errors of commission carry with them penalties as great, or greater, than those of omission. Increasing experience serves only to sharpen one's alertness during this stage, and there is no room for complacency in any case, however normal, until the placenta has been delivered for at least half an hour, with the uterus well retracted and with minimal bleeding.*

Ian Donald was a restless, ambitious and at times ruthless man, not above self-promotion to achieve his goals. He was, however, revered by his junior staff whose work he acknowledged in the preface to the third edition of his book: 'above all, I stand humbly in the debt of my junior colleagues, one of whose functions is continually to instruct me and save me from the abyss of seniority'.

Ian Donald had strong opinions on most things, particularly in the area of therapeutic abortion, to which he was strongly and vociferously opposed. He was appointed CBE in 1973, but many felt that higher honours were denied him because of his strongly expressed views. In October 1976 he retired to Paglesham, Essex, where he exercised his talents as an accomplished sailor, pianist and artist. His last years were plagued by progressive heart failure, and he died on

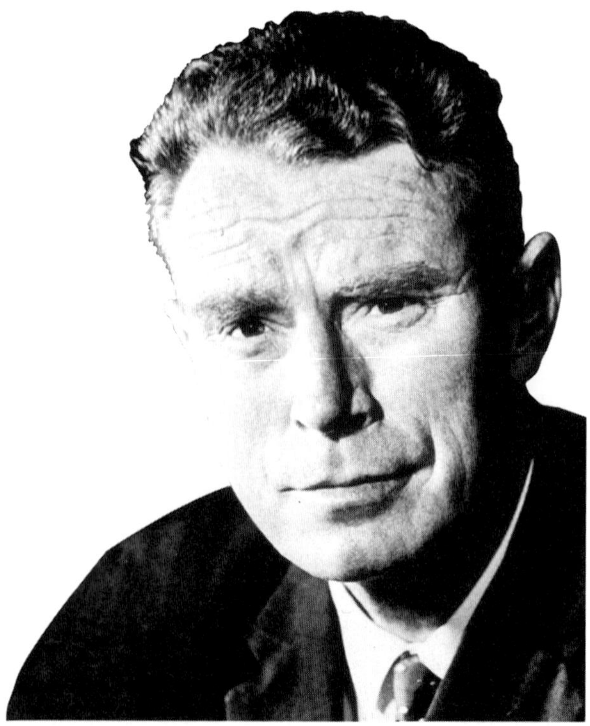

Ian Donald

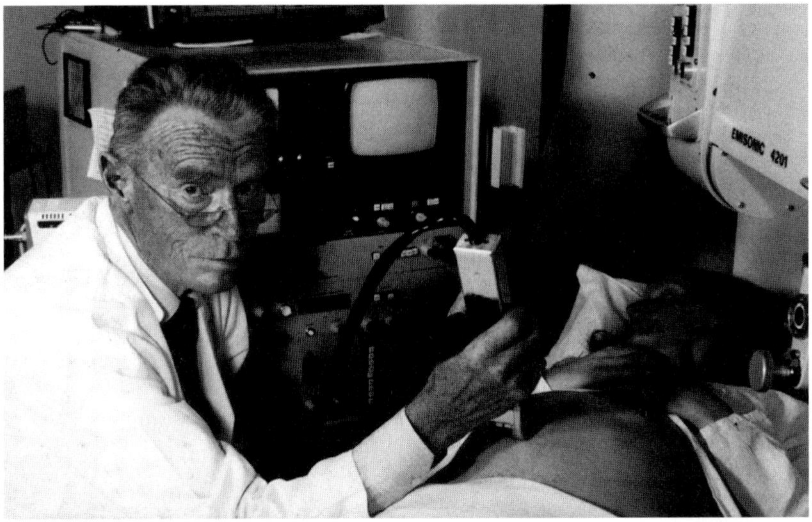

Ian Donald scans his daughter, Caroline

19 June 1987. At a memorial service held in the University of Glasgow Memorial Chapel, John Willocks, another of Donald's early workers in ultrasound, said, 'If you seek his memorial, look around you. In every maternity hospital you will see ultrasound in use. A great discovery by a great man'.

Selected Publications

Donald I., Lord J. Augmented respiration: studies in atelectasis neonatorum. *Lancet* 1953; 1: 9–17.

Donald I. *Practical Obstetric Problems*. London: Lloyd-Luke Ltd; 1955.

Donald I, MacVicar J, Brown TG. Investigation of abdominal masses by pulsed ultrasound. *Lancet* 1958; 1: 1188–94.

Bibliography References

88, 263, 272, 367, 415–417, 860, 1029, 1110, 1504, 1706–1708.

Donné, Alfred François (1801–1878)

Trichomonas Vaginalis

Alfred Donné was a medical student in Paris when he began his life-long interest in microscopy. The subject of his MD thesis was the microscopical aspect of 'Researches into blood molecules, pus and mucous, including the aqueous humor of the eye'. He later invented a collapsible microscope that could be carried in a coat pocket. In 1836, at the Paris Academy of Science, he presented his discovery of the protozoon *Trichomonas vaginalis:*

> *The animalcule is of a size double that of a human erythrocyte, or about the size of a pus cell, namely 1/40 mm in diameter. The body is round, but may elongate and assume diverse forms. At the anterior end is a long flagellum-like appendage, very thin, which may wave back and forth with great rapidity. On the underpart are a number of very fine cilia that cause a rotating movement.*

Donné proposed the name *Trichomonas vaginalae* for this new genus. The name was later changed to *Trichomonas vaginalis* and for the next century was regarded as a harmless commensal in the vagina. It was not until almost a century later that it was established to be a sexually transmitted infection.

Alfred François Donné was born in the small town of Noyen, 25 km north of Paris. At the insistence of his family he took a law degree in Paris, but he then immediately enrolled as a medical student, graduating in 1831. He did his clinical work at the Charité Hospital, Paris. After some initial opposition, his position

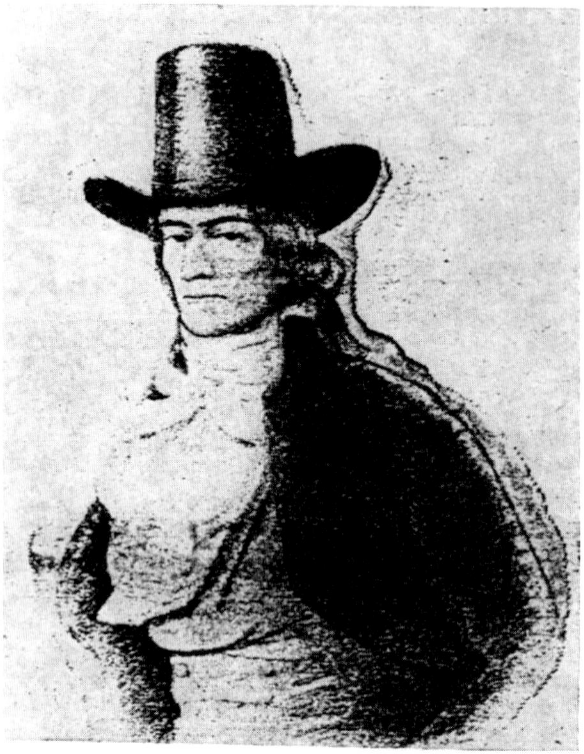

Alfred François Donné

as a pioneer and teacher of microscopy was established and he was appointed Inspector General of Medicine at the University of Paris. In 1842 he described the 'third corpuscle' or blood platelets. In 1844 he wrote a text on the use of the microscope, *Cours de microscopie,* and in it he described the leucocytosis of leukaemia.

In 1855 Donné was appointed rector of the University of Montpellier. He retired from this position in 1875 and returned to Paris. He died of a cardiovascular accident on 7 March 1878.

Selected Publications

Donné AF. Animalcules observés dans les matières purulentes et les produits des sécretions des organes génitaux de l'homme et de la femme. *C R Acad Sci (Paris)* 1836; 3: 385–6.

Donné AF. De l'origine des globules du sang, de leur mode de formation et de leur fin. *C R Acad Sci (Paris)* 1842; 14: 366–8.

Donné AF. *Cours de microscopie.* Paris: Ballière; 1844.

Bibliography References

209, 386, 440, 677, 715, 1603.

Doppler, Christian Andreas (1803–1853)

Doppler Effect

Born on 29 November 1803 in Salzburg, Austria, the second son of a master stonemason, Doppler's mathematical abilities and poor health, despite early signs of promise in stonemasonry, dictated his education in mathematics and physics at the Polytechnic Institute in Vienna. He returned to Salzburg three years later to complete his studies in science and philosophy. Frustrated by his inability to land a teaching job, he was on the verge of emigrating to the United States of America in 1835 when he was appointed professor of elementary mathematics and accounting at the State Secondary School in Prague. In 1841 he was appointed professor of mathematics and practical geometry at the State Technical Institute of Prague, and there he enunciated his Doppler principle. Doppler first presented his theory, unsupported by experimental data, on 25 May 1842, to the Royal Bohemian Society of Prague. His lecture, 'On the coloured light of the double stars and certain other stars of the heavens', postulated that the colour perceived by the eye depends on the frequency of the light pulsations that stimulate it. If the observer moves towards or away from the light source the frequency of pulsations will increase or decrease accordingly. To explain his theory Doppler used the analogy of a ship:

> *which steers directly against the approaching waves and will, in the same time, meet a greater number and much stronger waves than a ship at rest, and even more so than one which moves along in the direction of the waves. Why cannot what applies to the waves of water also, with necessary modifications, be accepted for the air and ether waves?*

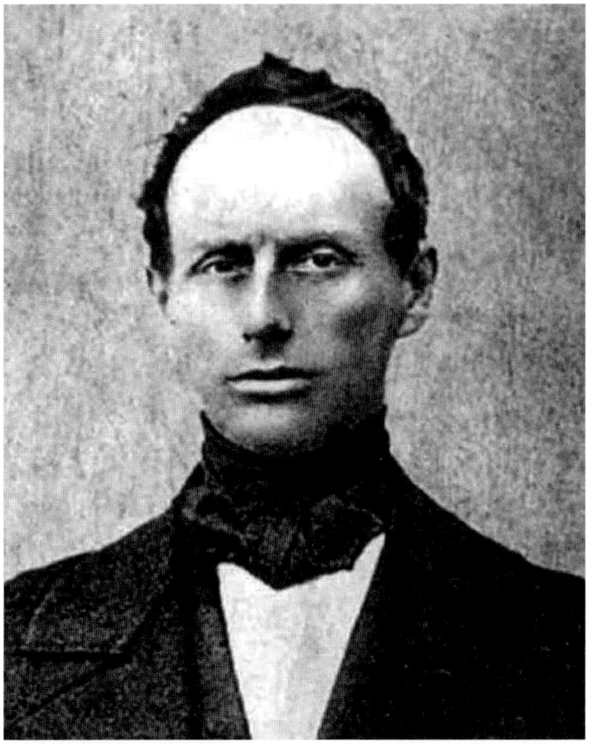

Christian Andreas Doppler

The first experimental confirmation of the acoustical Doppler effect was carried out by Christophorus Buys Ballot (1817–1890) of Utrecht in 1845, using a train drawing an open car with several trumpeters.

Doppler recognised that the effect applied to both light and sound. The principle is used daily, not only in medical ultrasound diagnosis, but in police radar speed traps and in global positioning systems (GPS).

In 1850 Doppler was appointed professor of experimental physics at the University of Vienna. Among his students was Gregor Mendel (1822–1884), the father of modern genetics. Suffering from pulmonary tuberculosis, Doppler went to Venice in November, 1852, hoping to recover in a warmer climate. There he died at 5 a.m. on 17 March 1853 in the arms of his wife, Mathilda. They had five children. Doppler's first name is often incorrectly recorded as Johann Christian but he was baptised Christian Andreas, after the name of the nearest male saint, St Andreas, on whose day he was born.

Selected Publications

Buys Ballot CHD. Akustische Versuche auf der Niederländischen Eisenbahn nebst gelegentlichen. Bemerkungen zur Theorie des Hrn. Prof Doppler. *Pogg Ann* 1845; 66: 321–51.

Doppler C. Über das farbige licht der Dopplesterne und einiger anderer gestirne des Himmels. *Böhmischen Gesellschaft der Wissenschaften* 1843; 2: 465–82.

Bibliography References

150, 505–507, 789, 1172, 1687.

Douglas, James (1675–1742)

Pouch of Douglas

James Douglas was born in Baads, 12 miles west of Edinburgh. His family claimed descent from Robert the Bruce. He was one of 12 children, four of whom became Fellows of the Royal Society. His early education is unclear, but he received his MD from the University of Rheims in 1699, although there is no evidence he ever studied there. He moved to London in 1700, developing a large obstetric practice while carrying out his anatomical research. He became personal physician to Queen Caroline. Douglas was one of the first to give anatomy classes and to realise the importance of anatomy to the advancement of clinical medicine. His main contribution was an anatomical monograph on the peritoneum in which he describes the structure later known as the pouch of Douglas:

> *Where the peritonaeum leaves the foreside of the rectum, it makes an angle, and changes its course upwards and forwards over the bladder; and a little above this angle, there is a remarkable transverse stricture or semioval fold of the peritonaeum, which I have constantly observed for many years past, especially in women.*

His name was immortalised in the famous couplet from Alexander Pope's *Dunciad* (1742):

> There all the learn'd shall at the labour stand,
> And Douglas lend his soft, obstetric hand.

Other eponymous designations include the recto-uterine portion of the uterosacral ligaments, the 'folds of Douglas', and the linea semicircularis of the rectus sheath, the 'line of Douglas'.

Douglas was also an accomplished natural historian and botanist. He published a folio, *Arbor Yemensis Fructum Cofe Ferens,* on the coffee plant in 1727. His other literary endeavours included published works on Horace, grammar and pronunciation. Douglas encouraged William Hunter, who was his resident pupil in 1741. He died on 1 April 1742, and his widow gave lodging to both William and John Hunter in their early days in London. No known portrait of him exists.

Selected Publications

Douglas J. *A Description of the Peritonaeum and of That Part of the Membrana Cellularis Which Lies on its Outside.* London: J. Roberts; 1730.

Bibliography References

108, 192, 298, 406, 648, 1337, 1457, 1583, 1584.

Down, John Langdon (1828–1896)

Down's Syndrome

John Langdon Down was born in Torpoint, Cornwall to a father of Irish descent and a mother from an old Devon family. At 14 years of age he became an apprentice to his father, a local apothecary. He later studied medicine at the London Hospital qualifying in 1856. His liberal views, compassion and care for the mentally disabled led to his appointment, in 1858, as the medical superintendent of the Earlswood Asylum for Idiots at Redhill, Surrey. He published his classic description of 'mongolism' in 1866:

> *The hair is not black, as in the real Mongol, but of a brownish colour, straight and scanty. The face is flat and broad, and destitute of prominence. The cheeks are roundish, and extended laterally. The eyes are obliquely placed, and the internal canthi more than normally distant from one another. The palpebral fissure is very narrow. The forehead is wrinkled transversely from the constant assistance which the levatores palpebrarum derive from the occipito-frontalis muscle in the opening of the eyes. The lips are large and thick with transverse fissures. The tongue is long, thick, and is much roughened. The nose is small. The skin has a slight dirty yellowish tinge, and is deficient in elasticity, giving the appearance of being too large for the body.*

The nasal and skin characteristics in his description are now used as the basis for ultrasound markers in early intrauterine detection programmes.

In 1959 Jérôme Lejeune verified the chromosomal anomaly. Two years later, in a letter to the *Lancet*, an

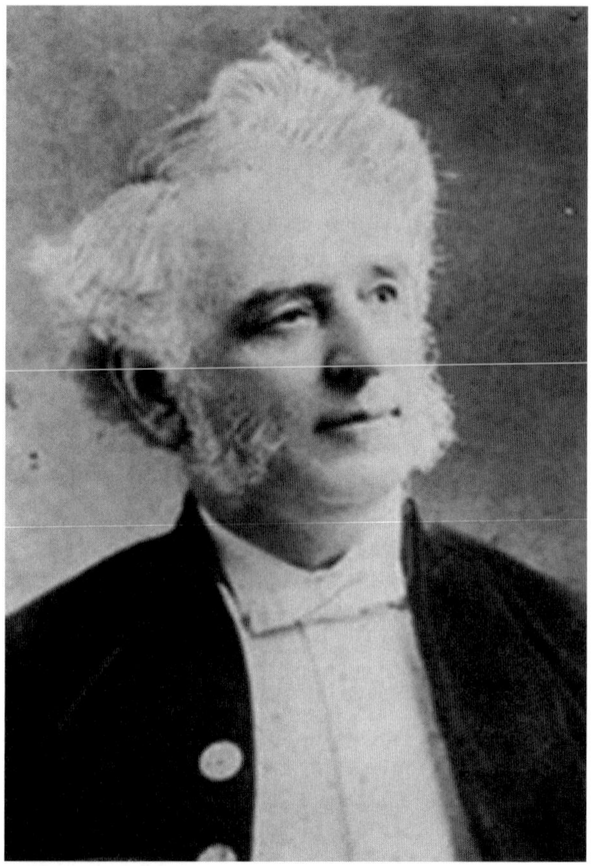

John Langdon Down

international group of scientists suggested that the racial word 'mongol' be discontinued and Down's (trisomy 21) syndrome be used instead. In addition, the Mongolian People's Republic complained to the World Health Organization that the term 'mongol' was inappropriate and demeaning to their country. Thus, in 1961, the term was dropped, and Down belatedly gained eponymous recognition. This was ironic justice, as Down had in fact described Frohlich's syndrome 40 years before Alfred Frohlich (1871–1953). He also delineated the Prader–Willi syndrome almost a century before Andra Prader and Heinrich Willi.

The Down's had four children, three sons and one daughter. Two of his sons became doctors. One, Reginald, succeeded his father at the institute and it was he who added the observation of the distinctive palmer crease in children with Down's syndrome. Reginald had three children, one of whom had Down's syndrome and lived to 65. In 1868, Down left Redhill and entered private practice in Harley Street, London. At the same time, with his wife he established a home for 'feeble-minded' children in Middlesex.

On 7 October 1896 John Langdon Down suddenly collapsed and died of an apparent heart attack, just as he was setting out for his office in Harley Street.

Selected Publications

Down JL. Observations on an ethnic classification of idiots. *London Hospital Reports* 1866; 3: 259–62.

Lejeune J. Study of the somatic chromosomes of nine mongoloid children. *CR Acad Sci (Paris)* 1959; 248: 1721–2.

Bibliography References

437, 438, 462, 745, 968, 1662, 1663, 1732.

Doyle, Joseph Bernard (1907–1992)

Doyle's Operation

Joseph Doyle first described his operation of paracervical uterine denervation for the relief of dysmenorrhoea to the New England Obstetrical and Gynecological Society on 27 October 1954. His procedure was done either abdominally or vaginally by clamping and dividing the uterosacral ligaments and then interposing peritoneum between the divided ends to prevent regrowth of the nerve endings. In 73 cases Doyle achieved satisfactory pain relief in 69 patients (94.5%). In discussing the failure of medical management and the relationship of primary dysmenorrhoea to anovulation, he said:

> *Accordingly, it seems hardly scientific or fair to relegate to a psychosomatic therapeutic nihilism those unfortunate women who do not happen to respond to the test of hormonal relief by the production of anovulatory menstruation.*

Despite his impressive results, Doyle's operation sank into obscurity. However, the principle was revived in the laparoscopic approach to division of the uterosacral ligaments by electrocautery or laser for relief of pelvic pain: laparoscopic uterine nerve ablation (LUNA).

James Bernard Doyle was born in Boston on 8 November 1907. He graduated from Harvard Medical School in 1932. As an assistant clinical professor in the department of obstetrics and gynaecology at Tufts Medical School, Boston, his academic interests were in fertility and uterine physiology. He worked at the Cambridge City and St Elizabeth Hospitals. He retired from obstetrics and gynaecology in 1966 and, with the encouragement of his psychiatrist son, took up the practice of psychiatry for the next 10 years. He died at Middlesex, Massachusetts on 6 April 1992.

Selected Publications

Doyle JB. Paracervical uterine denervation for dysmenorrhea. *Trans N Engl Obstet Gynecol Soc* 1954; 8: 143.

Doyle JB. Paracervical uterine denervation by transection of the cervical plexus for the relief of dysmenorrhea. *Am J Obstet Gynecol* 1955; 70: 1–16.

Bibliography References

1485.

Duchenne, Guillaume Benjamin Amand (1806–1875)

Erb–Duchenne Palsy/Duchenne's Muscular Dystrophy

Guillaume Duchenne was born in Boulogne to a family with a long seafaring tradition. He studied medicine in Paris under René Laennec (1781–1826), Guillaume Dupuytren (1777–1835), Léon Cruveilhier (1791–1874) and François Magendie (1783–1855), graduating in 1831. He practised in Boulogne for several years but returned to Paris after the death of his wife in childbirth and the subsequent alienation and separation from his only son by his wife's family. Known mainly for his description of progressive muscular dystrophy, he pioneered muscle biopsy in 1868, using what came to be called his 'histological harpoon'. In 1872 he described partial upper brachial plexus palsy in the newborn, two years before Wilhelm Erb's description in adults.

An unorthodox but gifted and tenacious clinical investigator, he remained on the periphery of the Parisian medical establishment, never holding a hospital or university appointment. He was a poor lecturer, but his writings were frequent and well received. Duchenne was often ridiculed for his rural and uncultured demeanour. However, he was befriended by Jean-Martin Charot (1825–1893) and Armand Trousseau (1801–1867), who recognised his talent. Charcot summed up his admiration when he said:

> *How is it that, one fine morning, Duchenne discovered a disease which probably existed in the time of Hippocrates?*

During his working life he was so preoccupied that he forgot appointments. Once, when invited to dinner, he arrived in formal dress eight days after the event.

Later in his life recognition came to Duchenne, but he was already secure in his legacy:

> *No, my only ambition is that I shall not die, living always in my works. There are those who have all honours to-day, but later they will be forgotten, while my work will still live.*

Duchenne was happily reunited with his son in 1862, when the latter took up the study of neurology in Paris. Tragically the son died from dementia praecox in 1871. Duchenne died in Paris on 17 September 1875 from a cerebral haemorrhage.

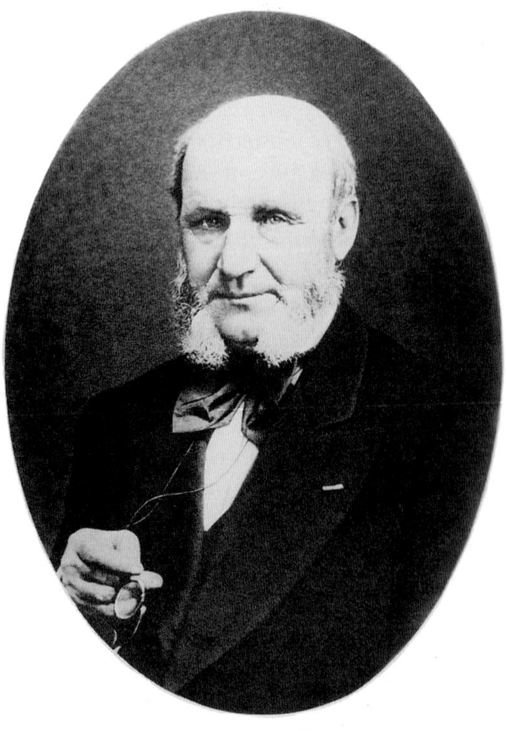

Guillaume Benjamin Amand Duchenne

Selected Publications

Duchenne GBA. *De l'electrisation localisée et de son application à la pathologie et à la thérapeutique*. 3rd edn. Paris: J. B. Baillière, 1872, p. 357.

Bibliography References

33, 302, 552, 648, 703, 806, 1283, 1312, 1649.

Duhrssen, Alfred (1862–1933)

Duhrssen's Incisions

A now obsolete chapter in obstetrics involved incision of the cervix to achieve vaginal delivery in the face of incomplete cervical dilatation. The procedure had been described off and on in the previous century, but it was the detailed report of 12 cases in 1890 by Alfred Duhrssen that linked his name to the procedure:

> *If one wishes to undertake delivery in a case of incomplete dilatation of the external os and to save the infant also, then all resistance must be made to disappear from the sides of the cervical rim. This can only result from incisions that extend to the vaginal attachment, and indeed four of them: two laterally, one anteriorly and one posteriorly . . . I never use a speculum, I cut while holding the cervical rim between the index and middle fingers of my left hand, using the ordinary Siebold scissors.*

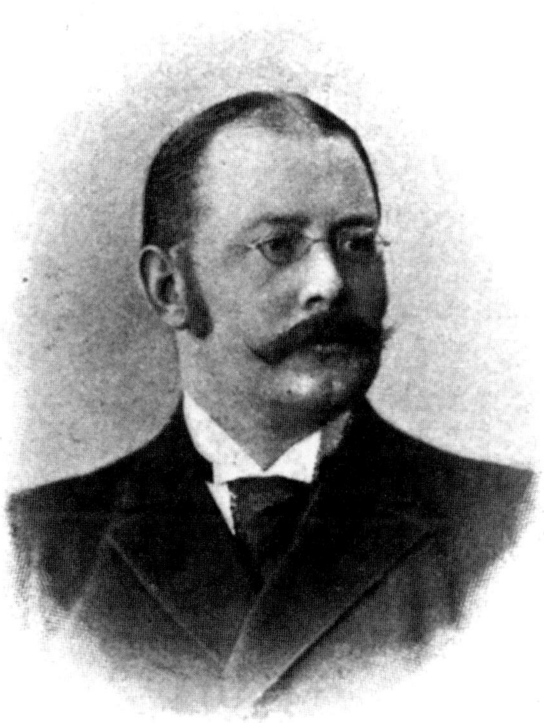

Alfred Duhrssen

Alfred Duhrssen was born in Heide, Germany to a medical family; his father, uncle and grandfather were physicians. He was educated in Marburg, Berlin and Königsberg and rose to the rank of professor, establishing his own Frauenklinik in Berlin. Duhrssen became a leader and proponent of the vaginal surgical approach to myomectomy and removal of the adnexa. He also advocated vaginal caesarean section on rare occasions. With his technique, the anterior and posterior cul-de-sacs were opened and the bladder dissected free. The cervix and lower uterine segment were then incised sufficiently to allow delivery of the infant by version or forceps extraction. This route of caesarean section was not embraced by others.

Duhrssen was an active man who participated in many outdoor sports. The later years of his life were marred by Parkinson's disease.

Selected Publications

Duhrssen A. Über den Werth der tiefen Cervix-und Scheiden-Damm-Einschnitte in der Geburtshülfe. *Arch Gynäkol* 1890; 37: 27–66.

Duhrssen A. Ein neuer Fall von vaginalen Kaiserschnitt. *Arch Gynäkol* 1896; 61: 548–64.

Bibliography References

32, 524, 548, 553, 648, 889, 983, 987, 1291, 1528.

Duncan, James Matthews (1826–1890)

Placental Separation/Duncan's Folds/Gestational Diabetes

Born in Aberdeen, the son of a shipping agent, Duncan qualified as a doctor of medicine at Aberdeen when he was 20 years old. He pursued further studies in Edinburgh and at the Hôtel Dieu in Paris. Upon return to Edinburgh he became a private assistant to James Young Simpson and with him took part in the famous after-dinner experiment with chloroform on 4 November 1847. Indeed, Duncan had the honour to be the first to slide beneath the table under the influence of chloroform.

He was a leading candidate to succeed Simpson as professor in Edinburgh, but to his great disappointment was not elected, Simpson's nephew being appointed instead. He later became lecturer in midwifery and physician-accoucheur at St Bartholomew's Hospital, London. Duncan lectured and wrote widely, applying a scientific basis to the problems of infertility and labour. He studied the mechanism of the third stage of labour and showed that, after separation, the placenta, if not interfered with, slides sideways from the uterus into the vagina (known as the Matthews Duncan method of placental separation). In contradicting Bernhard Schultze's previous teachings, he wrote:

> *The erroneous belief that the placenta generally descends presenting its foetal surface, seems to me to have arisen from observers not keeping in mind the very great frequency with which the natural mechanism of delivery of this cake is interfered with. I may say, that it is unfortunately the rule to interfere with this part of a natural mechanism of delivery. Such interference, generally carried out as it is by pulling the cord, produces an unnatural mechanism – inversion of the placenta.*

In the pre-insulin era, Duncan published the first series of 22 pregnancies in 15 diabetic women; four of the mothers died, as did seven of 19 viable fetuses. He made some observations that apply to what is now known as gestational diabetes:

> *Diabetes may occur only during pregnancy being absent at other times . . . Diabetes may cease with the termination of pregnancy recurring some time afterwards.*

He also recognised the association of maternal diabetes with fetal macrosomia: 'The dead foetus is sometimes described as enormous'.

Duncan outlined the formation of the lower uterine segment in labour as well as the association of hepatic disease with pernicious vomiting in pregnancy, later known as hyperemesis gravidarum. He coined the term 'missed abortion'. The folds of peritoneum on the post-partum uterus are known as Duncan's folds, following his description. He died while on holiday at Baden-Baden on 1 September 1890.

Queen Victoria sent a telegram of sympathy from Balmoral to Mrs Matthews Duncan:

> *I cannot say how shocked and deeply grieved I am at the terrible blow which has fallen upon you. The country and Europe at large have lost one of their most distinguished men and one who will be sorely missed.*
>
> *VR*

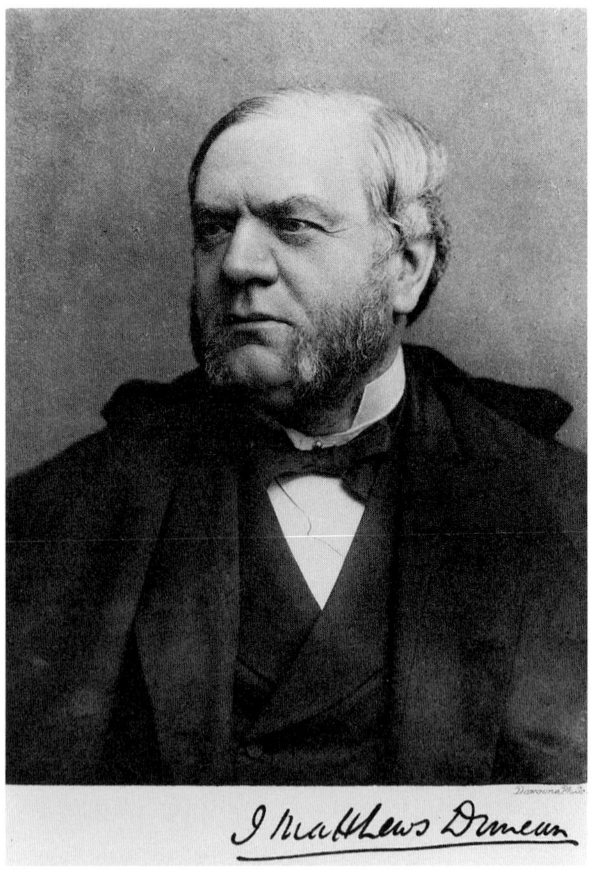

James Matthews Duncan

Selected Publications

Duncan JM. On the displacements of the uterus. *Edinb Med J* 1854; 81: 321–48.

Duncan JM. On the mechanism of the expulsion of the placenta. *Edinb Med J* 1871; 16: 899–903.

Duncan JM. Clinical Lecture on hepatic disease in gynaecology and obstetrics. *Med Times Gaz* 1879; 1: 57–9.

Duncan JM. On puerperal diabetes. *Trans Obstet Soc Lond* 1882; 24: 256–85.

Bibliography References

96, 422, 456, 582, 648, 822, 1182, 1577, 1595.

Dusée (d. 1734)

Dusée's Forceps

Regarded as the French connection in the early development of obstetric forceps, almost nothing is known of the Paris obstetrician Dusée, who left no written description of his forceps. Indeed, the first documented account was by the Edinburgh obstetrician, Alexander Butter, who obtained a pair of Dusée's forceps and gave the first description of them to the Medical Society of Edinburgh in 1733:

> *The forceps for taking hold of a Child's Head, when it is fallen so far down among the Bones of the Pelvis, that it cannot be pushed back into the Uterys, to be extracted by the Feet, and when it seems to make no Advances to the Birth by the Throws of the Mother, is scarce known in this Country, though Mr Chapman tells us, it was long made use of by Dr Chamberlane, who kept the form of it a secret, as Mr Chapman does also. I believe therefore that a sight of such an instrument which I had from M. Dusée who practices Midwifery at Paris, and who believes it to be his own Invention, would not be unacceptable to you, and the Publication of a Picture of it may be of some Use to some of your Readers.*

The forceps blades were solid. The shanks were flattened where they crossed and could be locked by a removable screw at two levels to accommodate high or low pelvic application. The cephalic curve of the blades was, as Butter described, 'made more concave in the middle than is necessary to fit them to the surface of the convex head of the child, in order, as M. Dusée said, to hinder them to compress the temporal arteries'.

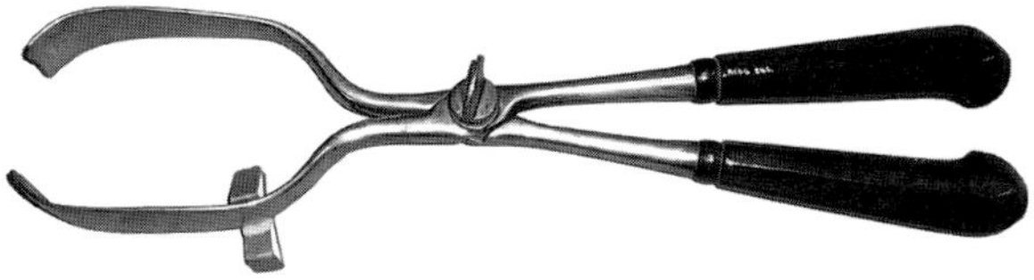

Dusée's forceps

This exaggerated cephalic curve and the cumbersome locking mechanism made the forceps unserviceable in practice. William Smellie tried them without success and wrote,

> *In order to avoid this loss of children which gave me great uneasiness, I procured a pair of French forceps, according to a draught published in the Medical Essays by Mr Butter, but found them so long, and so ill-contrived that they by no means answered the purpose for which they were intended.*

The Dutch obstetrician, Paulus De Wind, who was a pupil of Dusée but never observed him using the forceps, had a similar experience:

> *after returning to Zealand in the Netherlands I soon found by experience that it was unsuited for its purpose. It was far too large and I could not introduce it into the body of my patient.*

Dusée's important innovation was to cross and join the shanks of his forceps. However, although it was one of the first pair of obstetric forceps described, albeit not by the designer, the instrument proved unusable. Indeed, there is no record of Dusée ever using them himself.

Selected Publications

Butter A. The description of a forceps for extracting children by the head when lodged low in the pelvis of the mother. *Medical Essays and Observations Edinburgh* 1773; 3: 254.

Doran A. Dusée: his forceps and his contemporaries. *J Obstet Gynaecol Br Emp* 1912; 22: 121–41.

Doran A. Dusée, De Wind and Smellie: an addendum. *J Obstet Gynaecol Br Emp* 1912; 22: 203–7.

Bibliography References

347, 361, 399, 424, 425, 648, 721, 1260.

E

Erb, Wilhelm Heinrich (1840–1921)

Erb–Duchenne Palsy

Erb reported four cases of upper brachial plexus palsy involving cervical nerve roots five and six in 1874. His description involved adults: two cases from trauma, one due to metastatic cancer and one from unknown causes. In this publication, Erb acknowledged Guillaume Duchenne's earlier (1872) description of upper brachial plexus palsy in the newborn:

> *We find another group of similar cases of birth paralysis, which appears all too often in newborn infants and has been described by Duchenne . . . I have myself observed a case in an infant which had been delivered two months before after a version and subsequent extraction.*

Erb showed that the muscles involved were supplied by the fifth and sixth roots of the brachial plexus. He applied electrical stimulation at a point 2 cm above the clavicle and in front of the transverse process of the sixth cervical vertebra – Erb's point – and produced contraction of the muscles involved. He referred to brachial plexus palsy in the newborn as 'delivery paralysis', noting that it may be associated with obstetric manoeuvres:

> *Moderately energetic manipulation by the obstetrician can easily compress the roots of the brachial plexus and the plexus itself so that a more or less persistent paralysis ensues.*

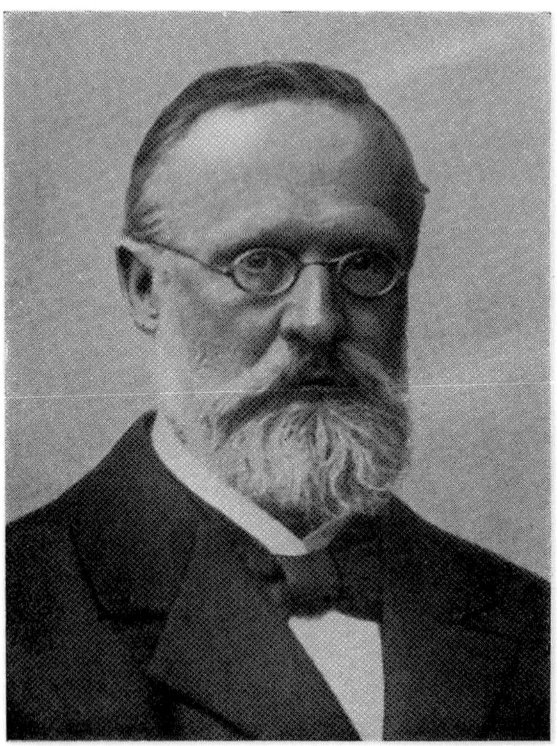

Wilhelm Heinrich Erb

The son of a forester, Erb was born in Winnweiler, Bavaria. He was greatly influenced by his teacher Nikolaus Friedreich (1825–1882) and eventually succeeded him as professor at Heidelberg in 1883. Erb was one of the pioneers of electrodiagnosis and electrotherapy in medicine and coined the term 'tendon reflex'. He recognised the association between syphilis and tabes many years before this was proven in the laboratory. He was not known for his sense of humour and had a brusque and, on occasions, ill-tempered manner. He instructed his students to pray each morning, 'O Lord let me not idle my life away today', his version of *carpe diem.* Erb was distressed by his country's downfall in the First World War, in which one of his four sons was killed on the western front. He collapsed while attending a concert of his favourite symphony, Beethoven's *Eroica*, and died soon after on 29 October 1921.

Selected Publications

Erb WH. Über eine eigenthümliche Localisation von Lähmungen in Plezus brachialis. *Verh Naturhis-med Verein Heidelb* 1874–77; 1: 130–6.

Bibliography References

33, 194, 363, 553, 648, 673, 703, 859, 968.

Estes, William Lawrence (1855–1940)

Estes' Operation

In the pre-antibiotic era of the early twentieth century, gonococcal pelvic inflammatory disease was sometimes treated with bilateral salpingectomy to remove the pyosalpinges. William Estes, chief surgeon of St Luke's Hospital in Bethlehem, Pennsylvania, developed an operation which attempted to preserve ovarian function and some potential for fertility in these cases:

> *Surgeons who are accustomed to see the conditions produced by the usual gonococcal and mixed infections in the pelves of women know that in a very large majority of cases, the tubes are in such condition that it would be extremely hazardous to attempt to save even a part of one of them, but the ovaries frequently have at least a small portion of their stroma not destroyed, nor seriously affected. The operation I wish to advocate and the method I wish to describe is adapted to the cases of salpingitis and salpingo-ovaritis, in which the whole of both tubes must be removed, and a portion, at least, of one or both ovaries must also be sacrificed.*

After removal of the tubes, Estes advised preserving the ovarian ligament 'with its small artery and the attachments to the broad ligament also if it can be done without leaving bad tissue behind'. He then cut the ovarian stroma:

> *... in such a pattern that it will fit into the oval concavity left in the horns of the uterus when the tubes are excised ... The stumps of the round ligament and broad ligaments are then brought into apposition with the sides of the uterus in such a way that the implanted segment of the ovary is entirely covered by the serous membrane of these ligaments.*

Estes first described the procedure in 1909, and in his later 1934 review reported 50 cases, all of whom preserved menstrual function and four of whom became pregnant, with two going to term. Estes did not claim originality for this procedure, citing others who had implanted ovaries through the uterine wall into the cavity of the uterus, notably Robert Tuttle Morris (1857–1945), professor of surgery at the New York Postgraduate Medical School.

William Estes was born on 28 November 1855, the only son of the third marriage of his plantation-owning father. He grew up on a plantation of several thousand acres in Tennessee with 150 slaves. He was educated at home and at the local schools and entered Bethel College in Russellville, Kentucky at the age of 16. In 1874 he attended the medical department of the University of Virginia and graduated MD in 1877. Up to this point his medical education was mainly theoretical. He moved to New York City Medical College and attended clinics and operating sessions largely as an observer. He served a two-year internship at Mount Sinai Hospital and finished there in 1880. During this period of training he gained experience in gynaecological and general surgery. In 1881 he became the first superintendent, director and chief surgeon of the newly built St Luke's Hospital in South Bethlehem, Pennsylvania. There he remained and established a busy surgical service and also founded one of the first schools of nursing in the country.

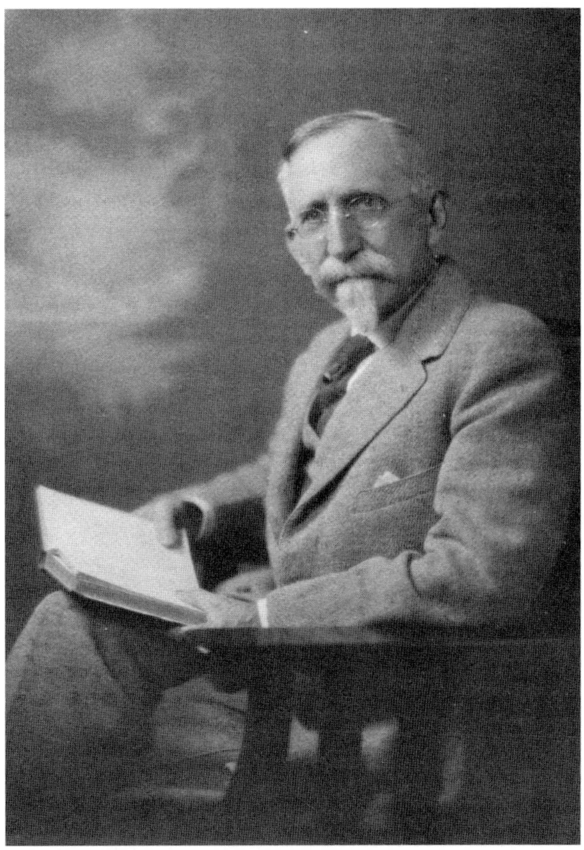

William Lawrence Estes

He retired as surgeon-in-chief in 1920 but remained as an active surgeon for another 14 years. He died in 1940 and was succeeded by his surgeon son.

Selected Publications

Estes WL. A method of implanting ovarian tissue in order to maintain ovarian function. *Penn Med J* 1909: 13: 610–13.

Estes WL. Further results with ovarian implantation. *JAMA* 1924; 83: 674–8.

Estes WL, Heitmeyer PL. Incidence of pregnancy following ovarian implantation. *Am J Surg* 1934; 24: 563–81.

Morris RT. *Lectures on Appendicitis and Notes on Other Subjects.* New York, NY: G. R. Putnam's Sons; 1895.

Bibliography References

530, 1415.

Euler, Ulf Svante von (1905–1983) Bergström, Karl Sune Detlof (1916–2004)

Prostaglandins

The first demonstrations that seminal fluid caused contraction of smooth muscle were by Raphael Kurzrok and Charles Lieb in New York and Maurice Goldblatt in England. Ulf von Euler was a young physiologist from Sweden, working for six months in the laboratory of Henry Dale in London, when he found a substance in the extracts of rabbit intestine that caused contraction of an isolated jejunum preparation. Initially they were unable to isolate the substance and called it 'substance P' (for preparation). He returned to the pharmacology department of the Karolinska Institute, in Stockholm, Sweden, and continued work on biologically active substances. In 1934 he isolated a lipid in ram's semen that caused both contraction and relaxation of smooth muscle. He named it prostaglandin because of its source in the prostate gland:

> *With regard to the nature of the active substance, it is dialysable and soluble in water, alcohol, acetone, ether and chloroform. The substance is unstable at high temperatures, more so in alkali than in acid. Cataphoresis experiments have shown that the active substance has acid properties. In order to make reference more convenient, and since it is clear that this substance is different from other autopharmacologic substances it has been preliminarily called 'prostaglandin'.*

In 1945 von Euler gave Sune Bergström, a young biochemist at the Karolinska, some prostaglandin extracts to purify. After an initial delay, Bergström amassed a large team of research chemists and began the long and tedious work necessary to identify the constituents of the prostaglandin extract. By the late

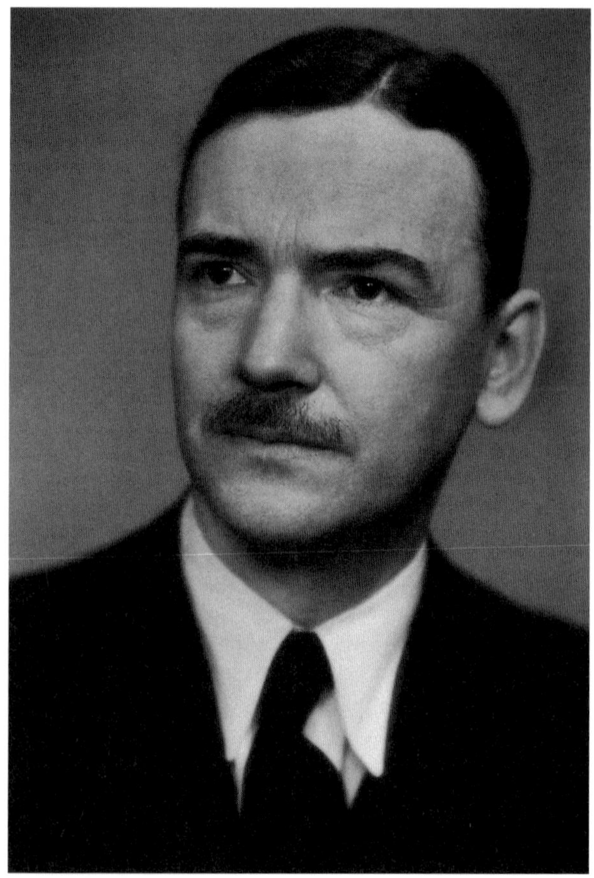

Ulf Svante von Euler

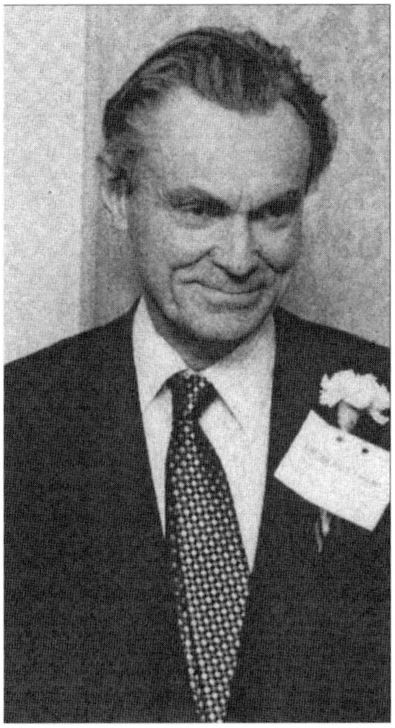

Karl Sune Detlof Bergström

1950s and the 1960s they identified six different prostaglandins and their chemical structure. The clinical application of prostaglandin and anti-prostaglandin drugs followed soon after.

Ulf von Euler's father, Hans von Euler (1873–1964), came from Augsburg, Germany, and shared the Nobel Prize for chemistry in 1929. Ulf von Euler was to emulate his father and share the Nobel Prize for physiology in 1970. He was professor and director of physiology at the Karolinska Institute until his retirement in 1971. He was decorated with the Swedish Order of the North Star.

Sune Bergström was a biochemist trained at the Karolinska Institute in Stockholm, where he also received his MD. After fellowships in London, New York and Basel, he was appointed professor of physiological chemistry at the University of Lund in 1947. He was recalled to the Karolinska Institute and appointed successively, professor of chemistry (1958), dean of the medical faculty (1963) and rector (1969). He worked with the World Health Organization and through them helped to promote the clinical application of the prostaglandin compounds. In 1982 he shared the Nobel Prize for physiology. He died on 15 August 2004 following a stroke.

Selected Publications

Euler US von. Zur Kenntnis der pharmakologischen Wirkungen der Nativsekreten und Extrakten männlicher accessorischer Geschlechtsdrüsen. *Arch Exp Path Pharmak* 1934; 175: 78–84.

Euler US von. On the vasodilating and plain muscle stimulating substances from accessory genital glands in man and certain animals (prostaglandin and vesiglandin). *J Physiol* 1936; 88: 213–4.

Bergström S, Sjovall J. The isolation of prostaglandin F from sheep prostate glands. *Acta Chemica Scand* 1960; 14: 1693–1700.

Bergström S, Sjovall J. The isolation of prostaglandin E from sheep prostate glands. *Acta Chemica Scand* 1960; 14: 1701–5.

Bibliography References

93, 94, 157, 531, 576, 856, 1012, 1106, 1266, 1330, 1374, 1452, 1727.

F

Fallopius, Gabriel (1523–1562)

Fallopian Tubes

One of the most illustrious anatomists of the sixteenth century, Gabriel Fallopius, gave the first complete description of the human oviducts in 1561. He named the tubes the uteri tuba or trumpets of the uterus:

That slender and narrow seminal duct rises, fibrous and pale, from the horns of the uterus itself; becomes, when it has gone a little bit away, appreciably broader, and curls like a branch until it comes near the end, then losing the horn-like curl, and becomes very broad, has a distinct

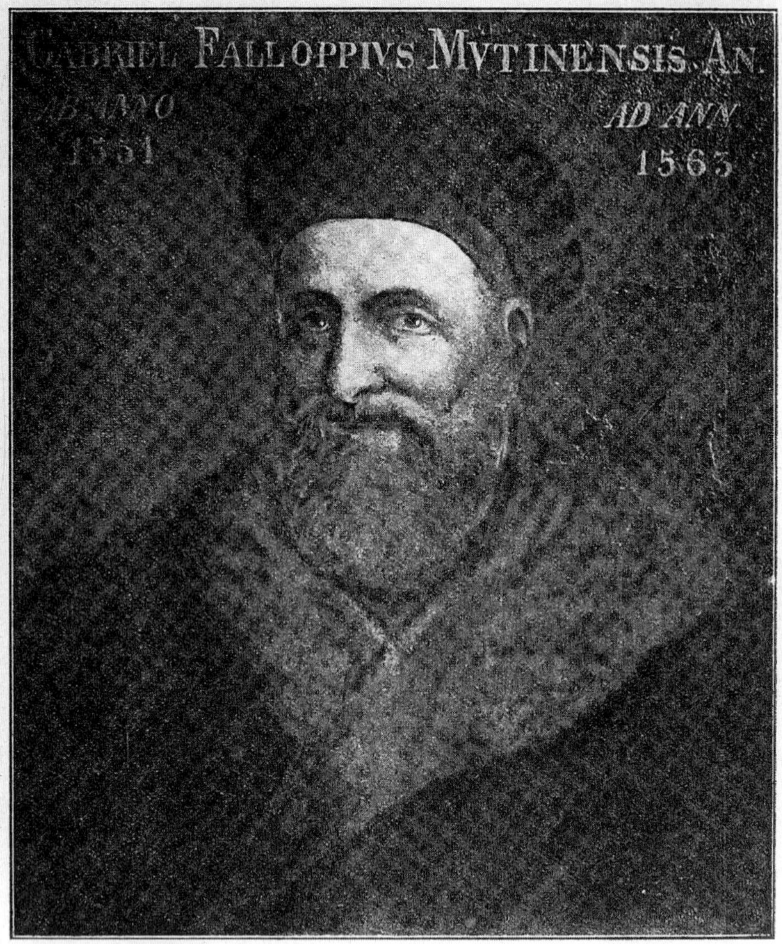

GABRIELE FALLOPPIO

DA UN RITRATTO AD OLIO. ESISTENTE NELL' ISTITUTO ANATOMICO

Gabriel Fallopius

extremity which appears fibrous and fleshy through its red colour, and its end is torn and ragged like the fringe of well-worn garments, and it has a wide orifice which lies always closed through the ends of the fringe falling together; and if these be carefully separated and opened out, they resemble the orifice of a brass trumpet.

Gabriel Fallopius was born to a noble Italian family in Modena. He initially studied theology and held an ecclesiastical appointment in the cathedral at his home town. He resigned to study medicine and became a favourite pupil of Vesalius. After his first appointment as professor of anatomy at the University of Pisa, he succeeded Vesalius as professor of anatomy, surgery and botany at Padua, also having charge of the botanical gardens. He made numerous contributions to anatomy, including the words vagina, placenta and corpus luteum as applied to the ovary. He described the inguinal ligament before François Poupart. Along with Caspar Bartholin, his is one of the few names that has become so entrenched in the anatomical lexicon that it is spelt without a capital.

Selected Publications

Fallopius G. *Observationes anatomicae*. Venice: Marco Antonio Ulmum; 1561, p. 221.

Bibliography References

406, 552, 557, 648, 968, 1197, 1343.

Farre, Arthur (1811–1887)

Farre's White Line

The line of attachment between the peritoneum of the mesovarium and the body of the ovary was first described by Farre in Todd's *Cyclopaedia of Anatomy and Physiology* in 1859. The abrupt transition between the two, the germinal cuboidal epithelium of the ovary and the flat mesothelium of the peritoneum, appears as a white line at the hilum of the ovary.

Arthur Farre was born in London. He studied medicine at Cambridge and St Bartholomew's Hospital, London. He became professor of midwifery at King's College, London and obstetric physician extraordinary to Queen Victoria.

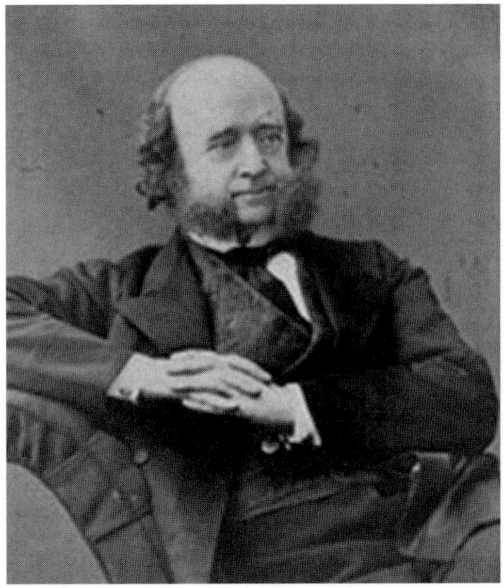

Arthur Farre

Selected Publications

Farre A. The Uterus and its Appendages. In: Todd RE (ed.) *Cyclopaedia of Anatomy and Physiology*. (Suppl Vol.) 1859, p. 548.

Bibliography References

406, 867, 1290, 1715.

Ferguson, James Haig (1863–1934)

Haig Ferguson's Forceps

Haig Ferguson modified Simpson's obstetric forceps by shortening the handles and placing slots in the middle of the fenestrae to allow the application of traction tapes. He originally presented his forceps design to the Edinburgh Obstetrical Society in 1911 and published his experience with the instrument in 1926:

> *The traction tapes are threaded through eyelet holes which are made at the level of the middle of the fenestra in each blade. The attachment of the tapes to the blades is practically therefore at the level of the biparietal diameter of the head (opposite the parietal eminences)at a height where axis-traction rods cannot attain to. This high traction on the head through the tapes tends markedly to increase flexion, which is a further advantage.*

The result was a popular and widely used instrument.

James Haig Ferguson, a son of the manse, was born in Fossoway, Scotland. He took his medical education in Edinburgh, graduating in 1884. After many years in general practice he specialised in obstetrics and gynaecology with appointments at the Royal Infirmary and Royal Maternity Hospital in Edinburgh. One of the first to recognise the need for

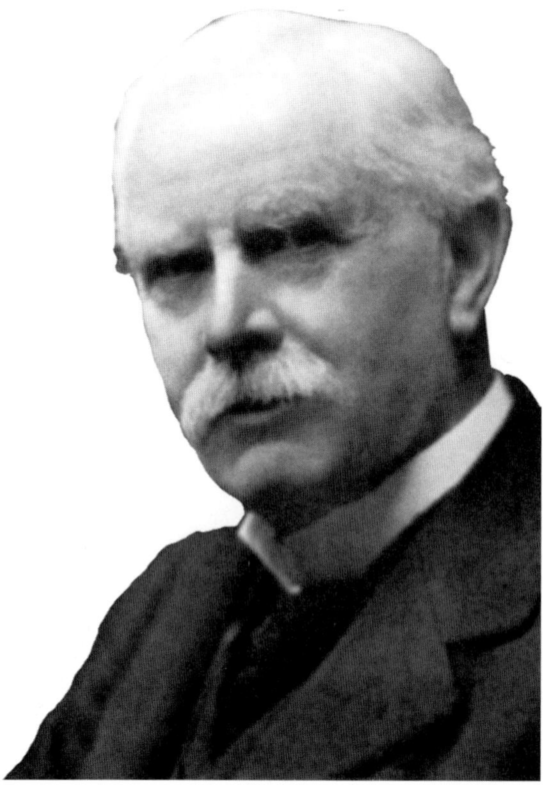

James Haig Ferguson

antenatal care, Ferguson opened a hostel for antenatal patients next door to the Edinburgh Royal Maternity Hospital in 1899. He became president of the Royal College of Physicians of Edinburgh. On his mother's side he was related to Field Marshal Earl Haig. He died at home on 2 May 1934.

Selected Publications

Ferguson JH. A simple and improved modification of the midwifery forceps. *Trans Edin Obstet Soc* 1925–6; 46: 78–92.

Bibliography References

361, 399, 721, 822, 959, 1183, 1285, 1420.

Ferguson, James Kenneth Wallace (1907–1999)

Ferguson's Reflex

In 1941 Ferguson published his experimental work in rabbits, showing that cervical and vaginal dilatation produced the release of oxytocin from the posterior pituitary via stimulation of a nervous pathway. He concluded that 'afferent impulses from the lumbo-sacral cord are important in maintaining a tonic secretion of oxytocic hormone'. He went on to state:

> *Certain phenomena of parturition in the human may be interpreted rather plausibly in view of the findings of this paper. It is generally observed that labour pains increase in frequency and strength as the cervix dilates. They reach their maximum in the second stage when the cervix is fully dilated. It is plausible to suppose that in the human, as in the rabbit, stretching the cervix may augment the secretion of oxytocin. This may explain why a dilating bag or rimming of the cervix is so effective for inducing labour. Rupture of the membranes, forcing the presenting part against the cervix, may achieve the same result more slowly. Involuntary 'bearing down' in the human is*

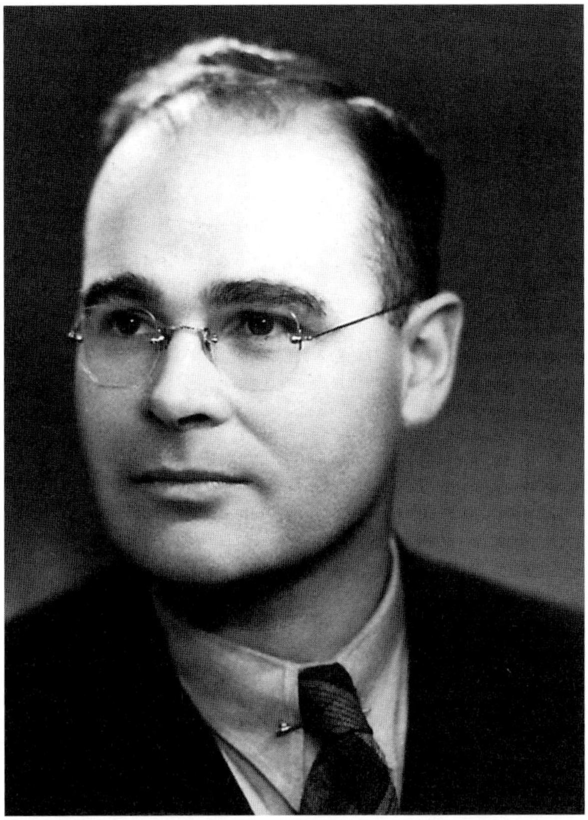

James Kenneth Wallace Ferguson

characteristic of the second stage of labour when the fetus is stretching the vagina: thus the adequate stimulus for bearing down may be the same in the human as in the rabbit.

This utero-pituitary reflex became known as 'Ferguson's reflex' and retains its clinical relevance in modern obstetrics when epidural anaesthesia blocks the reflex, stopping the normal physiological increase in oxytocin release during the second stage of labour.

James Kenneth Wallace Ferguson, a Canadian physician/scientist, was born in in Tamsui, Formosa (now Taiwan), on 19 March 1907, the son of a medical missionary. He received his MA in physiology and MD degrees from the University of Toronto. In 1934 he spent a year as a National Research Council fellow in the laboratory of Sir Joseph Barcroft in Cambridge. He became professor of pharmacology at the University of Toronto and later director of the Connaught Medical Research Laboratories in Toronto during the development and introduction of polio vaccines. He was awarded the MBE in 1945 by King George VI for his work in developing a non-freezing oxygen mask for the RAF North Atlantic Ferry Command during the Second World War.

Ferguson retired in 1972 and as professor emeritus remained active, visiting the department of pharmacology at the University of Toronto well into the 1990s. He died in December 1999.

Selected Publications

Ferguson JWK. A study of the motility of the intact uterus at term. *Surg Gynecol Obstet* 1941; 73: 359–66.

Bibliography References

75, 76, 91.

Ferguson, John Creery (1802–1865)

Fetal Heart Auscultation

In November 1827 a 22-year-old woman attended the Dublin General Dispensary complaining of indigestion. She saw the clinic physician, John Creery Ferguson, who applied his recently acquired stethoscopic skills and became the first to hear the fetal heart in Ireland and Britain. He later published his observations in the short-lived journal, *Dublin Medical Transactions*:

She told me her menses were regular and that her abdomen which I observed to be enlarged was so only occasionally. Indeed such was the excellent arrangement of the dyspeptic symptoms which she stated herself to labour under that she completely blind-folded me. However on her third visit . . . I employed the stethoscope . . . The patient received the news with extreme indignation . . . had I not positive evidence of my senses to confirm the opinion I had expressed I should have felt extremely uncomfortable.

He had learned fetal heart auscultation from Jacques Kergaradec and René Laennec during a period of study in Paris in 1827. As a physician, Ferguson's use of the stethoscope was limited to establishing the diagnosis of pregnancy. He introduced it to his obstetrical colleague Robert Collins (1800–1868), Master of the Rotunda Hospital, who enthusiastically grasped its potential. He encouraged its detailed study by his assistant master, Evory Kennedy.

John Creery Ferguson was the son of an apothecary and born in Tandragee, Northern Ireland. The family moved to Dublin and Ferguson graduated MB from Trinity College in 1827. During his student years he also spent time in Edinburgh and Paris. He flourished in Dublin medical circles and became professor of medicine at Apothecaries Hall in 1832 and professor of the practice of medicine at Trinity College Dublin in 1846. He held this position until 1850, when he was appointed the foundation professor of medicine at the new Queen's College of Belfast.

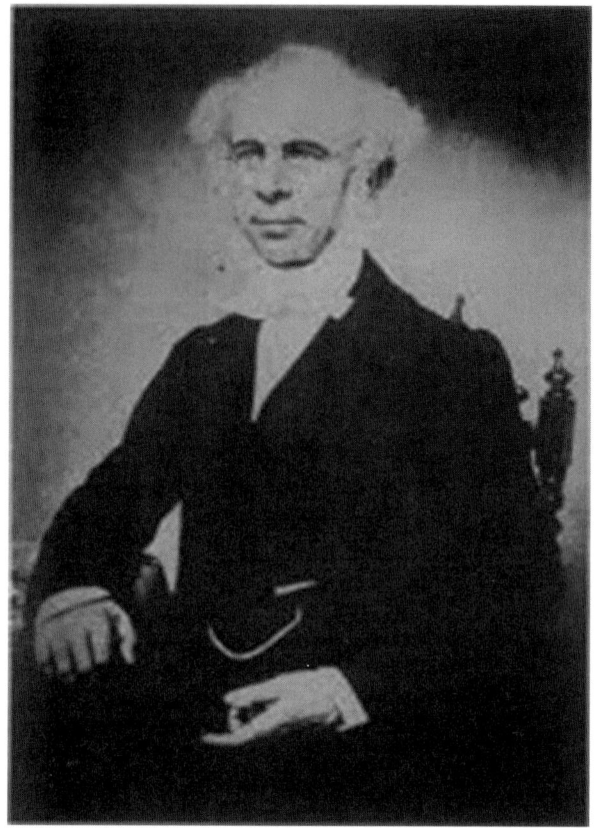

John Creery Ferguson

Selected Publications

Ferguson JC. Auscultation, the only unequivocal evidence of pregnancy, with cases. *Dub Med Trans* 1830; 1: 64.

Bibliography References

1126, 1211, 1212.

Filshie, Gilbert Marcus (b. 1941)

Filshie Clip

While he was still doing his postgraduate training in obstetrics and gynaecology, Marcus Filshie became involved in research on birth control, which was to become a life-long interest. Working under the guidance of Professor Sultan Karim in London, he carried out some of the first studies using prostaglandins for early pregnancy termination. He continued this work with Karim at the Mulago Hospital, Makerere University,

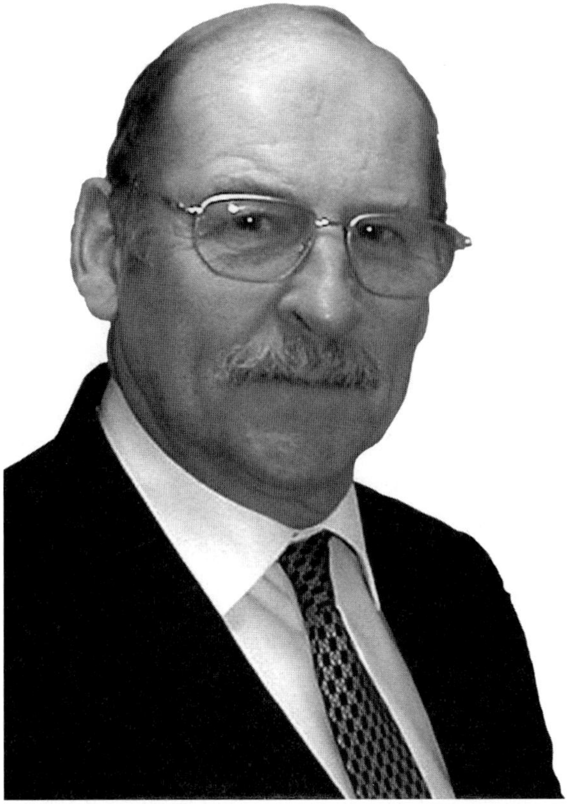

Gilbert Marcus Filshie

Uganda. There he also developed outpatient suction curettage for incomplete miscarriage. Some of his early work was sponsored by the Simon Population Trust, and they offered to fund further research into methods of birth control. Filshie decided to look into simpler techniques for tubal ligation. Working with Don Casey, Chairman of the Simon Population Trust, Filshie suggested a metal clip, the jaws of which would be lined with silicone rubber to remove any dead space and prevent recannalisation. Initial trials were carried out in pigs in 1974, and the first cases in humans were performed in 1975. During the developmental stage, a number of different clips were designed, along with an applicator for use via laparoscopy. The width of the clip, as applied to a tube was 4 mm, the dimensions being similar to a Hulka clip. Filshie felt that its advantage was the simplicity of the clip design and applicator. Appropriate randomised trials were undertaken in the late 1970s, and the final model was produced in 1982. In 1978 Don Casey suggested the clip be called the Filshie clip. Laparoscopic sterilisation using the Filshie clip has proved to be very popular, and by 2017 more than five million pairs had been used worldwide.

Marcus Filshie was born on 21 December 1941. He attended school at Leeds and then entered medical school at the University of London, qualifying in 1966. His postgraduate training in obstetrics and gynaecology was undertaken in London at the King's College and Queen Charlotte's Hospitals. In 1972 he spent a year as senior lecturer at Makerere University in Uganda. He returned in 1973 to a position as lecturer in Obstetrics and Gynaecology at Nottingham University Medical School. He remained in Nottingham and in 1987 was appointed reader in the university department. In 2014, through the Royal College of Obstetricians and Gynaecologists (RCOG), he established and funded the Marcus Filshie Fellowship, which supports an RCOG trainee to work in Uganda for six months.

Selected Publications

Filshie GM, Casey D, Johnson IR, Oats JJ, Lamming GE. A new silastic/tantalum clip for female sterilization. *Br J Obstet Gynaecol* 1977; 84: 236–7.

Filshie GM, Casey D, Pogmore JR, Dutton AG, Symonds EM, Peake AB. The titanium/silicone rubber clip for female sterilization. *Br J Obstet Gynaecol* 1981; 88: 655–62.

Karim SM, Filshie GM. Therapeutic abortion using prostaglandins F2. *Lancet* 1970; 1: 157.

Bibliography References

168, 263, 1190.

Foley, Frederick Eugene Basil (1891–1966)

Foley Catheter

Relief from urinary retention by urethral catheterisation has been undertaken since recorded history. In the beginning, hollow plant stems or feather quills were used. Metal and clay catheters have been in use since the first and second centuries AD. These were particularly suitable for the short female urethra. Attempts to produce flexible catheters involved animal skins stuck together with glue. The first serviceable flexible catheters were produced with the discovery of elastic gum in the eighteenth century, followed by vulcanised rubber catheters in the early nineteenth century. Many patients with chronic urinary retention were taught to catheterise themselves four times a day, and some did so successfully for many years. The first urethral balloon catheter designed for long-term retention was invented in 1853 by the French surgeon JF Reybard. He devised a rubber catheter with a balloon made of pig or sheep caecum. The balloon was inflated with air or water through a separate channel running within the lumen of the rubber catheter.

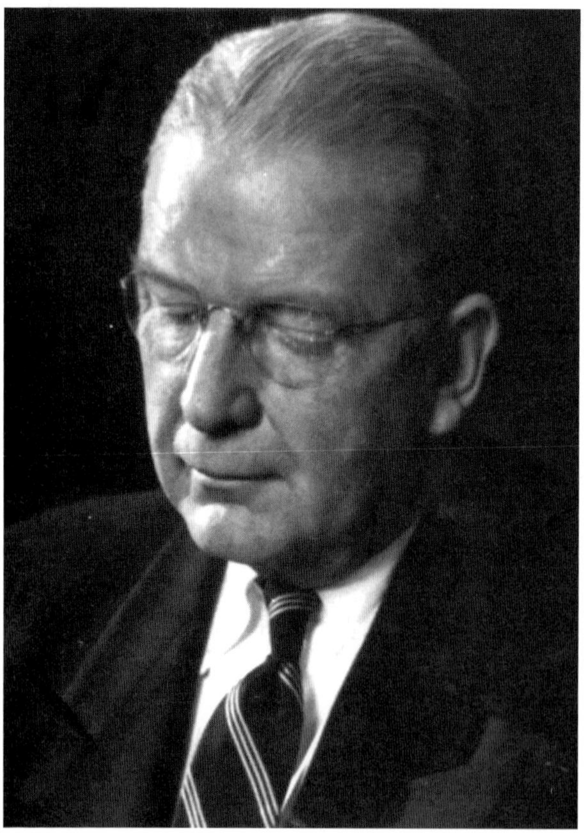

Frederick Eugene Basil Foley

On 25 October 1928, Frederick Foley, a urologist in St Paul, Minnesota, read a paper before the Chicago Urological Society on cystoscopic prostatectomy. The paper was mainly about a new cystoscopic instrument to resect the enlarged prostate gland. However, within this paper was reference to a 'hemostatic bag catheter' which was 'devised by the writer in 1927'. This consisted of an ordinary soft rubber catheter with a balloon sleeve of rubber surrounding the shaft just below the eye at the catheter tip. A smaller diameter rubber catheter ran within the lumen of the larger catheter and through a small perforation in the wall into the cavity of the balloon, which could therefore be distended by fluid injected through the small catheter. Foley designed this catheter for two purposes: to provide haemostatic tamponade to the excised prostatic bed and for continuous drainage of the bladder:

> *From this early experience with the hemostatic bag catheter it was at once evident that a modified form of the device would make an ideal self-retaining indwelling catheter for routine use in constant drainage of the bladder. It was felt that no existing form of 'self-retaining' catheter was actually self-retaining and certainly none of them was eminently satisfactory. The prospect was that the proposed device would give positive self-retention, comfort to the patient and completely satisfactory performance to say nothing of the urologic blessing of relief from adhesive tape fixation.*

By the early 1930s, working with the American Cystoscope Makers Inc., Foley produced the first integral catheter with the balloon channel incorporated into the wall of the catheter. The catheter was now made of latex rubber which was much less irritating than red rubber; 'also it has appeared that latex is tolerated by the urethral mucosa better than the ordinary red rubber catheter'. Thus was born the catheter that has become ubiquitous across all medical specialties in the past 80 years.

Frederick Foley was born in St Cloud, Minnesota. He took his undergraduate degree at Yale in 1914, as a language major, and received his MD from the Johns Hopkins School of Medicine in 1918. He undertook surgical training for two years at Johns Hopkins and for another year at the Peter Brigham Hospital, Boston. He moved back to his home state and practised urology in St Paul, Minnesota. In 1936 he applied for a patent on his fully developed catheter, only to find that the Davol Rubber Company had already received a patent four months earlier. After a number of appeals and reversals of decisions, Foley ultimately lost the patent application. However, across the eponymous world of the urinary catheter his name is used hundreds of times each day. Frederick Foley died of lung cancer in 1966.

Selected Publications

Foley FEB. Cystoscopic prostatectomy: a new procedure and instrument. *J Urol* 1929; 21: 289–308.

Foley FEB. A hemostatic bag catheter: a one-piece latex rubber structure for control of bleeding and constant drainage following prostatic resection. *J Urol* 1937; 36: 134–9.

Foley FEB. A self-retaining bag catheter: for use as an indwelling catheter for constant drainage of the bladder. *J Urol* 1937; 36: 140–3.

Reybard JF. *Traité pratique des rétrécissements du canal de l'uretre*. Paris: Labe; 1853.

Bibliography References

266, 843, 845, 1155.

Fothergill, William Edward (1865–1926)

Manchester Repair Operation/Fothergill's Points and Stitch

Born in Southampton to a Quaker family of Yorkshire descent, with six generations of doctors, William Fothergill was raised in Darlington, England. He took his medical degree at Edinburgh University in 1893 and later worked at St Mary's Hospital, Manchester. He modified Archibald Donald's operation for uterine prolapse. This became known as the Fothergill operation, but later, as Donald's pioneering contribution was recognised, it was called the Manchester operation. Indeed, in Donald's 1908 paper describing his technique, he acknowledges Fothergill's production of the diagrams that 'were drawn during the performance of the operation'. In the Manchester operation Fothergill described four points to be picked up by forceps: one just below the urethral orifice, two slightly posterolateral to the cervix on both sides and one in the midline of the posterior fornix over the apex of the pouch of Douglas. These four points were then joined by an incision to start the operation. The Fothergill stitch involved suturing the stumps of Mackenrodt's ligaments anterior to the excised cervical stump to promote support of the cervix and antevert the uterus.

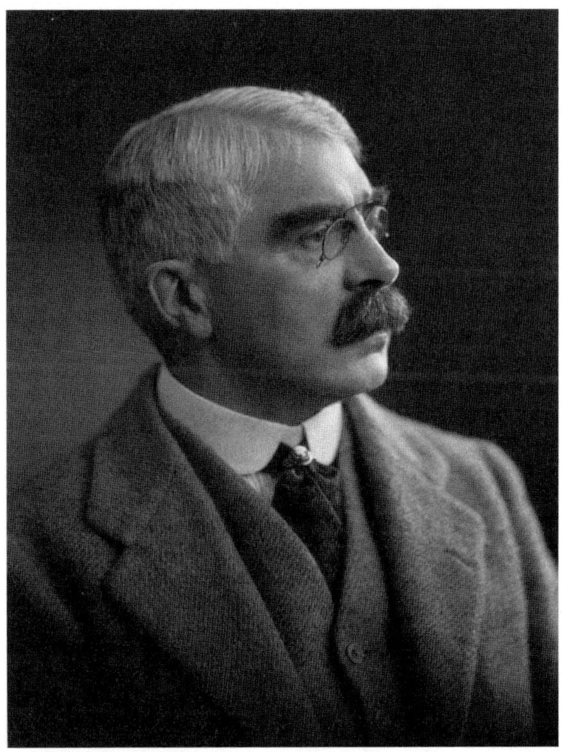

William Edward Fothergill

Fothergill was a firm believer in gynaecologists having an obstetrical training. As he wrote in the introduction of his book, *Manual of Diseases of*

Women, 'no one who has not in one way or another become a good obstetrician can ever hope to understand the diseases of women'.

Fothergill succeeded Donald as professor of obstetrics and gynaecology at Manchester University in 1920. He died shortly after giving a speech at the Glasgow University Club.

Selected Publications

Fothergill WE. Clinical demonstration of an operation for prolapse uteri complicated by hypertrophy of the cervix. *BMJ* 1913; 1: 762–3.

Fothergill WE. Anterior colporrhaphy and its combination with amputation of the cervix as a single operation. *J Obstet Gynaecol Br Emp* 1915; 27: 146–7.

Bibliography References

501, 524, 574, 822.

Fracastoro, Girolamo (1478–1553)

Syphilis

Born in Verona into a noble family, Girolamo Fracastoro studied mathematics, philosophy and medicine at the University of Padua, where he was a fellow student with Nicolaus Copernicus. Fracastoro introduced the name 'syphilis' in his poem, *Syphilis sive de morbo Gallico* (Syphilis or the French Disease), written in Latin hexameter, composed over a 20-year period and published in 1530. The poem described the tribulations of a shepherd called Syphilis who, for impious behaviour, was smitten with the disease by Apollo. It also covered the origins, prevention and treatment of the disease and ran to 1,300 verses. This work brought Fracastoro international fame and was published in several languages and editions. Gradually the name 'syphilis' came to replace the former term *morbus Gallicus*.

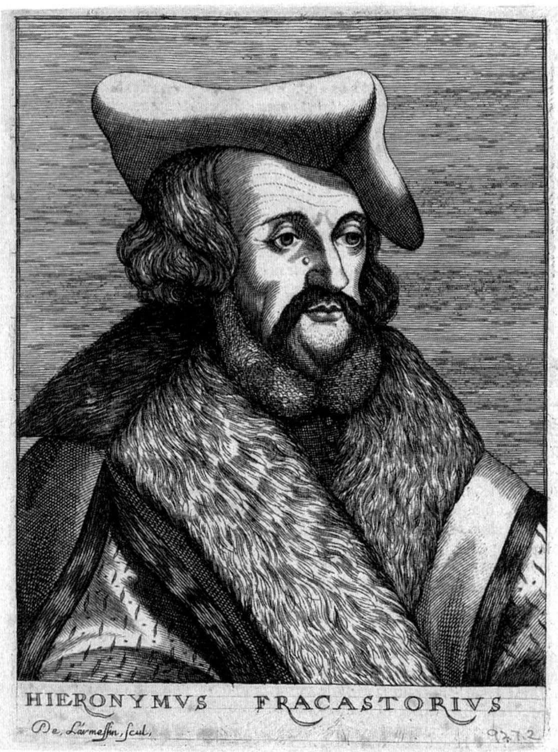

Girolamo Fracastoro

Girolamo Fracastoro is said to have been born with partially fused lips requiring surgical separation. As an infant he is also reputed to have survived within the arms of his mother when she was struck and killed by a lightning bolt. Fracastoro became a physician of high repute and was personal physician to the Bishop of Verona.

The poem which brought him so much acclaim was a relatively light-hearted work. He wrote many scientific articles, and his *Treatise on Contagion*, published in 1546, came close to explaining bacterial infection. His sensible advice to the citizens of Verona during a typhoid epidemic was to 'boil your water and bury your dung'. He died from a stroke on 6 August 1553.

Selected Publications

Fracastoro G. *Syphilis sive de morbo Gallico*. Venice; 1530.

Bibliography References

109, 255, 648, 747, 974, 1072, 1080, 1417, 1549, 1742.

Friedman, Emanuel A. (b. 1926)

Friedman Curve

In the 1940s, in the German literature, a number of studies by Wolf, Koller and Zimmer were published on the graphic representation of cervical dilatation during labour. All of these studies were centred on the influence of rupture of the membranes on the progress of cervical dilatation. None of the studies followed the progression of labour from start to delivery. Indeed, at this time there was not even agreement on the standard measurement for assessing cervical dilatation; frequently used measures were fingerbreadths or the diameter of various coins of various realms.

In 1954 Emanuel A Friedman, then a resident at the Sloane Hospital for Women and the College of Physicians and Surgeons of Columbia University, published his first paper on the graphic analysis of labour. This was followed the next year by his analysis of 500 primigravid labours. As Friedman was later to recount:

> *It was during the long night of June 10, 1953, that the too-frequent periodic examinations I made on the first patients studied, immediately revealed the now familiar characteristic sigmoid curve of normal cervical dilatation. Since that time, extensive study has revealed that the rate of change, within the limits of acceptable error, is specific for each patient and undergoes predictable alterations during the course of normal labor.*

Friedman went on to develop labour curves for primigravid and multiparous women by plotting cervical dilatation against time in labour, taking time zero as the onset of regular contractions. He divided the first stage of labour into the latent phase, during which the cervix dilated slowly, and the active phase, when dilatation was rapid. The active phase was subdivided into the acceleration phase (as the rate of dilatation increased), the phase of maximum slope (the maximum rate of dilatation) and the deceleration phase (at 8–9 cm the dilatation rate slowed slightly and the rate of fetal descent increased). He defined normal and abnormal rates for each of these phases in both primigravid and multiparous women. He divided the abnormal or non-progressive labours into three groups, which he felt allowed the most accurate diagnosis and rationale management: prolonged latent phase, protraction disorders (protracted dilatation and protracted descent) and arrest disorders (arrest of dilatation or arrest of descent). He defined the clinical associations and causes within each of these three groups, promoting more rational diagnosis and management of non-progressive labours.

As Friedman was to note some 20 years after his first study:

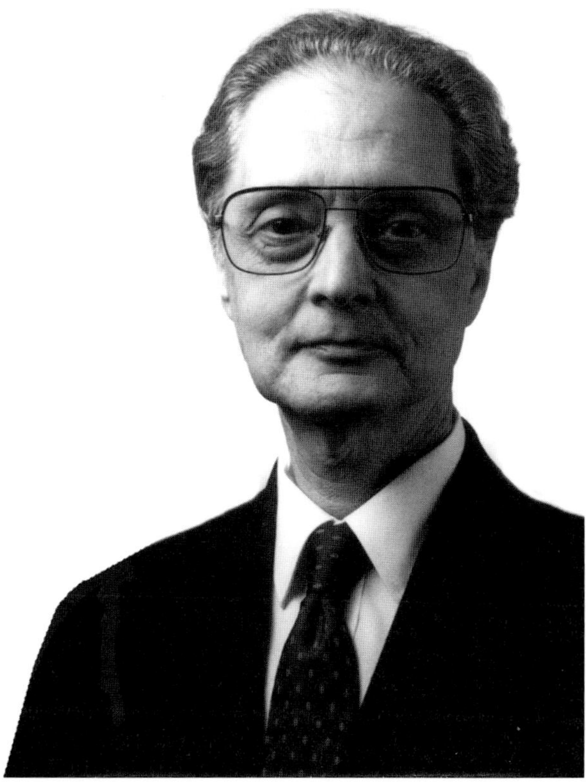

Emanuel A Friedman

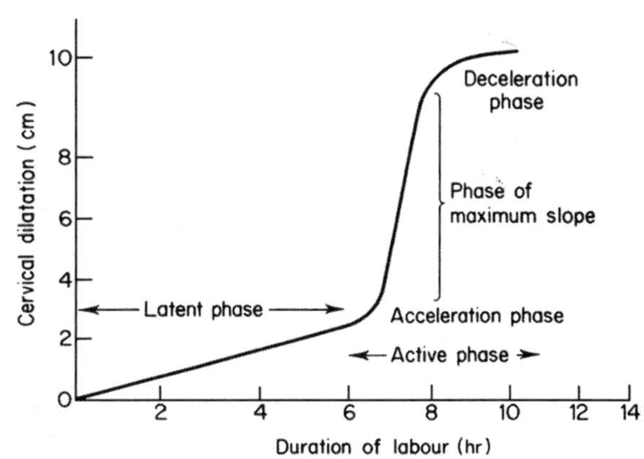

Friedman curve

We now have at hand utilitarian and objective means of evaluating labor in progress and of diagnosing abnormalities of labor as they arise. Given a definitive diagnosis of a specific labor pattern disorder, the appropriate program of management can be applied and pursued, thereby optimizing the outcome from mother and baby. In this way we can more readily fulfill our stated objectives in obstetrics of delivering a healthy baby of a healthy mother.

The simplicity and logic of Friedman's graphic representation of labour became known as the 'Friedman curve'. This graphic representation of labour, or variations of it, has been adopted worldwide in labour partograms. In correspondence with this author Friedman noted that he never calls the labour curve by his own name, 'because I feel the Good Lord made them; I merely described them'. While others, notably Hugh Philpott and Kieran O'Driscoll, have modified Friedman's partograph, they all pay tribute to his seminal work.

Mannie Friedman was born on 9 June 1926 in New York City. After service in the US Navy during the Second World War, he took his BA at Brooklyn College, New York, in 1947 and his MD in 1951 at Columbia University College of Physicians and Surgeons. It was during his time as a college student that he adopted the factitious letter 'A' as his middle name, having not been assigned a middle name at birth. Early on in his studies he was summoned to the dean's office to be told that he was to be dismissed for consistently failing his courses. It turned out that there were three Emanuel Friedmans in the class and he was being confused with another failing student. Luckily this was discovered, and each of the Friedmans were assigned a different middle initial to ensure that this error would not recur. Being the first in line he was assigned the letter 'A', the same letter grade he had received in his exam. He retained the middle initial thereafter.

After medical qualification he spent a year as an intern at the Bellevue Hospital in New York and then five years as a resident in the Columbia University Hospitals, mostly at the Sloane Hospital for Women. He remained as a junior faculty member at Columbia University until he was appointed, in 1963, as professor and chairman of the department of obstetrics and gynaecology at Chicago Medical School. From 1969 to 1990 he worked at the Harvard Medical School in Boston, becoming chairman of the department from 1971 to 1976. In the 1980s, he was one of the first to teach that the risks of mid-pelvic forceps delivery to the baby made this an unacceptable method of delivery.

He retired in 1990, returned to his home city and worked part-time teaching and facilitating the research of junior members at the Albert Einstein College of Medicine in New York. Although he is best known for his work on the graphic analysis of labour, his academic output was prodigious, with more than 500 publications.

Selected Publications

Friedman EA. The graphic analysis of labor. *Am J Obstet Gynecol* 1954; 68: 1568–75.

Friedman EA. The primigravid labor: a graphicostatistical analysis. *Obstet Gynecol* 1955; 6: 567–89.

Friedman EA. Labor management updated. *J Reprod Med* 1978; 20: 59–60.

Friedman EA, Acker DB. Use of midforceps and associated risks. *Am J Obstet Gynecol* 1987; 156: 764–6.

Bibliography References

583, 923, 1218, 1323, 1485.

G

Gardner, Herman L. (1912–1982)

Gardnerella Vaginalis

Herman Gardner was a Texan first and last. He was born in Fort Worth, Texas in 1912 and graduated MD in 1937 from the University of Texas at Galveston. He set up a practice of obstetrics and gynaecology in Houston and remained there for 38 years until his retirement in 1977. He also served as clinical professor at Baylor College of Medicine in Houston. It was here that he teamed up with Charles Dukes of the department of microbiology and began his long-term study of vaginitis. When Gardner began his studies, what is now known as 'bacterial vaginosis' was called non-specific vaginitis. In 1954 Gardner and Dukes published a preliminary report in *Science* in which they stated, 'we have isolated a new bacterium that appears to be the causative agent in the vast majority of so-called "non-specific vaginitides"'. They followed this the next year with a full report in the *American Journal of Obstetrics and Gynecology*. The clinical observations were made by Gardner on 1181 women in his own practice and the bacteriological studies were carried out by Dukes:

> *It has been a long-standing observation of one of us (HLG) that the majority of bacterial vaginitides show on microscopic examination solid fields of small pleomorphic gram-negative bacilli. During several years prior to the present investigation, vaginal material had been sporadically submitted to clinical laboratories for culture. The reports were extremely variable and in no way supported the contention that a single organism was responsible . . . This time a large variety of highly enriched media were used and incubations made under various oxygen and carbon dioxide tensions. At the end of 48 hours, a 10 percent sheep blood agar plate, incubated under reduced oxygen tension, was found to contain thousands of minute transparent colonies which could be detected only by reflected light. A smear from these colonies showed bacilli similar to those seen on the direct smear. After finding the identical organism in pure culture in 13 of the next 14 patients considered as having bacterial vaginitis, it appeared that a specific etiological agent had been found to explain the majority of 'non-specific' bacterial vaginitides We have assigned the name Haemophilus vaginalis to the newly isolated bacillus.*

Thus, the name of this condition became *Haemophilus vaginalis* vaginitis. In 1963 the name of the organism was changed to *Corynebacterium vaginale*, because of physiochemical differences from the *Haemophilus* species. Herman Gardner was honoured in 1980 when the name of the organism was changed to *Gardnerella vaginalis*. In 1984 the term 'bacterial vaginosis' was established to describe the presence of increased discharge associated with a complex alteration in vaginal bacterial flora without an inflammatory reaction.

Herman Gardner was an involved leader in many professional associations and, among other roles, served as President of the Texas Association of Obstetricians and Gynecologists, the Central Association of Obstetricians and Gynecologists and the International Society for the Study of Vulvar Disease. In recognition of his work he received many honours, including the Quadrennial Prize from the Royal Belgium Society of Obstetricians and Gynaecologists. In addition to family and community interests, he had a cattle breeding ranch, was president of the International Brangus Breeders Association and was involved with the Houston Livestock Show and Rodeo. He died in Houston on Christmas Eve 1982. The Herman Gardner Memorial Lecture is given at the Biennial Conference on Diseases of the Vulva and Vagina.

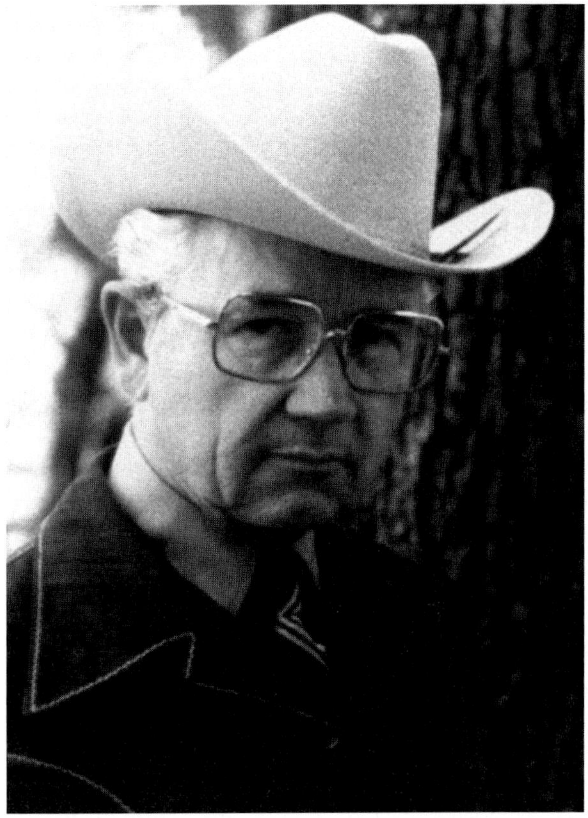

Herman L Gardner

Selected Publications

Gardner HL, Dukes CD. New etiologic agent in non-specific bacterial vaginitis. *Science* 1954; 120: 853.

Gardner HL, Dukes CD. *Haemophilus vaginalis* vaginitis. *Am J Obstet Gynecol* 1955; 69: 962–76.

Greenwood JR, Pickett MJ. Transfer of *Haemophilus vaginalis* Gardner and Dukes to a new genus *Gardnerella: G. Vaginalis (Gardner and Dukes). Int J System Bacteriol* 1980; 30: 170–8.

Mardh PA, Taylor-Robinson D. *Bacterial Vaginosis*. Uppsala, Stockholm: Almquist and Wiksell, 1984, pp. 259–60.

Zinnemann K, Turner GC. The taxonomic position of 'Haemophilus vaginitis' (Corynebacterium vaginale). *J Pathol Bacteriol* 1963;85: 213–9.

Gartner, Hermann Treschow (1785–1827)

Gartner's Duct

After the mesonephros develops into the fetal kidney, the mesonephric or Wolffian duct involutes. However, vestigial tubular remnants may be identified within the leaves of the broad ligament, the cervix and lateral walls of the vagina. These were first described in detail in the cow and sow by the Danish anatomist, Hermann Gartner, in 1822:

> *I have examined many uteri . . . I have generally found the same result, namely, a canal which begins on each side of the place where the vagina terminates in the cornu uteri, passes through a glandular body in the middle of the vagina, goes under the sphincter vesical, and perforates the vagina close beside the orifice of the urethra.*

Hermann Treschow Gartner was born in October 1785 at St Thomas, West Indies, then a Danish colony, where his father was a government official. The family returned to Copenhagen when young Gartner was 10 years old. He took medicine in Copenhagen graduating in 1807. He later studied in London and Edinburgh. He practised in Copenhagen and became surgeon to the Danish Army.

Gartner died in Copenhagen on 4 April 1827. No known portrait of him exists.

Selected Publications

Gartner H. An anatomical description of a glandular organ observed in the uterus of some lower animals (abstract). *Edin Med Surg J* 1824; 21: 460–3.

Bibliography References

406, 552, 605, 978, 1486.

Gaskin, Ina May (b. 1940)

Gaskin All-Fours Manoeuvre

Ina May Middleton was born in small-town Iowa on 8 March 1940 to parents with a strong work, education and protestant religious ethic. She took her MA in English studies. In San Francisco she met and married Stephen Gaskin, a teacher and Zen pastor. In 1970, along with 300 like-minded hippies, they set out on a cross-country tour in some 50 school buses that were converted to mobile homes. During the tour, 11 of the women had babies and Ina May Gaskin, based on having had one child herself, was considered the most qualified birth attendant.

The first delivery was conducted in one of the buses in a university parking lot. Gaskin was profoundly affected by the experience and 'felt a definite calling to be a midwife'. The caravan of buses ultimately reached Summerton, south of Nashville, Tennessee, where they established a commune, The Farm, on 1,000 acres of woodland and fields.

Within the commune Gaskin and a small group of potential midwives established The Farm Midwifery Center. With reading and support from local obstetricians they developed experience and proficiency, ultimately becoming certified professional midwives. Over the next 30 years they looked after some 2,000 pregnancies and delivered 95 per cent at home. Gaskin promoted low-intervention childbirth with maintenance of the skills necessary for assisted vaginal delivery of breech and twins, and the retention of certain techniques used by indigenous midwives in central and South America.

It was in this context, in 1976, that she adopted the all-fours manoeuvre for shoulder dystocia, having learned this from a midwife in Guatemala who in turn had observed it in Mayan Indians. Gaskin wrote of the all-fours manoeuvre in her book, *Spiritual Midwifery*, which went through four editions between 1976 and 2002:

> *Instead of the mother's coccyx being pushed towards the symphysis pubis in the way it is in the seated position, there is no pressure on the coccyx and the baby's weight is pushing on the symphysis pubis, thereby widening the anterior to posterior diameter a little.*

In the all-fours posture, the flexibility of the sacro-iliac joints may allow a 1–2 cm increase in the antero-posterior diameter of the pelvic inlet. In addition, gravity can help the posterior shoulder descend below the sacral promontory. With this technique the posterior shoulder is delivered first by gentle head traction.

In 1991, Gaskin collaborated with family physicians to have the manoeuvre published in the medical literature, with a report of 32 cases of shoulder dystocia, all of which had been resolved with the all-fours position. The manoeuvre has been adopted by obstetricians and incorporated into obstetric texts and national guidelines on shoulder dystocia. It has become a valuable additional technique for the beleaguered accoucheur faced with this complication.

Ina May Gaskin's work at The Farm Midwifery Center has been widely recognised. She received an honorary degree from Thames Valley University in London in 2009, and the Right Livelihood Award in 2011, 'for her whole life's work teaching and advocating safe, woman-centred childbirth methods that best promote the physical and mental health of mother and child'.

Selected Publications

Gaskin IM. Shoulder dystocia: controversies in management. *Birth Gazette*. 1988; 5: 14–17.

Meehan AL, Gaskin IM, Hunt P, Ball CA. A new (old) maneuver for the management of shoulder dystocia. *J Family Practice* 1991; 32: 625–9.

Bruner JP, Drummond SB, Meenan AL, Gaskin IM. All-fours maneuver for reducing shoulder dystocia during labor. *J Reprod Med* 1998; 43: 439–43.

Gaskin IM. *Spiritual Midwifery*. 4th edn. Summertown, TN: Book Publishing Company; 2002, p. 354.

Bibliography References

99, 115, 491, 662, 1385.

Giffard, William (d. 1731)

Obstetric Forceps/Breech Delivery

William Giffard, a surgeon and man-midwife working in London, was prominent among those responsible for the introduction of obstetric forceps into common use in England. The earliest recorded use, unsuccessful, of obstetric forceps was by Giffard on April 18 1726. He later reported a successful delivery using his 'extractor' on 28 June 1728:

> *... whereupon I passed my extractor and drew it with much difficulty forwards toward the labia, and then taking hold of the head on each side with my hands (which cannot be done whilst it lies in the vagina) I drew the shoulders out; the other parts readily followed ... This case proves, that a child presenting right, but sticking in the passage, may be brought alive (I won't say always) without either use of hooks, or lessening the head, contrary to the opinion of most former writers.*

These reports came from the records of 225 cases carefully collected by Giffard in his obstetric practice, much of it among the poor of London. This was edited and published by his physician friend and colleague, Edward Hody, in 1734, three years after Giffard's death. By right Giffard's name should be attached to the manoeuvre used to deliver the after-coming head of the breech, known eponymously as the Mauriceau–Smellie–Veit manoeuvre. Giffard described his technique in case report No. 13 on 6 April 1726:

> *I clapped one hand flat upon the breast, and with the other taking hold above the shoulders, drew towards me, but the head did not readily follow: I therefore passed my fingers up to the child's mouth, supporting the breast with my wrist and arm, and putting one finger into the mouth,*

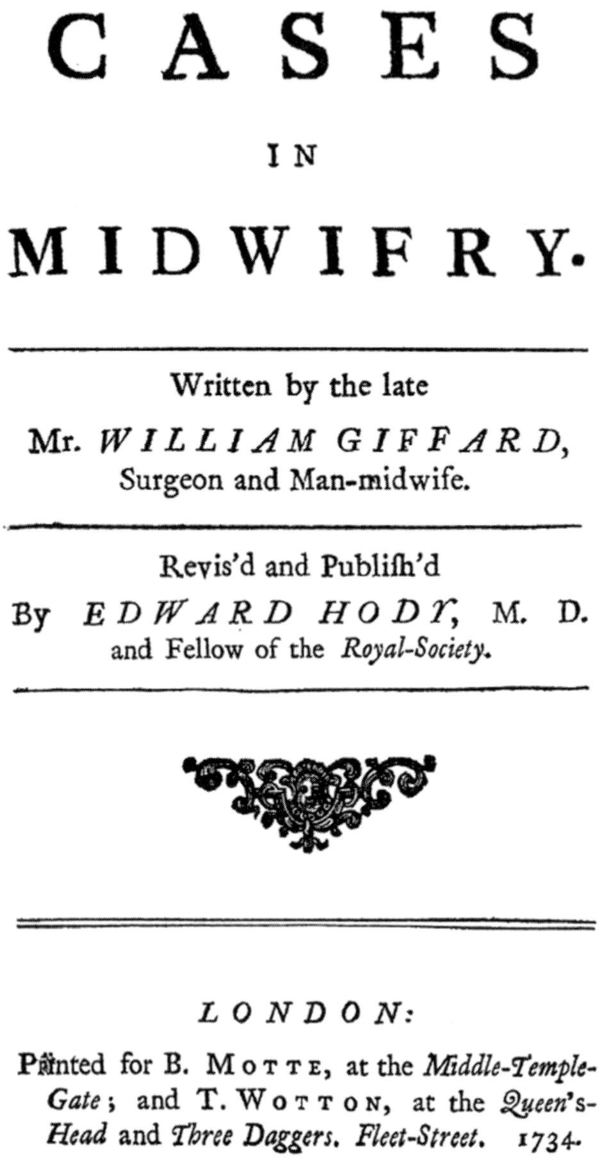

CASES

IN

MIDWIFRY.

Written by the late

Mr. *WILLIAM GIFFARD*,

Surgeon and Man-midwife.

Revis'd and Publiſh'd

By *EDWARD HODY*, M. D.

and Fellow of the *Royal-Society*.

LONDON:

Printed for B. Motte, at the *Middle-Temple-Gate*; and T. Wotton, at the *Queen*'s-*Head* and *Three Daggers*. *Fleet-Street*. 1734.

Title page of Giffard's *Cases in Midwifery*

and two others upon the cheeks, I pulled towards me, and at the same time drawing with my other hand above the shoulders, brought out the head.

Jacques Guillemeau, almost a century before, had advocated flexion of the aftercoming head with one or two fingers in the mouth, but the full manoeuvre with both hands was described by Giffard. François Mauriceau's technique advocated an assistant to pull on the legs. William Smellie adopted the same technique as Giffard. Aloys Gustav Veit (1824–1903) popularised the manoeuvre in Germany but contributed nothing else. Perhaps it is the lyrical roll of the triple eponym, 'Mauriceau–Smellie–Veit', that has ensured the erroneous, but enduring legacy.

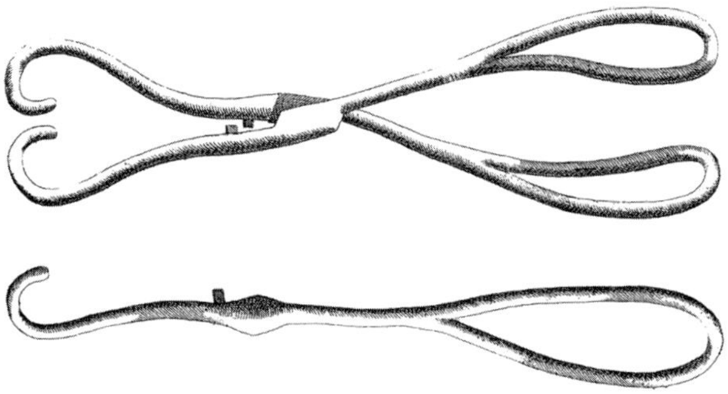

Illustration of William Giffard's 'extractor' in his *Cases in Midwifery*

According to his friend, Edward Hody, Giffard was 'a plain man, remarkable for an honest, frank behaviour, of strong judgement, skilful and experienced in his profession, and very charitable to the poor, averse to all kinds of flattery, and a generous and judicious practitioner'.

William Giffard retired to Brentwood, Essex and died there in 1731.

Selected Publications

Giffard W. *Cases in Midwifery*, revised and published by Edward Hody. London: Motte; 1734. Also published in: The Classics of Obstetrics and Gynecology Library. New York, NY: Gryphon Editions; 1995 (facsimile).

Veit G. Über die beste Methode zur Extraktion des nachfolgenden Kindeskopfes. *Greiswald Med Beitr* 1863; 2: 19.

Bibliography References

347, 361, 399, 503, 548, 648, 983, 1261, 1595, 1710.

Gigli, Leonardo (1863–1908)

Gigli's Saw

One of the more barbaric chapters of obstetrics involved attempts to overcome pelvic contraction by dividing the upper pubic ramus, known as pubiotomy, to enlarge the pelvic inlet. In the face of almost certain maternal death from caesarean section or loss of the infant from the destructive procedures necessary for vaginal delivery in cases of contracted pelvis, obstetricians searched for less lethal methods of assistance. Symphysiotomy enjoyed favour with some, but the mortality and morbidity were still considerable.

The first use of the chain saw in obstetrics was that of the Edinburgh obstetrician John Aitken in 1785. It consisted of jointed links like a watch chain with a serrated cutting surface on the concave side. A hook at each end accommodated a handle or a curved blunt needle for placement; the latter was then removed and a second handle attached. By pulling alternately on each handle the saw cut through the bone. Aitken used this to perform symphysiotomy and he also suggested pubiotomy. However, attempts to perform pubiotomy were frustrated by the crudeness of the chain-type saws. In the late nineteenth century, Leonardo Gigli, an Italian obstetrician working in Breslau, developed a fine (0.65 mm) string wire saw after extensive studies on cadavers.

The advantage of Gigli's design was that it was much finer and sharper and cut easily through bone. Aitken's saw tended to clog and blunt quickly. As Gigli wrote:

> *I thought I could simplify symphysiotomy by means of these wires and make its technique more reliable. An oblique cut through the os pubis, to the right or left of where the head lies . . . is much easier and much more certain than the median incision, because all the dangers of the latter are thereby avoided and its advantages preserved.*

Gigli went on to describe the preparatory suprapubic incision and placement of the saw by means of a needle guide:

> *Having thus applied the string saw, we can accomplish the division of the bone with a few strokes, easily and with great safety, as though the bone were not being sawed but cut with a knife. I have done this very rapidly with the string saw many times.*

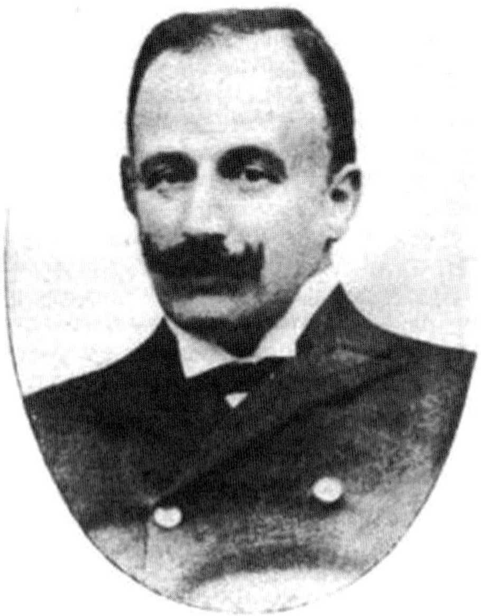

Leonardo Gigli

He added a suitable note of caution:

Although the instrument has now been brought to a stage of complete development, it is still the operator's responsibility to exercise special skill at all stages of the operation and to develop the dexterity necessary for manipulation of the saw.

Pubiotomy had limited popularity in Europe and marginal acceptance in the United States, where John Whitridge Williams was one of its supporters. However, by the 1920s, as the safety of caesarean section increased, it was abandoned in obstetrics and the saw bequeathed to orthopaedic and neurosurgical colleagues.

Leonardo Gigli was born in Sesto Fiorentino, Italy. He qualified in 1889, obtaining his MD from the University of Florence. After two years postgraduate training in Florence he travelled for further study to Paris, London and Breslau, where he developed his pubiotomy saw. Upon return to Florence in 1893 he gained a hospital appointment but his hopes for a teaching position at the University of Florence were denied. He was embittered by the opposition and criticism of his Florentine colleagues, despite his high reputation in Germany. Gigli died of pneumonia on 4 April 1908 just before his forty-fifth birthday.

Selected Publications

Gigli L. Della sezione della sinfisi con la sega in filo metallico (Drahtsager). *Ann Ostet Ginec* 1893; 15: 557–60.

Gigli L. Über ein neues Instrument zum Durchtrennen der Knochen, die Drahtsäge. *Zentralbl Chir* 1894; 21: 409–11.

Bibliography References

25, 205, 206, 614, 648, 692, 721, 846, 1261, 1280, 1430, 1486, 1646, 1728.

Gilliam, David Tod (1844–1923)

Gilliam's Uterine Ventrosuspension

Of the many operations devised to suspend the uterus in the late nineteenth and early twentieth century, the procedure described by Gilliam was one of the simplest and most effective. In his publication of 1900 he outlined: 'The basic principle of this operation is that of invagination of the proximal portion of the round ligaments into the abdominal wall . . .'. He achieved this by ligating the round ligament and pulling it through the peritoneum lateral to the rectus muscle. The ligated portion of each round ligament was then sutured to the anterior rectus sheath.

David Tod Gilliam was born in Hebron, Ohio on 3 April 1844. At the age of 17, he joined the army and served in the Civil War. He was wounded and

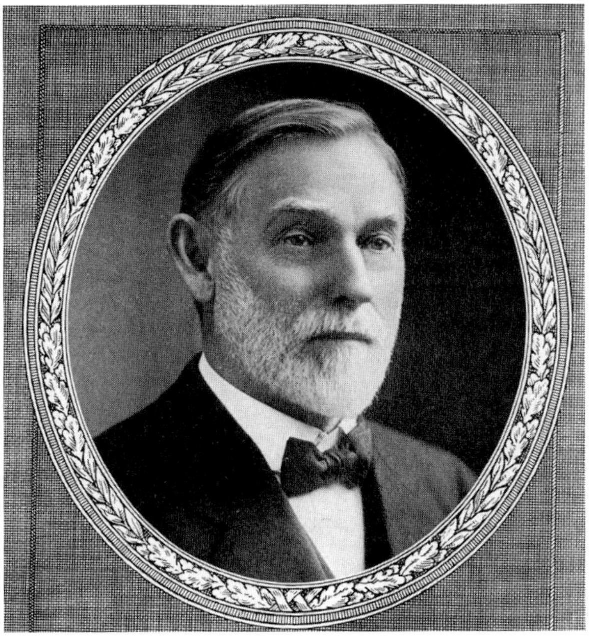

David Tod Gilliam

captured by the Confederates but later escaped. He entered medical school and graduated from the Cincinnati Medical College in 1871. After several years of general practice, he embarked upon a remarkable peripatetic academic career, becoming successively professor of pathology at Columbus Medical College in 1877, professor of physiology at Starling Medical College in 1879 and in 1885 professor of obstetrics and gynaecology at the same school. His clinical work was done at the St Anthony's and St Francis' Hospitals in Columbus, Ohio. Gilliam held high office as president of the Ohio State Medical Association and vice-president of the American Medical Association.

He died of a cerebral haemorrhage on 2 October 1923. His son and grandson also became surgeons.

Selected Publications

Gilliam DT. Round ligament ventrosuspension of the uterus: A new method. *Am J Obstet Dis Women Child* 1900; 41: 299–303.

Gilliam DT. *A Text-book of Practical Gynecology for Practitioners and Students.* 4th edn. Philadelphia, PA: FA Davis Co; 1911, pp. 222–6.

Bibliography References

330, 524, 619, 1237, 1485, 1749.

Goodell, William (1829–1894)

Goodell's Sign

William Goodell described softening of the cervix as an early sign of pregnancy:

> *If the cervix has the consistency of the tip of one's nose, pregnancy is unlikely. When the cervix is soft as one's lips, pregnancy is probable.*

William Goodell was born on 27 October 1829 in Malta, the son of a missionary. He was educated in the United States and graduated from Jefferson Medical College in 1854. He practised medicine for several years in Constantinople, where his parents worked, but left Turkey and returned to the United States in 1861. Goodell was the medical director of the Preston Retreat Lying-in Hospital in Philadelphia from its opening in 1866 until 1887. He introduced early post-partum ambulation, based on his observations in Turkey, where he noted that native women resumed full activity within hours of delivery without detriment. In 1870 he was appointed lecturer in obstetrics and diseases of women at the University of Pennsylvania, rising to clinical professor in 1874. His literary and lecturing talents were legendary in Philadelphia. He was a conservative surgeon and one of the first to employ Ignac Semmelweis' principles in the prevention of puerperal sepsis.

Goodell suffered from gout and, in his later years, from intractable insomnia. He died on his birthday in

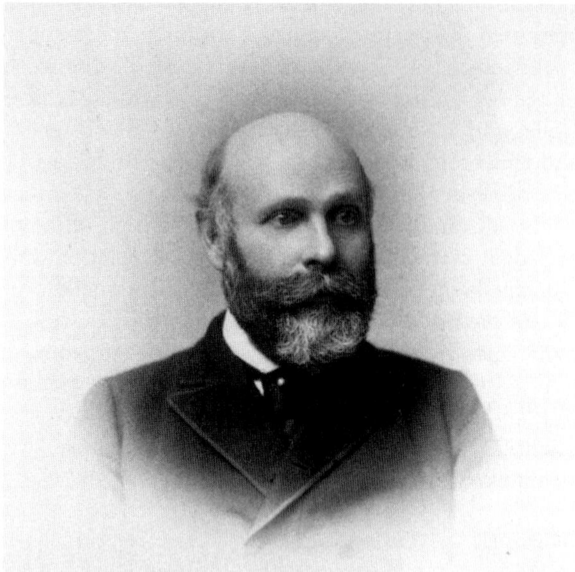

William Goodell

1894 following a stroke. The head of the department of obstetrics and gynecology at the University of Pennsylvania is the William Goodell Professor.

Selected Publications

Goodell W. *Lessons in Gynecology*. 3rd edn. Philadelphia, PA: F. A. Davis; 1889.

Bibliography References

98, 139, 634, 801, 1485.

Gordon, Alexander (1752–1799)

Puerperal Sepsis

It is to Ignac Semmelweis that the credit has been given for proving the contagious nature of puerperal fever and, in particular, the method of its prevention. However, 65 years before the publication of Semmelweis' epic work, Alexander Gordon of Aberdeen had clearly demonstrated the infective nature of puerperal fever in his *Treatise on the Epidemic Puerperal Fever of Aberdeen*, published in 1795. In observing two epidemics of erysipelas in 1787 and 1788 he found they occurred concomitantly with epidemics of puerperal fever:

> *That the cause of this disease was a specific contagion, or infection, I have unquestionable proof . . . this disease seized such women only, as were visited, or delivered, by a practitioner, or taken care of by a nurse, who had previously attended patients affected with the disease. In short, I had evident proofs of its infectious nature, and that the infection was as readily communicated as that of the small-pox, or measles and operated more speedily than any other infection with which I am acquainted.*
>
> *The midwife, who delivered No. 1. on the table, carried the infection to No. 2, the next women whom she delivered. The physician, who attended No. 1 and 2, carried the infection to No. 5 and 6, who were delivered by him and to many others.*
>
> *It is a disagreeable declaration for me to mention, that I myself was the means of carrying the infection to a great number of women.*

Gordon also suggested techniques for prevention, although, unlike Semmelweis, he did not report on the application of these methods:

> *The same means ought to be practised, for preventing the infection of the Puerperal Fever. The patient's apparel and bed-clothes ought, either to be burnt, or thoroughly purified; and the nurses and physicians who have attended patients affected with the Puerperal Fever, ought carefully to wash themselves, and to get their apparel properly fumigated, before it be put on again.*

Needless to say, Gordon's observations were not well received by the local midwives and

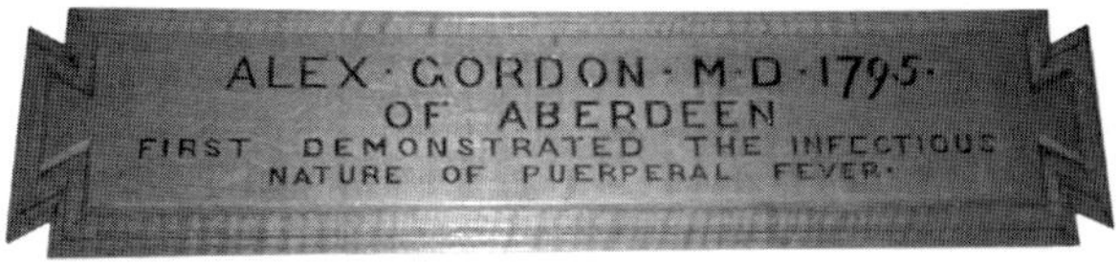
ALEX · GORDON · M·D ·1795·
OF ABERDEEN
FIRST DEMONSTRATED THE INFECTIOUS
NATURE OF PUERPERAL FEVER·

Plaque dedicated to Alexander Gordon at the Aberdeen Maternity Hospital

physician-accouchers. As he was to write in the preface to his *Treatise*:

> *The benevolent reader must observe, with displeasure, the ungenerous treatment which I met with from that very sex whose sufferings I was at so much pains to relieve; for, while I was using my best endeavors to mitigate the calamities of many miserable sufferers, several others were very busy traducing my character, who prompted by prejudice, very uncandidly proclaimed the deaths, and concealed the cures on purpose to raise an odium against my practice.*

Alexander Gordon, the son of a tenant farmer, was born in Miltown of Drum, Peterculter, near Aberdeen, Scotland. From these humble origins Gordon was sufficiently industrious to get his MA degree from Marischal College in Aberdeen in 1775. He then studied medicine at the Aberdeen Infirmary and Edinburgh University. After graduation he served for five years as surgeon's mate and then surgeon in the Royal Navy, thence to London for further training at the Middlesex Lying-in Dispensary and Westminster Hospital. Here he attended lectures by Thomas Denman, to whom he later dedicated his treatise. He returned to Aberdeen in 1785. In 1788 Gordon was awarded the MD from his home university. There he lectured to midwives and medical students and concentrated on obstetric practice. Shortly after publication of his treatise he was recalled for naval service and contracted tuberculosis. He died at the home of his twin brother, James, in Logie, Aberdeenshire. Alexander Gordon is buried at the West Kirk of St Nicholas in Aberdeen, part of which dates from the twelfth century.

Selected Publications

Gordon A. *A Treatise on the Epidemic Puerperal Fever of Aberdeen*. London: GG and J Robinson; 1795.

Bibliography References

51, 124, 275, 301, 377, 471, 648, 681, 822, 882, 939, 940, 946, 1049, 1203, 1228, 1518, 1590, 1595.

Graaf, Regnier de (1641–1673)

Graafian Follicle

Before the seventeenth century the mammalian egg was felt to arise from an amalgam of semen from the ovary passed down the fallopian tube and mixed with male semen in the uterus. Both Andreas Vesalius and Gabriel Fallopius described vesicles in the female testis, as the ovary was then called, but were unaware that these contained the ovum. Later the ovaries of birds were recognised as the organs of egg formation in that species. Nicholas Stenson (1638–1686), the Danish anatomist, Jan Swammerdam (1637–1680) and Johannes Van Horne (1621–1670) from Leyden independently deduced that the female testes (ovaries) were, as in the bird, the site of egg formation. However, these observations, made between 1666 and 1667, were not published. Swammerdam later attacked the veracity of de Graaf's work, to no avail.

In 1672 de Graaf described the ovarian follicles, their maturation and function:

> *Thus, the general function of the female testicles is to generate the ova, to nourish them, and to bring them to maturity, so that they serve the same purpose in women as the ovaries of birds. Hence, they should rather be called ovaries than testes because they show no similarity, either in form or contents, with the male testes.*

In the pre-microscopic era Karl von Baer described the individual ovum. De Graaf also described the corpus luteum, calling it the *substantia glandulosa*, but incorrectly felt it denoted conception based on his study of rabbits.

It is possible that de Graaf described the first case of congenital adrenal hyperplasia:

> *On the 27th June 1670, there was born at Delft an infant, whom, because of the malformation of its genital parts, its*

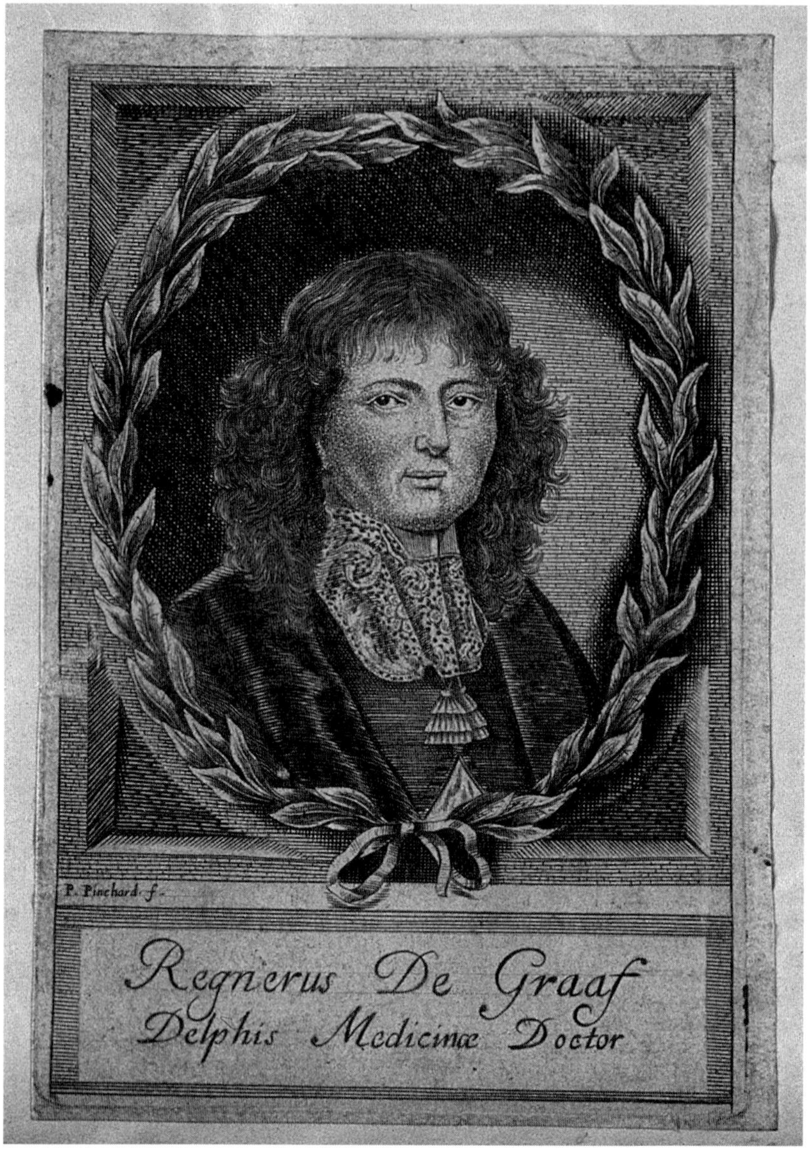

Regnier de Graaf

parents did not want distinguished with either a male or female name until they had consulted experts in the matter.

The infant was designated male (Cornelius) but died at 22 days of age, 'struck by a serious illness' (possibly salt depletion). After careful post-mortem dissection, de Graaf and his colleagues concluded, 'From what has been said it is more than clear that this infant was merely a girl with a huge clitoris'.

Regnier de Graaf was born in Schoonhaven, Holland. He took his medical training at Utrecht and Leyden with additional studies in France. He carried out physiological studies on pancreatic function, gaining him the MD from Leyden in 1663. In 1688 he published a detailed anatomical treatise on the male genital organs, followed four years later by his account of the ovary. In 1672 the chair of anatomy at Leyden became vacant but de Graaf was not appointed, possibly because he was Catholic. De

Graaf died of the plague in Delft when he was 32 years old.

Selected Publications

de Graaf R. *De mulierum organis generatoani inservientibus.* Leyden: Hackiana; 1672.

Jocelyn HD, Setchell BP. Regnier de Graaf on the human reproductive organs (English translation). *J Reprod Fertil* 1972; Suppl 17.

Bibliography References

251, 406, 548, 552, 606, 615, 648, 676, 689, 742, 873, 1031, 1102, 1371, 1469, 1703.

Gräfenberg, Ernst (1881–1957)

Gräfenberg Ring

Ernst Gräfenberg was born on 26 September 1881 in Adelebsen, Germany, a small town surrounded by hills, one of which was called Gräfen-Berg (Count's Hill). In the nineteenth century, when Jews were allowed to acquire family names, Gräfenberg's family took on the name of the hill. Gräfenberg took his medical studies in Munich and Göttingen, graduating in 1905. He initially studied ophthalmology but changed to obstetrics and gynaecology and worked under Herman Pfannenstiel at Kiel. In 1910 he entered gynaecological practice in Berlin and later became head of the gynaecology department of the Municipal Hospital in the Britz district of Berlin. This was a low-income community with many septic abortions. Gräfenberg was involved with the birth control movement from its early days and began investigating the intrauterine contraceptive device (IUCD) in 1920. Others from Germany, including Richard Richter and Karl Pust, had used the IUCD in the early 1900s, but Gräfenberg studied it most carefully. He first presented his method at a post graduate course organised by Margaret Sanger in December 1928.

Gräfenberg's original IUCD was made of silkworm gut and shaped like a star. He later changed it to a ring made of silver, which at that time contained 26 per cent copper, and found lower expulsion, pregnancy and infection rates. In his careful study he included endometrial biopsies, in conjunction with Robert Meyer, and found no inflammatory changes in the endometrium. He found that the tailless silver ring was least likely to cause infection.

The key to Gräfenberg's low infection rate was that his device was isolated in the uterine cavity, compared to the standard cervico-uterine devices that established a direct connection between the vagina and the uterine cavity. He said, 'I lay much stress upon the fact that in the method which I recommend no part of the device projects beyond the inner edge of the cervix'. In 1931 Gräfenberg reported on his experience with 1,500 silkworm and 600 silver rings. Most of the clinical aspects of IUCD use that are recommended today were established by Gräfenberg. He did however have some rather

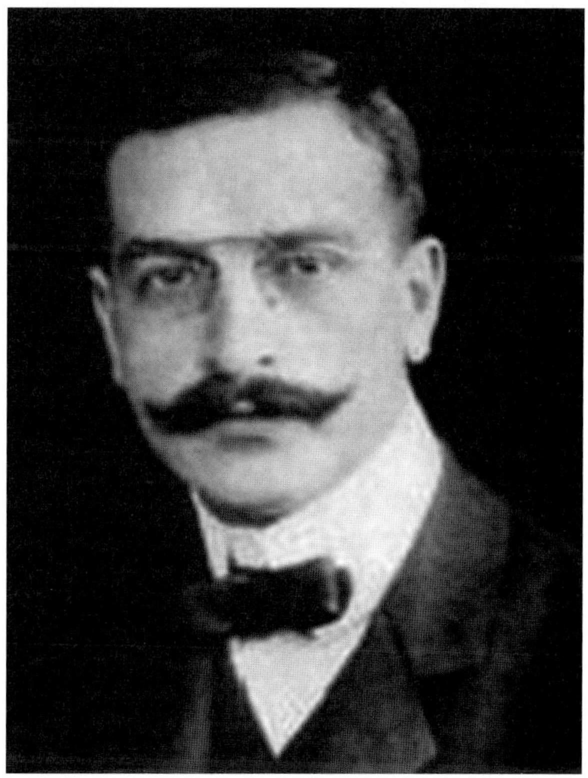

Ernst Gräfenberg

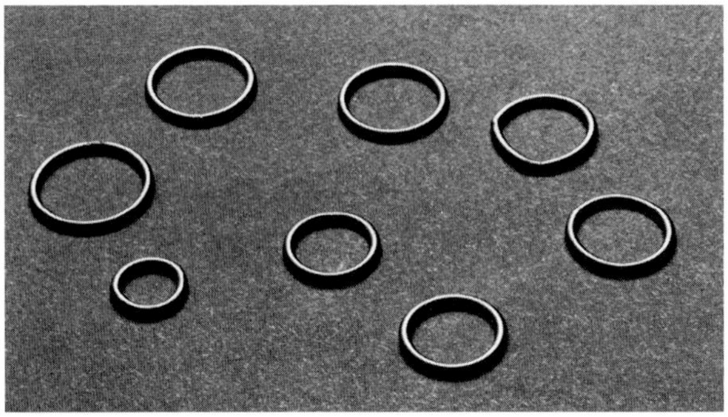

Gräfenberg rings

pointed observations on the characteristics of some couples, which if expressed nowadays would evoke harsh criticism:

> *Every method that affects the man is doomed to failure, for the man must not be balked in his pleasure, whereas the woman is always the one to suffer. We must also remember, however, that many women are lazy and stupid, and take no interest in protecting themselves. All these points must be taken into consideration.*

In the poisonous political climate of Germany in 1937, Gräfenberg was jailed. His long-standing friendship with Margaret Sanger saved him, as she was able to negotiate his release, after paying a ransom. He left Germany for the United States in 1940, to start again at the age of 60. For the first year he worked as a pathologist in Chicago, while he passed his American licensing examinations. He then settled in New York and built a large private practice; many of his patients were also German exiles. He worked at the Mount Sinai and Sydenham hospitals and the Margaret Sanger Research Bureau. During his years in New York Gräfenberg developed a stainless-steel ring but used it in comparative secrecy because of the prevailing medical opinion against the IUCD. Apparently, many celebrities sought this service, with both parties being assured of confidentiality.

Gräfenberg died from the effects of progressive Parkinson's disease on 28 October 1957. There was no announcement of his death in the medical journals. It was some years after his death before his enormous contribution to intrauterine contraception was accepted and recognised.

Selected Publications

Gräfenberg E. Intrauterine Methods: An Intrauterine Contraceptive Method. In: Sanger M, Stone HM (eds). *Proceedings of the Seventh International Birth Control Conference: The Practice of Contraception.* Baltimore, MD: Williams and Wilkins; 1931: pp. 33–47. Also published in: The Classics of Obstetrics and Gynecology Library. New York, NY: Gryphon Editions; 1992 (facsimile).

Pust K. Ein brauchbarer Frauenschutz. *Deutsche Med Wochenschr* 1923; 49: 952–3.

Richter R. Ein Mittel zus Verhutung der Konzeption. *Deutsche Med Wochenschr* 1909; 35: 1525.

Bibliography References

368, 504, 656, 886, 1366, 1486, 1576, 1599, 1614.

Graves, TW (c.1870)

Graves' Speculum

The vaginal speculum has been used since antiquity to diagnose and treat cervical and vaginal disorders. Of the bivalve variety, the one in most common use is the Graves speculum or a modification thereof. Other bivalve specula were devised by Marie Boivin in 1825 and Edward Gabriel Cusco (1819–1894). Cusco was an ingenious surgeon-inventor who worked at the Hôtel Dieu in Paris.

In 1878 Graves sent an illustration of his speculum design along with explanatory notes to the *New York Medical Journal.* In the notes he said,

> *I wish to state in the beginning that it is not original except in its arrangement, being a combination of the 'bivalve' and 'Sims' speculum with the addition of an extending (or rather distending) movement . . . the extension especially meet the requirements of the general practitioner, who, making his examination without aid, needs a reliable instrument that will accommodate itself to the variable dimensions of different vaginae . . .*

Almost nothing is known of TW Graves other than that he was a general practitioner in Woburn, Massachusetts.

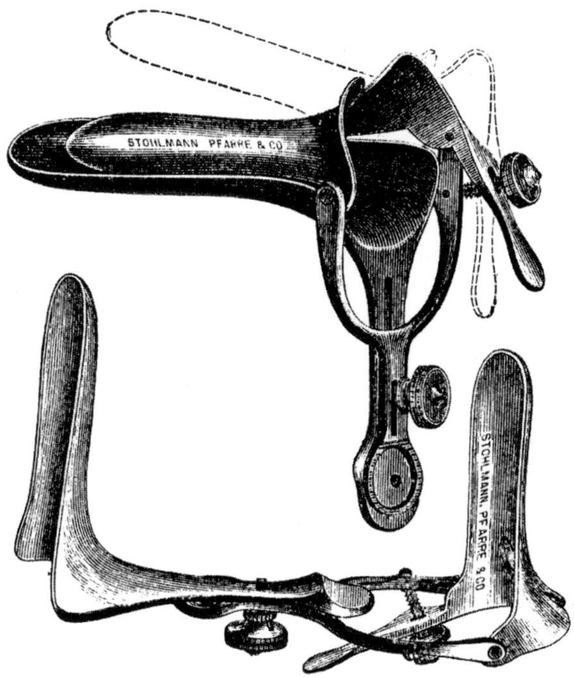

Graves' speculum

Selected Publications

Graves TW. A new vaginal speculum. *N Y Med J* 1878; 28: 506.

Bibliography References

1288, 1289, 1291.

Green-Armytage, Vivian Bartley (1882–1961)

Green-Armytage Forceps

Green-Armytage was, to some extent, one of the unheralded leaders of gynaecology in the first half of the twentieth century. He was born in Clifton, Bristol and received his medical degree from the University of Bristol in 1906. A year later he entered the Indian Medical Service and remained in that organisation for 25 years, apart from the First World War. During that conflict he was mentioned thrice in dispatches for gallantry, receiving the Mons Star and Legion of Honour, but no recognition from his homeland. He gained his MD in 1912 and the MRCP in 1917. In his earlier years he applied hypnosis to the practice of obstetrics and gynaecology.

In 1922 he was appointed professor of midwifery and gynaecology at the Medical College of Calcutta. There he gained a huge reputation as a clinician and teacher for his work at the Eden Hospital for Women in Calcutta. He returned to London in 1933 and was appointed to the West London Hospital and three years later to the British Postgraduate Medical School at Hammersmith. There was some resentment at his appointment, owing to his confident flair and willingness to challenge the London medical establishment. However, his manifest ability, particularly as a vaginal and infertility surgeon, ensured his increasing influence in British gynaecological circles. He attracted many local and overseas graduate students, and his operating theatre often resounded to applause from the observers of his surgical performances.

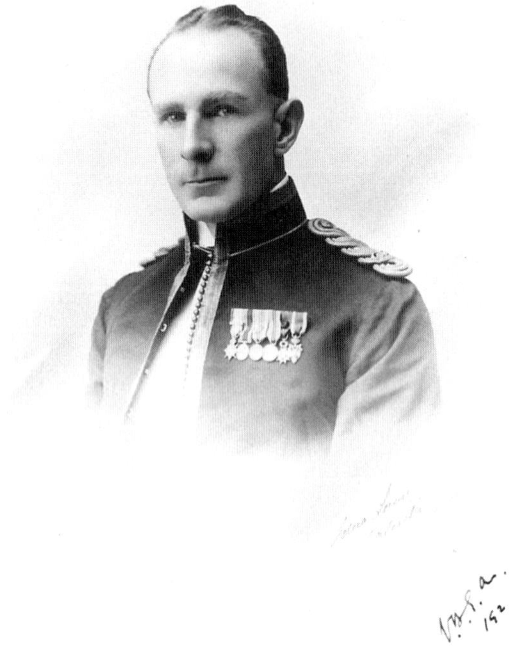

Vivian Bartley Green-Armytage

A founding fellow of the Royal College of Obstetricians and Gynaecologists, he was vice-president from 1949 to 1952. He also endowed a college travel fellowship, Anglo-American lectureship and the annual JY Simpson oration. He remained actively working, and in demand internationally as a lecturer and visiting surgeon, until three weeks before his final illness.

Green-Armytage is remembered eponymously for his atraumatic, broad-ended, haemostatic forceps to reduce blood loss from the sinuses in the cut edges of uterine muscle at caesarean section. He described them thus:

> *They are soft-springed and have transverse serrations. Four of them are applied to the lower, and four to the upper, edges of the incision. They do no injury and stop all oozing. Moreover, being so grooved they can be pulled upon, and so the lower edge is not lost after delivery in a welter of blood and liquor amnii.*

They are still unsurpassed for this purpose and remain in widespread use.

Selected Publications

Green-Armytage VB. In: Section of obstetrics and gynaecology. *Proc R Soc Med* 1936; 30: 557–9.

Bibliography References

97, 822, 1201.

Gregg, Norman McAlister (1892–1966)

Gregg's Triad (Rubella Embryopathy)

In the spring and summer of 1940 there was a severe epidemic of rubella in Australia. In 1941, Norman Gregg, senior ophthalmic surgeon at the Royal Alexandria Hospital for Children in Sydney observed 'in my own practice an unusual number of cases of congenital cataracts made their appearance'. After careful observation, history-taking and correspondence with colleagues in other parts of Australia, he suspected a common link with maternal rubella in early pregnancy. He presented his findings to the Ophthalmological Society of Australia in October 1941 and they were published in the transactions of the society later that year:

> *Although one was struck with the unusual appearance of the cataracts in the first few cases, it was only when similar cases continued to appear that serious thought was given to causation, the remarkable similarity of the opacities in the lens, the frequency of an accompanying affection of the heart and the widespread geographical incidence of the cases suggested there was some common factor in the production of the diseased condition, and suggested it was the result of some constitutional condition of toxic or infective nature rather than of a purely development defect.*

Gregg noted that the cataracts were usually 'obvious from birth and that many of the babies were also

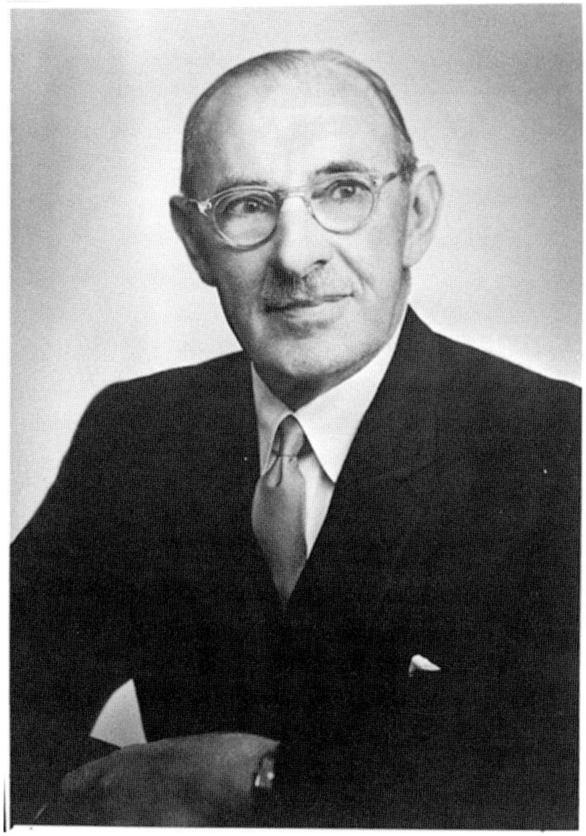

Norman McAlister Gregg

suffering from a congenital defect of the heart'. The third manifestation of the triad, deafness, only became known after two mothers, who had rubella in pregnancy, pointed out this finding in their children. This was subsequently confirmed by Gregg and others.

Norman McAlister Gregg was born in Sydney and became a medical graduate of the University of Sydney. He was a superb all-round athlete and represented New South Wales at cricket and tennis. Immediately after graduation he served in France for three years during the First World War and was awarded the Military Cross for gallantry in the field. He later took training in ophthalmology in London and Birmingham. Recognition of the significance of his work came slowly in the postwar years and he was knighted in 1953. Sir Norman Gregg died in his sleep in July 1966.

Selected Publications

Gregg N McA. Congenital cataract following German measles in the mother. *Trans Ophthalmol Soc Aust* 1941; 3: 35–46.

Gregg N McA. Further observations on congenital defects in infants following maternal rubella. *Trans Ophthalmol Soc Aust* 1944; 4: 119–31.

Bibliography References

212, 213, 407, 411, 567, 572, 658, 659, 704, 1196, 1675, 1732.

Guillemeau, Jacques (1550–1612)

Breech Delivery

Jacques Guillemeau was one of Ambroise Paré's favourite pupils and lived in the Paré home for eight years. He was born in Orléans, France into a family of surgeons and educated as a classical scholar before training with Paré. He acquired a great reputation as a surgeon and man-midwife, becoming surgeon to the Hôtel Dieu in Paris and to three kings of France.

In 1609 he published his midwifery text, *L'Heureux accouchement des femmes,* which was translated into English as *Childbirth or, The Happie Deliverie of Women* in 1612. In the second edition of this text is described the technique of putting one finger into the mouth of the infant during extraction of the aftercoming head in breech delivery. This method of flexing and thereby reducing the diameter of the head was developed by later obstetricians as the Mauriceau–Smellie–Viet manoeuvre.

In 1599 he saved the life of Paré's daughter, Anne Simon, who almost died from haemorrhage associated with placenta praevia. Guillemeau accelerated delivery using internal podalic version and breech extraction as taught to him by Paré. He later described this encounter in his book:

> *Madame Simon ... being near term was surprised by a great haemorrhage. Finding her nearly pulseless, with feeble voice and blanched lips, I made the prognosis to her*

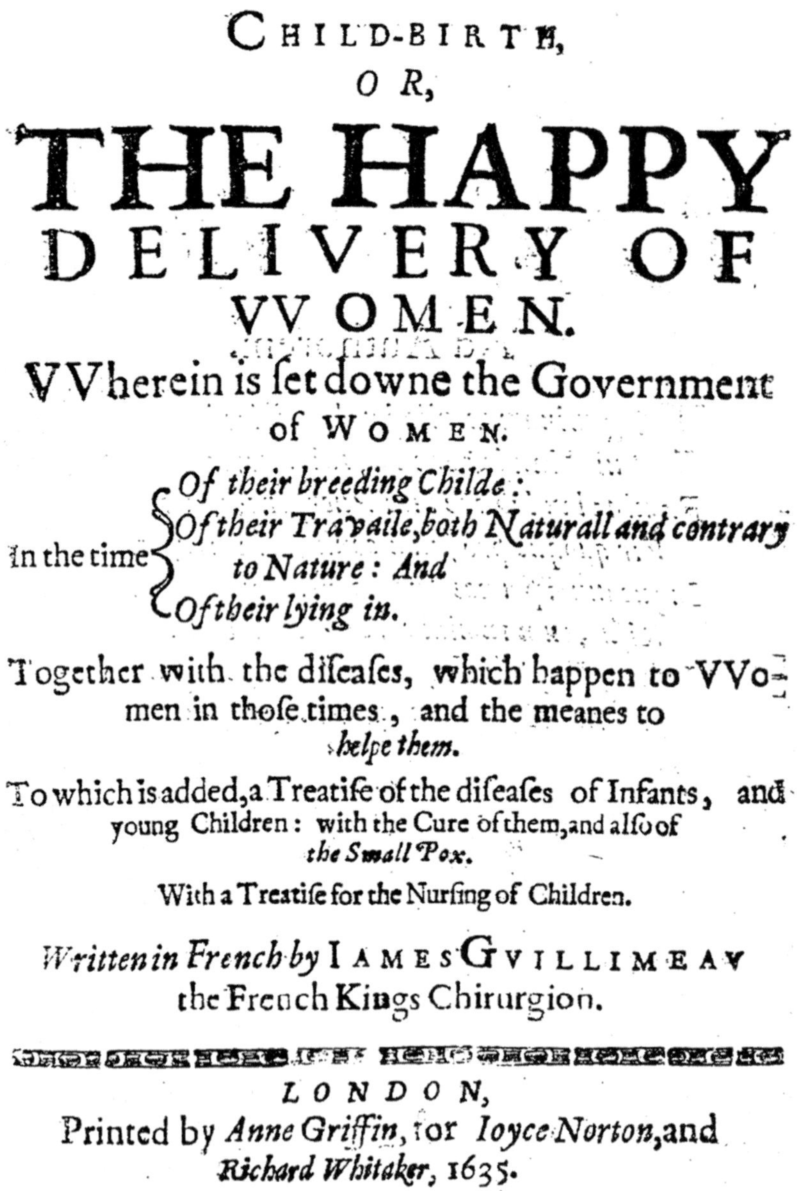

CHILD-BIRTH,
OR,
THE HAPPY
DELIVERY OF
VVOMEN.
VVherein is ſet downe the Government
of WOMEN.

In the time { Of their breeding Childe:
Of their Travaile, both Naturall and contrary
to Nature: And
Of their lying in.

Together with the diſeaſes, which happen to VVomen in thoſe times, and the meanes to
helpe them.

To which is added, a Treatiſe of the diſeaſes of Infants, and young Children: with the Cure of them, and alſo of
the Small Pox.

With a Treatiſe for the Nurſing of Children.

Written in French by IAMES GVILLIMEAV
the French Kings Chirurgion.

LONDON,
Printed by Anne Griffin, for Ioyce Norton, and
Richard Whitaker, 1635.

Title page of the 1635 English translation of Jacques Guillemeau's midwifery text

mother and her husband that her life was in great danger. The only way to save her was to deliver her immediately, the which I had seen practised by the late Monsieur Paré, her father, who caused me to do the like unto a gentlewoman of Madame de Senneterre. The mother and husband entreated me to save her and put the case in our hands. Thus promptly, following the advice of Messieurs the Physicians, she was happily delivered of a lively infant.

Jacques Guillemeau died in Paris on 3 March 1612.

Selected Publications

Guillemeau J. *L'Heureux accouchement des femmes.* Paris: Abraham Picard; 1609.

Guillemeau J. *The Happie Deliverie of Women.* London: Hatfield; 1612.

Bibliography References

159, 199, 359, 503, 548, 648, 983, 1261, 1408, 1486, 1588.

H

Halban, Josef (1870–1937)

Endometriosis

The last of the three main theories to explain the distribution of endometriosis was put forward by Josef Halban in 1924. He proposed that lymphatic and haematogenous spread explained extra-pelvic sites of endometriosis and, indeed, endometrial cells have been found in the pelvic lymphatics and blood vessels. Although the theories of John Sampson and Robert Meyer are thought to explain the majority of cases, the three hypotheses are not mutually exclusive and all may operate under certain circumstances.

Josef Halban was born, trained and died in Vienna. He was a busy gynaecological surgeon who also carried out basic research. He investigated ovarian function and the control of menstruation. From ovarian transplant experiments in animals he concluded that there was an internal secretion from the ovaries. He also postulated that the placenta had an endocrine function. He observed increased hair growth in pregnant women, sometimes called Halban's sign of pregnancy. He correlated short episodes of amenorrhoea with a cystic corpus luteum: Halban's disease or corpus luteum persistens.

Halban was a student of Friedrich Schauta and became a professor of gynaecology in 1909. His wife, Selma Kurz, was a noted singer in the Vienna opera.

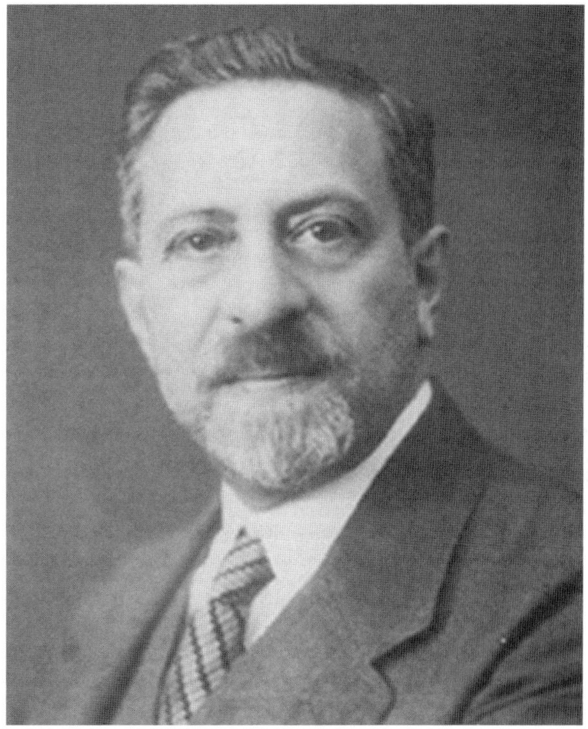

Josef Halban

Selected Publications

Halban J. Hysteroadenosis metastatica. Die lymphofene Genese der sogenannte Adenofibromatosis heterotopica. *Wien Klin Wochenschr* 1924; 37: 1205–10.

Bibliography References

356, 501, 542, 648, 1031, 1485.

Hallopeau, François Henri (1842–1919)

Lichen Sclerosus

The condition now known as lichen sclerosus started in its original description by Henri Hallopeau as *lichen plan atrophique*. This was changed to *lichen sclerosus et atrophicus* and, in 1976, the International Society for the Study of Vulvar Disease discarded the word *atrophicus* to render the modern name. Hallopeau's original observation, however, remains apt. The patient from which this description emanated was a 45-year-old woman, treated in L'Hôpital Saint Louis, Paris in February 1887:

> *'Lichen plan atrophique' begins with the formation of papules which are similar at first to those of ordinary lichen planus, although less highly coloured, and, which, like those, give rise to a sensation of pruritus, become pale, involute promptly and form, then, white spots with a cicatricial appearance which are remarkable for the presence of punctiform depressions; these eruptive elements become grouped and confluent in such a way that they produce plaques, several centimetres in diameter; their surface is checkered, and riddled with punctiform depressions; their contours are irregular; isolated papules are seen at their periphery, some discoloured and involuting, others still rose coloured and active. The eruption progresses by successive attacks.*

François Henri Hallopeau was born in Paris on 17 January 1842. He was a bright student, entered the Paris Medical School at the age of 24 and qualified second in his class three years later. In his early career he became expert in neurology and pathology. He worked in the Paris hospitals, including Tenon, Saint Antoine and latterly Saint Louis, at which hospital he developed his interest in dermatology. He was a prodigious worker and writer, with over 800 publications. Part of this output was facilitated by the fact that he slept poorly and often rose in the middle of the night to write. In addition to his description of lichen sclerosus he was the first to delineate *acrodermatitis continua*. He retired from his hospital appointment in 1907 but continued working as a consultant until, almost blind and barely able to walk, he was forced to give up a few months before his death in March 1919. As well as hard-working he was apparently an affable colleague and was known affectionately in his later years as *le Père Hallopeau*.

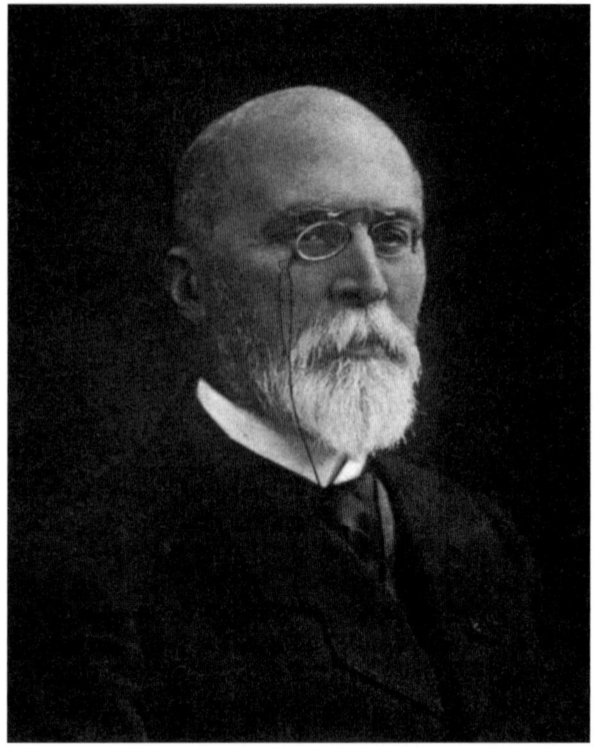

François Henri Hallopeau

Selected Publications

Hallopeau, H. Du lichen plan et particulièrement de sa form atrophique. *Union Médicale* 1887; 43: 729–33.

Bibliography References

118, 776, 1046, 1398, 1441.

Hamlin, Reginald Henry James (1908–1993) Hamlin, Catherine (b. 1923)

Obstetric Fistula

In the spectrum of good works in obstetrics and gynaecology, the contribution of Reginald and Catherine Hamlin must rate at or near the top. For almost half a century the Hamlins devoted themselves to the service of women with obstetric fistulae in Ethiopia. The forbears of both the Hamlins had a tradition of missionary service over at least three generations. Reginald Hamlin was born in 1908 at Napier, New Zealand, of English descent. As a child he had a good voice and was a member of the notable Christchurch Cathedral Choir. He had always wanted to do medicine but started his life as a teacher and then did an MA in history at Canterbury University. He qualified in medicine in 1941 from the Otago School of Medicine. He joined the New Zealand Navy in the Second World War and served in the Pacific arena. Catherine Hamlin was born in Sydney, Australia in 1924 of Anglo-Scots descent. She graduated in medicine from the University of Sydney in 1946. The Hamlins met while working at the Crown Street Women's Hospital in Sydney, where Reginald was the Medical Superintendent when Catherine Nicholson, as she then was, was appointed a resident in obstetrics and gynaecology. After marriage in 1952 they went to do further training in London and then worked in Hong Kong, before returning to the Adelaide Maternity and Children's Hospitals in Australia in 1956. Reg Hamlin was a considerable obstetrician and wrote an excellent book, *Clinical Diagnosis in Labour*, in 1959, with a second edition in 1965. In this book his admiration for two obstetricians shines through: William Smellie and Munro Kerr.

In 1959 the couple answered an advertisement to start a school of midwifery in the Princess Tsehi Hospital in Addis Ababa, Ethiopia. Within the first year they recognised that obstetric fistula was a major problem. They corresponded with known experts in the field, including Naguib Mahfouz, Heinrich Martius and Chassar Moir, and began surgical management of vesicovaginal fistulae with good success. In addition to their fistula, these women had often been cast out from the community and lain for weeks and often months in the fetal position in an attempt to heal, resulting in contractions of their hips and knees. They often had associated obstetric neuropathy causing foot drop. Reg Hamlin called them 'fistula pilgrims' because they often journeyed several hundred kilometres to get to the hospital for help. He summarised their plight as follows:

> *Mourning the still birth of their only child, incontinent of urine, ashamed of their offensiveness, often spurned by their husbands, homeless, unemployable, except in the fields, they endure, they exist, without friends and without hope. They bear their sorrows in silence and shame, their miseries, untreated, are utter, lonely and lifelong.*

After working for many years within the government hospital and treating hundreds of these women a year, the Hamlins realised they would have to concentrate their efforts and build a separate fistula hospital. They decided this would have to be independent, run by charitable donations, and treat only women with fistulae. After years of fundraising efforts, the Addis Ababa Fistula Hospital opened on 24 May 1975. Many of the women were in dire condition on arrival and often required months of rehabilitation before surgical treatment. The Hamlins organised orthopaedic and physiotherapy services to this end. No woman with a fistula was turned away, and after they were cured there was a celebration ceremony, which included each woman receiving a new dress. The Hamlins always advised women who were cured to have their next baby in hospital. The practicalities of this were often difficult in rural Ethiopia. Their guiding advice was 'when you feel the baby walking around in your stomach that is the time for you to start walking to the hospital'. By early in the twenty-first century the Hamlins had treated 20,000 women with obstetric fistula with a greater than

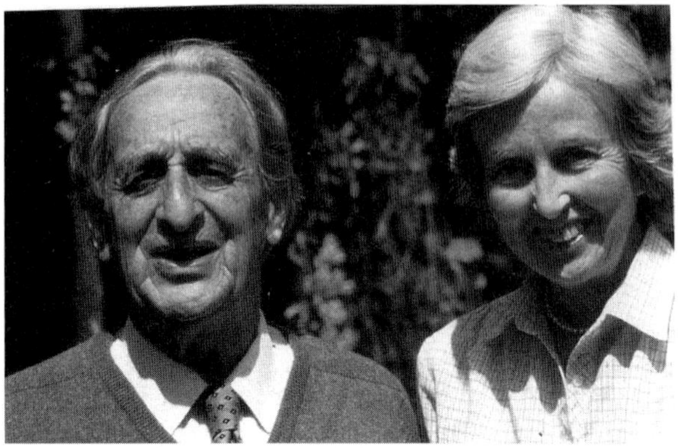

Reginald and Catherine Hamlin

90 per cent success rate. They developed services with visiting surgeons for complex cases. After many years of work, sustained by their religious faith, the Hamlins' achievements were acknowledged internationally. Reg Hamlin received the OBE from the Queen in 1965. Jointly the Hamlins received the Haile Selassie Humanity Prize and Gold Medal in 1971, the Honorary Gold Medal from the Royal College of Surgeons of England in 1989 and the Distinguished Service Award of the American College of Obstetricians and Gynecologists in 1992. In 1995 Catherine Hamlin was made a Companion of the Order of Australia, that country's highest award.

Reg Hamlin developed a fibrous sarcoma of his right leg, which was removed in 1991, followed by radiation treatment. This recurred within months and he was nursed at the Hamlins' home on the grounds of the hospital and died in the early hours of 5 August 1993. He was buried in the British War Graves Cemetery in Addis Ababa.

Catherine Hamlin carried on, and many of their trainees from Africa now staff the hospital, one of whom who has succeeded her as medical director. She concluded her book, *The Hospital by the River,* in 2001: 'I have written this book in the hope that the torch lit by Reg for the fistula pilgrims of Ethiopia and indeed of the world will burn even more brightly and that others will be inspired to stamp out this long-neglected and shameful maternal tragedy'.

Selected Publications

Hamlin RHJ. *Clinical Diagnosis in Labour.* Edinburgh and London: E&S Livingstone Ltd; 1959.

Hamlin RJ, Nicholson EC. Experiences in the treatment of 600 vaginal fistulas and in the management of 80 labours which have followed the repair of these injuries. *Ethiopian Med J* 1966; 4: 189–92.

Hamlin RJ, Nicholson EC. Reconstruction of the urethra totally destroyed in labour. *BMJ* 1969; 2: 147–50.

Hamlin C. *The Hospital by the River: A Story of Hope.* Sydney: Macmillan; 2001.

Bibliography References

686, 687, 725, 811, 1187, 1699, 1739, 1740.

Hanks, Horace Tracy (1837–1900)

Hanks' Cervical Dilators

Cervical dilators have been in use since the time of Hippocrates, when they were used to dilate the cervix to allow medications to be deposited into the uterus. Horace Hanks developed his cervical dilators in 1874, some five years before Alfred Hegar. His original dilators, as described in the *Medical Record* of 1875, were made of hard rubber with double-ended tapered tips. About six centimetres from each tip there was a circular raised collar to limit the depth of insertion. In 1877, before the Medical Society of the State of New York, Hanks presented 37 cases of dysmenorrhoea treated with his dilators. He argued that this method of treatment was less invasive than the commonly performed surgical incision of the internal cervical os. In answer to criticism that this was an old form of treatment, Hanks replied, 'dilatation in one form or another has been resorted to by different surgeons, but I claim originality in a *rapid* and *forcible* dilation,

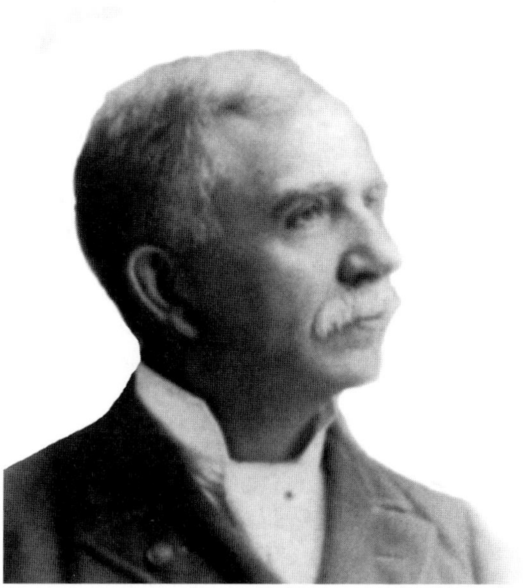

Horace Tracy Hanks

and the *forcible retroflexion* at the same time'. Hanks dilators were subsequently manufactured in metal and used widely throughout the United States.

Horace Hanks was born in East Randolph, Vermont on 27 June 1837. He studied medicine at the University of Vermont and Albany Medical College in New York, graduating MD from the latter institution in 1861. He served for one year as house surgeon in Albany City Hospital and became assistant surgeon to the 30th Regiment, New York State Volunteers in 1861 and served during a number of battles in the Civil War. After his military service he practised in Royalston, Massachusetts, but in 1868 he moved to New York, attended lectures at the College of Physicians and Surgeons and specialised in gynaecology. He ultimately became professor of diseases of women in the New York Postgraduate Medical School and Hospital. In declining health, he resigned in 1898 and died at his home in New York City on 18 November 1900.

Selected Publications

Hanks HT. New dilators for the cervical canal, or female urethra. *Med Rec* 1875; 7: 655.

Hanks HT. A new method of operation for the cure of anteflexion and the relief of its accompanying dysmenorrhea; with remarks and a tabulated report of thirty-seven cases. *Trans Med Soc NY* 1877; 10: 98–112.

Bibliography References

801, 1486, 1669.

Hart, Alfred Purvis (1888–1954)

Neonatal Exchange Transfusion

Although repeated perinatal loss due to 'familial icterus gravis' was well known in the early twentieth century, the exact pathogenesis of isoimmunisation and erythroblastosis fetalis was unknown. On 18 December 1924, Alfred Hart, paediatrician at the Toronto Hospital for Sick Children, was consulted on a healthy male newborn with a family history 'so remarkable that one was prepared for trouble'. Six previous infants had all been healthy at birth, developed progressive jaundice in 24 hours, and died within days. Hart felt that 'the condition was due to some unknown toxin circulating in the blood'. He wrote:

> *I felt that if something drastic was not done at once, the child was certainly going to die as the six other previous male babies had done. It was decided to do an exsanguination transfusion . . . in the hope of removing a sufficient amount of toxin to prevent the progress of the disease.*

Hart performed an exchange transfusion, taking 300 ml from the longitudinal sinus via the anterior fontanelle, and transfusing 335 ml into the left ankle saphenous vein. The donor was 'a healthy male unrelated to the family'. The infant's jaundice subsided and he continued to thrive. In seeking to remove the 'toxin', Hart stumbled upon the optimum treatment of exchange transfusion, although the exact pathophysiology of haemolytic disease of the newborn was not understood until 1941. Hart reported the case in the *Canadian Medical Association Journal*, but it was

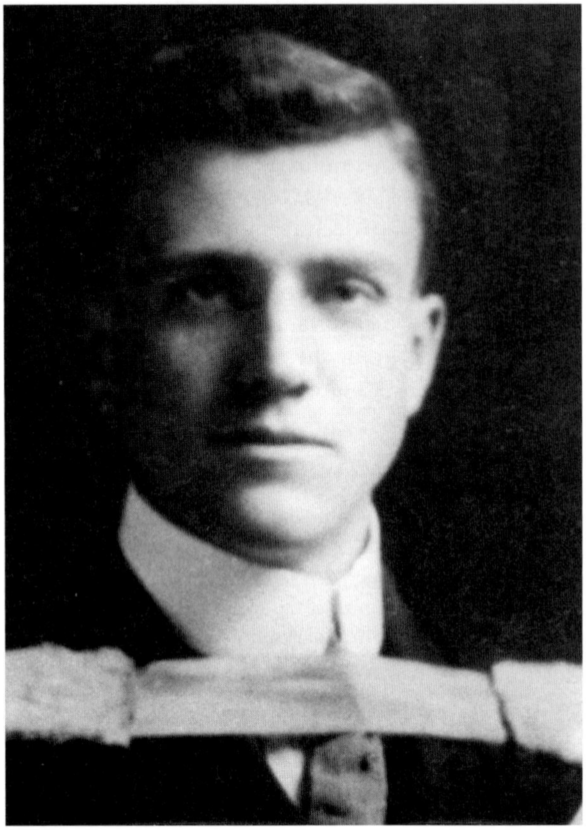
Alfred Purvis Hart

overlooked and 21 years would pass before Harry Wallerstein (1906–1993) successfully used the technique in New York. Later, Louis Diamond (1902–1999) of Boston established the use of the umbilical vein for exchange transfusion.

Alfred Purvis Hart was born in the farming community of Wilfred, Ontario. He graduated MB from the University of Toronto in 1911 and entered general practice in Bruce Mines, Ontario. In 1915, he went to England for paediatric training at the Great Ormond Street Children's Hospital, London. He joined the Imperial Forces in February 1916 as a Captain in the Royal Army Medical Corps. In March 1916, he was sent to France and mentioned in dispatches during two battles on the Somme. He was with the Royal Munster Fusiliers in their attack at Passchendaele in November 1917. He received the Military Cross in November 1919. The citation read, 'For great initiative, gallantry and devotion to duty at the Advanced Dressing Station, east of the church at Rejet-de-Beaulieu, during the exceptionally heavy bombardment on 4th November 1918. He repeatedly dressed wounded men and superintended the evacuation of casualties even when his dressing station was blown in by shell fire. He undoubtedly saved many lives'.

After demobilisation in 1919 he spent a further year at the Great Ormond Street Children's Hospital and returned to Canada in 1920. From 1921 he served as a paediatrician to the Hospital for Sick Children in Toronto and continued there for 30 years until his retirement in 1951. He maintained an interest in farming and was buried in the town of his birth.

Selected Publications

Diamond LK. Erythroblastosis foetalis or haemolytic disease of the newborn. *Proc R Soc Med* 1947; 40: 546–9.

Hart AP. Familial icterus gravis of the newborn and its treatment. *Can Med Assoc J* 1925; 15: 1008–11.

Wallerstein H. Treatment of severe erthroblastosis by simultaneous removal and replacement of the blood of the newborn infant. *Science* 1946; 103: 583–4.

Bibliography References

80, 82, 91, 175, 388, 389, 465, 1741, 1744.

Harvey, William (1578–1657)

Fetal Physiology

William Harvey is best known for his discovery of the circulation of the blood, which he first outlined in a lecture to the Royal College of Physicians in London in April 1616. He did not publish this, his most famous work, until 1628 when the first edition appeared in Latin: *Exercitio anatomica de motu cordis et sanguinis in animalibus.* The English edition, *On the Motion of the Heart and Blood in Animals,* did not follow until 1653.

William Harvey was born in Folkstone, England. He took his undergraduate degree at Caius College,

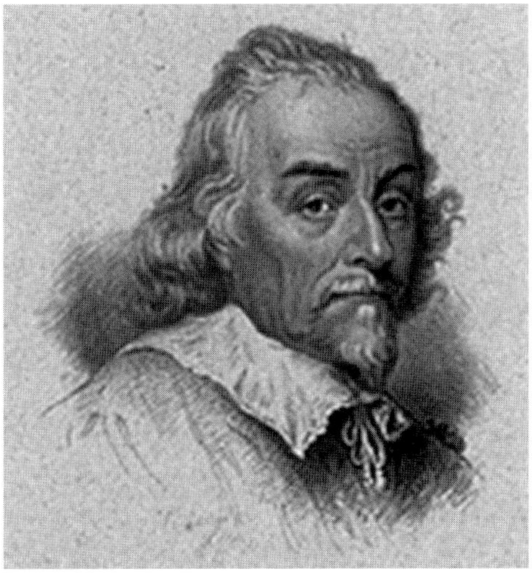

William Harvey

Cambridge in 1597. The following year he began medical studies at Padua and there was influenced by the great anatomist and embryologist, Hieronymous Fabricius (1537–1619). He was awarded his MD with distinction in 1602. Returning to England he was admitted to the membership of the Royal College of Physicians in 1604 and appointed Lumleian lecturer of the college in 1615. Harvey was appointed physician to James I and later to Charles I. His work on the circulation was scorned by many, but through his careful, observant and experimental approach he made enormous contributions to anatomy, physiology and clinical medicine:

> *. . . that no man can be truely called prudent, or knowing, who doth not by his own experience (attained by manifold remembrance, frequent sensation, and difficult observation) know things to be so. For without that we think only, or believe: and such a knowledge as that, is to be reputed other men's, rather than our own.*

He was loyal to Charles I, and during the civil war in 1642 left London for Oxford with the royal court. His house was ransacked and many of his papers lost.

Harvey retired from practice in 1646. However, in 1650 a friend persuaded him to release a manuscript that Harvey had worked on for 20 years. It was published in Latin the following year as, *Exercitationes de generatione animalium,* and in English in 1653, *Anatomical Exercitations Concerning the Generation of Living Creatures.* Much of this work contains his observations on fetal development in several animals, including the royal deer at Hampton Court. He also dissected many human embryos and fetuses. All his observations were made with the naked eye. He showed that there was no direct connection between the maternal and fetal blood vessels, as Giulio Arantius had demonstrated previously. Of the placenta he wrote:

> *In my opinion, then, the placenta has an office analogous to that of the liver and mamma . . . constituting the bond of union between the 'conception' and the uterus . . . served to concoct or digest the alible nutriment which proceedeth from the parent to support the foetus.*

He was aware of fetal activity in utero:

> *For he swimmeth in a water and moved himself to and fro . . . But the foetus so soon as it is born, aye before it is born, will suck . . . Wherefore he seems to be good at it of old and to have practised it in the womb.*

Included in his book was a section, *De partu* (Of Birth), which was the first English text on obstetrics and shows that Harvey had considerable clinical experience. He describes pseudocyesis, superfetation and eclampsia. His approach was conservative: 'childbirth is a natural process that requires no interference in the great majority of the cases'. Harvey also reported a remarkable case of early post-partum ambulation in a woman from Munster, Ireland in the early 1600s which, were it to get into the hands of modern hospital administrators, could lead to an even earlier post-partum hospital discharge policy:

> *There was a woman big with child, which followed her husband, who was a soldier in the army; and the army being daily in motion, was it seems forced to make a halt . . . whereupon the poor woman finding her labour come upon her, retired to the next thicket, and alone by herself without any midwife or other preparation brought forth twins: which she presently carried to the river, and there washed both herself and them; which done she wrapt her infants in a coarse cloth and tied them to her back, and that very day, marched along with the army 12 miles together, barefooted: and was never the worse for the matter.*

Harvey was married but had no children. He was described as being 'of the lowest stature, round faced . . . his hair was black as a raven, but quite white twenty years before he died'. His wife died in 1645 and he lived with his brothers, who were wealthy merchants. He suffered badly with gout. Although elected president of the Royal College of Physicians in 1654, he refused the position because of ill health. He woke on the morning of 3 June 1657, unable to speak. Bloodletting was unsuccessful and he died soon after, comforted by a large dose of opium.

Selected Publications

Harvey W. *Exercitationes de generatione animalium*. London; 1651.

Harvey W. *Anatomical Exercitations Concerning the Generation of Living Creatures*. London: James Young; 1653. Also published in: The Classics of Obstetrics and Gynecology Library. New York, NY: Gryphon Editions; 1991 (fascimile).

Bibliography References

26, 55, 72, 107, 347, 460, 606, 615, 648, 689, 755, 830, 969, 1023, 1031, 1102, 1139, 1196, 1214, 1494, 1665, 1671.

Harvie, John (c.1710–1770)

Management of the Third Stage of Labour

In his small book, *Practical Directions, Shewing a Method of Preserving the Perinaeum in Birth and Delivering the Placenta Without Violence*, published in 1767, John Harvie's advice on managing the perineum during delivery, while sensible, was not new. However, his views on the delivery of the placenta were, and he was the first to advocate external manual expression of the placenta. This he proposed within a much more conservative approach to the management of the third stage of labour. He outlined the two main schools of thought at that time:

> *The first, and perhaps the most general, method has been to deliver the placenta immediately after the child. To perform this, some have recommended an immediate introduction of the hand; others have advised pulling on the navel string; and some say that the woman should be brought to sneeze, cough or vomit.*
>
> *The second method is to leave this business principally to nature.*

Harvie favoured the second approach with the modification to be outlined later. He spoke against each of the immediate methods of placental delivery, claiming that the introduction of the hand into the uterus 'is attended with great pain and danger'. Pulling on the umbilical cord was, he said, 'extremely dangerous, and likely to produce an inversion of the uterus'. While 'the more usual consequences of being made to cough, sneeze or vomit are ... the blood is with force expelled from the vessels of the uterus'.

In general, Harvie advocated waiting for the placenta to deliver without interference. However, he said, 'There is another safe method of assisting nature in the delivery of the placenta', which he described as follows:

> *As soon as the child is committed to the care of the nurse let the accoucheur apply his hand upon the belly of the woman, which is then very loose, and he will readily feel the contracting uterus; then, having placed the flat of the hand over it, let him by a light and gentle pressure bring it downwards or towards the pubis and he will feel the uterus sensibly contracting and then feel it so reduced in size as to be certain the placenta is expelled. By this method he will seldom have anything to do afterwards but to help it through the os externum; if even so much remains undone ...*

Similar principles were followed by leading obstetricians in Dublin in 1781, which came to be known as the 'Dublin method' of managing the third stage. Almost a century later Carl Credé would describe a similar technique and receive the eponymous recognition.

John Harvie was a pupil of William Smellie and was married to the niece of Smellie's wife. When Smellie retired in 1759, Harvie inherited his teaching

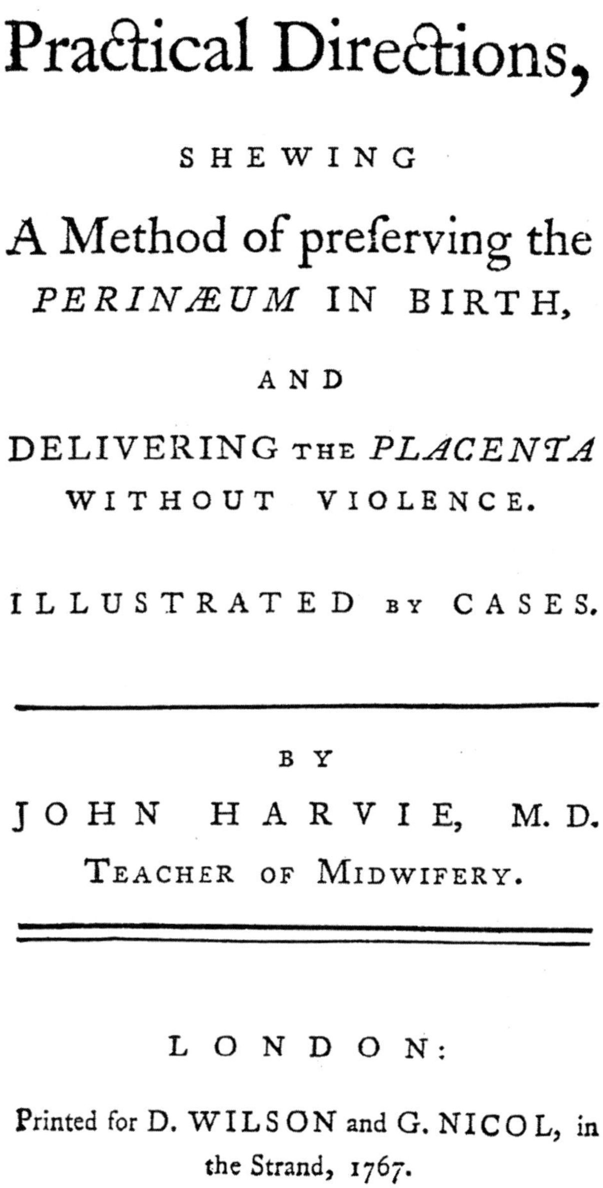

Practical Directions,

SHEWING

A Method of preserving the *PERINÆUM* IN BIRTH,

AND

DELIVERING THE *PLACENTA* WITHOUT VIOLENCE.

ILLUSTRATED BY CASES.

BY

JOHN HARVIE, M. D.

TEACHER OF MIDWIFERY.

LONDON:

Printed for D. WILSON and G. NICOL, in the Strand, 1767.

Title page of John Harvie's monograph

equipment and carried on his lectures in the same tradition. There must also have been a musical bond between the two men, for when Smellie died he left two flutes and most of his music to Harvie.

Selected Publications

Harvie J. *Practical Directions, Shewing a Method of Preserving the Perinaeum in Birth and Delivering the Placenta Without Violence*. London: D. Wilson and G. Nichol; 1767.

Bibliography References

822, 1495, 1595.

Haultain, Francis William Nicol (1861–1921)

Haultain's Operation for Uterine Inversion

Acute puerperal uterine inversion is a rare and, if not corrected, often fatal complication of labour. Occasionally in uncorrected cases the woman survives and chronic uterine inversion causes irregular bleeding and discomfort. A variety of non-surgical methods for replacement have been tried, including Aveling's repositor. When these fail, the vaginal surgical approaches of Pier Spinelli and Otto Küstner have been tried.

In 1901 Haultain reported a case of chronic uterine inversion in which all attempts to manipulate the uterus vaginally were met with brisk bleeding:

> *I made at this time a slight attempt to reduce the displacement but the bleeding was so copious I felt compelled to desist and plug the vagina as quickly as possible. On account of her enfeebled condition I did not feel justified in making further attempts at reduction from below and decided to attempt replacement from above, as I thought it would be done with a minimum blood loss.*

At laparotomy he found he still could not reduce the inversion, even with an assistant pushing from below while he pulled on the round ligaments and tried to dilate the constriction ring:

> *I therefore decided to cut through the constriction rim posteriorly . . . I continued my incision through the posterior uterine wall as it appeared through the slit till reduction was complete.*

This approach, while originally described in a case of chronic uterine inversion, has been used occasionally in neglected acute cases.

Francis William Nicol Haultain was born in Colombo, Ceylon, but received his schooling in Edinburgh. He graduated MB from Edinburgh in 1882 and spent some time touring medical centres in Austria and Germany. He returned to Edinburgh and established a specialist practice in obstetrics and gynaecology. He received his MD from Edinburgh University for a thesis on retroversion of the gravid uterus. Reputedly a fearless and dexterous surgeon,

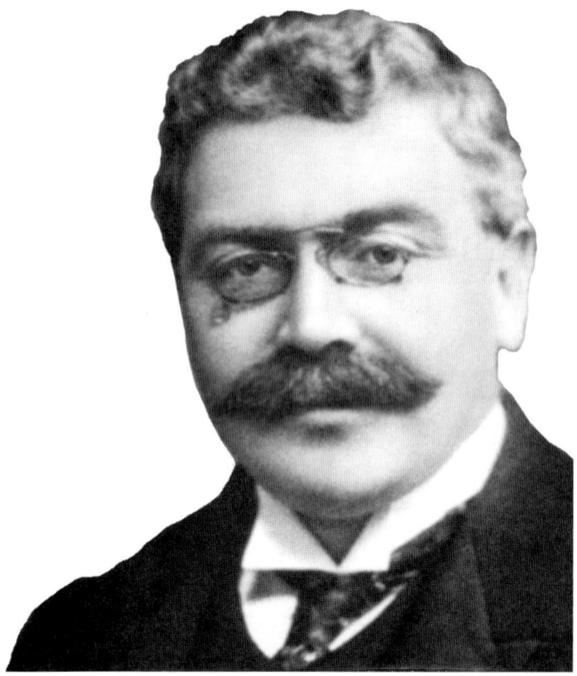

Francis William Nicol Haultain

Haultain held appointments at the Royal Maternity Hospital and Edinburgh Royal Infirmary, in addition to a large private practice. He was elected president of the Edinburgh Obstetrical Society in 1909. His son followed him into medicine and the specialty of obstetrics and gynaecology.

Selected Publications

Haultain FWN. The treatment of chronic uterine inversion by abdominal hysterotomy, with a successful case. *BMJ* 1901; 2: 974–6.

Bibliography References

648, 701, 822.

Hayward, George (1791–1863)

Vesicovaginal Fistula

Although John Mettauer performed the first surgical closure of a vesicovaginal fistula in North America, it was George Hayward who published the first report of his own successful case in 1839. Hayward's case was a 34-year-old woman who had suffered from a vesicovaginal fistula for the past 15 years following delivery of a stillborn infant after a labour lasting three days. Hayward cautioned the woman that the surgical results of attempted fistula closure were poor but that he 'regarded her case on the whole as a favourable one'. He performed the operation on 10 May 1839 in the presence of Walter Channing. With the patient in the lithotomy position he inserted a large bougie of polished whale bone through the urethra into the bladder to bring the fistulous opening into view. He excised the fistulous tract and dissected the bladder mucosa from the vaginal walls:

> *This was done partly with the view of increasing the chances of union by presenting a larger surface and partly to prevent the necessity of carrying needles through the bladder. I then introduced a needle, about one third of an inch from the edge of the wound, through the membrane of the vagina and cellular membrane beneath and brought it out at the opposite side at about an equal distance. Before the needle was drawn through, a second and third were introduced in the same way and this being found sufficient to close the orifice, they were carried through and the threads tightly tied.*

A silver catheter was placed in the bladder for continuous drainage and this was removed, cleaned and replaced each day. The silk sutures were removed after five days. After seven days the catheter was removed. The result was a complete cure. Between 1839 and 1851 Hayward operated on nine women with vesicovaginal fistula, with three complete successes and some improvement in five others.

George Hayward was born in Boston on 9 March 1791. He graduated from Harvard in 1809 and took his medical degree at Philadelphia in 1812. As was common in those days he undertook a tour of European centres, including some time observing the British surgeon Astley Cooper. He returned to Boston and worked as a surgeon at the Massachusetts General Hospital. He was closely involved with the introduction of ether anaesthesia in surgical practice and, indeed, performed the second operation under ether anaesthesia the day after the first procedure by Dr John Warren on 16 October 1846. He performed the first major operation under ether anaesthesia on

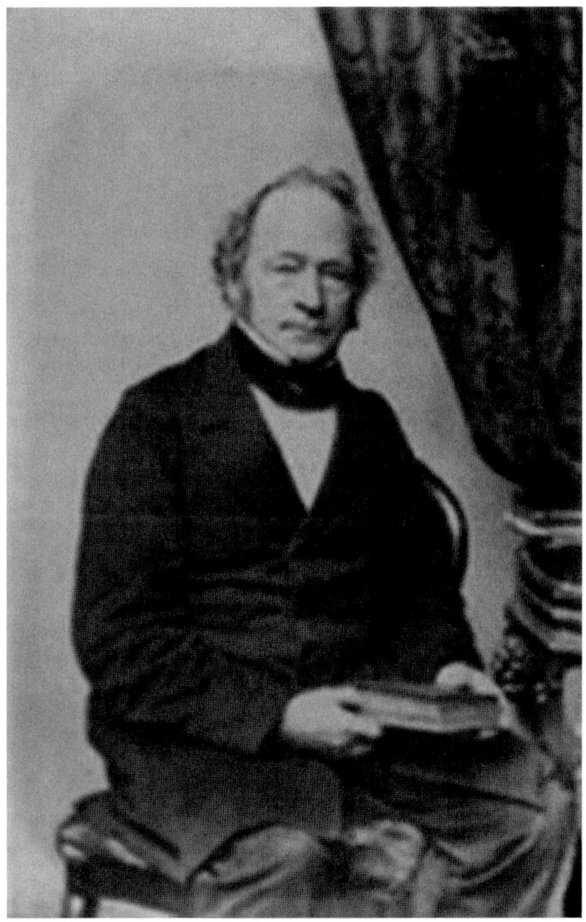

George Hayward

2 November 1846: a leg amputation. Although he was an academic professor of surgery at Harvard, he published sparingly and was a relatively quiet, self-effacing man.

Selected Publications

Hayward G. Case of vesicovaginal fistula, successfully treated by an operation. *Am J Med Sci* 1839; 24: 283–8.

Hayward G. Cases of vesicovaginal fistula treated by operation. *Boston Med Surg J* 1851; 44: 209–24.

Mettauer JP. Vesico-vaginal fistula. *Boston Med Surg J* 1840; 22: 154–5.

Bibliography References

285, 810, 811, 1485, 1656, 1739, 1740.

Heaney, Noble Sproat (1880–1955)

Vaginal Hysterectomy

When Noble Sproat Heaney was a premedical student, his favourite aunt died four days after a vaginal hysterectomy. Whether this played a role in his ultimate choice of career and led him to become a master vaginal surgeon is moot. Nonetheless, during the 1930s and 1940s, Heaney was to become one of the most influential proponents of vaginal hysterectomy in the United States. He decried the abandonment of vaginal hysterectomy and the reasons gynaecologists had been lured to the abdominal route:

> *Formerly vaginal hysterectomy was much in vogue but with the development of abdominal surgery and especially because of the over-emphasis placed upon so-called chronic lesions of the appendix, gynecologists gradually deserted the vaginal route in order to remove appendices, sever Jackson's membranes, stitch up prolapsed cecums, and do much other questionable surgery. Now that these conditions have been evaluated, and the harmlessness of most of these deviations has been established, a new race of gynecologists has been reared which has relatively little or no familiarity with the vaginal attack on pelvic lesions. It is the purpose of this paper to show again how low the mortality and morbidity of vaginal hysterectomy may be with the hope that this operation may find a place in the operative armamentarium of every gynecologist.*

In acquiring the skills for vaginal hysterectomy, he advised progression from easy to more difficult cases and advocated a policy of 'careful boldness'.

> *Those who persist in perfecting themselves in the technique of vaginal hysterectomy gradually disregard more and more of the contradictions so insistently laid down by those with little or no familiarity with the operation.*

Heaney devised a technique of vaginal hysterectomy based on his postgraduate training in Nebraska, Germany and Austria in the early twentieth century. His technique, or modification thereof, is still widely used. He also designed a number of instruments used in vaginal surgery; including the Heaney needle holder, clamp and retractor. His technique for closing the peritoneum, incorporating ligation of the vessels and ligaments is known as the 'Heaney stitch'.

Noble Sproat Heaney was born in a log cabin on a farm outside the small town of Mendon, Illinois. The home had been built by his grandfather when he emigrated to America from Ireland. It is said that the homestead was used to hide slaves fleeing from the southern states en route to the northern United States and Canada. His premedical education was carried out at Knox College, followed by graduation from Rush Medical College, Chicago in 1904. After his internship he spent one year as an assistant to Palmer Findley in Omaha, Nebraska. This was one of the ways to get specialist experience in the days before formal residency training. He then gained

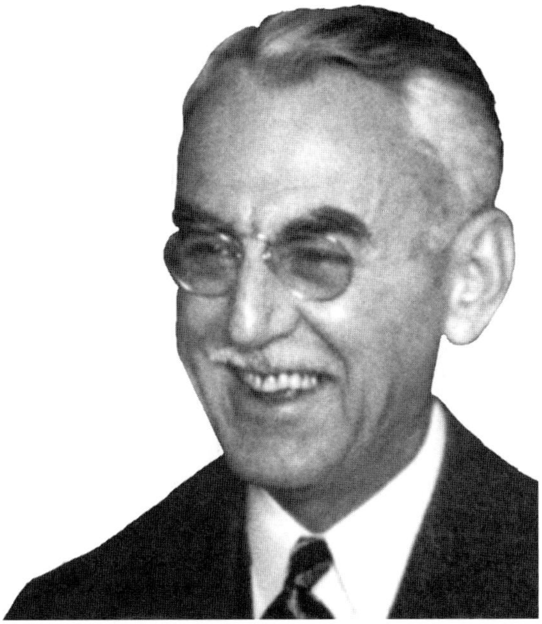

Noble Sproat Heaney

postgraduate experience at the Presbyterian Hospital, Chicago and at the University of Nebraska. Feeling that his training in vaginal surgery was inadequate, he went to Heidelberg and later worked with Ernst Wertheim in Vienna. He returned to Chicago in 1909 and from 1919 to 1946 was head of the department of gynaecology at the Presbyterian Hospital. He demanded loyalty and hard work from his junior staff. Heaney was an acknowledged master of vaginal hysterectomy and rarely operated without an appreciative audience. In 1938 he was elected president of the American Gynecological Society.

Heaney was proud of his humble farming roots, albeit with a slightly defensive attitude. For a time, he had a commercial dairy farm in Glen Ellyn, Illinois. He did not like or do much obstetrics and was at odds with Joseph DeLee. His uncle was called Noble, and Sproat, the name he went by, was his mother's maiden name. He was a heavy smoker and endured several operations for a gastric ulcer. In 1946 he moved to the warmth of California and practised for another five years at the Presbyterian and Hollywood Hospital in Los Angeles.

He died from cerebrovascular disease at his home in Los Angeles on 26 September 1955.

Selected Publications

Heaney NS. A report of 565 vaginal hysterectomies performed for benign pelvic disease. *Am J Obstet Gynecol* 1934; 28: 751–5.

Heaney NS. Vaginal hysterectomy - its indications and technique. *Am J Surg* 1940; 48: 284–8.

Bibliography References

19, 20, 97, 125, 163, 524, 706, 1291, 1485.

Hegar, Alfred (1830–1914)

Hegar's Dilators/Hegar's Sign

It is ironic that two of the best remembered eponyms, Hegar's sign and dilators, were first published by assistants working in Alfred Hegar's clinic in Freiburg. The first published description of Hegar's sign of early pregnancy was by Carl Reinl in 1884:

> *Last winter, in Professor Hegar's gynaecology clinic, I had the opportunity of acquainting myself with a new and excellent sign of the early months of pregnancy. This consists in the demonstration of an unusual softness, flexibility, and thinning of the lower uterine segment, that is, of the part directly above the insertion of the uterosacral ligaments . . . The pliability and laxness of*

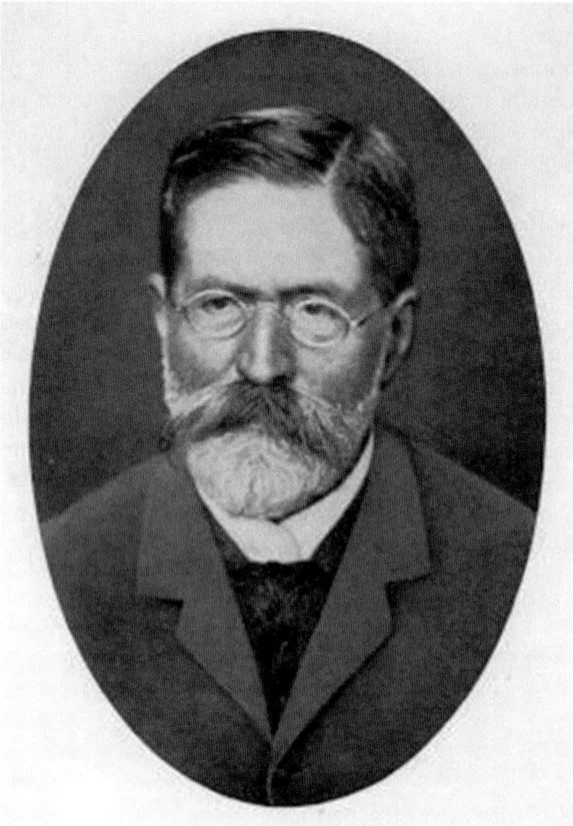

Alfred Hegar

these parts can be so extensive that one may be in doubt as to whether any connection exists between the cervix and the larger abdominal or pelvic mas . . . one has the impression that the cervix uteri ceases above, and that the upper swelling is something apart by itself . . . the more consistent cervix passes above into a softened mass, which then again joins with the harder swelling above.

It is not certain whether Reinl discovered the sign or was taught it by Hegar. However, Hegar's publication on the subject 11 years later suggests the latter.

Hegar was one of the first to use graduated sounds to dilate the cervix, before which laminaria tents were generally used. The earliest reference to these dilators was published by Tchoudowski who had observed their use in Hegar's clinic in 1879. Hegar's first description came with the publication of the second edition of his gynaecology text two years later:

> *We have used this method of dilatation many times in recent years and found it to be very satisfactory. That it has not been generally adopted as yet is probably due in large measure to unsatisfactory technique and imperfect instruments. One must have a large number of dilators at hand, each one of which that is introduced having only a slightly greater diameter than the previous one . . . The smallest dilator is 2 mm in diameter. The rest are graduated in diameters which increase progressively only 1 mm at a time'.*

Alfred Hegar, the son of a doctor, was born in Darmstadt, Germany. His medical studies were taken in Heidelberg, Berlin and Vienna. After qualification in 1852 he began practice in his home town, concentrating on obstetrics. From this source he published work on the pathology of early pregnancy loss. In 1864 he was appointed professor of obstetrics and gynaecology at Freiburg where he remained until he retired in 1904. He was a renowned pelvic surgeon.

Selected Publications

Hegar A, Kaltenbach R. *Die operative Gynäkologie*. 2nd edn. Erlangen: Enke; 1881.

Hegar A. Diagnose der frühesten Schwangerschaftsperiode. *Deutsche Med Wochenschr* 1895; 21: 565–7.

Reinl C. Ein neues sicheres diagnostischen Zeichen der Schwangerschaft in den ersten Monaten. *Prague Med Wochenschr* 1884; 9: 253–4.

Tchoudowski M. De la dilatation du canal cervical (d'après Hegar). *Arch Tocol* 1879; 6: 737–55.

Bibliography References

528, 553, 648, 1014, 1450, 1458, 1595.

Hesselbach, Franz Kaspar (1759–1816)

Hesselbach's Triangle

Hesselbach's triangle, described in 1806, is the area bounded by the inguinal ligament, the lateral margin of the rectus abdominus muscle and the inferior epigastric artery. In Hesselbach's original description, the lower border of the triangle was the pubic ramus and each of the lower angles were the sites of origin of direct inguinal and femoral herniae respectively. The modern relevance of this anatomical triangle is in the selection of a safe area for the introduction of cannulae in gynaecological laparoscopic surgery and in the classification and repair of inguinal hernia. In this context the identification of the obliterated umbilical arteries helps avoid the inferior epigastric vessels.

Franz Kaspar Hesselbach was born on 27 January 1758 in Hammelburg, Bavaria. He studied medicine in Würzburg, and such was his diligence in anatomical dissection that the professor of anatomy and surgery, Karl von Siebold (1736–1807), made him his private pupil. He ultimately succeeded von Siebold and became chief surgeon at the Julius Hospital in Würzburg. One of his students was Conrad Langenbeck. Hesselbach died on 24 July 1816.

Selected Publications

Hesselbach FK. *Anatomisch-chirugische Abhandlung über den Ursprung der Leistenbrüche.* Würzburg: Baumgärtner; 1806.

Bibliography References

8, 17, 149, 406, 552, 831, 1633.

Hicks, John Braxton (1823–1897)

Braxton Hicks Bipolar Version/Braxton Hicks Contractions

Internal podalic version and breech extraction, 'delivery by the art', was the method used to empty the uterus in cases of placenta praevia or eclampsia before the advent of caesarean section. It was also used to deliver the fetus in some cases of cephalopelvic disproportion and malpresentation. External version was promoted by Adolphe Pinard and others, but had more limited application.

In 1860 Braxton Hicks published his description of a combined method using both external and internal hands to turn the fetus (bipolar version):

> *Introduce the left hand, with the usual precautions, into the vagina, so far as to fairly touch the foetal head, even should it recede an inch . . . Having passed one or two fingers (if only one, let it be the middle finger) within the cervix, and resting them on the head, place the right hand on the left side of the breech at the fundus . . . Employ gentle pressure and slight impulsive movements on the fundus towards the left iliac fossa. In a very short time it will be found that the head is rising and at the same time the breech is descending . . . The foetus is now transverse; the knee will be opposite the os, and, the membranes being ruptured, it can be seized and brought into the vagina.*

He claimed that with less manipulation and force needed from the internal hand, the risk of uterine rupture was diminished and the procedure was not so painful for the patient. Another advantage he cited was for the doctor: 'the removal of the coat and baring of the arm of the operator' were unnecessary. Hicks was careful not to decry the standard technique of internal podalic version: 'I disclaim all intention of unnecessarily deprecating an exceedingly valuable and ancient operation – one which has saved numberless lives'.

Combined techniques of version had been advocated before by Marmaduke Wright, in cases of shoulder presentation, and by Justus Wigand. The advantage of Hicks' technique was that it could be performed with minimal cervical dilatation. Hicks recommended his technique for all cases in which podalic version was necessary. He especially advocated its use in cases of placenta praevia, in which the ability to turn the fetus with less manipulative trauma to the lower uterine segment and at low cervical dilatation was a great advantage. Once the fetal leg was grasped and brought down it provided tamponade to the placenta and bleeding site, with a dramatic reduction in blood loss. As he put it:

> *Anything which gave the practitioner some power of action was to be earnestly welcomed ... Turn, and if you employ the child as a plug the danger is over. Then wait for the pains, rally the powers in the interval and let nature, gently assisted, complete the delivery.*

Before this technique was introduced, obstetricians had two choices in a case of bleeding from placenta praevia: either resort to forcible dilatation of the cervix, *accouchement forcé*, or await spontaneous dilatation of the cervix. In either case the patient often succumbed to haemorrhage before the uterus could be emptied. Braxton Hicks' procedure allowed an early and relatively atraumatic method of reducing blood loss and accelerating delivery. Its widespread application significantly reduced maternal mortality until it was largely supplanted by the emergence of safe caesarean section.

Braxton Hicks' name endures in both the medical and lay lexicon because of his observation of uterine contractions during normal pregnancy:

> *But after many years' constant observation, I have ascertained it to be a fact that the uterus possesses the power and habit of spontaneously contracting and relaxing from a very early period of pregnancy, as early, indeed, as it is possible to recognise the difference of consistence – that is, from about the third month ...*
>
> *The consistency with which these contractions of the uterus have always occurred to me leaves no doubt on my mind but that it is a natural condition of pregnancy ...*
>
> *In a general way the pregnant woman is not conscious of the contractions of the uterus ... But occasionally it happens that the uterus is more than usually sensitive, and the contractions are accompanied by pain ...*

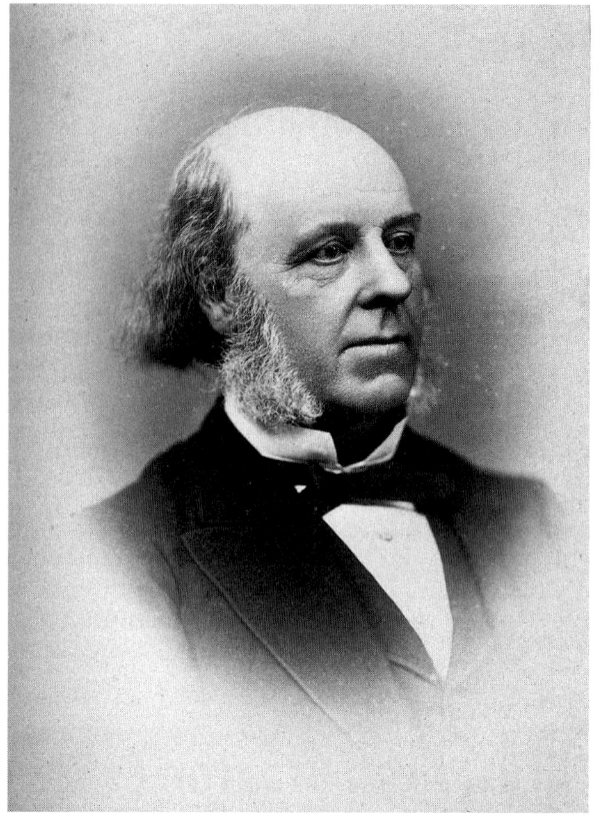
John Braxton Hicks

Braxton Hicks showed remarkable patience in making his observations with 'full contact of the hand continuously over a period from five to twenty minutes'. He wrote his paper after experience 'for the last six years and upwards'. He felt that the purpose of these contractions was to help the circulation of blood in the uterus and placenta and to 'adapt the position of the fetus to the form of the uterus'. He used the observation to help confirm the diagnosis of pregnancy.

John Braxton Hicks was born in Rye, England. He took his medical training at Guy's Hospital, receiving his degree in 1847. As a student he won a medal in the double skulls with the hospital rowing club. He entered general practice in the Tottenham district of London and later concentrated on obstetrics. In 1859 he was appointed assistant obstetric physician to Guy's Hospital. He ultimately became consulting obstetric physician to both Guy's and St Mary's hospitals. In 1871 he served as president of the Obstetrical Society of London. He published more than one hundred papers on medical topics, as well as other subjects, also being an authority on botany, entomology and Wedgwood pottery. He retired from practice in 1894. He died at home on 28 August 1897, three months after a prolonged bout of influenza. His attending physician wrote, 'Death was due to cardiac failure, the result of depreciated muscular fibre, most probably an influenzal sequela'.

Selected Publications

Hicks JB. On a new method of version in abnormal labour. *Lancet* 1860; 2: 28–30.

Hicks JB. On the contractions of the uterus throughout pregnancy: their physiological effects and their value in the diagnosis of pregnancy. *Trans Obstet Soc London* 1871; 13: 216–31.

Bibliography References

88, 333, 528, 648, 722, 723, 822, 918, 983, 1090, 1261, 1466, 1595, 1735.

Hillis, David Sweeney (1873–1942)

Hillis–DeLee Fetal Stethoscope/Mueller–Hillis Manoeuvre

The priority for invention of the obstetrical head stethoscope became a bitter and unresolved dispute between two of the most prominent obstetricians at the Chicago Lying-in Hospital: David Hillis and Joseph DeLee. This modification of the conventional stethoscope was worn on the head and allowed the doctor or midwife to listen to the fetal heart during the second stage of labour while keeping both hands free. Hillis noted:

> *Frequent observation of the fetal heart tones during the last part of the second stage of labor presents certain technical difficulties after the attendant is surgically prepared for the delivery. In breech labors in which the heart tones must be watched very carefully, it is always desirable and often necessary for the operator to observe the heart tones himself.*

Hillis acknowledged that DeLee had the original idea of a stethoscope that required no manual control but claimed he designed the instrument which he first reported in 1917. Five years later, DeLee published his description of a virtually identical instrument but always claimed he had spoken of and designed such a stethoscope before Hillis.

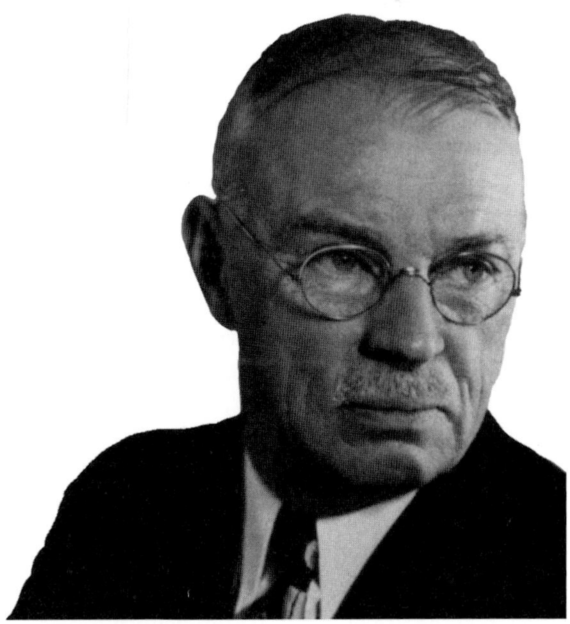

David Sweeney Hillis

David Sweeney Hillis was born in Chicago and graduated from Northwestern University Medical School in 1898. During the First World War, he served as a lieutenant-commander in the US Naval Reserve Medical Corps. He became professor of obstetrics at his alma mater and chairman of the obstetrical department at the Cook County Hospital. He also described a modification of Peter Mueller's technique to assess the relationship of the fetal head to the pelvis. With one finger placed on the fetal head *per vaginum*, the other hand pressed down on the uterine fundus to assess the degree of descent and likelihood of engagement in labour: the Mueller–Hillis manoeuvre.

Mueller's original description in 1886 involved an assistant applying the fundal pressure. Hillis died of lung cancer in the Passavant Memorial Hospital, Chicago on 9 November 1942.

Selected Publications

DeLee JB. Ein neues Stethoskop für die Geburtshilfe besonders geeignet. *Zentralbl Gynäkol* 1922; 46: 1688–9.

Hillis DS. Attachment for the stethoscope. *JAMA* 1917; 68: 910.

Hillis DS. Diagnosis of contracted pelvis by the impression method. *Surg Gynecol Obstet* 1930; 51: 857–94.

Mueller P. Über die Prognose der Geburt bei engen Becken. *Arch Gynäkol* 1886; 27: 311–3.

Bibliography References

536, 648, 1485, 1611.

Hinselmann, Hans (1884–1959)

Colposcopy

In the early part of the twentieth century, research in Austria and Germany led to the realisation that invasive cervical cancer was preceded by abnormalities in the cervical epithelium, which they called the 'carcinomatous surface coating'. Hans Hinselmann studied leukoplakia of the cervix, which was visible to the naked eye in some cases of early cervical cancer. To improve his scrutiny of the cervix he devised a lamp and magnifying glass. Working in collaboration with Leitz he developed the mobile binocular colposcope, which he first used in December 1924. Hinselmann was looking for non-palpable ulceration, which he felt was the way all early cancers started. Instead he found a variety of epithelial patterns reflecting pre-cancerous changes. Through years of study Hinselmann laid the foundations of clinical colposcopy and developed the use of acetic acid in delineating abnormal aceto-white epithelium. He described the mosaic pattern of dysplastic cervical epithelium.

Hans Hinselmann was born in Neumünster, Germany. After studies in Heidelberg and Kiel he received his MD from Kiel University in 1908. After postgraduate training in Jena and Bonn he became extraordinary professor of obstetrics and gynaecology at the University of Bonn in 1921. As well as his career-long study of colposcopy, Hinselmann investigated eclampsia and placental function. In 1925 he moved to Hamburg-Altona, Germany as head of the department of obstetrics and gynaecology. Hinselmann was intolerant of colleagues who did not accept his findings, and he clashed with Robert Meyer.

The Second World War was a bad time for Hinselmann. His two eldest sons were killed at the Battle of Stalingrad. One of his former students joined the SS and was chief physician at Auschwitz, where he continued his work on cervical biopsy and sent the samples to Hinselmann for histological evaluation. After the war, Hinselmann was jailed by a British military tribunal for the sterilisation of gypsy women, which had been carried out by assistants in his clinic. His sentence of three years was halved for health reasons. In 1949, discredited and without an

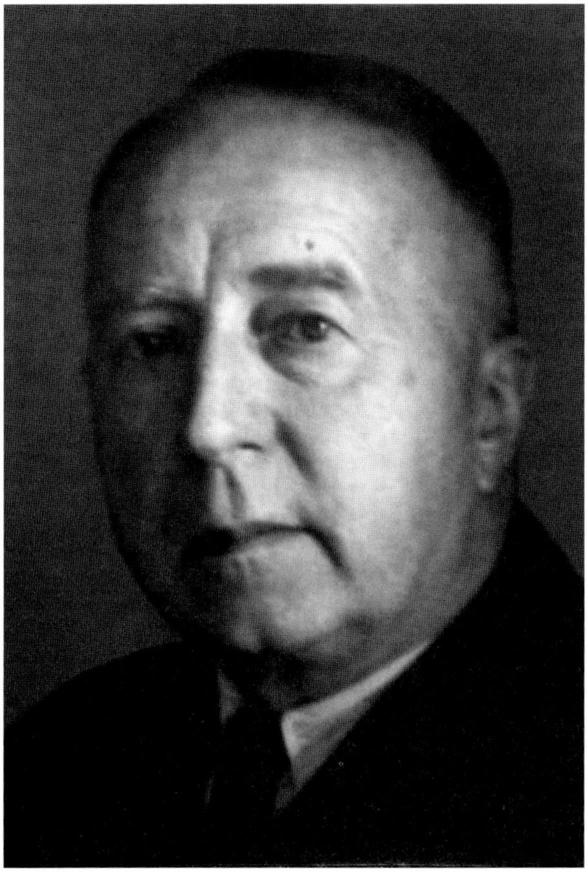

Hans Hinselmann

appointment, he established a pathology laboratory in his own home. He was rescued from obscurity by his former students and devotees in South America, where he made lecture tours in 1949, 1951 and 1957. He was awarded an honorary degree from the University of Brazil in 1957.

In 1959, after returning from a meeting in Zurich, he suffered a myocardial infarction. Visited at his home by a colleague, he said, 'Here you see me in my final hours'. True to his word he died soon after from a second infarct on 18 April 1959.

Selected Publications

Hinselmann H. Verbesserung der inspektionsmöglchkeiten von vulva, vagina und portio. *München Med Wochenschr* 1925; 72: 1733.

Bibliography References

383, 396, 964, 1242, 1365, 1622, 1676.

Hoboken, Nicolaas (1632–1678)

Folds of Hoboken

The umbilical arteries and vein do not contain valves. However, prominent intraluminal folds of the muscular walls, particularly of the arteries, were thought to have a valvular function. These structures were described by others, but Hoboken's full account in his publication, *Anatomia secundinae humanae,* secured his eponymous link. They are variously known as the folds, nodes or valves of Hoboken.

Nicolaas Hoboken was born in Utrecht, Holland, of German extraction. He gained his doctorate of philosophy in 1658, and his medical degree in 1662, from his home university. He became professor of

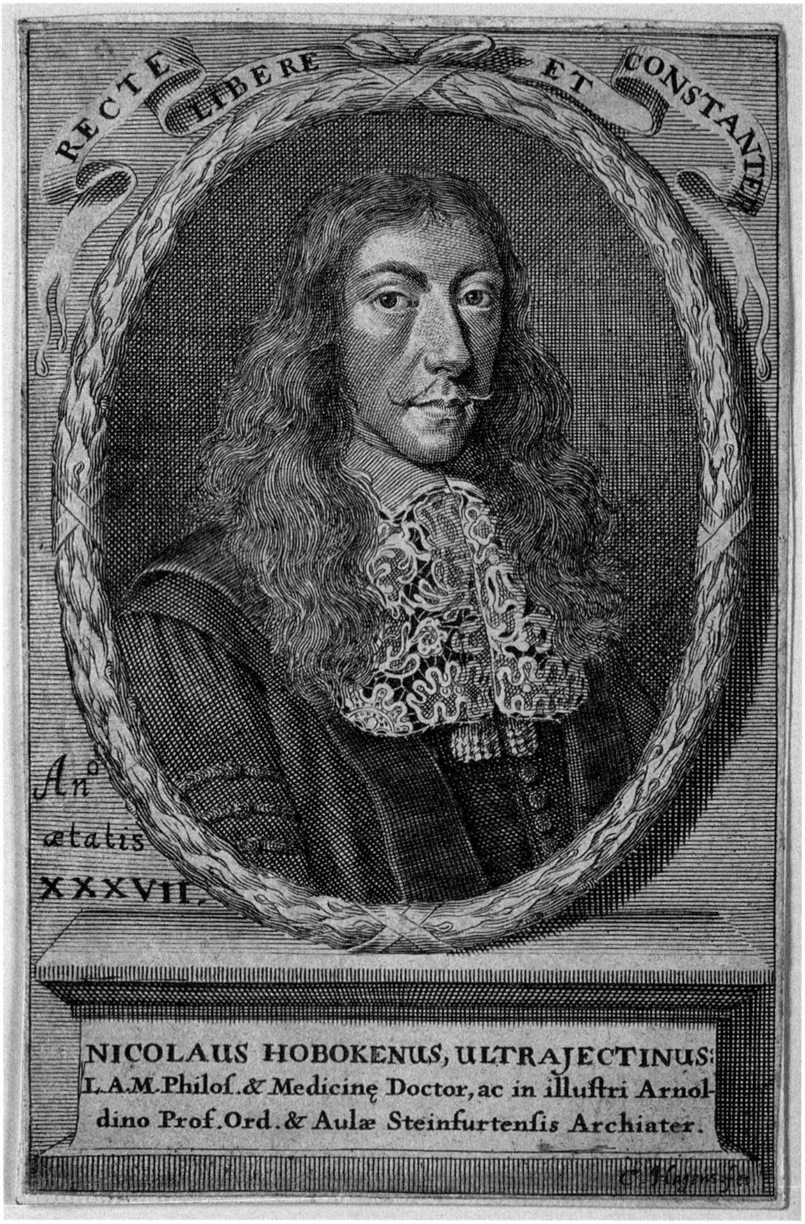
RECTE, LIBERE ET CONSTANTER
Anº
ætatis
XXXVII.
NICOLAUS HOBOKENUS, ULTRAJECTINUS:
I.A.M. Philoſ. & Medicinę Doctor, ac in illuſtri Arnol-
dino Prof. Ord. & Aulæ Steinfurtenſis Archiater.

Nicolaas Hoboken

medicine and mathematics at Steinfurt and later, in 1669, in Harderwyck. Hoboken was influenced by Nicholas Tulp, famous as the demonstrator in Rembrandt's 'Anatomy Lesson'.

Selected Publications

Hoboken N. *Anatomia secundinae humanae.*Utrecht: Joannes Ribbius; 1669.

Bibliography References

347, 406, 648.

Hodge, Hugh Lennox (1796–1873)

Hodge Pessary/Hodge Manoeuvre

The plethora of pessaries designed in the mid-nineteenth century must be viewed in the context of a time when surgical vaginal repair was virtually unavailable and uterine retroversion was believed to be the cause of many gynaecological woes. The innovation of the Hodge pessary was to change the shape from circular to oblong and add a double curve that followed the curvature of the vagina. One of Hodge's biographers described how the inspiration for the double-lever shape came about:

> *Sitting one evening in the University his eyes rested on the upright steel support designed to hold the shovel and tongs, which were kept in position by a steel hook, and as he studied its supporting curve, the longed-for illumination came and the lever pessary was the result.*

Hodge described his rationale as follows:

> *The important modification consists in making a ring oblong, instead of circular, and curved so as to correspond to the curvature of the vagina. Great advantages result from this form; the convexity of the curve being in contact with the posterior wall of the vagina, corresponds with more or less accuracy, to the curve of the rectum, perineum and sacrum.*

The double-curved S-shape of the pessary was designed to press against the uterosacral ligaments behind the cervix and promote anteversion of the uterus.

Hugh Lennox Hodge was born in Philadelphia, the grandson of a Scottish-Irish Presbyterian who emigrated to America in 1730. His father was an army surgeon who died when Hugh was barely two years old. He graduated in medicine from the University of Pennsylvania in 1818. After qualification he spent a year as a ship's surgeon on a voyage to India, where he gained experience in the cholera hospitals. He returned to Philadelphia, set up practice and lectured in anatomy and surgery. His eyesight began to fail and he switched his clinical endeavours to obstetrics. In 1835 he was appointed professor of obstetrics and diseases of women and children at the University of Pennsylvania. Hodge became a skilled and influential obstetrician, and many of his views on pelvic architecture and abnormal labour were ahead of his time. He described digital pressure on the fetal sinciput with succeeding contractions during labour to aid flexion and rotation of the occipito-posterior position: the 'Hodge manoeuvre'. He erred, however, in dismissing Oliver Holmes' theory of the contagiousness of puerperal fever. It is often written that he was opposed to anaesthesia in labour, but his views have been misinterpreted. Hodge's reservations lay with

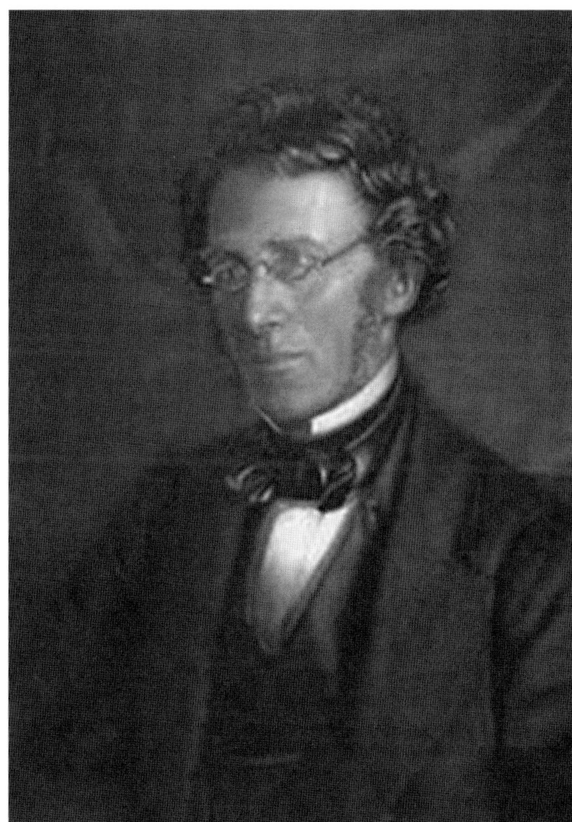

Hugh Lennox Hodge

the safety of chloroform and the indiscriminate use of complete anaesthesia as opposed to analgesia:

> *Often a slight anaesthetic influence may be sufficient to moderate without destroying sensibility, so that labour progresses regularly, without any considerable pain or disturbance ... The author, therefore, coincides in belief with those who insist that the patient ought not to be entirely unconscious ... There are a few cases of course, where complete anaesthesia may be essential.*

He resigned his chair in 1863 because of failing eyesight. Indeed, for the last 20 years of his life he could not read. After he retired he dictated from memory to an amanuensis his master work, *Principles and Practice of Obstetrics,* which became a classic among American obstetric texts. He had seven sons, one of whom became a surgeon and helped edit that work. Hugh Lennox Hodge succumbed to cardiac failure on 23 February 1873.

Selected Publications

Hodge HL. *On Diseases Peculiar to Women, Including Displacements of the Uterus.* Philadelphia, PA: Blanchard and Lea; 1860.

Hodge HL. *The Principles and Practice of Obstetrics.* Philadelphia, PA: Blanchard and Lea; 1864.

Bibliography References

99, 154, 376, 648, 729, 1407, 1419, 1596, 1597.

Hofbauer, Isford Isfred (1878–1961)

Hofbauer Cells

Characteristic cells of the stroma of the placenta resembling histiocytes were first described in detail by Hofbauer in 1905. He felt they had a 'digestive' function and might protect the fetus from infection. These have come to be called 'Hofbauer cells'.

Isford Isfred Hofbauer was born in Vienna of Austrian and Scandinavian parentage. Perhaps because of his Scandinavian first name, sometimes spelt Jsidro, he always signed himself simply 'J. Hofbauer'. He qualified in medicine at the University of Vienna, continuing with his postgraduate work under the tutelage of Friedrich Schauta and Ernst Wertheim. In 1909 he assumed the chair of obstetrics and gynaecology at the University of Königsberg. In 1924 John Whitridge Williams brought him to the Johns Hopkins Hospital in Baltimore to carry out research in pathology and the emerging field of endocrinology. He made many contributions to obstetrics, including the early introduction of posterior pituitary extract for haemorrhage and induction of labour. For augmentation of labour he advocated the intranasal application of pituitrin on cotton pledgets, so it could be quickly removed if uterine hyperstimulation occurred.

His arrogant, egotistical and aggressive personality ensured his departure from Baltimore after Williams' death in 1933. Hofbauer moved to Cincinnati, Ohio and finished his career there. In his later years it was said that, after speaking to a junior colleague, he would say: 'Go home and write in your diary that today you talked to Hofbauer'.

Selected Publications

Hofbauer J. *Grundzüge einer Biologie der Menschlichen Plazenta mit besonderer Berucksichtigung der Fragen der Fötalen Ernährung.* Vienna: Braumiller; 1905.

Hofbauer J. Hypophysenextract als wehenmittel. *Zentralbl Gynäkol* 1911; 35: 137–41.

Hofbauer J, Hoerner JK. The nasal application of pituitary extract for the induction of labor. *Am J Obstet Gynecol* 1927; 14: 137–48.

Bibliography References

536, 1485, 1520.

Holmes, Oliver Wendell (1809–1894)

Puerperal Sepsis

Oliver Wendell Holmes takes his place in obstetric history for his insight and literary expression rather than any direct contribution to the specialty, which he did not practice. At the meetings of the Boston Society for Medical Improvement in late 1842 and early 1843, several case reports of puerperal fever were presented. These suggested to at least one member of the society, Holmes, that the disease could be conveyed from the sick to the well. One report particularly impressed him:

> *The discussion was suggested by a case, reported at the preceding meeting, of a physician who made an examination of the body of a patient who had died with puerperal fever, and who himself died in less than a week, apparently in consequence of a wound received at the examination, having attended several women in confinement in the mean time, all of whom it was alleged, were attacked with puerperal fever.*
>
> *Whatever apprehensions and beliefs were entertained it was plain that a fuller knowledge of the facts relating to the subject would be acceptable to all present. I therefore felt it would be doing a good service to look into the best records I could find, and inquire of the most trustworthy practitioners I knew, to learn what experience had to teach in the matter . . .*

Holmes consulted the writings of, among others, Charles White, James Blundell, Edward Rigby junior and Alexander Gordon. To the latter he gave full credit for delineating the contagious nature of puerperal fever:

> *Gordon's expressions are so clear, his experience is given with such manly distinctness and disinterested honesty that it may be quoted as a model which might have been often followed with advantage.*

He also traced the reports and cases of local doctors. To this foundation of data, he added his logical and literary talents in presenting his paper to the society on 13 February 1843. This was published in the April edition of the *New England Quarterly Journal of Medicine and Surgery*, a publication with limited circulation. Holmes laid down eight guiding principles to prevent puerperal sepsis, including the link between physicians carrying out autopsies on septic cases and then attending obstetric patients:

> *If a physician is present at such autopsies, he should use a thorough ablution, change every article of dress, and allow twenty-four hours or more to elapse before attending to any case of midwifery. It may be well to extend the same caution to cases of simple peritonitis.*

Holmes' ideas had some effect locally but received little other attention until his position was vehemently attacked by one of the leading professors of obstetrics in Philadelphia, Charles Meigs (1792–1869). Hugh Hodge also disagreed with the theory, but with less vehemence. As a result, Holmes had his paper republished in 1855. Added to the work of Ignac Semmelweis and others in Europe, the contagious nature of puerperal fever and the means of its prevention came to be accepted. In a later tribute, EO Otis wrote, 'Some obstetricians had their suspicions but no authoritative voice had assembled all the evidence and then with the power of impassioned rhetoric drawn the inevitable conclusion that the disease was conveyed through the medium of the attending physician'.

Holmes himself wrote:

> *I held up to the professional public the damnable facts concerned with the conveyance of poison from one young mother's chamber to another's for doing which humble office I desire to be thankful that I ever lived though nothing else good should ever come into my life.*

Oliver Wendell Holmes was born in Cambridge, Massachusetts. He first studied law at Harvard but switched to medicine and graduated in 1829. He spent two years in Europe studying medicine, mainly in Paris. He was professor of anatomy and physiology at Dartmouth College from 1838 to 1840 and became professor of anatomy at Harvard Medical School from 1847 to 1882. At the time he wrote his

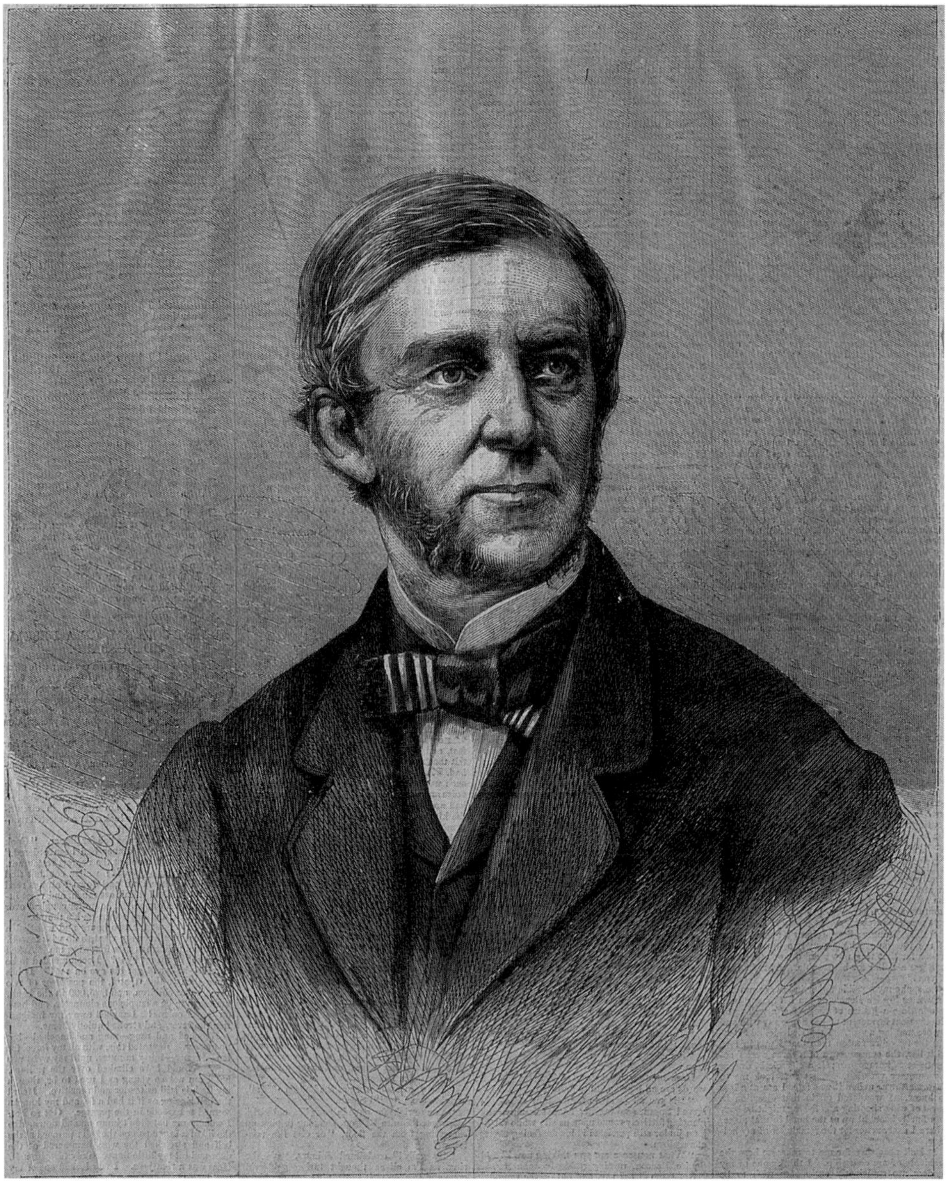

Oliver Wendell Holmes

essay on puerperal fever, he was in practice in Boston but held no other appointment. He became a celebrated essayist and poet. It was Holmes, in a letter to William Morton dated 21 November 1846, who first suggested the word 'anaesthesia' to describe the state induced by ether, the word having been previously applied to the pain-sparing qualities of the mandragora plant by the Greek physician, Pedacius Dioscoridies, in the first century. William Osler called Holmes 'the most successful combination which the world has ever seen of the physician and the man of letters'. Holmes described himself as a 'biped of exactly five feet three inches when standing in a pair of substantial shoes'.

Selected Publications

Holmes OW. Contagiousness of puerperal fever. *N Engl Quart J Med Surg* 1843; 1: 503.

Holmes OW. *Puerperal Fever as a Private Pestilence*. Boston, MA: Ticknor and Fields; 1855.

Bibliography References

110, 219, 301, 338, 487, 578, 648, 681, 683, 699, 708, 738, 938, 939, 1047, 1078, 1147, 1153, 1156, 1595.

Holmes, Rudolph Wieser (1870–1953)

Holmes' Uterine Packer

For two centuries, stimulating debate has rumbled around the pros and cons of uterine packing in the management of post-partum haemorrhage. The procedure has always been more popular in America than in Britain. As effective oxytocic drugs were developed, support for the practice declined, although it is still necessary on rare occasions. As one of the proponents put it, 'People will become uterine packers in the middle of the night when blood is flowing heavily'.

In the era before oxytocic drugs, a variety of instruments to facilitate uterine packing were developed. One of the most popular was devised by Rudolph Holmes of Chicago. It consisted of a two-centimetre diameter tube with an obturator to facilitate placement at the uterine fundus and an introducer to feed gauze along the tube:

> *The tube, with the obturator in place, is pushed up to the fundus uteri, guided by the left hand introduced into the lower uterine segment. The obturator is removed without withdrawing the hand from the vagina . . . the introducer is pushed home carrying the gauze with it . . . repeating the manoeuvre until the uterus and vagina are full. It is a useful expedient while packing to gently oscillate the distal end of the tube from side to side to throw the gauze in folds across the cavity . . . The most convenient gauze for tamponing by the introducer is a strip one-half yard wide and nearly twelve yards long: this gauze is folded into a strip about two inches wide. In cases of extreme atony full twelve yards may be introduced into the utero-vaginal tract; in other cases the amount will depend on the laxity of the uterus and roominess of the vagina.*

Uterine tamponade has recently enjoyed a resurgence in cases of haemorrhage unresponsive to oxytocic drugs, although balloon devices are often used rather than gauze.

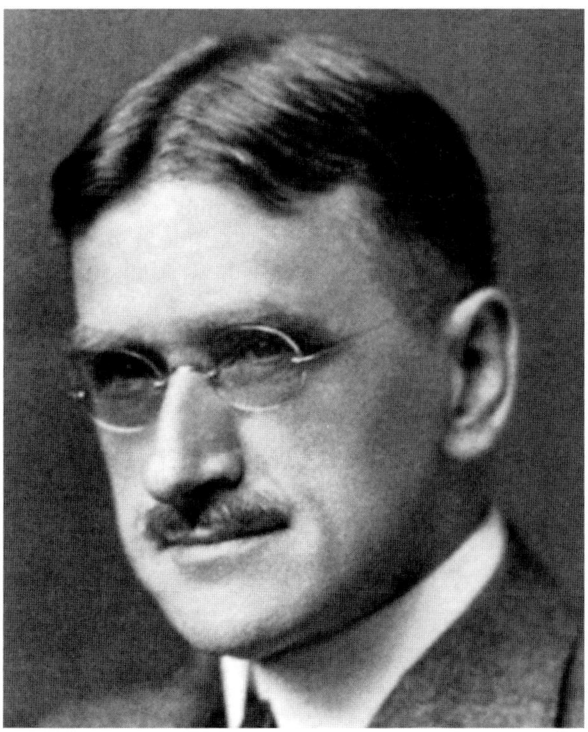

Rudolph Wieser Holmes

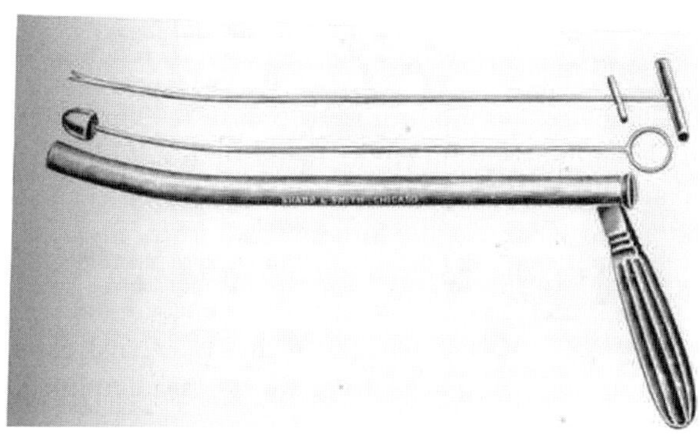

Holmes' uterine packer

Rudolph Wieser Holmes was born in Chicago and a medical graduate of Rush Medical College in 1893. He remained in Chicago all his professional life, ultimately becoming professor of obstetrics and gynaecology at his own university. He served as president of the Chicago Gynecological Society and the Central Association of Obstetricians and Gynecologists. He died in Charlottesville, Virginia on 25 April 1953.

Selected Publications

Holmes RW. A new method of tamponing the uterus post partum. *Am J Obstet Gynecol* 1902; 45: 245–50.

Bibliography References

536, 739, 801, 1156, 1356, 1561.

Hon, Edward Harry Gee (1917–2006)

Electronic Fetal Heart Rate Monitoring

In the summer of 1955, Edward Hon, then an obstetric resident at the Yale University Medical School, was asked by the department head to become involved in developing an electronic device to monitor the fetal heart rate. The choice was logical, as Hon had been trained in radio electronics before starting medical school. Earlier attempts at recording the fetal electrocardiograph (ECG) were masked by the superimposed maternal ECG and background noise. Hon and his co-worker Orvan Hess were able to 'cancel' the maternal ECG by electronic subtraction and thereby obtain a clear fetal heart rate tracing. In considering the clinical application of electronic fetal heart rate monitoring Hon wrote in 1957:

> *In addition to the 160,000 infant deaths associated with the birth process each year, there are a large number of infants afflicted with cerebral palsy and mental retardation. It is possible that these problems find a common basis in fetal anoxia.*
>
> *If significant gains are to be made in this area, a reliable means of accurately determining reversible 'fetal distress' must be found . . . It is hoped that the use of modern instrumentation methods may aid in the elucidation of clinical fetal distress.*

Hon used his monitor to record the fetal heart rate in labour and went on to define 'physiologic' and 'pathologic' bradycardias. In 1963 he developed a fetal scalp electrode, as did others, and from these the modern spiral scalp electrodes evolved.

By 1968 Hon had sufficient experience and data to relate three specific fetal heart rate patterns: early, variable and late decelerations to fetal head compression, umbilical cord compression and utero-placental insufficiency, respectively. The late deceleration pattern was the same as the type II dip described by Roberto Caldeyro-Barcia and the 'alarm dip' of Erich Saling. Hon's classification of fetal heart rate deceleration patterns has become accepted in clinical obstetrics.

Along with Caldeyro-Barcia in Uruguay, and de Haan, Hammacher, Kubli, Saling and Sureau in Europe, Hon was influential in having electronic fetal heart rate monitoring widely accepted into clinical practice. Hon's initial hopes of reducing perinatal mortality have been realised, although this cannot be attributed to fetal heart rate monitoring. His hope for a reduction in cerebral palsy has not, and it is now realised that most of these cases precede labour.

Edward Harry Gee Hon, the fifth of 11 children, was born in Canton, China on 12 January 1917. His family emigrated to Australia when he was a young boy, and his high school education was completed there. After this he worked for a time in his father's department store in Tenterfield, Australia. He then attended the Marconi School of Wireless in Sydney and received his diplomas in radio mechanics and technology. In 1945 he emigrated to the United States. He took his bachelor of science degree in physics from Union College, Nebraska and his MD in 1950 from Loma Linda University, California, graduating first in his class. His original intention was to return to China as a medical missionary.

He carried out residency training in pathology at Loma Linda and in obstetrics and gynaecology at Yale University. He remained on staff at Yale and during this time was supported by a Markle scholarship to carry out his basic research on electronic fetal heart rate monitoring. From 1960 to 1964 he was professor of obstetrics and gynaecology at Loma Linda University. He returned to Yale in 1964 to head the section of perinatal biology. In 1969 he moved back to California as professor of obstetrics and gynaecology at the University of Southern California in Los Angeles. He became professor emeritus in 1982 when he retired at age 65.

Hon started his final 'post-retirement' career as a research scientist at the Drew Postgraduate School in Los Angeles. Here he continued research into maternal cardiovascular changes in pregnancy with hypertension, premature labour and hyperemesis gravidarum. He undertook teaching and research trips to Australia, China and San Salvador. Hon received many honours in his lifetime, including Fellowship ad eundem of the Royal College of Obstetricians and Gynaecologists and the Distinguished Service Award of the American College of Obstetricians and Gynecologists. He was most proud to be awarded the Order of Australia in 1999, 'For service to medicine, particularly in the field of electronic foetal heart rate monitoring and for research in maternal monitoring in pregnancy'. Ed Hon continued working until he died in his sleep on 6 November 2006 at his home in Bradbury, California, just two months before his ninetieth birthday.

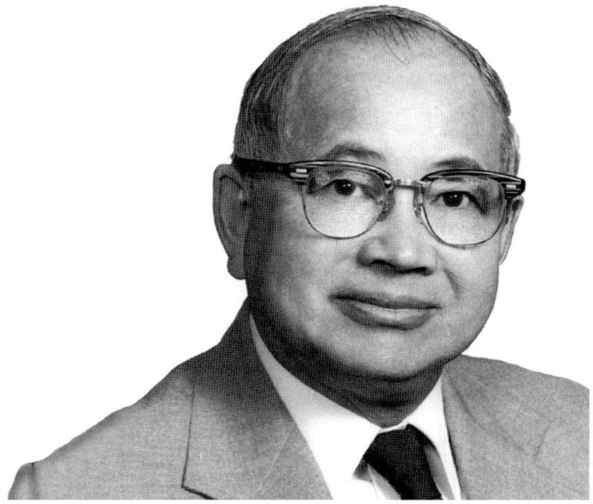
Edward Harry Gee Hon

Selected Publications

Hon EH, Hess OW. Instrumentation of fetal electrocardiology. *Science* 1957; 125: 553–4.

Hon EH. The electronic evaluation of the fetal heart rate: Preliminary report. *Am J Obstet Gynecol* 1958; 75: 1215–30.

Hon EH. Observations on 'pathologic' fetal bradycardia. *Am J Obstet Gynecol* 1959; 77: 1084–99.

Hon EH. The classification of fetal heart rate: a working classification. *Obstet Gynecol* 1963; 22: 137–46.

Hon EH. Electronic evaluation of the fetal heart rate and fetal electrocardiography (II). A vaginal electrode. *Am J Obstet Gynecol* 1963; 86: 772.

Hon EH. *An Atlas of Fetal Heart Rate Patterns.* New Haven, CT: Harty Press; 1968.

Bibliography References

635, 819, 916, 1536, 1731.

Hopkins, Harold Horace (1918–1994)

Fibre-Optic Endoscopy

If you look near the eye-piece on one of the most commonly used laparoscopes, you will see printed the name Hopkins. This is a tribute to Harold Hopkins, who was the English physicist largely responsible for applying fibre optics and his rod-lens system to endoscopy. One of the earliest suggestions of the application of fibre optics came from John Logie Baird (1888–1946), an electrical engineer from the West Coast of Scotland who, in 1926, suggested that an assembly of hollow glass rods might be 'an improved method and means of producing optical images' without the use of a lens. Logie did not pursue this option although he did take out a patent. Instead he made the major contribution to the development of television.

Harold Hopkins was a lecturer in the department of physics at the Imperial College of Science and Technology in London when, along with his research student Narinder Kapany, he published his paper on the potential use of bundles of fibre glass to replace the multiple lens system of current endoscopes:

> *An optical unit has been devised which will convey optical images on a flexible axis. The unit comprises a*

bundle of fibres of glass, or other transparent material, and it therefore appears appropriate to introduce the term 'fibrescope' to denote it. An obvious use of the unit is to replace the train of lenses employed in conventional endoscopes. The existing instruments of this kind, for example, cystoscopes, gastroscopes and bronchoscopes, etc, consist of a train of copying lenses and intermediate field lenses. They are either rigid or have only limited flexibility. Moreover, the image quality of these systems is poor . . . Even more important in this respect, however, is the need to use small relative aperatures for such instruments, this being necessary if acceptable definition is to be obtained with such large field curvature.

This paper was published in the January issue of *Nature* alongside a brief article from Abraham van Heel, the Dutch physicist from the Technical University of Delft in Holland. In his brief letter, van Heel suggested a similar application of glass fibre bundles. At the time he was working on a Dutch government contract to design a better submarine periscope.

In his paper Hopkins acknowledged the primacy of Baird. When Hopkins patented his rod-lens system in the late 1950s, the main potential market was for cystoscopes. However, none of the English or American companies were interested in developing this system. It was not until 1967 that an American surgeon interested in endoscopy introduced Hopkins to Karl Storz, a small manufacturer of medical instruments in Tuttingen, Germany. This collaboration with the rod-lens system and cold light fibre-optic illumination, was to revolutionise the design and production of endoscopes from the late 1960s.

Harold Horace Hopkins was born to a family of modest means in Leicester, England. He took his undergraduate degree at Leicester University in 1939. Early on in his career he worked with optics and soon mastered this field. In 1948 he was approached by the British Broadcasting Corporation and helped develop the television camera zoom lens for coverage of sporting events. He obtained his PhD in London in 1945 and in 1947 joined the department of physics at the Imperial College in London, where he rose from research fellow to lecturer and ultimately to reader. In 1967 he was appointed to a new chair as professor of applied physics at Reading University, where he remained until he retired in 1984. In his spare time Hopkins was an accomplished pianist, sailor and oenophile. Hopkins was regarded as one of the outstanding physicists of his generation. He died in Reading on 22 October 1994.

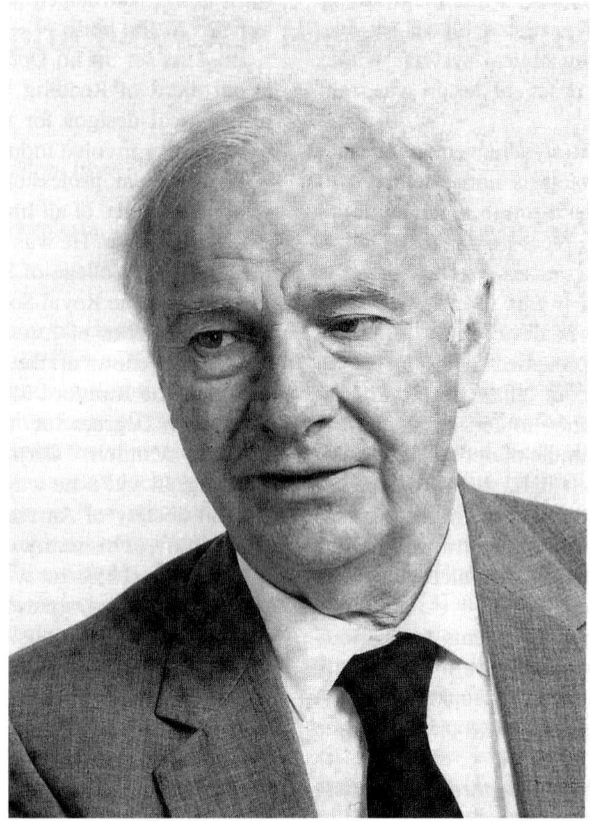

Harold Horace Hopkins

Selected Publications

Hopkins HH, Kapany NS. A flexible fibrescope, using static scanning. *Nature* 1954; 73: 39–41.

Van Heel ACS. A new method of transporting optical images without aberrations. *Nature* 1954; 73: 39.

Bibliography References

127, 128, 226, 297, 644, 711, 1111, 1315.

Houston, John (1802–1845)

Houston's Valves

It is an unlucky gynaecologist who comes into direct contact with Houston's valves of the rectum, lying as they do three or more inches from the anal margin. In his paper on the subject, Houston put forward his rationale for a clear understanding of the anatomy of the rectum as follows: 'The structure and arrangement of the mucous membrane of the rectum ought to be perfectly understood with a view towards the accurate diagnosis, or successful treatment of its diseases; particularly, in order to be able to introduce instruments with dexterity along its canal'. His detailed anatomical dissection and preparations led him to the following conclusions:

> *In the natural state, the tube of the gut does not form, as is usually conceived one smooth uninterrupted passage, devoid of any obstacles that might impede the entrance of bougies: it is on the contrary, made uneven in several places by certain valvular projections of its internal membrane, which standing across the passage, must frequently render the introduction of such instruments as a matter of considerable difficulty . . . The valves exist equally in the young and in the aged, in the male and in the female; but in different individuals there will be found some varieties as to their number and position. Three is the average number, although sometimes four, and sometimes only two are present in a marked degree. The position of the largest and most regular valve is about three inches from the anus opposite to the base of the bladder . . . The form of the valves is semilunar; their convex borders are fixed to the sides of the rectum, occupying in their attachments from one-third to one-half of the circumference of the gut. Their surfaces are sometimes horizontal but more usually they have a slightly oblique aspect, and their concave floating margins, which are defined and sharp, are generally directed a little upwards.*

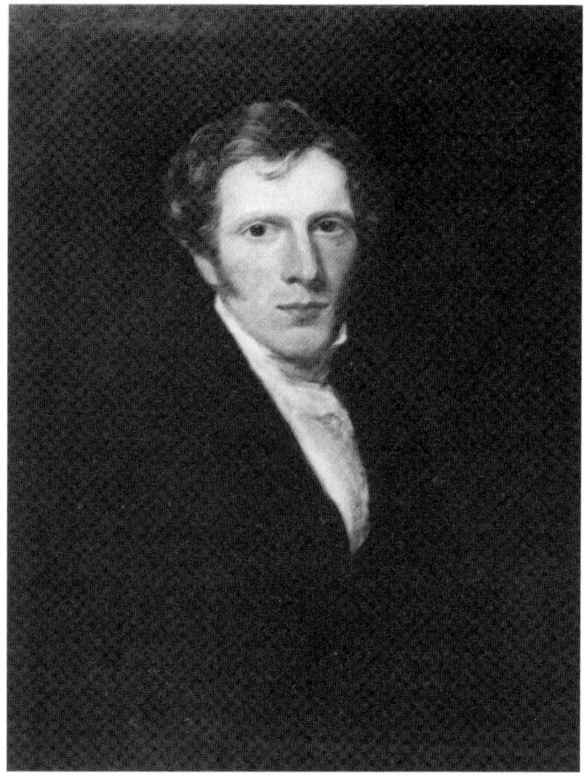

John Houston

John Houston, the son of a Presbyterian clergyman, was born in Northern Ireland in 1802. As a young boy he was adopted by his maternal uncle, a physician, who financed his education. He began his medical apprenticeship in 1819 with the surgeon John Shekleton, at the Royal College of Surgeons in Dublin. He finished his apprenticeship in 1824 and became a demonstrator of anatomy in the College of Physicians and Surgeons, and two years later acquired his MD at Edinburgh. He was a founder of the City of Dublin Hospital in 1832. This was a teaching hospital for the Royal College of Surgeons, and Houston had an active surgical practice there.

Houston was the first to introduce the microscope into Irish medicine. He used it to study the microscopy of tumours he had surgically removed. His observations led him to conclude that a degree of practical surgical staging might be feasible:

> *. . . there is a stage, in many cases of cancer in which the disease is strictly confined to the part, and in which it may be removed effectually by operation; but that when once, from a continuance of the affection, the system becomes influenced by it, a cure by such means is hopeless.*

Houston was a prodigious worker and built up an extensive anatomical and pathological museum, including the skull of a hippopotamus, which was later sold to the Queen's College of Belfast for £250. In April 1845 Houston collapsed while giving a lecture in Baggot Street Hospital. His collapse was accompanied by a violent headache and probably due to subarachnoid haemorrhage, from which he died two months later on 30 July 1845. It was generally thought that he had 'overworked' his brain.

Selected Publications

Houston J. Observations on the mucous membrane of the rectum. *Dublin Hosp Reports* 1830; 5: 158–65.

Houston J. *On the Microscopic Pathology of Cancer. Dublin Medical Press* 1844; 12: 5–8.

Bibliography References

220, 293, 294, 406, 952, 1126, 1693.

Houstoun, Robert (1678–1734)

Ovariotomy

Robert Houstoun was born in Glasgow, the eldest son of a surgeon-apothecary. He served an apprenticeship with his father and was registered as a surgeon-apothecary in 1698. For the next two years, he studied and worked at the Hôtel Dieu and Hôtel de la Charité in Paris, where he gained experience in surgery and obstetrics. He returned to Glasgow in 1701. In August of that year he was urged by a titled patient to aid a tenant's wife, 'who lay bedridden, of an uncommon disease, which no physician or surgeon who had seen her, could give any name to, or account for'. The patient was a 58-year-old woman called Margaret Millar, whom he found bedridden, weak, almost unable to eat and with difficulty breathing due to a 'monstrous' enlargement of her abdomen. She pleaded with Houstoun for relief. He explained the risks of operating to relieve the swelling, which in her desperation she accepted. Houston undertook the procedure then and there in the farmhouse:

> *I drew (I must confess) almost all my confidence from her sudden resolution, so that without loss of time I prepared what the place would allow and with an imposthume lancet laid open about an inch but finding nothing issue, I enlarged it two inches and even than nothing came forth but a little thin yellowish serum so I ventured to lay it open about two inches more. I was not a little startled to find only a glutinous substance bung up the orifice … I drew out about two yards in length of a substance thicker than any jellie or rather like glue … This was followed by nine full quarts of such matter … with several hydatides of various sizes containing a yellowish serum the least of them bigger than an orange with several large pieces of membranes which seemed to be part of the distended ovary. Then I squeezed out all I could and stitched up the wound in three places almost equidistant.*

Houstoun dressed the wound for the next eight days with compresses of French brandy, and to his delight, 'she mended apace to the admiration of everyone thereabouts'. She lived for another 13 years in good health.

The word 'ovariotomy' was first used by Charles Clay, after it was suggested to him by James Young Simpson. Strictly speaking the term came to be inaccurately used to describe the removal of an ovarian tumour, with or without conservation of residual ovarian tissue.

Debate has occurred off and on since then over precedence for the first ovariotomy: Houstoun or Ephraim McDowell over a century later in 1817. It is now generally accepted that McDowell did the first ovariotomy, as he removed the entire ovarian cyst and tied the pedicle. Houstoun's procedure was really incision and drainage. Nonetheless, both men were pioneers, and the courage and resolve of Houstoun, more than a century before McDowell, was remarkable.

Houstoun became successful in practice and in 1712 was awarded his MD after examination by the University of Glasgow. He later moved to London and in 1725 was elected a fellow of the Royal Society. He died in London on 15 May 1734, but his place of burial is unknown and there is no portrait of him.

Selected Publications

Houstoun R. An account of a dropsy in the left ovary of a woman, aged 58. Cured by a large incision made in the side of the abdomen. *Phil Trans* 1724–25: 33: 8–15.

Bibliography References

769, 822, 951, 961, 1252, 1496, 1497.

Hühner, Max (1873–1947)

Hühner's Postcoital Test

In 1888, Harry Sims, the son of Marion Sims, outlined the essential features of the postcoital test in a paper to the American Gynecological Society. Some of his report was based on the work of his father, who did much of the early investigation in this field. However, it was the detailed report of a large series in 1913 by the New York urologist, Max Hühner, that set the standard and caused it to become known as Hühner's test, although some call it the Sims–Hühner test. From his studies Hühner concluded:

> *If live spermatozoa are found in the cervical mucus we can at once absolve the husband from all responsibility. If dead spermatozoa are found in the cervical mucus it is safer to get a condom specimen to see whether the spermatozoa came out dead, or whether they were killed after they had entered the female by the secretions of the latter's genitals . . .*

Max Hühner was born in Berlin but moved to the United States and graduated from the College of Physicians and Surgeons of Columbia University in 1893. Following graduation, he did postgraduate work in Berlin and New York in urology and genito-urinary medicine. He served on the staff of the Bellevue and Mount Sinai hospitals in New York. Hühner was also an authority on Shakespearean literature and wrote a monograph entitled *Was Shakespeare an Angler?*

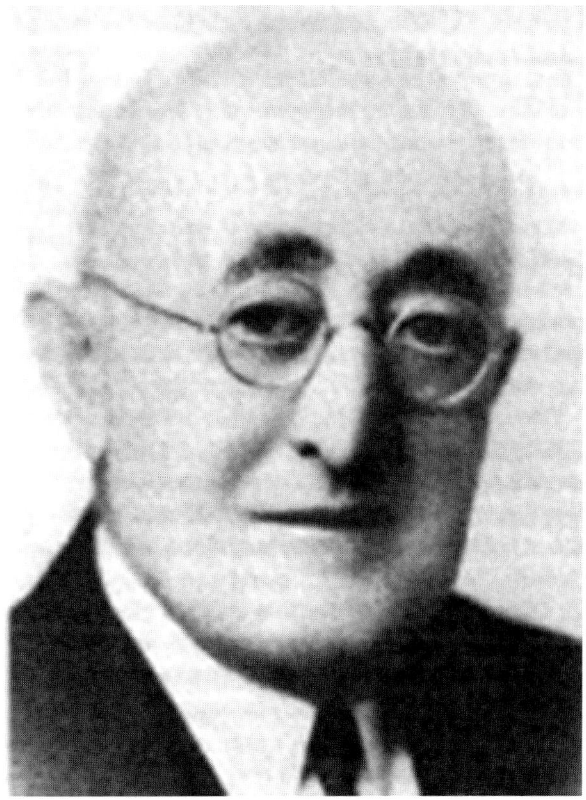

Max Hühner

Selected Publications

Hühner M. *Sterility in the male and female and its treatment*. New York, NY: Rebman; 1913.

Hühner M. The value of the spermatozoa test in sterility. *Urol Cutan Rev* 1914; 18: 587–92.

Bibliography References

751, 782, 1201, 1485, 1561.

Hulka, Jaroslav Fabian (1930–2014)

Hulka Clip/Hulka Tenaculum

By the late 1960s laparoscopic sterilisation using electocautery, pioneered by Raoul Palmer, was becoming established in gynaecological practice. However, the procedure was plagued with rare but serious burns to adjacent bowel. Jaroslav Hulka had recently taken up an appointment at the Carolina Population Centre of the University of North Carolina at Chapel Hill and turned his attention to the techniques of female sterilisation. He started with a hysteroscopic approach in rabbit and pig models but, despite a variety of media including coagulation, freezing, glue and silver nitrate, he found that the seal of the uterotubal junction was only temporary in too many cases to be effective. He redirected his efforts to the laparoscopic approach and in animal experiments with pigs tried a number of clips including tantalum, silver and stainless steel. However, he found that fistula formation through the crushed tissue occurred over time. He then became aware of a 2 mm wide spring, originally used for automatic weapons as an ammunition clip feeder, which had been tried unsuccessfully when incorporated into an intrauterine device. He made contact with George Clemens, a mechanical engineer in Chicago, and the two of them designed a clip with small teeth to maintain contact with the fallopian tube and incorporating the 2 mm spring to sustain closure of the clip. The material for the clip was a hard, non-yielding plastic, and the spring was made of stainless steel, gold plated to make it inert. The clips were tested on pigs in North Carolina and on monkeys in a primate colony in Puerto Rico. There were no pregnancies. The first human application of the clip was in November 1972 at the North Carolina Memorial Hospital. Clemens also designed a clip applicator, and these were distributed, along with clips, to a number of research centres throughout the world. In the first 1,000 cases the failure rate was 2 per cent, which was later found to be due to a tiny gap between the jaws of the clip, and this was corrected. The clip and applicator were manufactured by Wolfe Medical Instruments in Chicago.

In the course of his work on laparoscopic sterilisation, Hulka developed a tenaculum attached to a uterine sound. This facilitated mobilisation of the uterus to bring the fallopian tubes into the operative field. The Hulka clip was the first of the occlusive techniques to be developed as an alternative to electrocautery. It was to be followed by the Yoon falope ring and the Filshie clip.

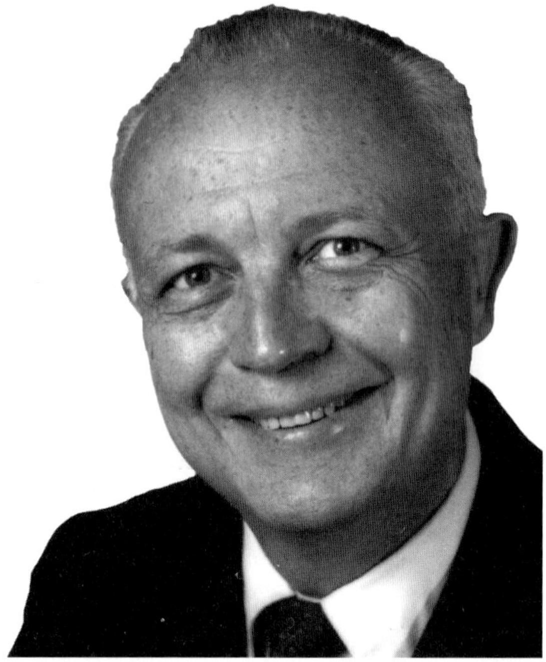
Jaroslav Fabian Hulka

Jaroslav Hulka was born in New York City on 29 September 1930. Both his parents, musicians from Czechoslovakia, were in New York on a Rockefeller Fellowship. Hulka grew up in New York, apart from one year in Prague. During his youth he studied the French horn at the Julliard School of Music in New York and also at the Prague Conservatory of Music. He graduated BA from Harvard College in 1952 and MD from the Columbia College of Physicians and Surgeons, New York in 1956. He served his residency in obstetrics and gynaecology at the Sloane Hospital for Women at the Columbia Presbyterian Medical Centre in New York. In 1961 he went to the University of Pittsburgh as assistant professor of obstetrics and gynecology. He moved to the University of North

Carolina at Chapel Hill in 1967 and worked in the Carolina Population Centre, the department of obstetrics and gynecology and the school of public health. In 1976 he was appointed full professor in both the department of obstetrics and gynecology and the school of public health, positions he held until 1996 when he became professor emeritus. He died at Chapel Hill on 24 November 2014.

Selected Publications

Hulka JF. Controlling tenaculum: an instrument for uterine mobilization. *Am J Obstet Gynecol* 1972; 115: 365–6.

Hulka JF, Omran KF. Comparative tubal occlusion: rigid and spring-loaded clips. *Fertil Steril* 1972: 23: 633–7.

Hulka JF, Fishburne JI, Mercer JP, Omran KF. Laparoscopic sterilization with a spring clip: a report of the first fifty cases. *Am J Obstet Gynecol* 1973; 116: 715–19.

Bibliography References

168, 368, 447, 1234, 1599.

Hunner, Guy LeRoy (1868–1957)

Hunner's Ulcer

Guy LeRoy Hunner was born on 6 December 1868 in Alma, Wisconsin. He was educated in the local public schools, graduated from high school in 1887 and then spent two years as a bookkeeper in his father's business, which included publishing and the wholesale grocery trade. This experience was enough to convince him to enter the University of Wisconsin, from which he received his bachelor of science degree in 1893. Later that year he entered the first medical class of the Johns Hopkins University and graduated MD in 1897. He carried out his residency training in gynaecology at Johns Hopkins under the supervision of Howard Kelly. In 1902 he joined the staff of the hospital, where he remained for the rest of his career. He was a pioneer in the application of urological investigation in gynaecology, particularly with the cystoscope. He made original contributions and a cystoscopic description of interstitial cystitis, which he called the 'illusive ulcer of the bladder'. This condition was eventually labelled 'Hunner's ulcer'.

In his initial paper, read at a meeting of the New England branch of the Urological Association in Boston on 30 November 1914, Hunner reported a number of cases of 'a rare type of bladder ulcer in women':

> *This group presents a strikingly uniform picture ... The tenderness and scar tissue contracture was so marked in most of the cases as to require thorough cocainizing and careful manipulation in order to do satisfactory cystoscopy ... In the neighborhood of this scar-looking*

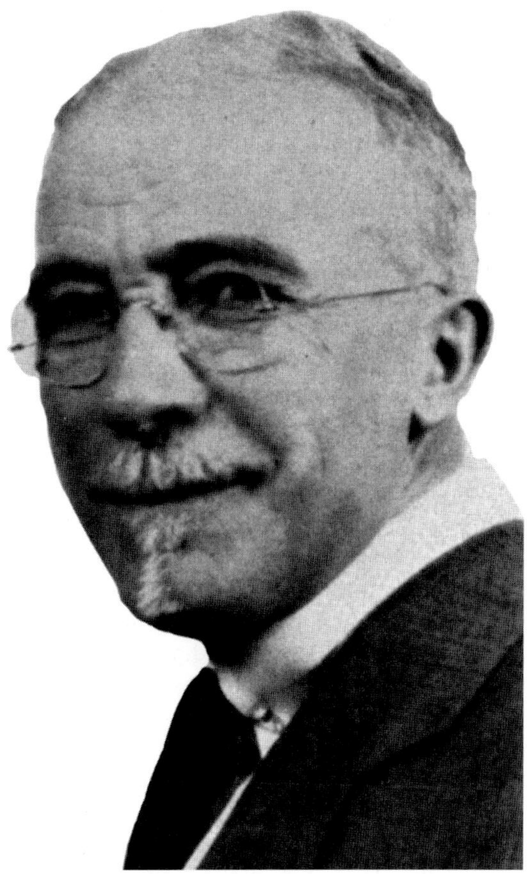

Guy LeRoy Hunner

area one sees one or more areas of hyperemia, which, on being touched with a dry cotton pledget, or with the end of speculum, bleed and first show their character as ulcers ... So far as I know there is no form of bladder inflammation or ulceration that has an absolutely characteristic clinical history or cystoscopic picture and the ulcer under discussion is no exception to the rule ... Our conclusion therefore is that a diagnosis of this peculiar form of bladder ulceration depends ultimately on its resistance to all ordinary forms of treatment ... My experience with this relatively small number of cases convinces me that excision is the treatment after one arrives at a diagnosis of this particular form of ulcer.

Ultimately, the condition came to be known as interstitial cystitis.

Hunner was regarded by his peers as a quiet, gentle, thoughtful man who was an excellent gynaecological surgeon. After retirement he lived on his farm on the Magothy River, 20 miles south of Baltimore, and remained physically active until his death at the age of 88 on 14 July 1957.

Selected Publications

Hunner GL. A rare type of bladder ulcer in women; a report of cases. *Boston Med Surg J* 1915; 172: 660–4.

Bibliography References

68, 535, 801, 1485.

Hunter, William (1718–1783)

Obstetric Anatomy/Hunter's Membrane

William Hunter was the lesser known of the two famous Hunter brothers. William, 10 years senior to his brother John, was cultured, well spoken and reflective. John was a robust, colourful and inspired investigator, whose contributions to the science of surgery are legend.

William Hunter was a practising physician and obstetrician, but it was as a teacher, particularly of anatomy, that he excelled. He regarded a good knowledge of anatomy as an essential basis for clinical medicine: 'Anatomy is the only solid foundation of medicine ... It discovers and ascertains truth, overturns superstition and vulgar error'. He felt he could do more good by teaching his art than by practising it: 'The influence of a teacher extends itself to the whole nation and descends to posterity'.

Undoubtedly, Hunter's *magnum opus* was his monumental production, *The Anatomy of the Human Gravid Uterus*, published in 1774. He worked on this book for almost 30 years and wisely employed the skilled Dutch artist Jan van Rymsdyk. From his drawings, engravers produced the 34 copper plates that are the basis of this beautiful work. Over the years 13 bodies were dissected as well as several abortions. All drawings were made from direct observation of the specimens. In this publication Hunter gave the first detailed description of the decidua, also known as 'Hunter's membrane':

The external membrane, or decidua, full of small branching veins which passed into it from the internal surface of the womb. At this place the vascular and opaque decidua was carefully removed: there was no appearance of injected veins upon the chorion, or in the amnion; both of which were so transparent that the childs skin could be seen distinctly through them.

William Hunter was born at Long Calderwood, seven miles from Glasgow, Scotland. At the age of 14 he went to Glasgow University where he spent the next five years. His father hoped he would become a minister, but after his early studies Hunter found he 'could not subscribe to the dogmatical articles of faith'. He applied for the position of schoolmaster is his home village but failed to get the appointment. He spent the next two years as an apprentice to Dr William Cullen (1710–1790) of nearby Hamilton. Cullen was later to become professor of medicine at both Glasgow and Edinburgh. In 1740 Hunter attended the lectures of Alexander Monro in Edinburgh, and the following year he left for London. Here he took up residence with William Smellie and later with James Douglas. He courted Douglas' daughter, Martha Jane, and they were betrothed, but she died in 1743 while Hunter was in Paris attending anatomy and surgery lectures. He never married saying, 'a man cannot have two loves, and my first and only love is to teach'.

Hunter later acknowledged the influence of Smellie:

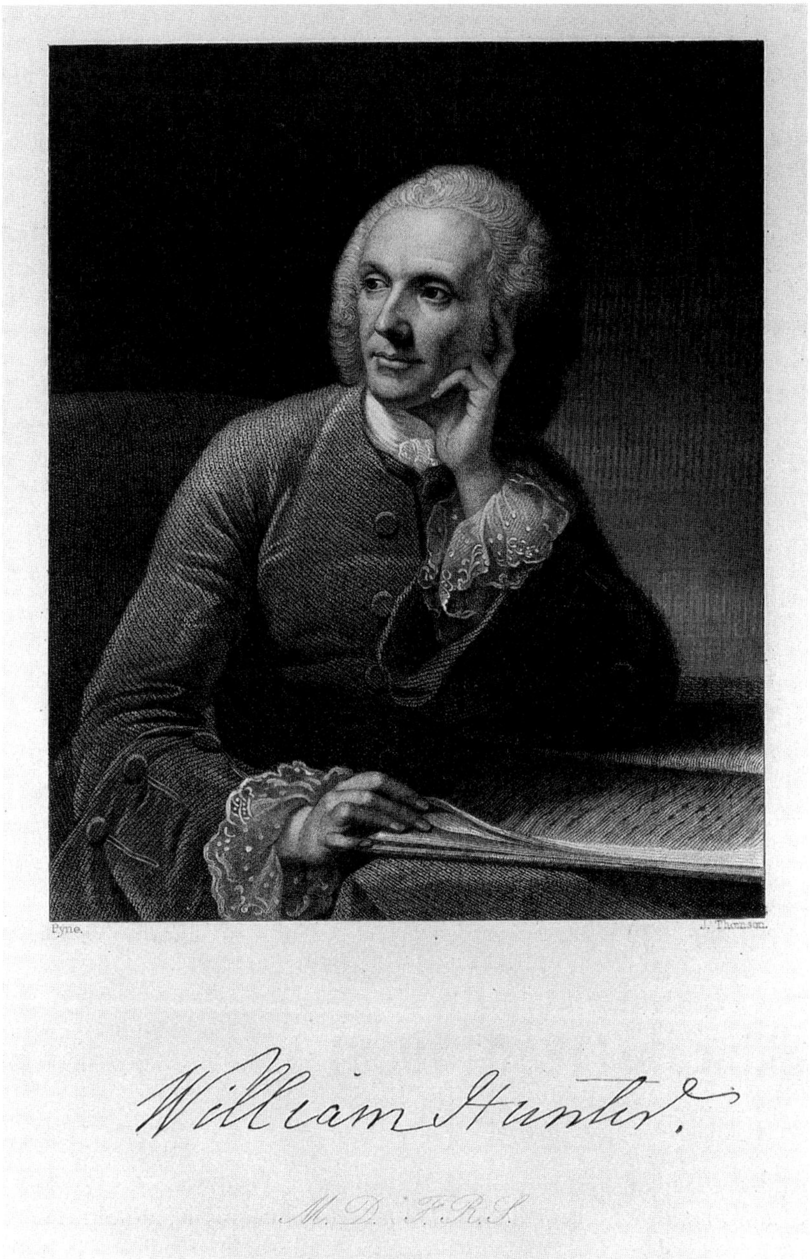

William Hunter

As I look back upon my life I see that my liking for midwifery began to take origin soon after I came to London, during the time I assisted Mr Smellie to prepare his lectures and accompanied him to assist his patients in the slums and rookeries around St Pauls.

In his early career Hunter did practice surgery but had a tendency to faint in that pre-anaesthetic era. Later his clinical work was as a physician and obstetrician. In 1768 he established the Great Windmill Street School of London, which became the premier private school for anatomical and surgical instruction. His reputation soared, and he became popular in the higher circles of society. He was appointed physician-accoucheur at the Middlesex Hospital in 1748, surgeon-accoucheur to the British Lying-In Hospital in 1749 and professor of anatomy at the Royal Academy of Arts in 1768. He was called to attend Queen Charlotte in her confinement in 1762 and was appointed as her physician extraordinary in 1764, 'charged with entire responsibility for the health of the Queen as a childbearing lady'. He delivered her of the future King George IV. At that time man-midwives were known as 'nightmen' and Hunter was called the 'Queen's Scotch Nightman'.

Hunter was a very conservative obstetrician and spoke against the excessive use of forceps, feeling that 'the forceps (midwifery instruments in general I fear) upon the whole, has done more harm than good'. He also spoke against the common practice of immediate delivery of the placenta by cord traction or manual extraction: 'the hurrying away the placenta is just as bad as hurrying on the labour, and forcing away the placenta is a terrible practice'. Smellie was to credit Hunter with changing his own management of the third stage of labour to this more conservative approach.

Hunter published many original observations on other aspects of medicine. He also built up a huge and comprehensive museum and library, not all of it confined to medical material. In addition to an extensive anatomical and pathological specimen collection, he had a library of more than ten thousand volumes and manuscripts on all fields of learning. These, along with his wide collection of shells, coins and paintings, he bequeathed to the University of Glasgow, where they currently reside in various departments.

Even a superficial review shows Hunter's life to be one of phenomenal productivity. He was troubled by gout in his later years, despite abstemious living. He was unwell when he insisted on delivering his usual introductory lecture to the surgery course on Thursday 20 March 1783 and fainted towards the end of his presentation. In the last hours of his life he said to his friend, Charles Coombe, 'But there is little that can be done, and my weakness gets worse. If I had strength enough left to hold a pen, I would write how pleasant and easy a thing it is to die', which he did on Sunday 30 March 1783.

The historian Harvey Graham said of William Hunter, 'He did as much for midwifery as his brother John did for surgery. Each of them entered a despised craft and did much to help convert it to an accepted branch of the art and science of medicine'.

Selected Publications

Hunter W. *The Anatomy of the Human Gravid Uterus.* Birmingham: John Baskerville; 1774. Also published in: The Classics of Obstetrics and Gynecology Library. Birmingham: Gryphon Editions; 1991 (facsimile).

Bibliography References

28, 63, 108, 189–191, 208, 248, 306, 310, 454, 472, 577, 648, 749, 760, 761, 867, 999, 1034, 1076, 1079, 1140, 1177, 1337, 1418, 1508, 1567, 1601, 1602, 1607, 1610.

Huntington, James Lincoln (1880–1968)

Huntington's Operation for Uterine Inversion

In 1921 James Huntington presented the topic of acute uterine inversion to the Surgical Fortnightly gathering in Boston. He began with these remarks:

> *This phenomenon so fearful in its consequences, so sudden and so rare, is nearly as much a puzzle today as it was in the dark ages of medicine. For this reason it is the bounded duty of every obstetrician, promptly and fearlessly, to report with the utmost frankness and care every case that comes within his practice.*

He went on to describe a case of acute uterine inversion in which manual replacement failed and the bleeding was so heavy that blood transfusion was required. He resorted to laparotomy and outlined the findings and his management:

> *Immediate laparotomy decided upon without further attempts from below. Patient almost pulseless … Peritoneal cavity opened, and what proved to be the lower uterine segment with appendages drawn into the crater presented at the wound. A thick bite of the uterus was seized with Allis forceps in the median line just inside the crater. With moderate traction it was brought above the ring, and a bite seized lower down, and so bit by bit the uterus was drawn back through the ring.*

Thus was born Huntington's operation for acute uterine inversion. Seven years later, along with two

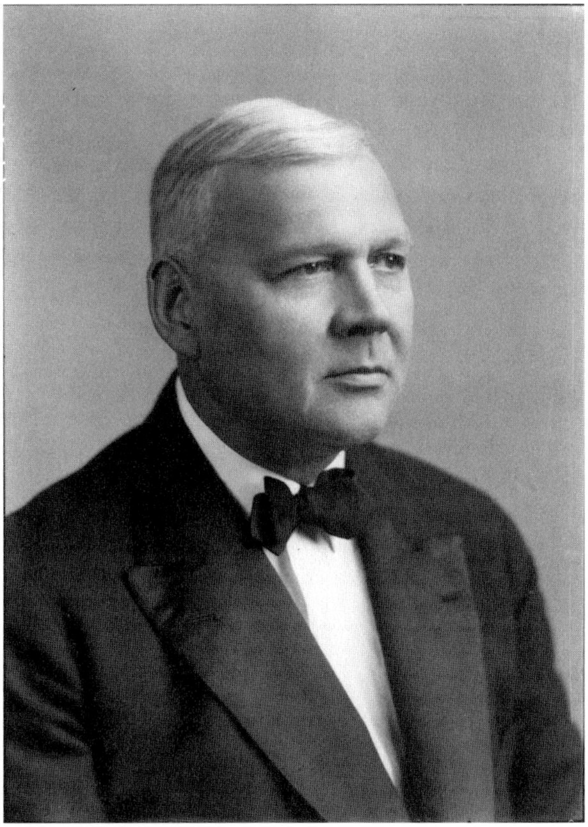

James Lincoln Huntington

colleagues, he reported a series of five successful cases using this technique.

James Lincoln Huntington was born in Malden, Massachusetts on 30 March 1880. He graduated MD from Harvard in 1906 and took postgraduate training in obstetrics and gynaecology in Boston. In 1910 he visited a number of European clinics. He worked at the Boston Lying-in and Cambridge hospitals. He was an early supporter of organised antenatal care but opposed to midwives.

Selected Publications

Huntington JL. Acute inversion of the uterus. *Boston Med J* 1921; 184: 376–80.

Huntington JL, Irving FC, Kellogg FS. Abdominal reposition in acute inversion of the puerperal uterus. *Am J Obstet Gynecol* 1928; 15: 34–40.

Bibliography References

536, 754, 1485.

I

Irving, Frederick Carpenter (1883–1957)

Irving Tubal Ligation

In an attempt to reduce the failure rate of the Madlener and, to a lesser extent, the Pomeroy sterilisation techniques, Frederick Irving devised an almost foolproof procedure in 1924. He later modified his technique and in 1950 reported 814 cases without failure. His procedure involved ligating and dividing the tube about 3 cm from the cornu, turning back the proximal portion of the tube and burying it in the cornual myometrium.

Frederick Carpenter Irving, known as Fritz to his friends, was born in Gouverneur, New York. He graduated from the Harvard Medical School in 1910. In the First World War he served as a medical officer with the United States Army in France and Italy. In 1931 he was appointed professor of obstetrics and gynaecology in Harvard Medical School and chief of obstetrics at the Boston Lying-in Hospital.

Fritz Irving was a progressive thinker and did much to develop links with paediatrics in his hospital and promote a perinatal focus to improve outcome. He was not above the occasional cynical observation

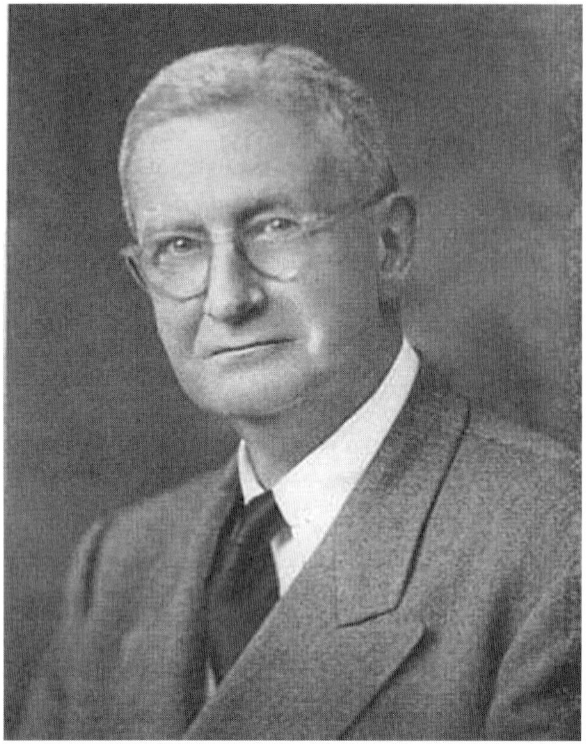

Frederick Carpenter Irving

when commenting on the prevalence of hysterectomy: 'a woman who completes the menopause with her uterus in situ is not only possessed of an unusual degree of elusiveness, but she will also be an object of curiosity among her friends'.

The author, John Irving, is Fritz Irving's grandson. In his best-selling novel, *Cider House Rules*, the central theme of which is therapeutic abortion in early twentieth-century America, John Irving acknowledges the influence of his grandfather and his book, *Safe Deliverance.*

Fritz Irving retired in 1951 and moved to the warmer climes of Florida, where he died on Christmas Eve, 1957.

Selected Publications

Irving FC. A new method of insuring sterility following cesarean section. *Am J Obstet Gynecol* 1924; 8: 335–7.

Irving FC. Tubal sterilization. *Am J Obstet Gynecol* 1950; 60: 1101–9.

Irving FC. *Safe Deliverance.* Boston, MA: Houghton Mifflin Company; 1942.

Bibliography References

168, 447, 1277, 1410, 1485, 1647.

J

Jacquemin, Étienne Joseph (1796–1872)

Jacquemin's Sign

The violet-blue discoloration of the introitus and vagina as a sign of early pregnancy is usually attributed to James Chadwick. In truth, the credit should go to Étienne Jacquemin, who described the sign 50 years earlier, as Chadwick acknowledged in his own paper on the subject. Jacquemin was a prison medical officer in Mazas, and part of his duties was to inspect and look after the prostitutes. An astute observer, he noted the colour change and went on to carefully examine and record his findings in over 4,000 pregnant women. He did not publish his results but reported them to his chief of staff, Dr Alexandre Parent-Duchatelet (1790–1836). In 1837, Parent-Duchatelet published the second edition of his book, *De la prostitution dans la ville de Paris*, and in it recorded and acknowledged Jacquemin's observations: 'a change of colour in the mucous membrane of the vagina to a violet hue, like the dregs of red wine'.

To help confuse the eponymous lineage, the like-named French obstetrician, Jean Marie Jacquemier, noted and correctly acknowledged Jacquemin's work in his obstetrical publication of 1846. The confusion between the similarly named French men was started and perpetuated in the most authoritative American textbook, *William's Obstetrics*. Thus, Jacquemin's contribution was attributed to Jacquemier.

Étienne Joseph Jacquemin was the son of a doctor and received his MD in 1822. He entered the prison medical service and eventually became chief medical officer at the prison of Mazas, which position he held until his death at 76 years of age.

Selected Publications

Parent-Duchatelet AJB. *De la prostitution dans la ville de Paris*. 2nd edn. Paris; 1837: 217–8.

Bibliography References

625, 648, 1014.

Joseph, Sister Mary (1856–1939)

Sister Mary Joseph's Nodule

Metastatic spread of cancer to the umbilicus is not common but can occur with any intra-abdominal malignancy. In women, gynaecological cancer, particularly ovarian cancer, is the most common primary site. Horatio Storer described such a case in 1864. Working at St Mary's Hospital in Rochester, Minnesota, Sister Mary Joseph acted as first surgical assistant to Dr William Mayo from 1890 to 1915. She observed a number of cases before laparotomy in which a hard or ulcerated umbilical nodule was present and noted that in all of these cases there was widespread metastatic disease from the primary intra-abdominal tumour, usually stomach or ovary. She brought this to the attention of Dr William Mayo, and he always acknowledged that it was Sister Joseph who had brought this sign to his notice. His only publication on the topic came in the proceedings of staff meetings of the Mayo Clinic in 1928, in which he wrote:

> *Before such a patient is admitted to x-ray examination and other tests . . . in order to protect the patient's time, strength and pocket book, whether there is visible or palpable evidence of metastatic extension which would at once make the diagnosis and prognosis clear, often this can be done speedily and with very little discomfort to the patient . . . in many doubtful cases, examination and palpation of the umbilicus will reveal that it is hard and infiltrated, perhaps not prominently.*

In 1949, Hamilton Bailey, in the eleventh edition of his *Demonstrations of Physical Signs in Clinical Surgery*, included this sign and wrote, 'Sister Joseph of the Mayo Clinic imparted this clinical observation to the late Dr William Mayo'. This attribution in such an influential text served to secure the eponym as Sister Mary Joseph's nodule.

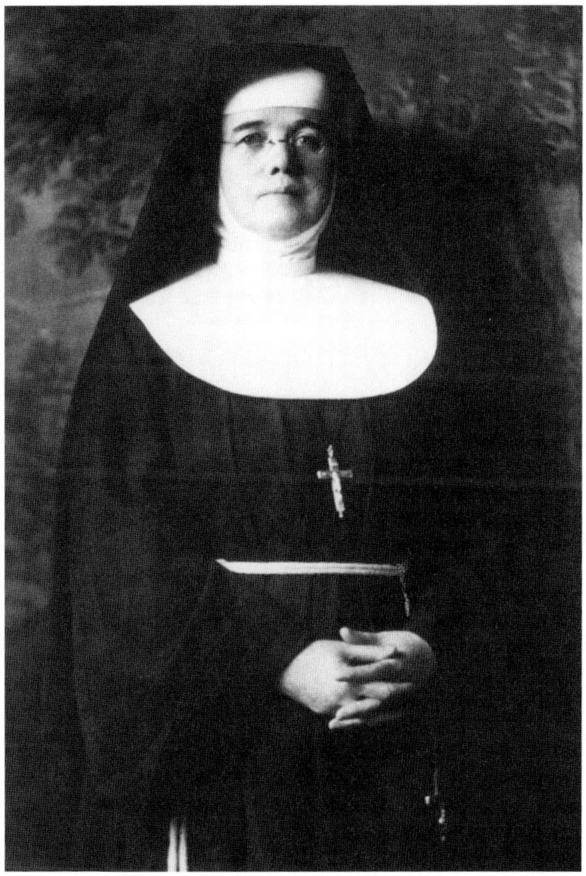

Sister Mary Joseph

Sister Mary Joseph was born Julia Dempsey on 14 May 1856 in Salamanca, New York. When she was young her family moved to Haverhill, Minnesota. In 1878 she entered the Order of St Francis of the Congregation of

Our Lady of Lourdes, recently established in Rochester, Minnesota. She became Sister Mary Joseph and spent her early years teaching in parochial schools in Ohio.

In September 1889 St Mary's Hospital was funded and opened by the Sisters of St Francis in Rochester. In November of that year, Sister Mary Joseph was assigned to St Mary's Hospital and taught nursing by a graduate nurse, Edith Graham, who was later to become the wife of Dr Charles Mayo. After six weeks' training, Sister Mary Joseph was made head nurse and, in addition to her administrative duties, was from 1890 to 1915 the first surgical assistant to Dr William Mayo. In 1892 she was appointed Superintendent of St Mary's Hospital and held this position until her death on 29 March 1939. She guided the growth of St Mary's Hospital from a 40-bed facility to a fully equipped modern hospital with 600 beds. Her skill as a surgical assistant was legend.

As the reputation of the Mayo brothers increased, visiting surgeons were in frequent attendance. Sister Joseph's technical skill was such that, while William Mayo was answering questions, she would frequently carry on with the operation. In his tribute to Sister Joseph after her death, William Mayo wrote, 'Her surgical judgment as to condition of the patient before, during and after operation was equal to that of any medical man of whom I have knowledge. Of all the splendid surgical assistants I have had, she easily ranks first'. Ironically, within four months of her death the two Mayo brothers, with whom she had worked for 50 years, died: Charles in May and William in July 1939.

Selected Publications

Bailey H. *Demonstrations of Physical Signs in Clinical Surgery* (11th edn). Bristol: John Wright and Sons Ltd; 1949.

Mayo WJ. Metastasis in cancer. *Proceedings of the Staff Meetings at the Mayo Clinic* 1928; 3: 327.

Storer H. Circumscribed tumour of the umbilical closely simulating umbilical hernia. *Boston Med Surg J* 1864; 19: 73.

Bibliography References

4, 566, 825, 1009, 1524.

K

Keep, Nathan Cooley (1800–1875)

Ether Analgesia in Labour

Following the successful administration of ether by the dentist William Morton (1819–1868) for a surgical procedure at the Massachusetts Hospital in Boston on 16 October 1846, James Young Simpson of Edinburgh first used ether analgesia in obstetrics on 19 January 1847. Nathan Cooley Keep, a Boston physician and dentist, was the first person in America to use ether for pain relief in labour. His patient, whom he did not identify in his report, was Fanny Appleton Longfellow, second wife of the poet Henry Wadsworth Longfellow:

> *The patient was in good health and in labor of her third child . . . her pains, which had been light but regular, becoming severe, the vapor of ether was inhaled by the nose, and exhaled by the mouth. The patient had no difficulty in taking the vapor in this manner from the reservoir, without any valvular apparatus. In the course of twenty minutes, four pains had occurred without suffering, the vapor of ether being administered between each pain. Consciousness was unimpaired and labor not retarded . . . From the commencement of the inhalation to the close of the labor, 30 minutes. Number of inhalations five. No unpleasant symptoms occurred, and the result was highly satisfactory.*

Keep had already considerable experience in the administration of ether for surgical operations and dentistry. Indeed, on the date he administered ether to Mrs Longfellow, Wednesday 7 April 1847, there was published in the *Boston Medical and Surgical Journal* Keep's article on the use of ether in more than 200 cases of surgery and dentistry. His short communication to the editor of that journal on the administration of ether in labour was dated 10 April 1847 and published in the journal one week after the event (14 April 1847).

In his personal journal of Wednesday 7 April 1847 Henry Longfellow wrote:

> *Fanny heroically inhaled the vapor of sulphuric ether, the great nepenthe, and all the pain of labor ceased, though the labor itself went on and seemed accelerated. This is the first trial of ether at such time in this country. It has been completely successful. While under the influence of the vapor, there was no loss of consciousness, no pain. All ended happily.*

In her own correspondence Fanny Longfellow wrote, 'I was never better or got through a confinement so completely'. Sadly, she was later to die after accidentally setting her dress on fire.

Nathan Cooley Keep's forebears came from Northamptonshire in England. His great-great-great-grandfather, John Keep, had republican tendencies which precipitated his hasty exit from England to Springfield, Massachusetts in 1644. Nathan Cooley Keep was born in Longmeadow, Massachusetts on 13 December 1800. At the age of 15, after basic education at the town school, he became an apprentice to a jeweller in Newark, New Jersey. He changed tack and in 1821 went to Boston as an apprentice in dentistry. In his spare time, he attended Harvard Medical School and graduated MD in 1827. However, his clinical practice was largely limited to dentistry, in which he introduced several technical innovations. Nathan Keep shared his laboratory with William Morton, and it is likely that Keep contributed more than is generally acknowledged to the early application of ether in both dentistry and surgery. Throughout his career, Keep campaigned for dentistry to be recognised as a medical specialty requiring a university education. He was the founding president of the Massachusetts Dental Society and vice-president of the American Association of Dental Surgeons. After many years of lobbying, Harvard University established the first university affiliated dental school in 1867. One year later Keep was appointed the first dean of the dental faculty at Harvard University, and in 1870 the university awarded him an honorary doctorate in dental medicine. He died in Boston at the age of 74 years.

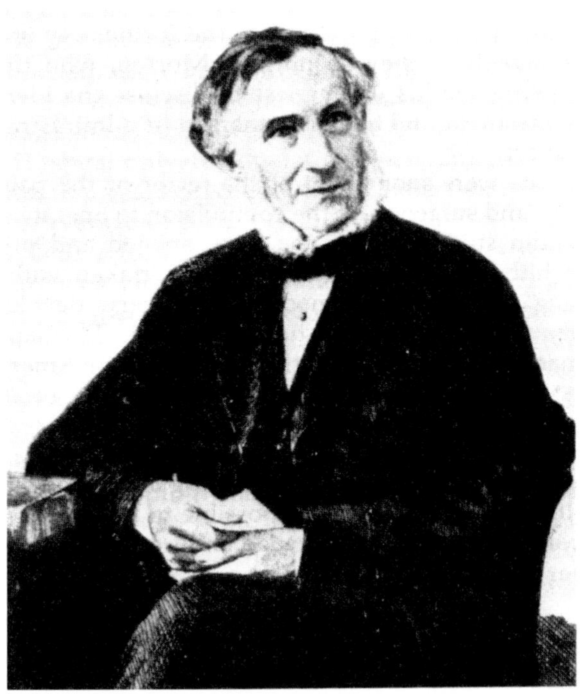

Nathan Cooley Keep

Selected Publications

Keep NC. The letheon administered in a case of labor. *Boston Med Surg J* 1847; 36: 226.

Keep NC. Inhalation of the ethereal vapor for mitigating human suffering in surgical operations and acute diseases. *Boston Med Surg J* 1847; 36: 199–201.

Wagenknecht E (ed.) *Mrs Longfellow: Selected Letters and Journals of Fanny Appleton Longfellow (1817–1861).* New York, NY: Longmans, Green and Co; 1956, pp. 129–30.

Bibliography References

252, 253, 287, 300, 446, 799, 802, 803, 1217, 1222, 1597, 1653.

Kegel, Arnold Henry (1894–1972)

Kegel's Exercises

Arnold Kegel devoted much of his professional life to research in restoration of pelvic floor function following the trauma of childbirth. He noted two types of damage:

> *When muscles and fascias are subjected to excessive tension during childbirth, two types of injury may result: (1) actual laceration and separation of the muscles and*

fascias and (2) separation of individual muscle cells from the motor nerves by which they are innervated.

He therefore argued that a two-pronged approach was required to counteract this damage:

It is not enough, therefore, to approximate the margins of lacerated muscles and fascias and suture them in place. Such a procedure will ordinarily lead to a restoration of the gross form of the perineal structures but will not in itself bring about a return to normal function. In some way, re-innervation of muscle cells must be accomplished and the injured muscle cells must again be educated to function.

In reviewing the paucity of information on exercise to restore pelvic muscle function, he noted one communication from a South African colleague:

One report of interest is that of Van Skolkvik, who observed unusually firm perinea among a tribe of natives in South Africa. He found that it was the duty of the midwife, who was usually the mother or mother-in-law, to see that the young mother recovered perineal strength after childbirth. Exercise by contraction of the vaginal muscles on distended fingers, was begun several days after birth and was continued periodically for several weeks, until the desired result was obtained.

Kegel therefore set about applying the principle of pelvic muscle exercise in clinical practice:

For the past fifteen years I have experimented with various means of exercising the perineal muscles. Any active exercise must be directed primarily toward drawing in the perineum. Only the exceptional woman, however, will continue the exercise long enough to produce results on mere instruction to do this. Many women, in addition, have no 'awareness of function' and, unless provided with some way of knowing whether or not they are being successful, soon become discouraged or are unwilling to make even an initial attempt at exercise.

Thus, Kegel designed a 'perineometer' consisting of a pneumatic vaginal cone attached to a manometer. With this, the woman could gauge the strength of her pelvic floor contractions and follow the improvement over time.

The popularity of Kegel's exercises has waxed and waned over the half century since their introduction. Modern urogynaecological studies have confirmed their value. The extent of acceptance into both medical and lay practice can be seen by the incorporation of the name Kegel into the language. Thus, in some circles, women may be told 'to Kegel' or that 'Kegeling' is good for them.

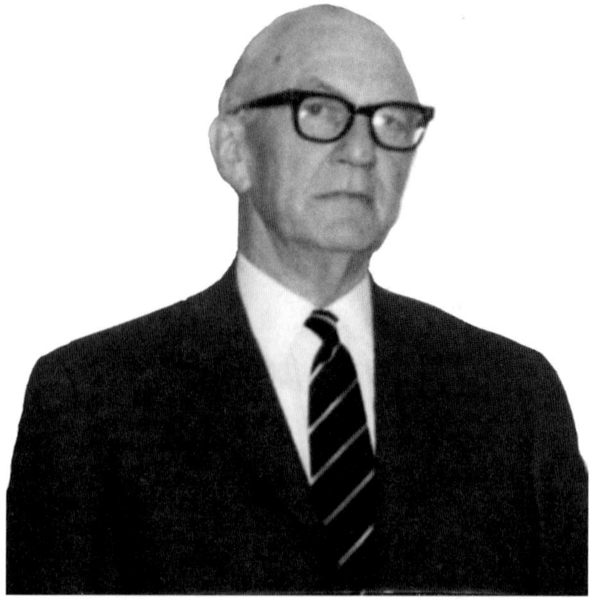

Arnold Henry Kegel

Arnold Henry Kegel was born in Lansing, Iowa and graduated from the Loyola University School of Medicine, Chicago in 1916. He was a clinical professor of obstetrics and gynaecology at the Hollywood Presbyterian Hospital and University of Southern California Medical School at Los Angeles. He died of coronary artery disease on 1 March 1972.

Selected Publications

Kegel AH. Progressive resistance exercise in the functional restoration of the perineal muscles. *Am J Obstet Gynecol* 1948; 56: 238–48.

Bibliography References

524, 803, 1485.

Kehrer, Ferdinand Adolf (1837–1914)

Transverse Lower-Segment Caesarean Section

In the development of the modern technique of transverse lower-segment caesarean section, Ferdinand Kehrer's contribution is frequently overlooked. He performed the first transverse lower-segment caesarean section at 5 a.m. on 15 September 1881 in a cottage in the village of Meckelsheim, near Heidelberg in Germany. He was assisted by a midwife and a general practitioner, who gave the anaesthetic. The 26-year-old patient had been in labour for 30 hours with a contracted pelvis due to osteomalacia. Some idea of the conditions under which Kehrer operated, using Listerian principles, are revealed in his description:

> *Preliminary preparations were then made. Two hanging lamps, one stand lamp and several candle-sticks were assembled, a small table was made ready with a stool at the end of it to support the legs, the instruments laid out in carbolic water, and the hand spray fitted up. Chloroform was administered and the patient brought to the table. The genitalia were shaved, the abdominal wall and thighs washed with carbolic solution, the vagina douched and then packed with a swab wrung out of the same solution ... The uterine wall was divided a little above the floor of the uterovesical pouch, the infant's left ear then presenting in the wound. The latter was now enlarged laterally at far as the round ligaments on either side. The head was delivered by applying the fingers of both hands as one would use the forceps. The placenta was extracted by drawing on the cord.*

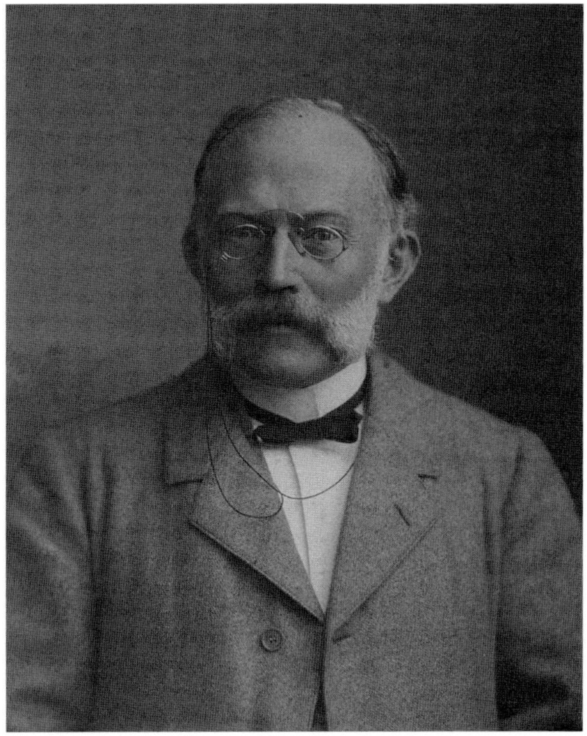
Ferdinand Adolf Kehrer

Kehrer felt that the transverse placement of the incision in the lower part of the uterus would be less likely to gape and that at this level the peritoneal layer could be separated from the uterine muscle. He placed great importance on the 'doppelnaht' (double layer) closure of the two separate layers of muscle and peritoneum to help contain any leakage of septic material from the uterus. He sutured the muscle layer with six interrupted silk sutures and then carefully sutured the peritoneal layer separately, also with interrupted silk sutures. He was later to propose that the peritoneal suture be continuous. Both the mother and her female infant survived. Kehrer performed a second caesarean section on 13 November 1881; the mother died, although the infant survived.

Ferdinand Kehrer did his early obstetrics with Ferdinand Ritgen in Giessen. He then moved as professor of obstetrics to Heidelberg, where he did his work on caesarean section. Kehrer's operative description is almost the same as the modern procedure, and he should be regarded as the founder of the transverse lower-segment caesarean section. He published the procedure in 1882, at almost exactly the same time as Sanger's classical upper-segment operation. In fact, Sanger's publication was theoretical, and his technique was not performed until May 1882. However, Sanger's method held sway until the 1920s, when Munro Kerr and others reintroduced the transverse lower-segment incision into the mainstream of obstetrics.

Selected Publications

Kehrer FA. Über ein modificirtes Verfahren beim Kaiserschnitte. *Arch Gynäkol* 1882; 19: 177–209.

Bibliography References

99, 102, 351, 541, 548, 553, 648, 987, 1085, 1205, 1261, 1333, 1486, 1631, 1734.

Kelly, Howard Atwood (1858–1943)

Anterior Repair

Howard Atwood Kelly was the youngest of the 'Big Four' foundation professors at the Johns Hopkins University School of Medicine. These included the three Williams: Osler (1849–1919) in medicine, Halstead (1852–1922) in surgery and Welch (1850–1934) in pathology, along with Kelly, who was appointed when he was only 31 years old. All four achieved lasting international recognition.

Kelly was born in Camden, New Jersey. His father served with the Pennsylvania Volunteers in the American Civil War. Thus, Kelly was strongly influenced by his mother during his early childhood. Two of her interests, the Bible and natural history, also became Kelly's life-long pursuits. He received a formal and disciplined school education at Faire's Classical Institute in Philadelphia. At 15 years of age he entered the University of Pennsylvania and took a four-year arts degree, graduating in 1877. He then entered the medical faculty and graduated MD in 1882. During the third year of medical school he studied with such intensity that he developed incapacitating insomnia and had to take a year off. To restore his health, he worked as a ranch hand in Colorado.

Kelly did his internship in the Episcopal Hospital of Kensington in the poor district of Philadelphia. He later set up practice in the same area and began to concentrate on surgery and gynaecology. He developed his surgical skills by putting in much additional dissection work. On one occasion when he was an intern, Kelly looked after a woman who died from kidney failure. Believing that permission for autopsy would not be granted, he slipped into the morgue at night and removed the kidneys via the vaginal vault. Starting in 1886 he made several study trips to Britain and Germany and worked with Max Sänger, Rudolph Virchow and Karl Pawlik. In 1887 he founded the Kensington Hospital for Women and began the serious study of urological conditions, stimulated by the work of Pawlik.

About this time, William Osler moved from Montreal to Philadelphia. He was very impressed with Kelly, whose surgical skill was widely recognised as being extraordinary. Through Osler's influence he was appointed assistant professor at the University of Pennsylvania in 1888. This was short-lived, as one year later Osler, having moved to Johns Hopkins, orchestrated Kelly's appointment to the new chair of obstetrics and gynaecology. Kelly did not like obstetrics and from the outset sought to separate gynaecology from obstetrics. This he achieved in 1899, with the appointment of John Whitridge Williams as professor and head of obstetrics.

Kelly was a major influence in establishing the emerging specialty of gynaecology. His two-volume text, *Operative Gynecology*, set the standard for content, writing and illustration. As he wrote in the preface:

> *Gynecology is so young a science, and many of its surgical procedures are as yet so incompletely developed, and I think the best service a gynecologist can render his specialty is to record accurately his own experiences. Scientific accuracy is especially necessary in gynecology, in which the discovery of anesthesia and the perfection of an aseptic technique have rendered operations safe which a few years ago would have been necessarily fatal. It is comparatively easy now to open the abdomen; it is no easier than it ever was to combat the causes of disease.*

Kelly devised the simple air cystoscope by placing the patient in the knee-chest position and allowing air to distend the urinary bladder. Thus, he was able to see and catheterise the ureteric orifices. He was led to this improvisation by accidently dropping the instrument and breaking the lens. He devised wax-tipped catheters upon which scratch marks might be detected to confirm the presence of stone. The Kelly clamp he designed remains in common use.

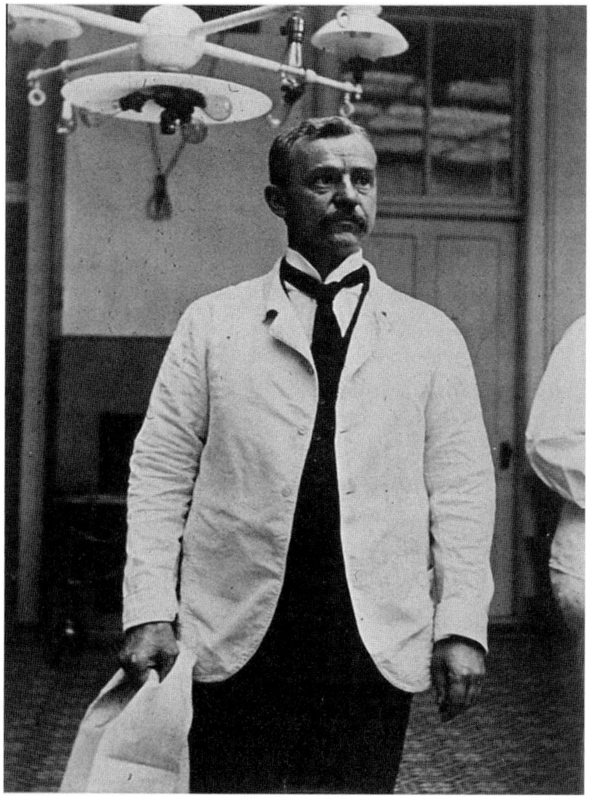

Howard Atwood Kelly

It was in 1913 that Kelly first described the 'Kelly plication stitch'. This mattress stitch is placed at the urethrovesical junction to plicate the pubo-cervical fascia. The resultant elevation of the urethrovesical junction was the essential component of the anterior repair for treatment of urinary stress incontinence.

Kelly's work rate and concentration were prodigious. He lectured and published extensively, as well as carrying a large and lucrative private practice. However, he did spend the summer months at his cottage on Ahmic Lake in Ontario, where he did much of his writing. His colleague Thomas Cullen also had a summer cottage on the same lake. Kelly's early interests, learned at the knee of his mother, were sustained. He became an expert and published widely on herpetology and mycology. A Bible scholar, he could read Hebrew and Greek, and he preached often. Many of his sermons and writings were against alcohol, tobacco, prostitution and political corruption.

He resigned from the chair at Johns Hopkins in 1919 when it was decreed that department heads could not do private practice. On one of his trips to Germany he met and married his wife. They had nine children, were together for 54 years and died within hours of each other.

Selected Publications

Kelly HA. The examination of the female bladder and the catheterization of the ureters under direct inspection. *Bull Johns Hopkins Hosp* 1893; 4: 101–5.

Kelly HA. *Operative Gynecology*. 2 vols. New York, NY: D. Appleton & Co; 1898. Also published in: The Classics of Obstetrics and Gynecology. New York, NY: Gryphon Editions; 1992 (facsimile).

Kelly HA. Incontinence of urine in women. *Urol Cutan Rev* 1913; 17: 15–16.

Bibliography References

21, 214, 269, 313, 329, 365, 621, 640, 648, 697, 782, 814, 934, 1098, 1314, 1382, 1570.

Kelsey, Frances Oldham (1914–2015)

Thalidomide Embryopathy

It was a Canadian physician/pharmacist who blocked the licensing of thalidomide in the United States and prevented the potential disaster of thousands of cases of a severe congenital abnormality.

Frances Oldham was born in Vancouver Island, Canada on 24 July 1914 to a Scottish mother and a British military father. Her mother sent her to a boys' school in Victoria, British Columbia, insisting that she get as good an education as her brother. She gained her bachelor's and master's degrees in science and pharmacology at McGill University in Montreal. In 1936 she took up a research position in the pharmacology department at the University of Chicago, completing her PhD in 1938 and remaining on the teaching faculty. She also enrolled as a medical student and completed her MD in 1950. During her time in Chicago, she met and married a fellow pharmacologist, Ellis Kelsey, and had two daughters.

Ellis Kelsey was appointed head of pharmacology at the University of South Dakota in the small town of Vermillion, South Dakota. Frances Kelsey worked as a family doctor there, and also found work as an editorial associate for the American Medical Association (AMA). In this capacity she edited manuscripts submitted to the journal and noted that many papers were mainly 'testimonials' of drugs submitted by physicians with no supporting science or data. This was to strike a relevant chord in her later work at the Food and Drug Administration (FDA)

In 1960 the Kelseys moved to Washington DC, where Ellis was appointed special assistant to the surgeon general. Frances Kelsey applied for and got a job as a medical officer at the FDA with a mandate to review new drug applications.

Thalidomide was introduced into the market in Germany by the company Chemie Grünenthal in 1957 as 'Contergan'. It was a sedative with virtually no potential for a fatal overdose, in contrast to the alternative barbiturates. As such, it was sold over the counter. It also turned out to be an effective antiemetic for pregnancy sickness. Thalidomide was marketed in the United Kingdom by Distillers Company as 'Distaval' and in Canada by the pharmaceutical company Richardson-Merrell as 'Kevadon'. However, Richardson-Merrell was anxious to break into the biggest market of all: the United States. But first they had to get the approval of the FDA and prove 'that the drug was safe before it could be marketed'. For many new drug applications, this was merely a rubber-stamp approval. The application was submitted on 8 September 1960 and was assigned to Frances Kelsey, who had been in office only a few weeks. The senior staff felt this would be an easy introduction for her, as the drug was already licensed in more than 20 countries. Kelsey, however, was not impressed with the paucity of legitimate scientific studies and lack of clinical data. From her previous work with AMA journal submissions, she recognised the names of some of the physicians who provided glowing testimonials of the drug's benefits; she regarded them as dishonest pharmaceutical hacks. To the surprise and annoyance of the company, Kelsey withheld approval and requested further studies.

Richardson-Merrell planned to launch the drug in the United States in March 1961. As the deadline approached they applied increasing personal and professional pressure on Kelsey, but she stood her ground, and the launch of the drug was postponed to November 1961. In early 1961 Kelsey saw a letter to the *British Medical Journal* that reported cases of peripheral neuritis with chronic use of thalidomide. She found out that Richardson-Merrell had been aware of this report and withheld it from their latest application to the FDA. This deceit hardened Kelsey's resolve to block the application. She pointed out that, if the drug caused neuritis in adults, what effect might it have on the fetus; she demanded further evidence with supporting data. Throughout 1961 she held firm against sustained pressure, including accusations of libel.

In November 1961, a German paediatrician, Widukind Lenz (1919–1995), reported cases of babies born with rare congenital limb abnormalities (phocomelia) at a paediatric conference in Germany. One month later, the *Lancet* published a letter from an Australian obstetrician, William McBride (b. 1927), in which he reported a 20 per cent incidence of severe limb anomalies in babies born to mothers who had taken thalidomide during pregnancy. Lenz informed the Grünenthal company and they withdrew the drug, after pressure from government officials. Grünenthal notified Richardson-Merrell in late November 1961, and they subsequently withdrew their application from the FDA, although they declared that 'they didn't really believe it'.

Ultimately, there were more than 5,000 children that survived with thalidomide embryopathy involving multiple anomalies but with phocomelia as the main manifestation. In the United States there were a limited number of cases; some pills had been released early by the company to doctors for 'clinical trials'.

Frances Kelsey's stubborn and principled stand over 15 months had saved the United States from the tragic consequences of the worst drug-induced cases of embryopathy in history. Recognition of her accomplishment came in August 1962, when President John F. Kennedy awarded her the highest civilian honour in the United States: the President's Award for Distinguished Federal Civilian Service. The citation read:

> *Her exceptional judgement in evaluating a new drug for safety for human use has prevented a major tragedy of birth deformities in the United States. Through high ability and steadfast confidence in her professional decision she has made an outstanding contribution to the protection of the health of the American people.*

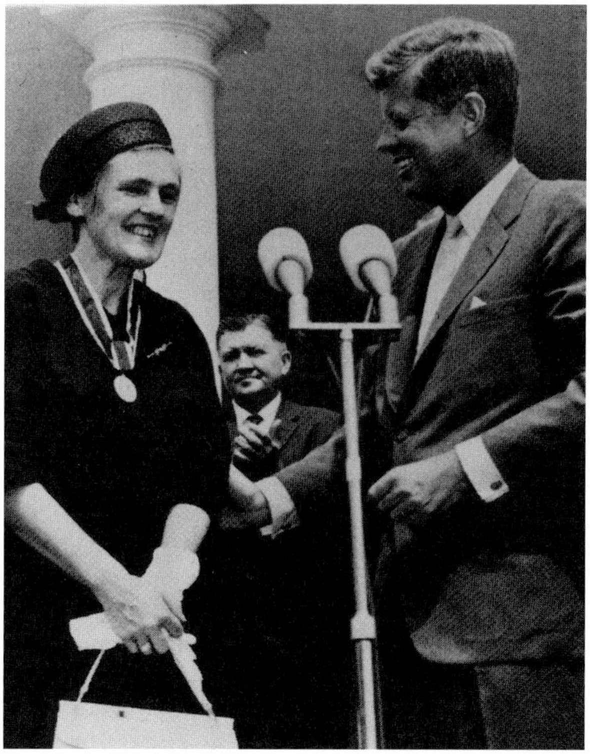

Francis Oldham Kelsey

Frances Kelsey remained at the FDA until she retired at the age of 90 in 2005. In 2014 she moved from Washington DC back to Canada to live with her daughter in London, Ontario. She died on 7 August 2015 at the age of 101, shortly after receiving the Order of Canada.

Ironically, thalidomide has found pharmacological redemption to the extent that it was serendipitously found to resolve erythema nodosum leprosum, the skin lesion of leprosy. Its immunomodulatory and anti-angiogenic actions have been effective in suppressing some rare skin disorders, and treatment trials of Kaposi's sarcoma, multiple myeloma and other cancers have been promising.

Selected Publications

McBride WG. Thalidomide and congenital abnormalities. *Lancet* 1961; 2: 1358.

Lenz W. Thalidomide and congenital abnormalities. *Lancet* 1962; 1: 45.

Bibliography References

352, 357, 816, 890, 966, 1013, 1016, 1195, 1513.

Kennedy, Evory (1806–1886)

Fetal Heart Auscultation

Auscultation of the fetal heart was slow to find acceptance in Britain and Ireland after its introduction by John Ferguson and Robert Collins (1800–1868). Evory Kennedy, while assistant master to Collins at the Rotunda Hospital in Dublin, studied the clinical application of the stethoscope in obstetrics and in 1833 published the first comprehensive monograph on the subject in English. One reason for its slow development can be found in the attitude exemplified by the influential James Hamilton (1767–1839), professor of midwifery at Edinburgh, when he challenged Collins' acceptance of fetal heart auscultation: 'Does he propose to apply the stethoscope to the naked belly of a woman, for if so, he may be assured that in this part of the world at least, such a proposal would be indignantly rejected by every young or old practitioner of reputed respectability'.

Kennedy's book was the result of five years' experience with fetal heart auscultation in the wards of the Rotunda Hospital. The text was widely read, and an American edition was published in 1843. He noted the influence of fetal movement and uterine contractions on the fetal heart rate:

> *The foetal pulsation is much more frequent than the maternal pulse . . . being about 130 or 140 in the minute; however, it is not necessarily observed to beat always at this rate . . . This variation may depend upon a variety of inherent vital causes in the foetus . . . An obvious explanation, however, is muscular action on the part of the foetus; and we shall very generally observe the pulsation of the foetal heart increased in frequency after*

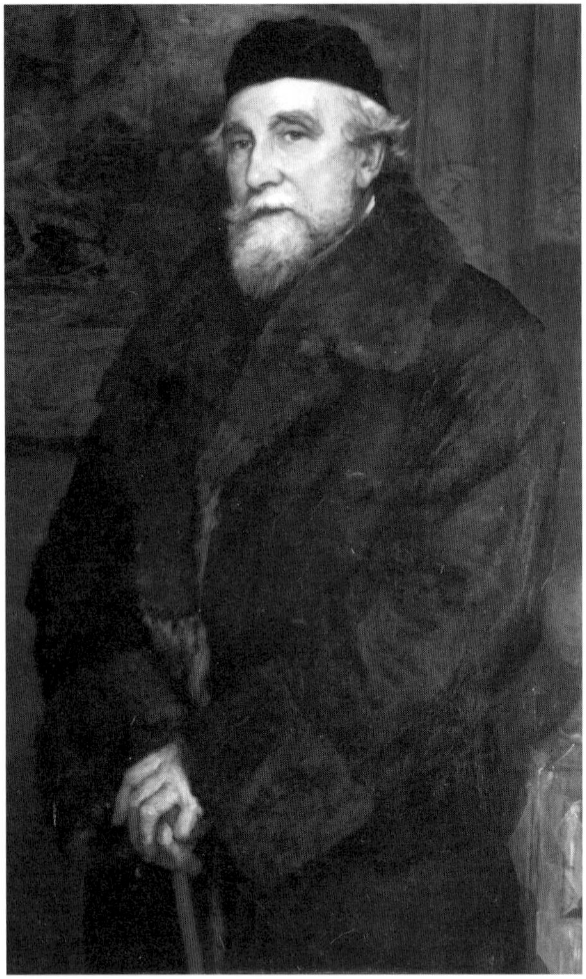

Evory Kennedy

such. The external cause, which we shall find most frequently to operate on the foetal circulation, is uterine action, particularly when long continued, as in labour.

In dismissing the contention of those who believed the passage of meconium was a sign of fetal death, Kennedy said, 'it merits no confidence whatever, as a proof of the death of the foetus'.

Evory Kennedy, a son of the manse, was born in Carndonagh, Donegal. He was the godson and namesake of a prominent Dublin obstetrician, Thomas Evory, who was Master of the Rotunda Hospital from 1793 to 1800. Kennedy followed in his godfather's footsteps by training in Edinburgh and gaining his MD (with a thesis on puerperal fever in 1827). Upon return to Dublin he was appointed assistant master to Collins and succeeded him as Master of the Rotunda Hospital in 1833 for the usual seven-year term. Following the death of Professor James Hamilton in Edinburgh, Kennedy applied for the vacant chair. The two main contenders were Kennedy and James Young Simpson. After a spirited campaign from both men, Simpson was elected by one vote. Kennedy remained prominent in Dublin medical circles, founded the Obstetrical Society of Dublin and twice served as its president. He spent his years of retirement from medical practice as Deputy Lieutenant of County Dublin and a Justice of the Peace, in which roles he campaigned vigorously against alcoholism.

Selected Publications

Kennedy E. *Observations on Obstetric Auscultation.* Dublin: Longman; 1833.

US edn 1843. Also published in: The Classics of Obstetrics and Gynecology Library. New York, NY: Gryphon Editions; 1994 (facsimile).

Bibliography References

668, 818, 819, 1126, 1211, 1213.

Kergaradec, Jacques Alexandre Le Jumeau (1787–1877)

Fetal Heart Auscultation

The first reported auscultation of the fetal heart was in 1818 by the Geneva surgeon, François Issac Mayor (1779–1854), although in France, c.1650, Phillipe Le Goust wrote a poem ridiculing his colleague Marsac for claiming to have heard the fetal heart beating 'like a mill-clapper'. However, it was Kergaradec, a colleague of René Laennec, who first used the stethoscope to systematically study the fetal heart sounds. Initially Kergaradec was listening for evidence of the fetus splashing in the amniotic fluid. However, his training with Laennec led him to identify the more rapid fetal heart rate as distinct from the maternal

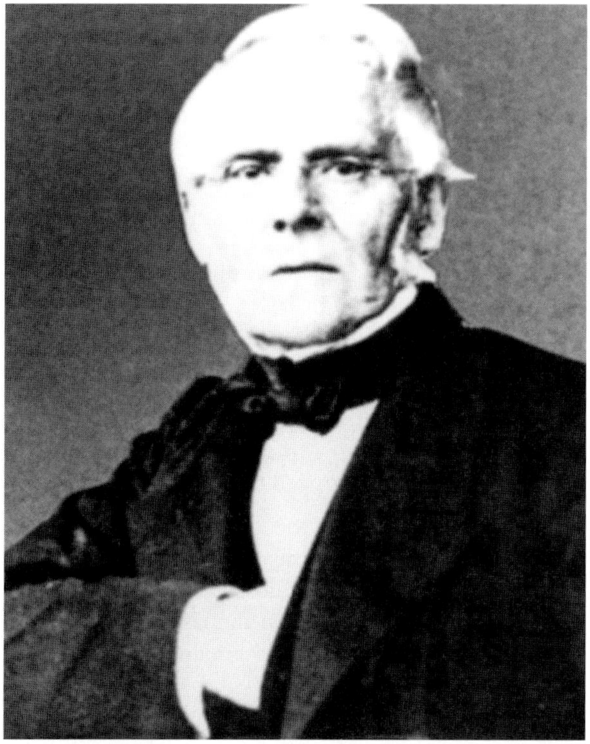

Jacques Alexandre Le Jumeau Kergaradec

pulse. Kergaradec reported his findings to the Paris Academy of Medicine on 26 December 1821 and published his work the following year. As he wrote:

> *One day whilst examining a patient near term and trying to follow the movements of the fetus with the stethoscope I was suddenly aware of a sound that I had not noticed before; it was like the ticking of a watch. At first I thought I was mistaken, but I was able to repeat the observation over and over again. On counting the beats I found that these occurred 143–148 times per minute and the patient's pulse was only 72 per minute.*

He subsequently described the placental souffle. At that time the only application of the knowledge was to confirm that the fetus was alive. However, Kergaradec foresaw future potential when he asked, 'Will it not be possible to judge the state of health or disease of the fetus from the variations that occur in the beat of the fetal heart?'

Kergaradec was later informed of Mayor's earlier observation, of which he was unaware. Mayor's report was limited to an abstract in the monthly record of the University of Geneva:

> *. . . by applying the ear to the mother's belly; if the child is alive you hear quite clearly the beats of its heart and you easily distinguish them from the mother's pulse.*

Jacques Alexandre Le Jumeau, Vicomte de Kergaradec, one of nine children, was born in Morlaix, Brittany to an ancient and noble family. His father fell foul of the Revolution, was forced to flee the country when Jacques Alexandre was only five and died in exile at St Petersburg. Jacques Alexandre's mother was imprisoned, and the family was brought up by the maternal grandparents. When he was seven years old, Kergaradec and his four brothers, as the sons of an aristocrat, were arrested and only saved from the guillotine when the excesses of the Revolution ended. At 11 years of age he began his medical apprenticeship at the Military Hospital of Morlaix. In 1802, by now a seasoned medical veteran at 15 years of age, he entered the school of medicine in Paris, graduating in 1809.

Laennec confirmed and acknowledged Kergaradec's work and included the monograph in the second edition of his work on auscultation.

Selected Publications

Le Jumeau JA. Vicomte de Kergaradec. *Mémoire sur l'auscultation, appliquée a l'étude de la grossesse.* Paris: Méquiquon-Marvis; 1822.

Mayor F. *Bibliothèque universelle des sciences et arts.* Geneva 1818: 9: 249.

Bibliography References

648, 668, 1210, 1211, 1261, 1521, 1522, 1536, 1595.

Kerr, John Martin Munro (1868–1960)

Lower-Segment Caesarean Section/Operative Obstetrics Text

One of the great advances in operative obstetrics was the development of the lower-segment caesarean section, as opposed to the classical upper-segment variety with its risk of subsequent rupture. Munro Kerr was the first person in the United Kingdom to realise the superiority of the lower-segment approach and a major influence in changing practice away from the classical uterine incision. In outlining the advantages of the lower-segment incision, he wrote:

> *I make no claims to originality as regards the incision, and I recommend it only because I believe the cicatrix that results will be less liable to rupture. The advantages of the incision are that one cuts through a less vascular area ... In the second place, it is thin and consequently the surfaces can be readily brought together ... The third advantage, and it is a very important one, is that the wound in this area is at rest during the early days of the puerperium. Lastly, there is great advantage that owing to the fact that the lower segment does not become fully stretched until labour is well advanced the scar is in a safer region than the ordinary longitudinal one.*

Munro Kerr was born in Glasgow, the son of a shipowner. He was educated at Glasgow Academy and Glasgow University, from which he graduated in medicine in 1890. He held resident hospital posts in Scotland as well as studying overseas in Berlin, Dublin and Vienna. Upon return to Glasgow he occupied a number of staff positions, including the Muirhead Chair of Obstetrics and Gynaecology, until his appointment as Regius Professor at Glasgow University in 1927.

Munro Kerr gained enormous experience as an obstetrician with the large volume of abnormal obstetrics in Glasgow at that time. He used this background to write his text on operative obstetrics, first published in 1908 under the title *Operative Midwifery*. Written in a clear, at times conversational style, and filled with clinical anecdotes, this classic text has been continued by successive authors since his death, and the centenary edition was published in 2007.

He was an excellent clinical teacher with a dramatic flair, who often wore a monocle. Munro Kerr received many academic honours and much international recognition. At the age of 87 he accepted the invitation of the Glasgow Obstetrical and Gynaecological Society to deliver the first William Hunter Memorial Lecture.

Munro Kerr began promoting the transverse lower-segment incision in 1921. Acceptance was slow, particularly in Britain, although he later had an ally in McIntosh Marshall of Liverpool. Long after his retirement, his achievement in gaining acceptance of the low transverse incision was acknowledged at the 12th British Congress of Obstetrics and Gynaecology, held in London in 1948. Invited to the lecture stage to receive the plaudits of the audience, he rose and dramatically raised his arms and declared, 'Alleluia! The strife is o'er, the battle done'.

When Munro Kerr was in the last year of his life, he was visited by his former student Dugald Baird.

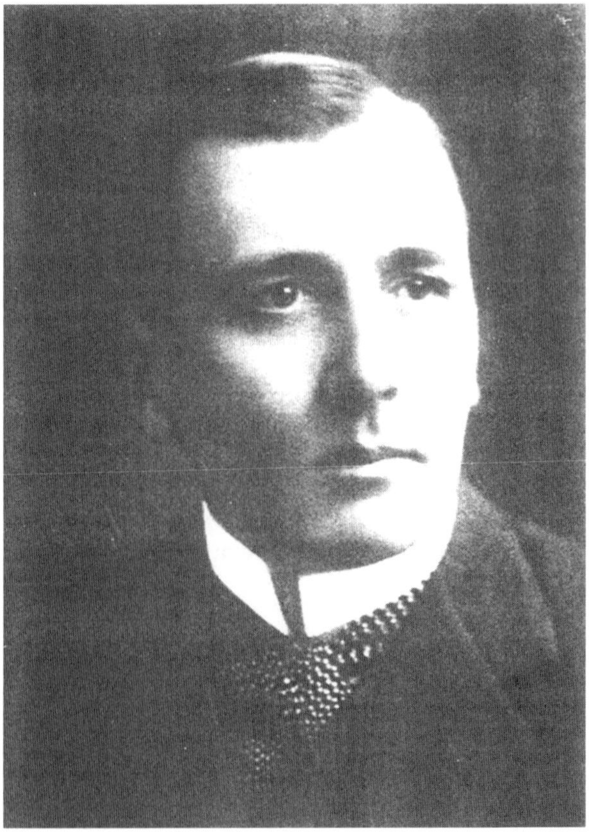

John Martin Munro Kerr

The discussion turned to death, and Munro Kerr said, 'I'd like to go out on the first tee at Killemont, put a ball down, hit a real beauty down the first fairway and then drop'. He died the following year at the age of 92 in Canterbury, where he had retired.

Selected Publications

Kerr JMM. *Operative Midwifery*. London: Ballière Tindall; 1908.

Kerr JMM. The lower uterine segment incision in conservative caesarean section. *J Obstet Gynaecol Br Emp* 1921; 28: 475–87.

Kerr JMM. The technic of cesarean section, with special reference to the lower uterine segment incision. *Am J Obstet Gynecol* 1926; 12: 729–34.

Bibliography References

99, 102, 273, 648, 753, 822–824, 950, 987, 1183, 1205, 1333, 1631, 1706, 1728, 1734.

Keyes, Edward Lawrence (1843–1925)

Keyes' Punch

The cutaneous punch, widely used in the diagnosis of vulval disease to remove tiny circular sections of skin for histological examination, is known as Keyes' punch. Keyes described his first use of the punch in a lecture to the New York Dermatological Society on 26 January 1887 that was published later that year:

> *In the summer of 1879, a young gentleman, living as a neighbor in the country, which discharging some piece of fireworks, blew his face full of specks of partly burnt powder. I was called upon by the father to remove this disfigurement, which was very considerable.*

Using the conventional methods of the time, Keyes cleaned and treated the wounds on several occasions but was unable to rid all the scars of the powder's blue tint:

> *Finding at last, when the little wounds had all healed, that my patient was marked in an unseemly manner, I determined to eradicate the numerous points of disfigurement, by entirely taking away the portion of integument involved in the colored scar. To do this I devised a number of small cutaneous trephines, or punches, as they may be called, with a sharp cutting edge; the diameter of the cutting edge varying from one millimetre upwards . . . The result of this trifling operation was admirable. The little bloody pits in the skin were allowed to fill with coagulated blood, and left without any dressing, as the bleeding promptly ceased. One year after the operation . . . The scars were practically invisible'.*

Shortly after this publication, Dr BA Watson, a surgeon at the New Jersey City Charity Hospital, wrote a letter to the editor pointing out his priority for the cutaneous punch. He had published two papers 10 years before using his own 'discotome' for exactly the same purpose. Keyes, who was apparently an honest and gentle man wrote back a letter, published by the editor, saying:

> *Dear Doctor: I am entirely unconscious of ever having seen either of the articles referred to above, but it is only*

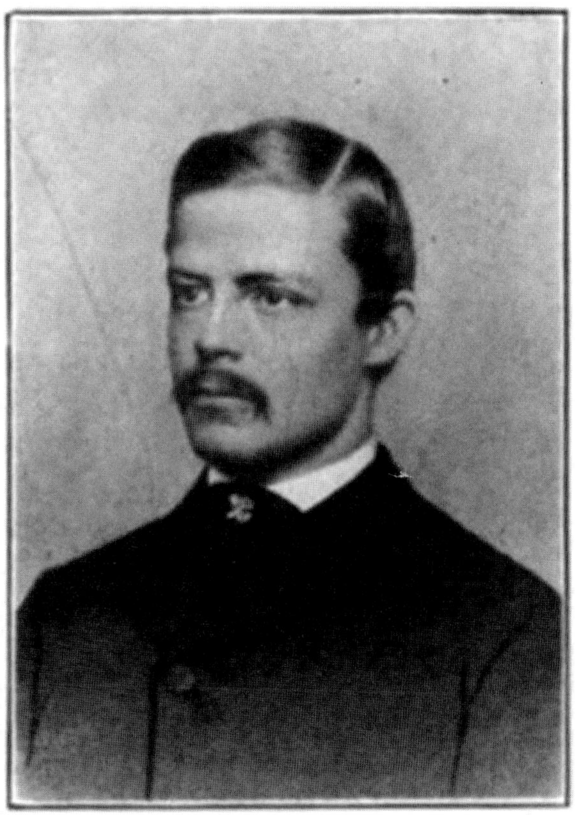

Edward Lawrence Keyes

just to Dr Watson that he should have the credit of priority if he wishes it, and the publication in your Journal of his letter with mine will give it to him. Yours etc., E. L. Keyes.

Edward Lawrence Keyes graduated from New York University in 1866, followed by further studies in dermatology and syphilology in Paris. One of his main interests was urology, and he became professor of genito-urinary surgery, syphilology and dermatology at the Bellevue Hospital Medical College, New York in 1881.

Selected Publications

Keyes EL. The cutaneous punch. *J Cutan Genitourin Dis* 1887; 5: 98–101.

Watson BA. New instruments: discotome. *Med Record (NY)* 1878; 14: 78.

Watson BA. Gunpowder disfigurements. *St Louis Med Surg J* 1878; 35: 145–8.

Bibliography References

270, 326, 1510.

Kielland, Christian Casper Gabriel (1871–1941)

Kielland's Forceps

Christian Kielland designed straight forceps without a pelvic curve to facilitate delivery from the mid-pelvis in cases of malrotation: occipito-transverse and occipito-posterior positions of the fetal head. Kielland argued that conventional forceps with a pelvic curve were impossible to apply correctly to the incompletely rotated head in the mid or upper pelvis. He reasoned, 'In such cases attempts to apply the forceps in any way other than over the brow and occiput are usually unsuccessful' and pointed out the fetal dangers of this type of application.

Kielland laid down very precise rules for the use of his forceps. When these were followed in the era of upper- and mid-pelvis assisted delivery, good results were obtained in many centres. Kielland's forceps have also been used with good effect for face presentation and the aftercoming head of the breech. They continue to be used in a dwindling number of hospitals throughout the world.

Christian Kielland came from a two-century lineage of Norwegian ship owners. He was born in Zululand, South Africa, where his father worked in a missionary station. The family returned to Norway when young Christian was three years old. He was educated in Oslo and graduated in medicine from the Universitas Regia Fredrickiana in 1899. After extra training in obstetrics, he took up private practice in Oslo and in 1915 was appointed to the university clinic. In 1910 Kielland spent three months in the gynaecology department of the Rigshospitalet in Copenhagen. It was there he first demonstrated his new forceps. In the ensuing years he made several visits to medical clinics in Germany, and after demonstrating his forceps at a meeting of the Munich Gynaecological Society, the first brief publication of his forceps appeared. The following year Kielland published a full description of his forceps and the rules for their

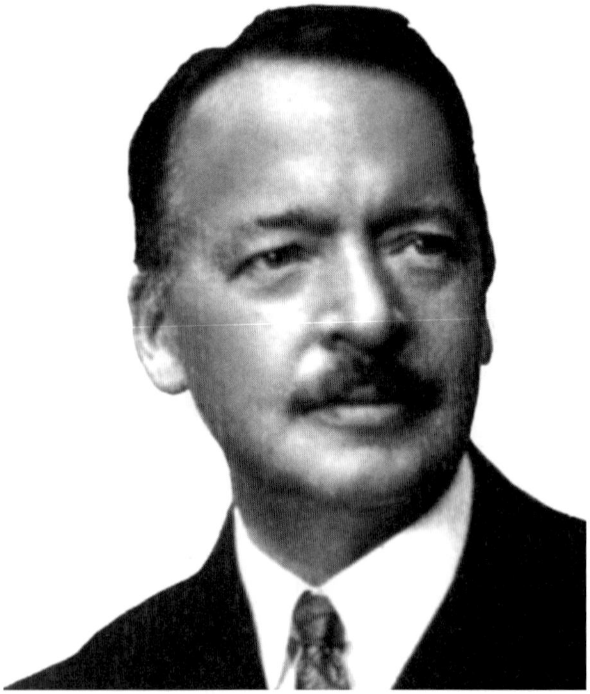

Christian Caspar Gabriel Kielland

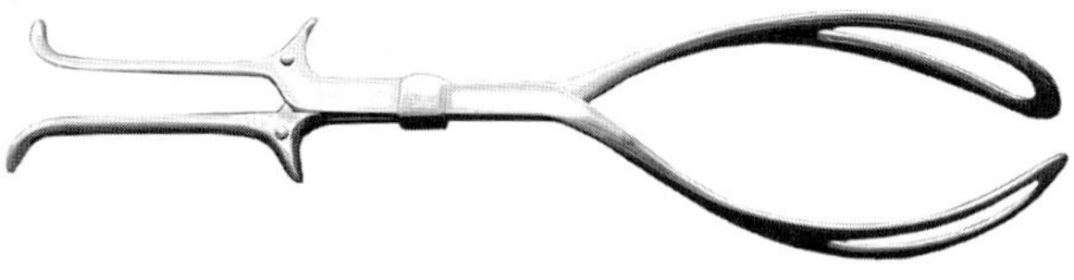

Kielland's forceps

application, based on their use in 352 deliveries he had conducted over the previous seven years.

Kielland's forceps were gradually adopted throughout the world, although not to a great extent in his home country. He visited both England and the United States to demonstrate his forceps. Kielland continued obstetric practice from his own clinic in Oslo until he died from a cerebrovascular accident on 18 March 1941.

Selected Publications

Kielland C. Eine neue Form und Einführungsweise der Geburtszange, stets biparietal an den kindlichen Schädel gelegt. *München Med Wochenschr* 1915; 62: 923.

Kielland C. Über die Anlegung der Zange am nicht rotierten Kopf mit Beschreibung eines neuen zangenmodelles und einer neuen Anglegungsmenthode. *Mschr Geburtsh Gynäkol* 1916; 43: 48–78.

Bibliography References

99, 361, 399, 451, 483, 648, 721, 1132, 1168, 1170, 1261, 1285.

Kimball, Gilman (1804–1892)

Subtotal Abdominal Hysterectomy

The first subtotal abdominal hysterectomies were performed by Charles Clay and AM Heath of Manchester on 17 and 21 November 1843, respectively. Both patients died. On 25 June 1853, Walter Burnham of Lowell, Massachusetts performed the first subtotal abdominal hysterectomy in which the patient survived. In all of these cases the laparotomy was carried out for what was thought to be a large ovarian cyst. When each surgeon entered the abdomen, they found that they were confronted with a large fibroid uterus that could not be returned to the abdominal cavity and were therefore forced to perform hysterectomy.

The first planned subtotal abdominal hysterectomy for uterine fibroids was carried out by Gilman Kimball, also of Lowell, Massachusetts. The woman in question had a uterine fibroid the size of a 'pregnancy six months advanced'. The size of the uterus was not the cause of the patient's distress but the associated menorrhagia was considered life-threatening: 'Every month a large quantity of blood is lost, reducing the patient extremely, even hazarding her life'. The patient's physicians consulted Kimball, who felt that:

> *Rather than give up the case as utterly hopeless, I would propose, as a last resort, the removal of the uterus itself . . . extraordinary and hazardous as this suggestion seemed, the feeling was unanimously and unhesitatingly expressed by everyone present at the consultation, that this procedure offered the only possible chance of saving the patient from impending death. This conclusion was no sooner made known to the patient, that it was readily consented to – both she and her husband claiming that a chance of life by an operation however small that chance might be, was better than the certainty of a speedy death.*

On that same day, 1 September 1853, the patient was anaesthetised with chloroform and 'an incision was made through the linea alba directly over the most prominent portion of the tumor'.

Kimball's plan was to reduce the size of the uterus by performing myomectomy, or as he put it 'see what could be done by way of enucleating the diseased portion of it – thus reducing its bulk so as to allow its being drawn out through a comparatively small opening'. This he achieved:

> *The uterus becoming at once greatly diminished in bulk, it was readily drawn out from the abdominal cavity, comfortably with the plan adopted in the outset, and placed in the hands of an assistant. A straight, double-armed needle was now passed through the organ in an antero-posterior direction, as low down as the supposed point of its junction with the neck, this part being, of course, left intact as regards its relation with the vagina. By this plan of appropriating to each lateral half a separate ligature, there was no great difficulty in making sure against all chance of subsequent haemorrhage; a consideration of great importance in view of what may otherwise be very liable to happen.*

The patient recovered well and, other than some 'inconvenience' from the uterine ligatures extruding through the abdominal incision (as was the practice at that time to avoid sepsis), she returned to full activity. Kimball acknowledged that on two previous occasions he had performed hysterectomy, thinking he was dealing with an ovarian cyst and that both patients had died: 'I should consider myself unjust, and culpably indifferent to my professional obligations, were I to withhold the fact that in two other instances of uterine extirpation, I have had the misfortune to lose my patients'.

Gilman Kimball was born in Newchester, New Hampshire, in 1804. He graduated MD from Dartmouth College in 1826. He was later awarded an honorary MD from both Williams College, in 1837, and Yale College, in 1856. He served in the American Civil War as brigade surgeon and medical director for General Butler. He was professor of surgery at the Berkshire Medical Institute and in the Vermont Medical College. At the time of the operation described above he was surgeon to the Lowell Hospital in Lowell, Massachusetts. He was elected to Fellowship of the American Gynecological Society in 1877 and was President of that Society in 1883. He died in his eighty-eighth year in 1892.

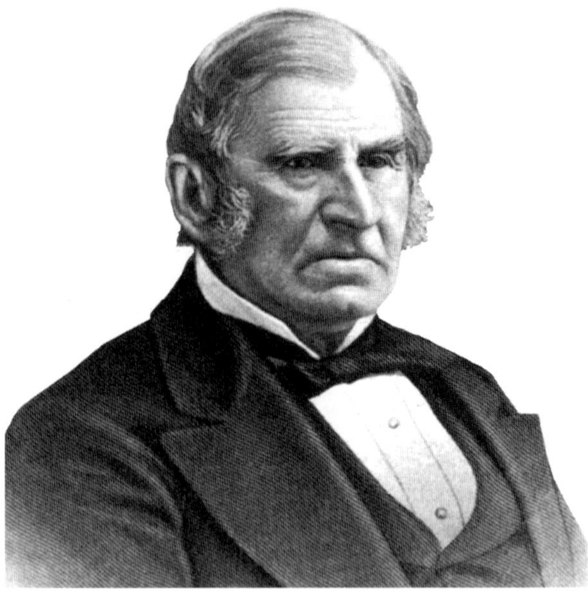

Gilman Kimball

Selected Publications

Kimball G. Successful case of extirpation of the uterus. *Boston Med Surg J* 1855; 52: 249–55.

Bibliography References

97, 125, 345, 362, 678, 690, 691, 810, 1001, 1291, 1485.

Kiwisch, Franz Ritter von Rotterau (1814–1852)

Prague Manoeuvre

Franz Kiwisch was born on 30 April 1814 in Klattau, Bohemia (then part of the Austrian empire). He obtained his medical degree in Prague in 1837 and travelled in Germany, France, Denmark and England. He was made district medical officer at Bydzow in 1842 and became docent of gynaecology. In 1845 he was appointed *Ordinarius* of obstetrics and gynaecology at Würzburg, where he was a highly respected teacher and clinician.

Through his influence, a method of delivering the aftercoming head of the breech was widely used and became known as the Prague manoeuvre. In this, the attendant grasps the legs of the infant with one hand and places the first and second fingers of the other hand over the shoulders on each side of the neck. With downward traction, the infant's head is extended over the perineum as the legs are swept in an arc towards the mother's abdomen. In cases in which the infant's body has delivered but the head has been allowed to descend occipito-posterior, the so-called reverse Prague manoeuvre may succeed in delivering the head. This had been described by Benjamin Pugh a century before.

Kiwisch returned to Prague in 1850 as professor of obstetrics and gynaecology. Sadly, his health failed soon after and he ultimately succumbed to tuberculosis of the lungs and spine at the age of 38.

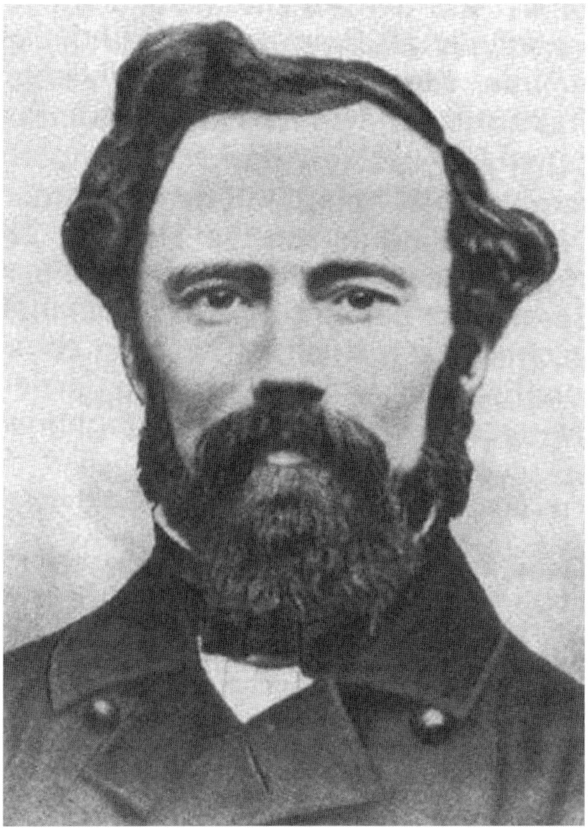

Franz Ritter von Rotterau Kiwisch

Selected Publications

Kiwisch F. *Beiträge zur Geburtskunde*. Würzburg: I Abth; 1846: 69.

Bibliography References

541, 542, 648, 673, 841.

Kleihauer, Enno (1927–2017) Betke, Klaus Hermann (1914–2011)

Kleihauer–Betke Test

In 1957, Kleihauer and Betke introduced their simple technique for detecting fetal haemoglobin in red cells. Sixty years later, the Kleihauer–Betke test remains in use, and their original paper is one of the most frequently quoted medical publications. As a young postgraduate student, Erno Kleihauer, working in paediatric haematology under the guidance of Klaus Betke, was doing a research project on the red cell properties of newborns and infants. An essential requirement was the ability to distinguish between fetal and adult haemoglobin in individual erythrocytes. As Betke was to write later:

In our search to find a method for the differentiation of Hb A and Hb F in the red cells of a blood smear I remembered a paper of E G Schenk from 1930 (Arch. exp. Path. Pharm. 150, p. 160) who had found that denatured adult haemoglobin is much more rapidly digested by pepsin than newborn haemoglobin. So we 'digested' fixed blood smears with pepsin, and in fact, it worked. Evaluating the best pH for the procedure, Enno Kleihauer ran also a blank of the acid buffer without pepsin, and this produced even better results.

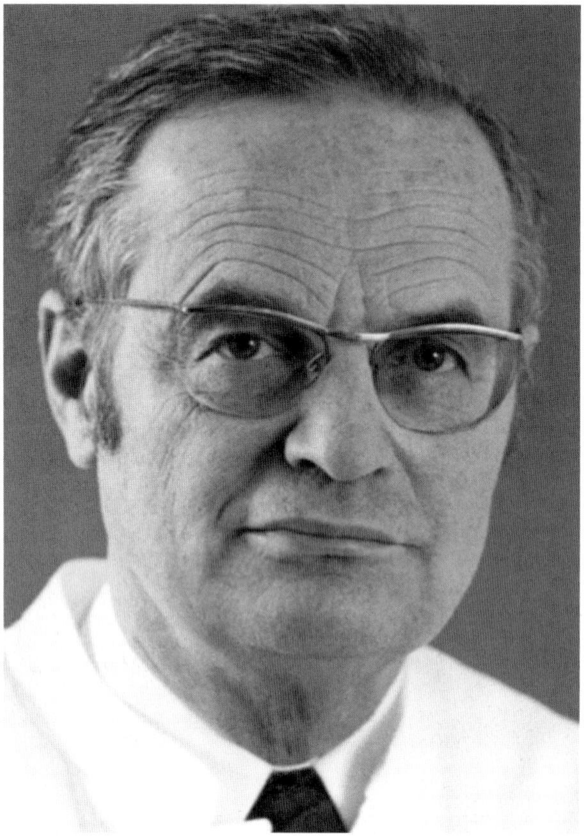

Klaus Hermann Betke

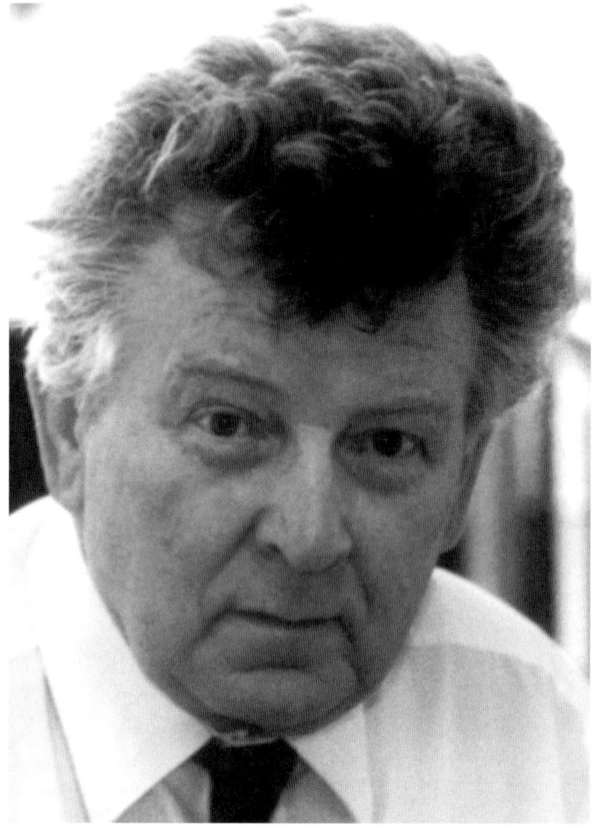

Enno Kleihauer

In their first publication, the second author, Dr Hildegard Braun, was responsible for the electron microscopy. As they wrote in their 1957 report:

> *In digestion experiments with fixed blood smears we noticed that with pepsin the blood pigment of erythrocytes of adults is dissolved faster than in erythrocytes of the newborn. The further examination of this phenomenon shows that pepsin is not necessary and the separation of alcohol fixed blood smears will occur with citric acid phosphate at pH 3.4–3.6.*

Thus was born the simple and reproducible acid elution test to differentiate adult from fetal red blood cells. The test has been of great importance in the diagnosis and management of haemoglobinopathies, as well as fetomaternal and maternal-fetal transfusions. It was first applied to the study of rhesus immunisation in 1959 by the Winnipeg group in Canada. Alvin Zipursky and his colleagues used the test to detect fetal cells in the maternal circulation just after delivery and found that 'transplacental haemorrhage of fetal blood is rather common'. The test became one of the foundations in the development of methods for preventing rhesus sensitisation.

Enno Kleihauer was born in Pewsum, Germany. He studied medicine at the universities in Hamburg and Freiburg, receiving his MD from Freiburg in 1956. He specialised in paediatrics and haematology, working with Betke in Freiburg, Tübingen and Munich. In 1966 he spent a year as a National Institute of Health research fellow in biochemistry at the University of Georgia. In 1969 he became director of the Ulm University Children's Clinic, which position he held until he retired in 1995.

Klaus Hermann Betke was born in Munich. He studied medicine in Freiburg, Königsberg and Berlin, qualifying in 1940. He was called upon to serve as a medical officer during the Second World War and towards the end was briefly an American prisoner of war. Betke trained as a paediatrician at the university departments in Würzburg, Erlangen and Freiburg. It was when he was a lecturer in Freiburg that he and Kleihauer carried out their work. He was successively head of the university department of paediatrics at Tübingen (1961–1967) and Munich (1967–1983).

Betke and Kleihauer were able to celebrate the fiftieth anniversary of their test at 93 and 80 years respectively. Both men lived into their ninth decade: Betke died aged 96 and Kleihauer in his ninetieth year.

Selected Publications

Kleihauer E, Braun H, Betke K. Demonstration von fetalem Hämoglobin in den Erythrocyten eines Blutausstrichs. *Klin Wochenschr* 1957; 35: 637–8.

Betke K, Kleihauer E. Fetaler und bleibender Blutfarbstoff in Erythrocyten und Erythroblasten von menschlichen Feten und Neugeborenen. *Blut* 1958; 4: 241–4.

Zipursky A, Hull A, White FD, Israels LG. Foetal erythrocytes in the maternal circulation. *Lancet* 1959; 1: 451–2.

Bibliography References

82, 458, 849, 1625, 1741, 1744, 1748.

Klikovich, Stanislav Casimirovicz (1853–1910)

Nitrous Oxide and Oxygen Analgesia

After the identification of nitrous oxide in 1772 by Joseph Priestly (1733–1804) and clinical research by Sir Humphrey Davey (1778–1829) in the 1790s, the use of nitrous oxide largely degenerated into a source of amusement at ‘laughing gas’ parties. However, in the mid-nineteenth century, its application in dental anaesthesia emerged. It became apparent that prolonged use of nitrous oxide led to hypoxia and for safety it must be mixed with oxygen. While nitrous oxide had been used sporadically for childbirth, it was Klikovich who first systematically studied the mixture of 80 per cent nitrous oxide and 20 per cent oxygen for analgesia during labour. He recorded his results with 25 women in labour, and most of his advice on the clinical administration remains relevant:

> *The woman should be coached to exhale deeply and then inhale as much gas as possible, because the effect appears faster when the gas remains in the lungs for a longer period of time. It is important to begin the first anaesthesia early in order to attain good pain relief; a late start will prevent the deep inhalation and, thus, render the effect incomplete . . . Thereafter, the inhalation is begun at one-half to one minute prior to the anticipated next contraction. Two to five breaths of the gas mixture usually suffice to produce the desired effect.*

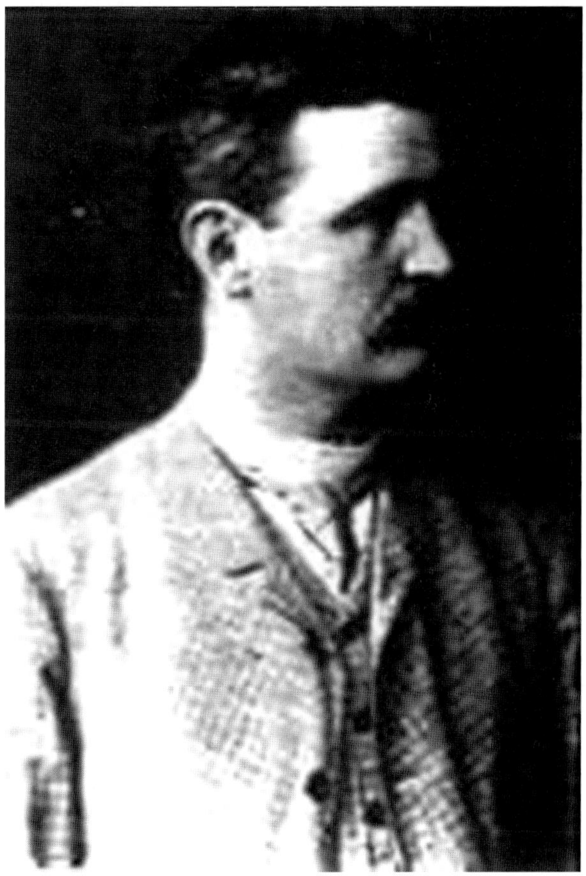

Stanislav Casimirovicz Klikovich

His careful clinical observations showed no ill effects and no alteration in uterine activity. The latter point he confirmed scientifically by quantitating uterine pressure in three parturients using a catheter with a balloon passed through the cervix and attached to a manometer.

Stanislav Casimirovicz Klikovich was born to Polish parents in Wilno, then part of Russian-occupied

Poland. In 1876 he qualified at the Academy of Medicine and Surgery in St Petersburg. For the next five years he worked at the St Petersburg Clinic of Internal Diseases under the guidance of Professor Sergei Botkin. There he performed extensive research on nitrous oxide and was awarded his MD in 1881. After this he returned to his home province of Wilno as a military doctor and then spent two years visiting clinics in Europe, including those of Robert Koch and Rudolph Virchow. He returned to Russia in 1886 and, in the disruptive political climate of the time, fulfilled a number of positions as lecturer and military physician. He died in Kazan at 56 years of age from the effects of a stroke.

Selected Publications

Klikovich S. Über das Stickstoffoxydul als Anaestheticum bei Geburten. *Arch Gynäkol* 1881; 18: 81–108.

Bibliography References

74, 457, 585, 997, 1293, 1336, 1439, 1440, 1584, 1685.

Klumpke, Augusta (1859–1927)

Klumpke's Paralysis

Augusta Klumpke was only 26 years old and an extern student at the University of Paris when she published her paper describing the rarer form of brachial plexus palsy involving damage to the lower nerve roots, C8 and T1, and the oculo-pupillary signs from paralysis of the cervical sympathetic. The latter she confirmed by experiments on dogs.

Augusta Klumpke was born in San Francisco but at 11 years of age, when her parents separated, moved to Lausanne, Switzerland with her mother and sisters. She was one of four sisters, all accomplished in the arts or sciences. When she tried to enrol as a medical student at the University of Paris, she was opposed by much of the faculty, particularly the head of neurology, Professor Alfred Vulpian (1826–1887). With persistence she gained admission and became the first female extern and then intern in the hospital, ironically on Vulpian's ward.

She received her MD in 1889. In 1888 she married the brilliant neurologist, Joseph Jules Dejerine (1849–1917), with whom she co-authored a classic two-volume text, *Anatomy of the Nervous System*, in 1898. Klumpke became an accomplished neurologist with a substantial bibliography. During and after the First World War she did much work on the treatment and rehabilitation of soldiers with neurological injuries. In 1921 her contributions were recognised with her appointment as an officer of the Legion of Honour. She had one daughter, who also became a physician. Augusta Klumpke died on 5 November 1927 and was buried beside her husband at the Père Lachaise churchyard in Paris.

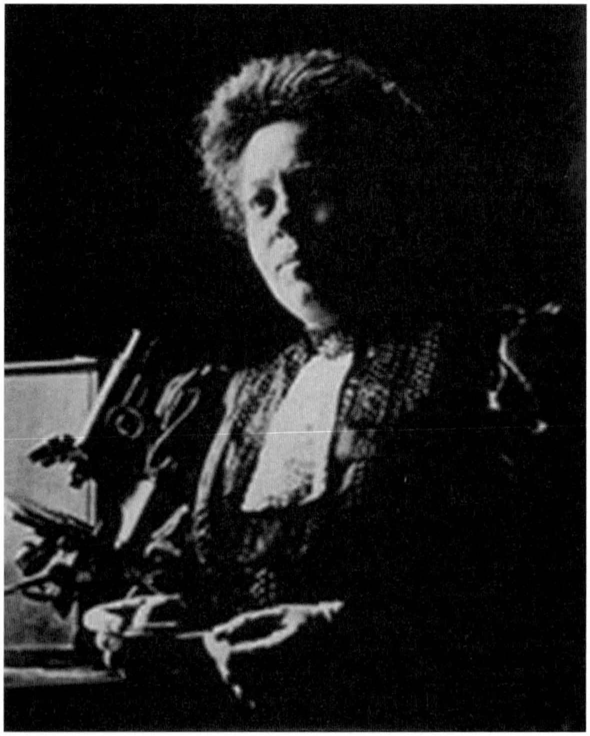

Augusta Klumpke

Selected Publications

Klumpke A. Contribution à l'études des paralysies radiculaires. *Rev Méd* 1885; 5: 591–616.

Bibliography References

8, 33, 778, 968, 1348, 1485, 1500.

Kobelt, Georg Ludwig (1804–1857)

Kobelt's Tubules

The mesonephric remnant, composed of tiny vestigial tubules, runs within the peritoneal folds between the ovary and tube. These are called the epoophoron or Kobelt's tubules and were described earlier by Johann Christian Rosenmüller (1771–1820). Kobelt also described the veins in the bulbs of the subclitoral vestibule, sometimes referred to as Kobelt's network.

Georg Ludwig Kobelt was born on 12 March 1804 in Baden. Initially he studied law at the University of Heidelberg but changed to medicine and qualified in 1833. In 1837 he made a medical tour of France, Holland and Great Britain. He was appointed professor of anatomy at the University of Freiburg in 1847. After several years of ill health, he died on 18 May 1857.

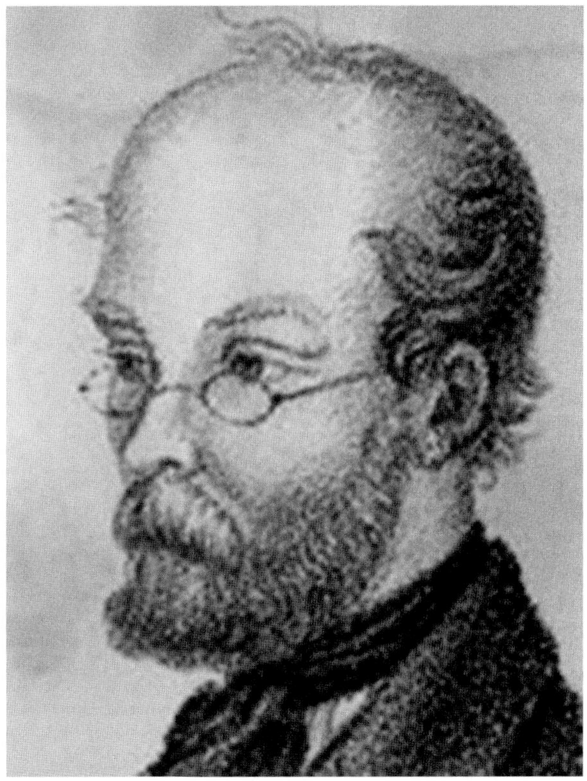

Georg Ludwig Kobelt

Selected Publications

Kobelt GL. *Die Männlichen und weiblichen Wollust-organe des Menschen und einer Saugetiere in Anatamisch-Physiologischer beziehung Untersieht und Dargestellt.* Freiburg; 1844.

Bibliography References

406, 1480, 1486.

Kristeller, Samuel (1820–1900)

Kristeller's Manoeuvre

In 1867, at a time when malpresentations and obstructed labour were usually managed by intrauterine manipulation, extraction and forceps delivery, Samuel Kristeller presented a preliminary report on his method of external manual compression to assist delivery. In advocating his technique for dealing with inadequate uterine action or dystocia, he wrote:

> *I recommended a number of external manipulations ('handgriffe') which must be performed in a systematic fashion. I have used this manoeuvre in a large number of deliveries for different indications . . . and became convinced that this manoeuvre is appropriate, without damaging effect, and in most cases very useful . . . Hence I now believe I can recommend the manoeuvre to my colleagues.*

Kristeller's manoeuvre involved encircling the upper and lateral portions of the uterus with the palms of the hands and, facing caudad, exerting rotatory movements with increasing pressure up to a sustained firm push for 5–8 seconds downwards to the pelvic brim. This was repeated up to 30 times with rest intervals of 1–3 minutes between compressions. It could be used with minor modifications in breech or cephalic presentation, the first or second stage of labour, and with or without anaesthesia. Kristeller felt his manoeuvre induced stronger uterine contractions as well as physical descent of the presenting part. He claimed that, by reducing the need for manual or forceps extraction of the fetus, it diminished the associated trauma.

He also developed a pair of obstetric forceps with a device to measure the extraction force, Kristeller's dynamometrical forceps. This was achieved by a spiral spring in the handle which was compressed with traction and reflected the amount of this compressive force on a scale on the surface of the handle. In so doing, Kristeller was one of the first to attempt an objective measurement of the forces of forceps extraction.

Samuel Kristeller was born in the province of Posen, Germany. He received his MD from the University of Berlin in 1843. He was the first Jewish physician to be appointed to a government position in Preussen. In 1851 he returned to Berlin and became *privat dozent* in gynaecology at the University of Berlin in 1860. He died on 15 July 1900.

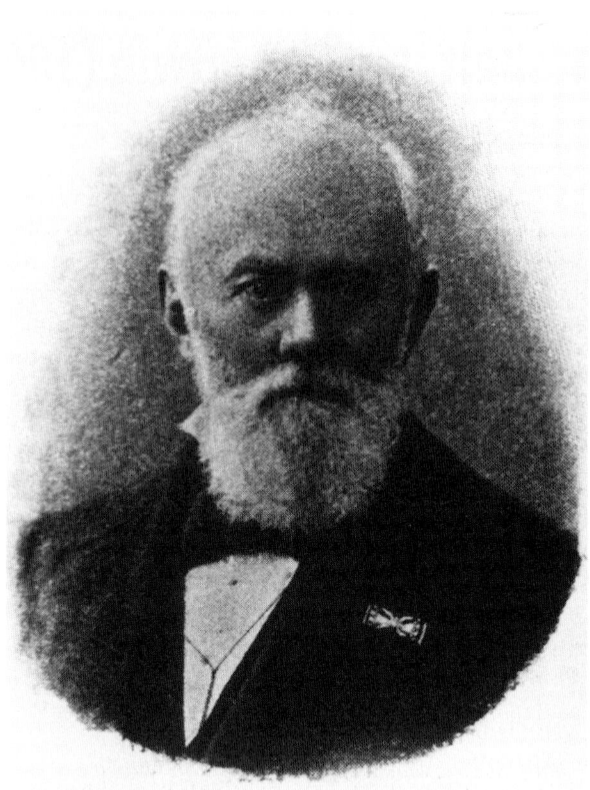

Samuel Kristeller

Selected Publications

Kristeller S. Dynamometrisch Vorrichtung an der Geburtszange. *Mschr Geburtsch* 1861; 27: 166–75.

Kristeller S. Neues Entbindungsverfahren unter Anwendung von äusseren Handgriffen: Vorläufige Mittheilung. *Berl Klin Wochenschr* 1867; 6: 56–9.

Bibliography References

113, 116, 361, 428, 541, 542, 553, 648, 721, 1039, 1261, 1654, 1668.

Krukenberg, Freidrich Ernst (1871–1946)

Krukenberg's Tumour

The modern criteria for Krukenberg's tumour vary among pathologists and differ from Krukenberg's original conclusions. In 1896 he reported six cases of bilateral ovarian tumours with a distinctive histological pattern:

> *In the cellular proliferation, round swollen cells with finely vacuolated cytoplasm, often distinctly mucin-producing, appear chiefly in the form of smaller or large clusters . . . The peculiar character that is given to the tumour through the appearance of the large swollen tumour cells . . . might then be expressed with the least possible prejudicial addition as 'mucocellulare'.*

Krukenberg believed the tumours to be of primary ovarian origin. This is now felt to be rarely, if ever, the case. Some pathologists define Krukenberg tumours as bilateral ovarian metastases with a primary in the gastrointestinal tract. Others confirm the diagnosis if the ovarian metastases have the typical mucin-secreting, 'signet-ring' cells, irrespective of the primary site.

Friedrich Ernst Krukenberg was born in Halle, Germany, the youngest of seven children to a family of some legal and medical renown. He carried out his pathological studies on ovarian tumours in Marburg when he was 24 years of age, and this formed the basis of his MD thesis. After his initial foray into gynaecological pathology, Krukenberg moved as far as he could from the pelvis to become an ophthalmologist in his home town of Halle.

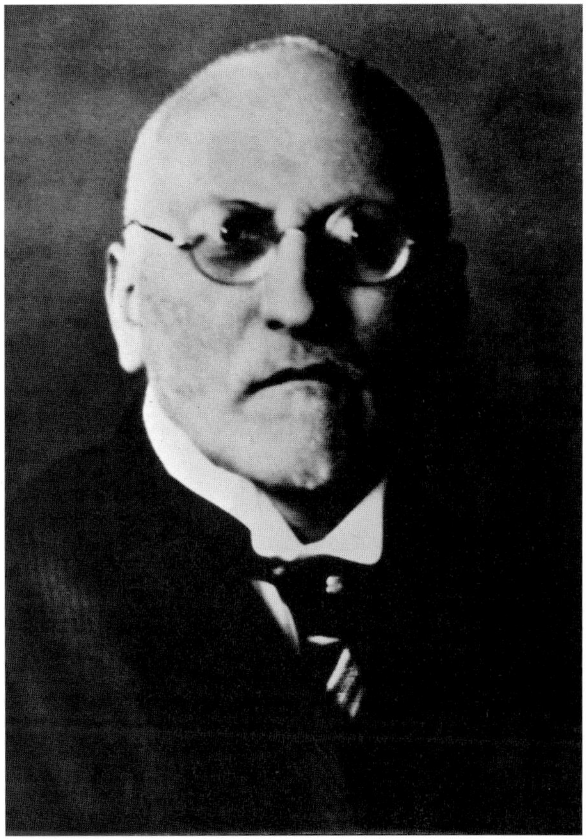

Friedrich Ernst Krukenberg

Selected Publications

Krukenberg F. Über das Fibrosarcoma ovarii mucocellulare (carcinomatodes). *Arch Gynäkol* 1896; 50: 287–321.

Bibliography References

552, 562, 700, 857, 1459.

Küstner, Otto Ernst (1848–1931)

Küstner's Operation

In contrast to Pier Spinelli, Otto Ernst Küstner developed a posterior vaginal approach to chronic uterine inversion. He made a transverse incision in the pouch of Douglas and through this opening inserted one finger into the funnel of the inverted uterus. He then incised the posterior wall of the uterus

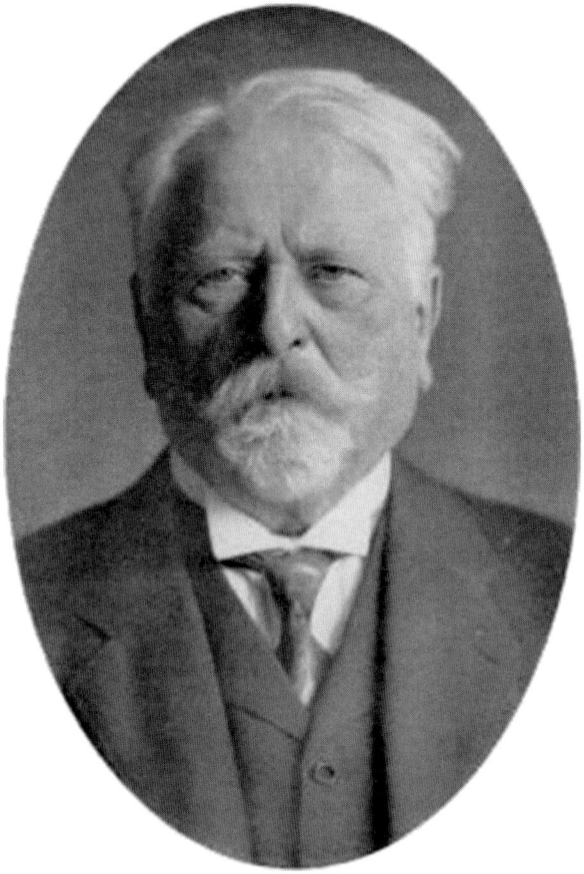

Otto Ernst Küstner

and the cervical constriction ring, allowing replacement of the uterine fundus. The procedure was completed by suture of the uterine incision and the pouch of Douglas.

Otto Ernst Küstner was born in Trossin, Germany. He did his medical training in Leipzig, Berlin and Halle. Virchow was one of his teachers. His postgraduate training was done in Vienna. He visited London and observed Spencer Wells performing ovariotomy. He travelled widely and wrote a gynaecology text that went into several editions. He became professor of obstetrics and gynaecology in Göttingen in 1887 and at Breslau in 1893. His work included the development of lower-segment caesarean section, X-ray pelvimetry, abdominal incisions and early ambulation post partum. Küstner became Dean of Medicine at Breslau in 1914. He had four sons, one of whom died of diphtheria and one who did obstetrics and gynaecology.

Selected Publications

Küstner O. *Zentralbl Gynäkol* 1893; 41: 17.

Bibliography References

119, 648, 1205, 1480, 1503, 1631, 1734.

L

Landsteiner, Karl (1868–1943)

Blood Groups

In a footnote to his paper of 1900 on the agglutinating effects of blood serum, Karl Landsteiner noted what he felt was a physiological property: 'The blood of some human beings destroys the red cells of other human beings'. Working with his own blood and that of his laboratory assistants, he separated the plasma and red cell components. Mixing the plasma of one with the red cells of another, he noted either no reaction or the clumping of red cells. Adding blood samples from other volunteers, he eventually identified three types of human blood: A, B and C (later called O). He published this work in 1901. One year later, two of his assistants, Alfred von Decastello (1872–1960) and Adriano Sturli (1876–1964), identified the fourth group, AB.

This landmark discovery set up the possibility of safe transfusion. In 1910 Emil Von Dungern (1876–1961) and Ludwig Hirszfeld (1884–1954) postulated the inheritance of blood groups. In 1914, the discovery by Richard Lewinshon (1895–1961) that adding citrate to blood prevented coagulation provided the last practical requirement for blood banking.

After his move from Vienna to New York, Landsteiner continued his work, developing immune sera in animals by the injection of red cells from other species. Working with Alexander Wiener (1907–1976), he produced rabbit serum with antibodies to the red cells of the Rhesus monkey. When this rabbit serum was mixed with human red cells, 85 per cent agglutinated (Rhesus positive) and 15 per cent did not (Rhesus negative). Thus was discovered one of the common reasons for transfusion reactions despite ABO compatible grouping. In 1941 Philip Levine (1900–1987) and his colleagues established the pathogenesis of haemolytic disease of the newborn as due to immunisation of the Rh-negative mother by her Rh-positive fetus, with its Rh antigen inherited from the father.

Karl Landsteiner was born in Baden, the son of a well-known journalist and newspaper publisher, who died when Karl was only six years old. He graduated in medicine from the University of Vienna in 1891. After additional postgraduate training in chemistry at a number of European universities, he started work at the Institute of Hygiene in 1896 and later in the Pathological-Anatomical Institute at the University of Vienna. It was here he did his work on the ABO blood group system. In 1919, as life in Vienna deteriorated following the First World War, Landsteiner left for Holland and for three years worked at the RK Ziekenhaus, a small hospital in The Hague. In 1922 he moved to the United States and an appointment at the Rockefeller Institute in New York. He became a United States citizen in 1929. In 1930 he received the Nobel Prize for his discovery of blood groups.

Landsteiner was a shy but critical scientist and teacher. He insisted that his assistants repeat all important experiments in front of him. He became cantankerous in his senior years. He was also an excellent pianist but sold his piano to avoid disturbing his neighbours.

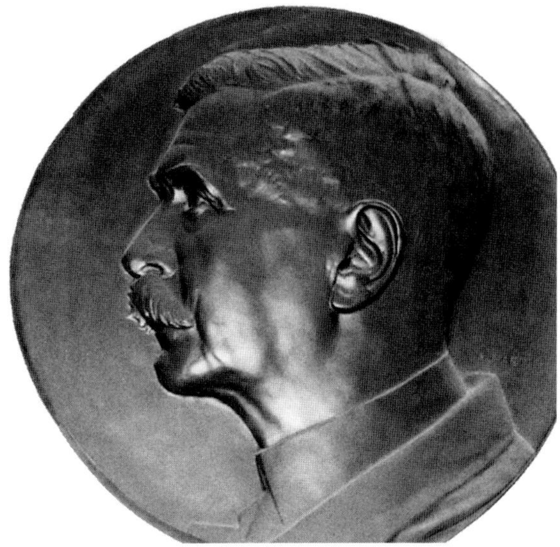

Karl Landsteiner

Landsteiner died two days following a coronary thrombosis suffered while working in his laboratory. At the unveiling of the Landsteiner memorial in the arcades at the University of Vienna in 1961, it was said: 'Whenever a blood transfusion is performed in the world . . . Karl Landsteiner is virtually present'.

Selected Publications

Landsteiner K. Zur Kenntnis der antifermentativen, lytischen und agglutinierenden Wirkungen des Blutserums und der Lymphe. *Zentralbl Bakt* 1900; 27: 357–62.

Landsteiner K. Über Agglutinationserscheinungen normalen menschlichen Blutes. *Wein Klin Wochenschr* 1901; 14: 1132–4.

von Decastello A, Sturli A. Über die Isoagglutinine im Serum gesunder und kranker Menschen. *Münch med Wochenschr* 1902, 49: 1090–5.

Landsteiner K, Wiener AS. An agglutinable factor in human blood recognised by immune sera for Rhesus blood. *Proc Soc Exp Biol NY* 1940; 43: 223–5.

Levine P, Burnham L, Katzin EM, Vogel P. The role of isoimmunization in the pathogenesis of erythroblastosis fetalis. *Am J Obstet Gynecol* 1941; 42: 925–37.

Bibliography References

34, 545, 870, 871, 899, 1057, 1262, 1378, 1493, 1509, 1672, 1690, 1741, 1745, 1748.

Langenbeck, Conrad Johann Martin (1776–1851)

Vaginal Hysterectomy

Early surgical attempts to deal with uterine prolapse, chronic uterine inversion and cervical cancer were limited to amputation of the cervix and part of the lower uterine corpus. In April 1812, the Italian surgeon GB Palletta of Milan inadvertently performed a vaginal hysterectomy while planning to do only a high cervical amputation. The patient died three days later.

In 1813, Conrad Langenbeck carried out the first planned and successful vaginal hysterectomy in a multiparous, 50-year-old woman with an ulcerated, possibly cancerous cervix. He performed this feat without anaesthesia or assistance. A surgical colleague was present but, suffering from gout, was unable to rise from his chair to assist. At one point, Langenbeck was left clutching the bleeding area in his left hand and holding one end of a ligature in his teeth while tying the other end with his right hand. By now desperately in need of assistance, Langenbeck exhorted his colleague, 'Sir, could you just try and limp over here', to which his hapless, gout-stricken assistant replied, 'I cannot'. Langenbeck dissected carefully so as not to open the peritoneal cavity, and it is likely that he left a thin portion of the uterine fundus. There was considerable haemorrhage, but the patient survived, her revival apparently aided by splashing cold water on her face. His claim to have removed the uterus without entering the peritoneal cavity was doubted. After the operation, the specimen was lost and his putative assistant died, allowing no independent confirmation of his achievement until the patient died 26 years later and a post mortem vindicated Langenbeck.

Conrad Johann Martin Langenbeck was professor of anatomy and surgery in Göttingen and surgeon-general of the Hanoverian Army. He was one of the most accomplished surgeons of his era. He was said to have been such a swift operator that a visiting colleague, turning to take a pinch of snuff, missed his performance of a shoulder amputation – some snuff, some surgeon!

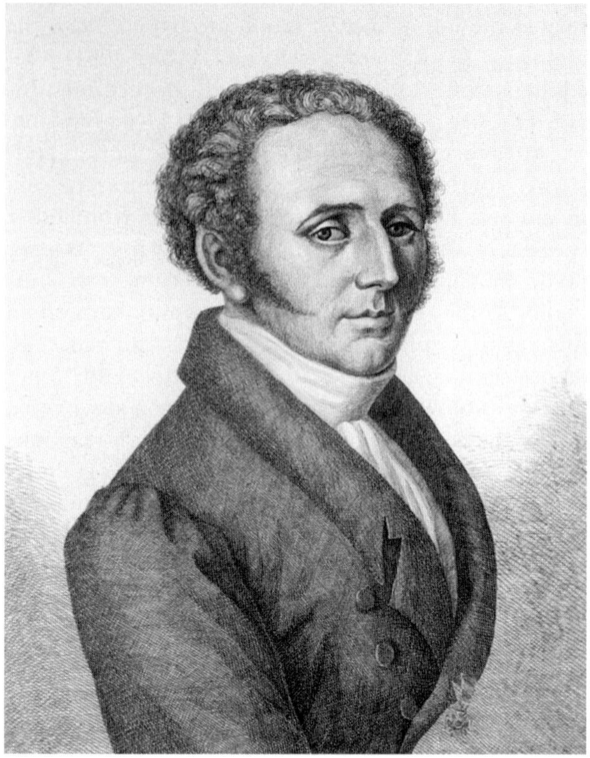

Conrad Johann Martin Langenbeck

Selected Publications

Langenbeck CJM. Geschichte einer von mir glücklich verichteten extirpation der ganger gebärmutter. *Bibioth Chir Ophth Hanover* 1817; 1: 557.

Bibliography References

97, 125, 204, 526, 597, 648, 1001, 1291, 1292, 1370, 1538, 1539.

Langer, Carl Ritter von Edenburg (1819–1887)

Langer's Lines

The natural cleavage lines of the skin are dictated by the orientation of the subcutaneous connective tissue and were first described in detail by Carl Langer in 1862. He was led to this observation when, using a sharp awl, he punched circular holes in the skin of cadavers and they became elliptical. These are known to all surgeons as the ideal line of incision to provide optimum skin healing.

Carl Langer was born in Vienna. He studied in Prague under Joseph Hyrtl (1810–1894). He became professor of zoology in Budapest in 1851. In 1856 he was appointed professor of anatomy at the Joseph's Academy for Military Medicine, and in 1870 he assumed the same position at the University of Vienna. He also served as dean of the faculty from 1871 to 1874 and as chancellor from 1875 to 1876.

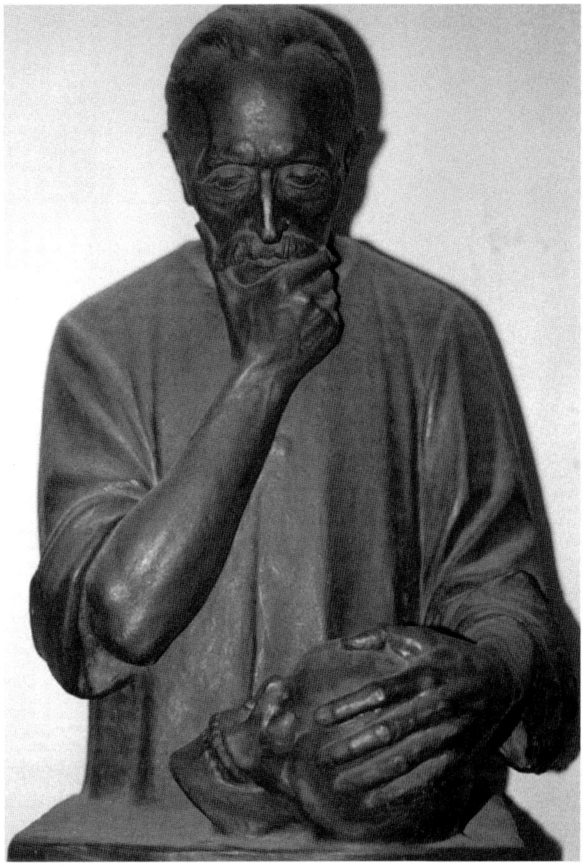

Carl Ritter von Edenberg Langer

Selected Publications

Langer K. Zur anatomie und physiologie der haut: über die spaltbarkeit der cutis. *Sber Akad Wiss Wien* 1862; 44: 19–46.

Bibliography References

495, 552, 968.

Langhans, Theodor (1839–1915)

Langhans' Layer (Cytotrophoblast)

It was Theodor Langhans who first differentiated the two types of epithelium covering the chorionic villi: the syncytiotrophoblast, or syncytium, and the cytotrophoblast, or Langhans' layer.

Theodor Langhans was born in Usingen, Germany. He took his medical training in the universities of Berlin, Göttingen and Heidelberg. His teachers included Rudolph Virchow (1821–1902) and Jakob Henle (1809–1885). He carried out his studies on the placenta in the pathological institute in Marburg and also described the giant cell in tuberculosis, known as Langhans' giant cell. In 1872 he was

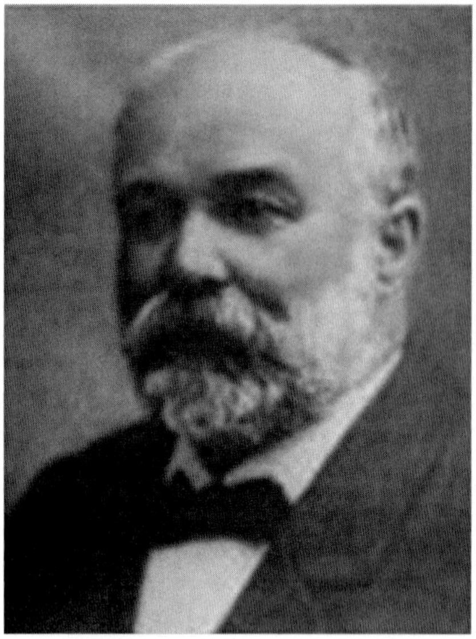

Theodor Langhans

appointed professor of pathological anatomy in Bern, which position he held with distinction for 40 years. In 1887, one of his students, Raissa Nitabuch, described the eosinophilic, fibrinoid deposition between the trophoblast and decidua: Nitabuch's layer.

Selected Publications

Langhans T. Untersuchungen über die menschlichen Placenta. *Arch Anat Physiol, Anat Abth* 1877: 188–267.

Nitabuch R. *Beiträge zur Kenntnis der menschlichen Placenta.* Berne; 1887.

Bibliography References

406, 872, 968, 1480.

Latzko, Wilhelm (1863–1945)

Latzko Repair of Vesicovaginal Fistula/Latzko's Sign

In 1914 Wilhelm Latzko described a technique for the vaginal closure of vesicovaginal fistula following hysterectomy. With modification, it remains in use today, having the twin advantages of simplicity and a high rate of success. Latzko's procedure was itself a modification of that proposed by Gustav Simon (1824–1876) of Germany in 1856, although it was developed for obstetric fistulae. Using the vaginal approach, Latzko dissected off the vaginal skin surrounding the fistula. He did not excise the fistulous tract but carefully prepared a bladder-vaginal base of tissue, which he closed over the fistula with successive inverted layers of sutures. In so doing, the upper 2–3 cm of vagina is obliterated over the fistula. He described the technique as follows:

Owing to the anatomy of the parts, the upper or posterior edge of the fistula always coincides with the transverse firm scar in the vault of the vagina. A circular area of vaginal mucosa is denuded from both the anterior and posterior vaginal walls for a distance of 1½ cm. from the fistula opening, thus removing all vaginal mucosa up to the opening of the fistula.

No vaginal mucous membrane is allowed to remain between the edges of the incision and the fistulous opening.

Sagittal sutures are now placed from above downward to co-apt the raw surfaces on either side of the fistulous opening . . . The posterior portion of the fistula is now closed. The remaining segment disappears after tying the second row of sagittally placed sutures. Closure of the anterior and posterior margins of the vaginal wound terminates the operation.

In 1942 he reported a series of 31 cases with 29 successful closures, most of which followed radical hysterectomy for cervical cancer.

Wilhelm Latzko was born in Vienna and graduated in medicine from the University of Vienna in

1886. He undertook postgraduate training there in both surgery and obstetrics and gynaecology. He became director of gynaecology at the Wiedener Krankenhaus and professor of obstetrics and gynaecology at the University of Vienna. Family commitments also occupied his time, and he served as temporary editor of a weekly newspaper and manager of a light bulb factory, both family-owned businesses.

In 1939, Nazi domination caused his emigration to Buenos Aires, with a subsequent move to New York. There he acted as a consultant to the Margaret Hague Hospital in Jersey City and the New York Beth Israel Hospital. He died in the latter hospital of cirrhosis and cancer of the liver.

Latzko's main contribution to obstetrics was the development of a technique for extraperitoneal caesarean section to reduce the risk of postoperative peritonitis. The very rare presentation of cancer of the fallopian tube with a palpable adnexal mass and a watery vaginal discharge, *hydrops tubae profluens*, is sometimes known as Latzko's sign.

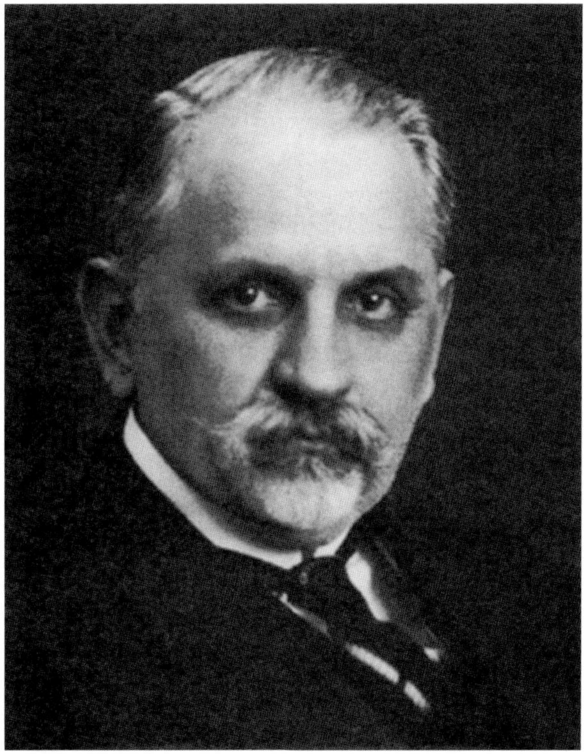

Wilhelm Latzko

Selected Publications

Latzko W. Über den extraperitoneal Kaiserschnitt. *Zentrabl Gynäkol* 1909; 33: 275–82.

Latzko W. Behandlung Hochsitzender blasen und Mastdarmscheidenfisteln nach Uterusextipatian mit hohem Schedienverschluss. *Zentralbl Gynäkol* 1914; 38: 906.

Latzko W. Postoperative vesicovaginal fistulas: genesis and therapy. *Am J Surg* 1942; 58: 211–28.

Bibliography References

536, 648, 801, 876, 1205, 1480.

Lazard, Edmond Meyer (1876–1969)

Magnesium Sulphate for Eclampsia

For centuries, eclamptic convulsions have represented one of the greatest threats to both mother and infant. William Hunter said that only two emergencies ever scared him: acute haemorrhage and puerperal convulsions. In the early part of the twentieth century, the treatment had not changed a great deal in 200 years. The condition that preceded eclamptic convulsions was known as toxaemia and was felt to be due to the retention of unknown toxins. Treatment was therefore directed at eliminating such toxins by 'bleeding and purging'. This was achieved by phlebotomy, usually removing about 500 ml of blood, and by the administration of purgatives such as croton oil or castor oil, augmented by stomach and colonic lavage with glucose and soda.

On 14 October 1924, Edmond Lazard, the senior attending obstetrician at Los Angeles General Hospital, read a paper before the Los Angeles Obstetric Society: *A Preliminary Report on the Intravenous Use of Magnesium Sulphate in Puerperal Eclampsia*, subsequently published in the *American Journal of Obstetrics and Gynecology*. He reported the use of intravenous magnesium sulphate to control eclamptic convulsions in 17 women:

> *Our experience in the few cases here reported has been so uniformly successful, that we feel it is worthy of further and more extensive trial and we are making this preliminary report in the hope that more extensive experience may bear out our impression that in the intravenous administration of magnesium sulphate, we have at our disposal a means not only of controlling the convulsions of eclampsia, but an efficient treatment of the toxemia itself . . . The treatment as developed at the Los Angeles General Hospital, consists of the intravenous administration of 20 c.c. of a 10 percent solution of magnesium sulphate as soon after the first observed convulsions as possible. Eliminative measures, such as phlebotomy, stomach lavage, administration of castor oil, colonic flushings with glucose and soda are carried out as in the treatment of any toxemic conditions. We are coming to feel more and more strongly, however, that the best results can be obtained by the least handling of the patient, consistent with obtaining the desired results . . . Our previous mortality in this class of severe eclamptics has been about thirty percent while in this series it was 5.8 percent . . . From our experience, I am disposed to try the intravenous use of magnesium sulphates in cases of pre-eclamptic toxemia which do not improve under the usual treatment in the hope that the toxemia can be controlled and the pregnancy carried to spontaneous labour without the supravention of an eclamptic attack.*

Lazard acknowledged that it was one of his interns, a Dr Emil Bogen, who had suggested the use of intravenous magnesium sulphate to control eclamptic convulsions in May 1924. Nine years later Lazard published his experience with 575 cases, of which 225 were eclamptic and 350 severe pre-eclamptic.

Lazard's treatment was almost uniformly accepted in the United States and became the standard initial treatment for severe pre-eclampsia and eclampsia. It was not used to the same extent outside the United States, where a variety of anticonvulsant and hypotensive treatments were used. It was not until 70 years after Lazard's initial report that the Eclampsia Trial Collaborative Group demonstrated that magnesium sulphate was associated with a lower risk of recurrent convulsions and maternal mortality when compared with the other standard anticonvulsants.

Edmond Lazard was born on 20 March 1876. He graduated MD from the University of Southern California. He became an obstetrician and gynaecologist and practised at the Los Angeles General Hospital, later the Los Angeles County Hospital. In his era Lazard was one of the most extensively trained obstetricians and gynaecologists in the Los Angeles district. He did a one-year internship in Kings County Hospital, Los Angeles and then spent three years training in various clinics and hospitals in Dresden (with Christian Leopold), Munich, Vienna and Paris. He was a founding member of the Los Angeles Obstetrical and Gynecological Society and served as its second president from 1915 to 1916. In 1939 he was elected president of the California Medical Association.

Lazard was youthful in appearance and apparently grew a moustache and small beard to appear more mature to his patients. One of his former students described him as follows: 'My initial impression was a dapper physician dressed in formal tailored clothes with gold rimmed glasses and steel grey moustache and goatee. He was always courteous, kind and helpful, never too busy for a word of instruction or encouragement to his students or staff. I never heard him utter a cross word nor witnessed him do an unkind deed'. Edmond Lazard died on 30 October 1969.

Selected Publications

Eclampsia Trial Collaborative Group: Which anticonvulsant for women with eclampsia? Evidence from the Collaborative Eclampsia Trial. *Lancet* 1995; 345: 1455–63.

Lazard EM. A preliminary report on the intravenous use of magnesium sulphate in puerperal eclampsia. *Am J Obstet Gynecol* 1925; 9: 178–88.

Lazard EM. An analysis of 575 cases of eclamptic and pre-eclamptic toxemias treated by intravenous injections of magnesium sulphate. *Am J Obstet Gynecol* 1933; 26: 647–56.

Bibliography References

268, 395, 791, 995, 1485.

Lee, Robert (1793–1877) Frankenhauser, Ferdinand (1832–1894)

Lee–Frankenhauser Plexus

It was not until 17 June 1841, when Robert Lee presented his findings to the Royal Society of London, that an adequate description of uterine innervation was forthcoming. Lee made his initial discovery on 8 April 1838 while dissecting a gravid uterus of seven months' gestation:

> *The uterus and its appendages are wholly supplied with nerves from the great sympathetic and sacral nerves. At the bifurcation of the aorta, the right and left cords of the great sympathetic nerve unite upon the anterior part of the aorta, and form the aortic plexus. This plexus divides into the right and left hypogastric nerves, which soon subdivide into a number of branches to form the right and left hypogastric plexus. Each of these plexuses, having the trunk of the hypogastric nerve continued through its centre, after giving off branches to the ureter, peritoneum, rectum, and trunks of the uterine blood-vessels, descends to the side of the cervix, and there terminates in a great ganglion, which, from its situation and relations, may be called the hypogastric ganglion, or utero-cervical ganglion.*

Ferdinand Frankenhauser published a more detailed description of the nervous plexus and ganglia 20 years later. Both men therefore provided the eponymous legacy, the Lee–Frankenhauser plexus.

Robert Lee was born in Melrose, Scotland and received his medical degree from Edinburgh University in 1814. He undertook further studies in Paris and London. In 1834 he briefly held the Regius chair of midwifery at the University of Glasgow. However, not being a Glasgow man, he was made to feel so unwelcome that he resigned within a few weeks of his appointment. In his letter of resignation he wrote, 'I feel the deepest regret that I should have given your Lordship so much trouble about an office, which I am certain no individual, however distinguished his rank in the profession may be, will hold with comfort who has not been a resident in Glasgow'.

Lee then returned to London and worked for the next 30 years at St George's Hospital. He spent seven years dissecting the nerves and ganglia of the uterus. A disgruntled former student of Lee's attempted to diminish his discovery by destroying and misrepresenting some of his anatomical preparations. The subsequent scandal led to the resignation of the president of the Royal Society and vindication for Lee.

Ferdinand Frankenhauser's early life and medical training are obscure. He became professor of obstetrics and gynaecology at Zurich in 1872 and remained there until 1888. His later years were marred by depression.

Selected Publications

Frankenhauser F. *Die Nerven der Gebaermutter und ihre Endigung in den Glatten Muskelfasern.* Jena: F.Mauke; 1867.

Lee R. *On the ganglia and other nervous structures of the uterus. Philosophical Transactions.* London: Richard and John E Taylor; 1842.

Bibliography References

406, 434, 435, 648, 822, 883, 977, 1480.

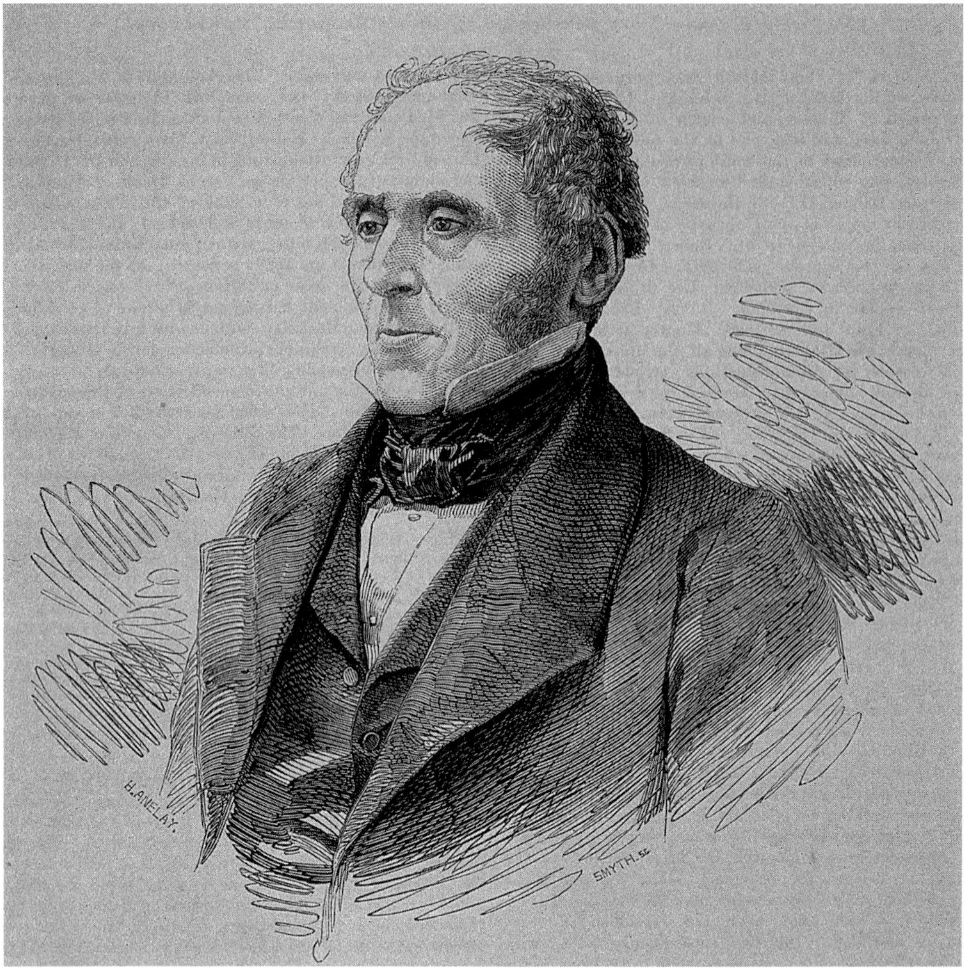

Robert Lee

Leeuwenhoek, Antonj van (1632–1723)

Microscopic Description of Spermatozoa

Antonj van Leeuwenhoek was born in Delft, Holland, the son of a basketmaker. At 16 years of age he was sent to Amsterdam to learn the trade of linen draper. He returned to Delft six years later and set up his own business. Despite this background, he became the most innovative and observant microscopist of his era. He was also a qualified surveyor and the official district wine-gauger. When not engaged in these tasks, he retired to his study, or closet, as he called it. There he perfected a technique, which he never divulged, for grinding and polishing his own lenses. With these he investigated everything and anything he could subject to microscopic scrutiny.

To some extent, Leeuwenhoek's limited education was an advantage. Unable to read Latin, he brought a fresh, unbiased mind to his work, unfettered by the prevailing unscientific biological literature. He was the first to describe 'animalcules' (bacteria and protozoa), red blood cells and striations on muscle fibres. He also gave the first description of animalcules, or spermatozoa, in semen. He believed that the spermatozoon represented the complete fetus, though admitted he could not substantiate this microscopically. In describing his findings, he used a grain of sand as the standard for size comparison. Leeuwenhoek's first description of spermatozoa was in 1677:

I have diverse times examined the same matter (human semen) from a healthy man . . . and I have seen so great a number of living creatures in it, that sometimes more than a thousand were moving about in an amount of material the size of a grain of sand. These animalcules were smaller than the corpuscles which impart a red colour to the blood; so that I judge a million of them not equal in size to a large grain of sand. Their bodies were rounded, but blunt in front and running to a point behind, and transparent, and with the thickness of about one twenty-fifth that of the body; so that I can best liken them in form to a small earth nut with a long tail. The animalcules moved forward with a snake-like motion of the tail, as eels do when swimming in water.

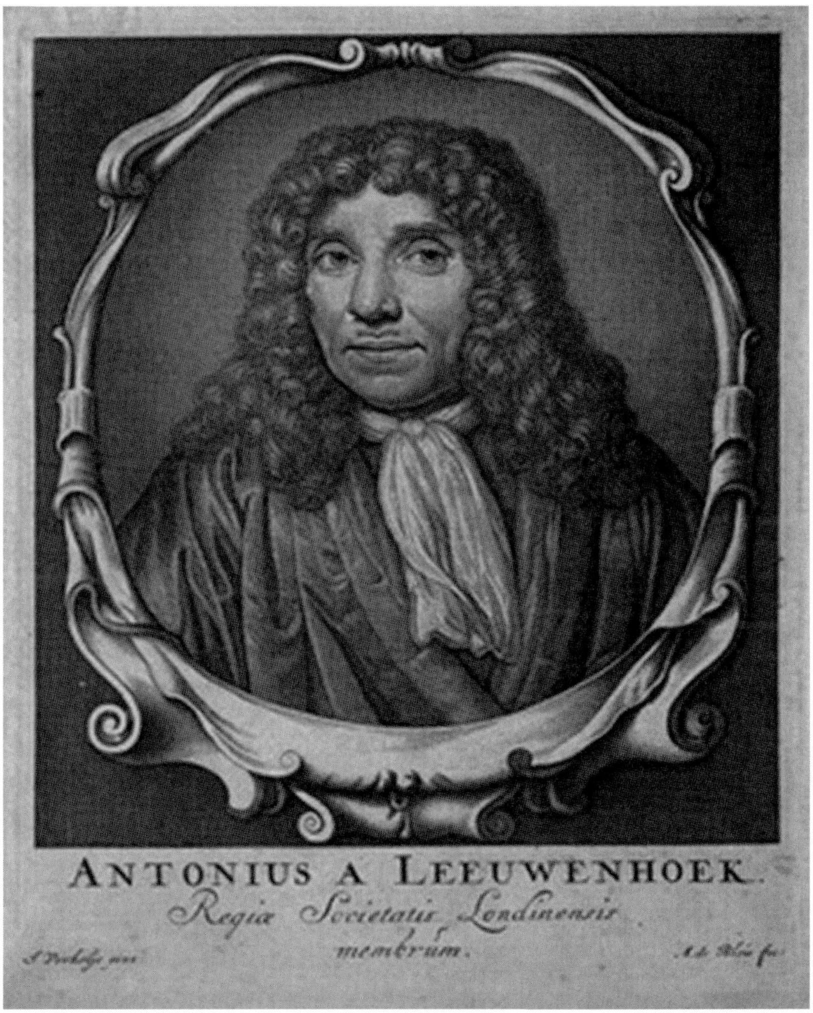

Antonj van Leeuwenhoek

Leeuwenhoek must also have been a very swift microscopist, as his standard for examining fresh semen was exacting: 'not liquified after the lapse of some minutes, but immediately after ejaculation, before six beats of the pulse had intervened'. He was also aware of potential criticism: 'What I describe here was not obtained by any sinful contrivance on my part, but the observations were made upon the excess with which nature provided me in my conjugal relations'.

His inquisitive enthusiasm extended to an attempt to observe the explosion of gunpowder under the microscope, which almost led to him becoming the world's first blind microscopist.

Leeuwenhoek was befriended by Regnier de Graaf, who brought his work to the attention of the Royal Society of London. It was well received, and Leeuwenhoek subsequently bombarded the society with his observations. In all, he wrote 308 letters to the Society detailing his observations, most of which were published. In 1680 he was elected a fellow of the Royal Society, a signal honour for one without scientific background or academic appointment. When he died, Leeuwenhoek bequeathed 26 of his microscopes to the Royal Society in London. One of these was found to have a magnifying power of 160, while another in his personal collection a power of 270. Unfortunately, most of these were lost in a fire at the residence of one of the society's members. Of his critics he wrote:

> *I am well aware that these, my writings, will not be accepted by some . . . but such things don't worry me; I know I'm in the right.*

To a large extent he was secure in this statement. To other than his critics he was sometimes known as the 'Delphic oracle'.

Selected Publications

Leeuwenhoek A. *Opera omnia seu arcana naturae.* Leyden; 1792.

Bibliography References

55, 180–182, 250, 404, 570, 744, 833, 1165, 1230, 1296, 1309, 1516, 1550, 1671.

Le Fort, Léon Clément (1829–1893)

Le Fort Operation

During the nineteenth century, even with the advent of anaesthesia, extensive surgical procedures were still attended by considerable morbidity and mortality. Surgical attempts to relieve marked uterine prolapse focused on partial occlusion of the lower vagina to block descent of the uterus. Otto von Spiegelberg and Alfred Hegar, among others, devised operations based on this principle. In 1877 Léon Le Fort described his own procedure of partial colpocleisis, which was so simple and safe that it continues to find limited application in the elderly and high-risk patient. In appraising the available operations in 1876 Le Fort wrote:

> *Procedures less dangerous and easily performed but ineffective, or else effective but hard to perform . . . carrying dangers for the patient, such were the alternatives offered me by surgery when, on November 10, 1876, there consulted me at the Beaujon Hospital a woman of 49 years, a laundress by trade, suffering from complete prolapse of the uterus . . . The patient asked to be relieved of her infirmity and preferred any kind of operation to the need of wearing a bandage.*

As he assessed the potential for simple surgical correction of uterine prolapse he proposed:

> *Evidently, if one could keep the vaginal walls in contact with each other, thus preventing one of them from going forward and the other backward, he could prevent prolapse completely. This is what I sought to do, striving to make the contact intimate and permanent and to restore the anterior and posterior vaginal walls to the same level in reuniting them by suture.*

Léon Clément Le Fort was born in Lille, France. Initially he entered his father's clothing business but

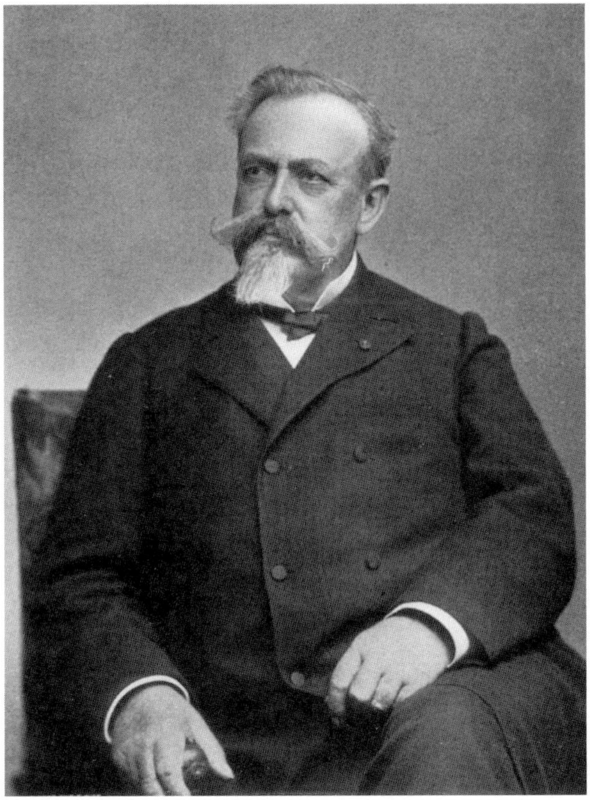

Léon Clément Le Fort

disliked this intensely and withdrew after one year. He was soon called up for military duty and served in the army's sanitary corps for two years during the Franco-Prussian War. Here he developed his feeling for medicine and enrolled as a student in Paris. His interests were legion, and he published significant work on the anatomy of the pulmonary circulation, puerperal sepsis, hysterectomy and chloroform anaesthesia. In 1873 he succeeded Charles Denonvilliers as professor of surgery in Paris as well as surgeon at the Hôtel Dieu. Le Fort was a committed civil libertarian and narrowly escaped arrest when he took part in a citizens' revolt while a medical student. In his senior years he spoke in defence of women accused of prostitution, saying, 'Pour protéger une femme qui peut être injustement accusée, je demande des juges'.

Selected Publications

Le Fort L. Nouveau procédeé pour la guérison du prolapsus utérin. *Bull Gén de Thérap* 1877; 92: 337–44.

Bibliography References

1086, 1473, 1480.

Lembert, Antoine (1802–1851)

Lembert Suture

Antoine Lembert, a Parisian surgeon, was not involved in obstetrics and gynaecology and his relevance to the specialty is oblique but vital. Perforce in gynaecology we may enter the bowel, usually inadvertently. If so, we can thank Lembert for devising the simple suture for its closure. This involves a single inverting suture, including all layers except the mucosa. When introduced, Lembert's technique became the standard method of bowel closure and anastomosis, revolutionising bowel surgery.

Lembert's senior colleague, Guillaume Dupuytren (1777–1835), devised a crushing clamp to approximate portions of bowel. He used this to aid closure of the artificial anus left as the result of a sloughed coil of herniated gangrenous bowel in a strangulated hernia. Lembert studied the intestinal walls at autopsy after this treatment. He found that the approximated peritoneal surfaces of the bowel formed an early watertight bond and reasoned that only these surfaces of divided bowel need be sutured together. He thus proposed the seromuscular suture excluding the mucosa. He outlined his rationale and its potential use:

> *A method which is based upon the property, which serous membranes possess of adhering together by means of inflammatory adhesions ... This method is equally applicable to all solutions of continuity of the intestine and even of the stomach, its technique will be the same though it may assume a different form.*

Ten years after Lembert's publication, Johan Friedrich Dieffenbach (1792–1847) of Berlin was the first to use and acknowledge Lembert's technique. The case was a 50-year-old man with a strangulated hernia in which 7 cm of gangrenous small bowel had to be resected. He described his method of reanastamosis:

> *Then I sutured the ends of the intestine by a special suture; the stitch was first inserted two lines from the free edge and always carried transversely across the gap so that the suture placed in the muscular layer brought together only the peritoneal surfaces in accordance with the teaching of Lembert. The mucosa was not sutured but its edges were inverted all the way round.*

Lembert was a modest man, and in his treatise gave excessive recognition to his teacher Dupuytren. The idea for the seromuscular suture was Lembert's alone. Antoine Lembert was born in Nancy on 10 April 1802. He studied and practised medicine and surgery in Paris, where he was also epidemiologist to the Seine Département. He died in Paris in 1851 from cancer of the stomach.

Selected Publications

Dieffenbach J. *Wochenschr des Heilkunde.* 1839, p. 401.

Lembert A. Mémoire sur l'entéroraphie avec la description d'un procédé nouveau pour pratique cette operation chirugicale. *Rep Gén Anat Physiol Path* 1826; 2: 100–7. English translation: Study on intestinal suture with a description of a new procedure for performing this surgical operation. *Dis Colon Rectum* 1988; 31: 489–94.

Bibliography References

149, 203, 309, 381, 647, 1030, 1659.

Leopold, Christian Gerhard (1846–1912)

Leopold's Manoeuvres

Towards the end of the nineteenth century, an understanding of the mechanism of spread of puerperal infection caused many obstetricians to turn from vaginal examination to abdominal palpation. One of the most ardent proponents of this change was Christian Gerhard Leopold. In 1890, with his colleague ME Pantzer, he published a paper stressing the dangers of vaginal examination and outlining a method of abdominal palpation to reduce the necessity for vaginal assessment. He described four 'manipulations' that came to be called Leopold's manoeuvres. Before the examination started he advised:

> *It is proper to cover the face of the person loosely with some light clean linen ... This is to be done especially when idle students stand about as spectators ... For the first three manoeuvres the examiner faces the patient. In the first the fundus is palpated with the tips of the fingers to ascertain the pole of the fetus. The second manoeuvre uses the flat of the hands and palms to determine the position of the fetal back and limbs. The thumb and middle finger of one hand grasps and identifies the presenting part just above the symphysis pubis as the third move. For the fourth manoeuvre the examiner faces the patients' feet, and, with the tips of the first three fingers of both hands, presses down beside the presenting part to determine the degree of engagement.*

The four manoeuvres still form the basis of obstetric abdominal palpation taught today.

Christian Gerhard Leopold was born in Meerane, Germany, the son of a doctor. He received his medical degree from the University of Leipzig in 1870 and immediately spent a year with the German Army in the Franco-Prussian War. He then toured medical centres in Vienna, London and Edinburgh. He returned in 1873 to be appointed assistant to Carl Credé. Later he married Credé's daughter, which did not hinder his career development. In 1883 he became chief of the Dresden Lying-in Hospital. He published

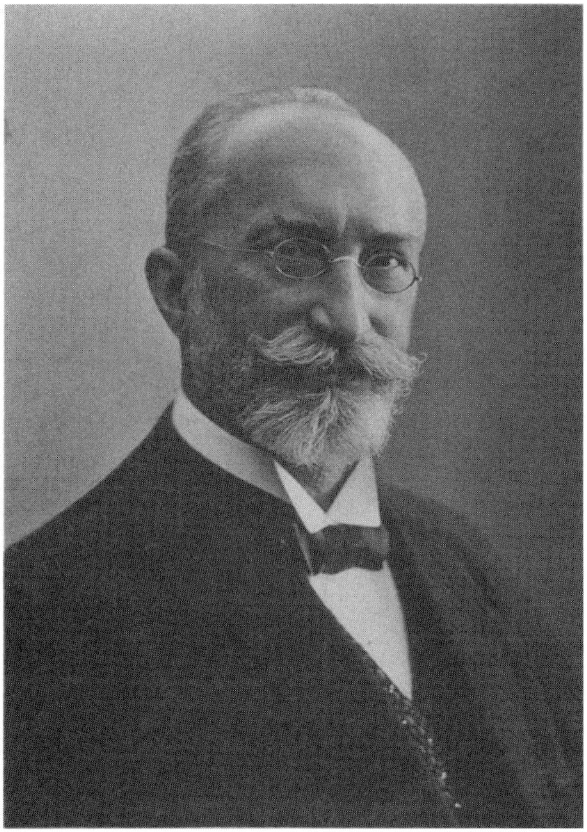

Christian Gerhard Leopold

extensively and co-authored a number of texts with Credé, ultimately succeeding him as editor of *Archiv für Gynäkologie* in 1892.

Selected Publications

Credé C, Leopold G. The obstetric examination. A short guide for physicians, students of medicine, midwives and students in midwifery. (English translation by JC Edgar.) *New York J Gynecol Obstet* 1892; 2: 1129–44.

Leopold G, Pantzer ME. Die Beschränkung der inneren und die grösstmögliche Verwerthung der äusseren Untersuchung in der Geburtshülfe. *Arch Gynäkol* 1890; 38: 330–66.

Bibliography References

548, 648, 892, 1408, 1480.

Lever, John Charles Weaver (1811–1859)

Proteinuria and Eclampsia

In his observation of 14 women with eclampsia, John Lever, lecturer in midwifery at Guy's Hospital, noted a similarity with patients suffering from chronic glomerulonephritis. This led him to 'examine the condition of her urine', and become the first to find albuminuria in an eclamptic women:

> *To settle this point, I have carefully examined the urine in every case of puerperal convulsions that has since come under my notice . . . and in every case, but one, the urine has been found to be albuminous at the time of the convulsions.*

The single case without albuminuria was found to have meningitis at post-mortem examination. Lever went on to clarify the association by testing the urine of 'upwards of fifty women' in labour:

> *. . . the result has been, that in no cases have I detected albumen, except in those in which there have been convulsions, or in which symptoms have presented themselves and which are readily recognised as the precursors of puerperal fits.*

James Young Simpson also made the connection between albuminuria and eclampsia about the same

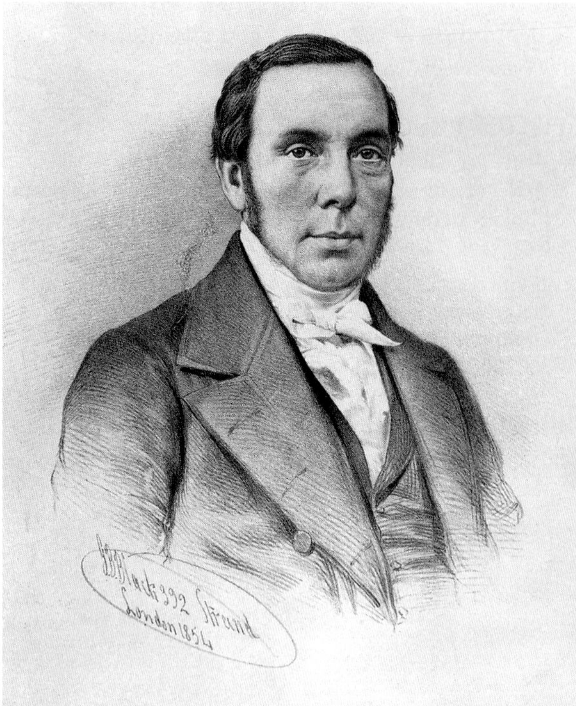

John Charles Weaver Lever

time, although his brief observation on one case was published one month after that of Lever.

John Charles Weaver Lever was born in Plumstead, England. After a medical apprenticeship in Woolwich he became a student at Guy's Hospital in 1832, qualifying two years later. While attending lectures, he walked to and from Woolwich each day, a distance of 20 miles. He developed a successful obstetric practice and in 1845 was appointed lecturer in midwifery at Guy's Hospital, where his lectures were described as 'clear and forcible'. His private practice became so extensive that his carriage, with its red wheels and borderings, was known in south London as 'Lever's fire engine'.

Selected Publications

Lever JCW. Cases of puerperal convulsions with remarks. *Guy's Hosp Rep London* 1843; 2: 495–517.

Simpson JY. Contributions to the pathology and treatment of diseases of the uterus. *Lond Edin Mon J Med Sci* 1843; 3: 547.

Bibliography References

347, 648, 898, 937, 1261.

Levret, André (1703 –1780)

Obstetric Forceps

André Levret followed François Mauriceau as one of the most influential French obstetricians of the eighteenth century. His careful study of the pelvis led him to devise forceps with a pelvic curve. He presented these at a meeting of the Academy of Sciences in Paris in 1747 and used them for the first time the following year. It seems likely that Levret and William Smellie independently conceived and designed the pelvic curve. Indeed, in many ways Levret, with his clear understanding and innovation, was the French counterpart of Smellie. In contrast to standard teaching, Levret advocated earlier caesarean section in selected cases of absolute dystocia. He made pertinent observations on the diagnosis and management of placenta praevia and was the first to introduce the term *accouchement forcé* for forcible dilatation of the cervix in such cases.

André Levret was born and educated in Paris. With a private income from a wealthy patron, he moved in the higher levels of Parisian society. He was also an accomplished surgeon, invented many instruments and was elected to membership of the Royal Academy of Surgery in Paris. His confidence and humour are shown in his response when summoned to attend the labour of the Dauphiness, mother of the future Louis XVI. Reputedly, a lady-in-waiting said to him, 'You must be pleased, Monsieur Levret, to deliver the Dauphine. That will make your reputation'. To which he replied, 'If my reputation were not already made, I should not be here'.

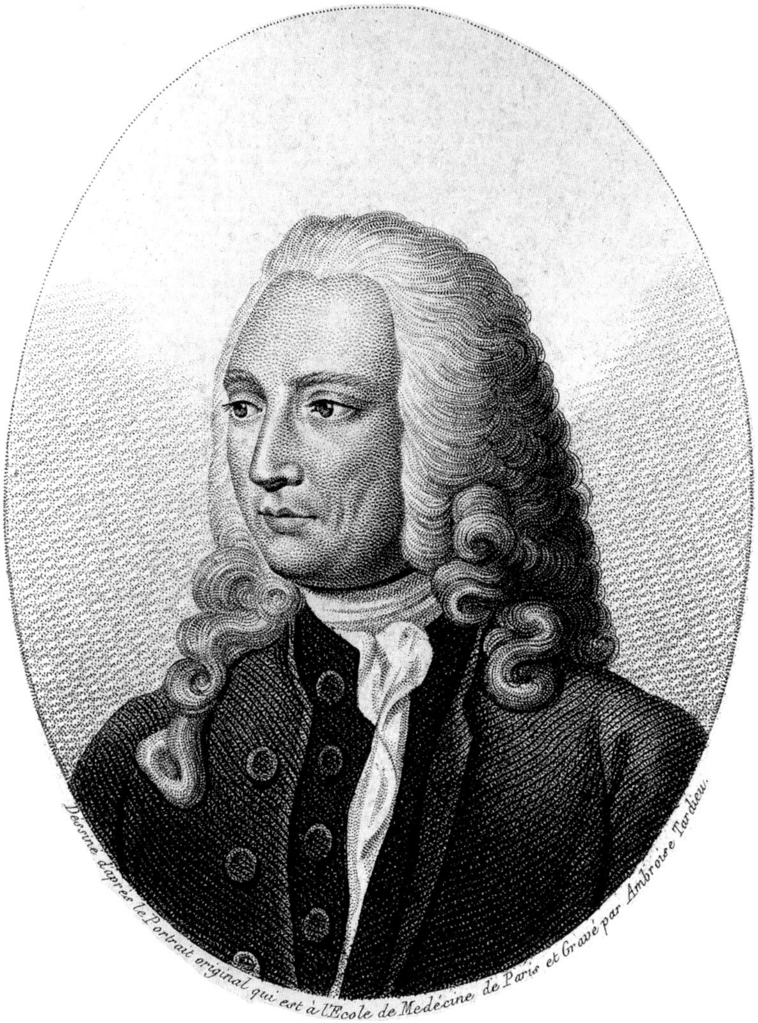
Dessiné d'après le Portrait original qui est à l'Ecole de Medécine de Paris et Gravé par Ambroise Tardieu.

André Levret

Selected Publications

Levret A. *Observations sur les causes et les accidens de plusieurs accouchemens laboreux*. Paris: Osmont; 1747.

Levret A. *L'Art des accouchements*. Paris: Le Prieur; 1761.

Bibliography References

44, 99, 298, 399, 423, 427, 451, 609, 676, 718, 721, 746, 899, 983, 1420, 1516, 1575, 1595, 1712, 1728.

Liggins, Graham Collingwood (1926–2010)

Antenatal Corticosteroids and Neonatal Respiratory Distress

Few Antarctic seals have had a home visit from an obstetrician during pregnancy, let alone from a future knight of the realm; an extreme example, perhaps, of community-centred maternity care. Such was the case in the 1980s when Graham Liggins, as part of a study of fetal adaptation to hypoxia in diving seals, had to perform bimanual examinations to confirm pregnancy in the Weddell seals under scrutiny. Most of his basic research, however, was carried out on the more accessible sheep in New Zealand.

It was in the late 1960s, during research into the initiation of labour in sheep, when Liggins noted that lambs delivered prematurely lived longer if they had been exposed antenatally to corticosteroids. Thus, with his paediatrician colleague Ross Howie (1933–2017), he undertook a prospective randomised controlled trial comparing maternal administration of betamethasone to a weak glucocorticoid in threatened premature labour. This showed a significant reduction in neonatal respiratory distress in infants born at less than 32 weeks gestation and treated for more than 24 hours. Furthermore, the neonatal death rate was reduced from 14.1% to 3.2% in the control and treatment groups respectively:

> *The results of the trial support the hypothesis that in humans, as in experimental animals previously studied, glucocorticoid administration to the fetus accelerates lung maturation ...*
>
> *How the glucocorticoid acts remains to be determined. The apparent promptness of the effect, even in the most immature fetuses, may be in part due to release of surfactant already stored within the alveolar epithelium ...*
>
> *Our findings have implications for the pathogenesis of RDS [respiratory distress syndrome], suggesting that alveolar atelectasis is the result rather than the cause of surfactant deficiency, and that the deficiency is primary rather than secondary, at least in those cases occurring in infants of less than 32 weeks' gestation.*

This work was subsequently confirmed in several trials with a concomitantly noted reduction in the incidence of intraventricular haemorrhage and necrotising enterocolitis. The potential for reduction of intraventricular haemorrhage had been noted by Liggins and Howie:

> *Contrary to expectations, death from intraventricular cerebral haemorrhage in the most immature infants of the treated group did not occur whereas this disorder was found in four infants of the control group. The difference is not statistically significant but nevertheless raises the possibility that RDS predisposes to intraventricular haemorrhage and that prophylaxis of neonatal respiratory disorders may reduce the incidence of the intracranial disorder.*

The impact of this evidence-based treatment in clinical perinatology has been enormous. Liggins' main achievement in basic research was to demonstrate that in the sheep it is the fetus and not the mother that initiates parturition. Throughout the 1970s and 1980s he made many original contributions to the understanding of the endocrine role in physiological preparation for birth, fetal pulmonary development and growth, and the control of fetal respiratory movements.

Graham Collingwood Liggins was born in Thames, New Zealand. He took his medical degree at the University of Otago. After two years in general practice in Hamilton, New Zealand he spent six years in England doing obstetrics and gynaecology at Newcastle-upon-Tyne and Gateshead. He returned to New Zealand in 1960 to appointments as senior lecturer and associate professor of obstetrics and gynaecology at the University of Auckland. In 1971 he became professor of obstetrics and gynaecological endocrinology. During this time he was a senior research fellow of the New Zealand Medical Research Council in the postgraduate school at Auckland. In 1987 he became emeritus professor and honorary senior research fellow, as well as director of the Research Centre in Reproductive Medicine. Liggins' consistent and considerable achievements have received widespread recognition, including a knighthood in 1991. The Liggins Institute at the University of Auckland is named after him. He died on 24 August 2010.

Sir Graham Liggins was always known to his friends and associates as 'Mont' Liggins. The origin of Mont apparently goes back to the days of his childhood and his fondness for a comic strip character called Monty the Mouse.

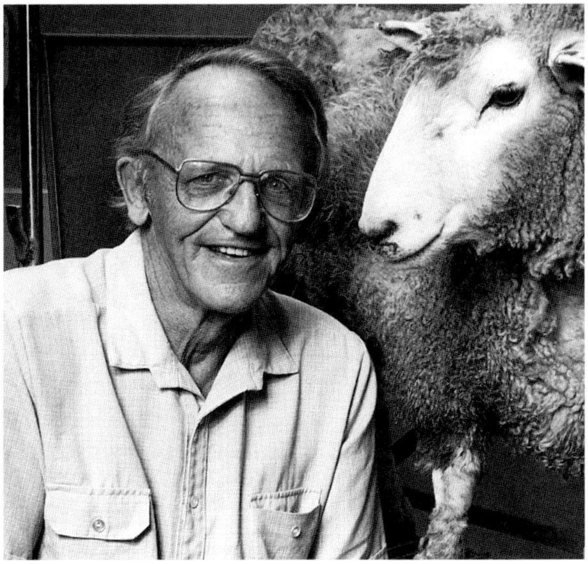

Graham Collingwood Liggins

Selected Publications

Liggins GC. Premature delivery of foetal lambs infused with glucocorticoids. *J Endocrinol* 1969; 45: 515–23.

Liggins GC, Howie RN. A controlled trial of antepartum gluocorticoid treatment for prevention of the respiratory distress syndrome in premature infants. *Pediatrics* 1972; 50: 515–25.

Bibliography References

369, 528, 1215.

Liley, Albert William (1929–1983)

Intrauterine Fetal Transfusion/Liley's Zones

Following the initial work of Douglas Bevis showing the relationship between elevated amniotic fluid bilirubin levels and haemolytic disease of the newborn, Liley systematically studied amniotic fluid in rhesus-immunised pregnancies. Using the spectrophotometer to measure bilirubin levels by optical density readings, he studied 101 immunised pregnancies with serial amniocentesis and developed a graph that allowed interpretation into three prognostic zones, 'Liley's zones'. Based on this graph Liley predicted when the fetus might die in utero before 32–34 weeks gestation, the earliest at which it was then realistic to consider early delivery and neonatal exchange transfusion with a reasonable chance of survival.

In 1963, Liley reported the first successful case of intrauterine fetal transfusion. The patient had two previous stillbirths due to rhesus immunisation, and the amniotic fluid suggested a severely affected fetus in this pregnancy. After discussion with a visiting doctor from Africa, who told him about the simple technique of intraperitoneal blood transfusion for children with severe sickle cell anaemia, Liley decided that the intraperitoneal route would be feasible in the fetus. As he reported:

> *It is apparent that timely discovery and selection of these cases is critical, and only amniotic-fluid analysis can provide the necessary precision . . . The aim of the exercise is simply to arrest deterioration if possible and gain a few extra weeks of gestation so that the skilled paediatric care of severe haemolytic disease is not nullified by gross prematurity.*

After two transfusions using a sixteen-gauge Tuohy needle to gain access and place an epidural catheter in the fetal peritoneal cavity, a normal male infant was delivered by caesarean section. In his report Liley tells of three previous cases of unsuccessful fetal transfusions, all involving hydropic fetuses.

Shortly after this publication, other centres took up the technique. With the development of ultrasound, the procedure has been refined and modified, so that the route of transfusion is now directly intravascular via the umbilical blood vessels.

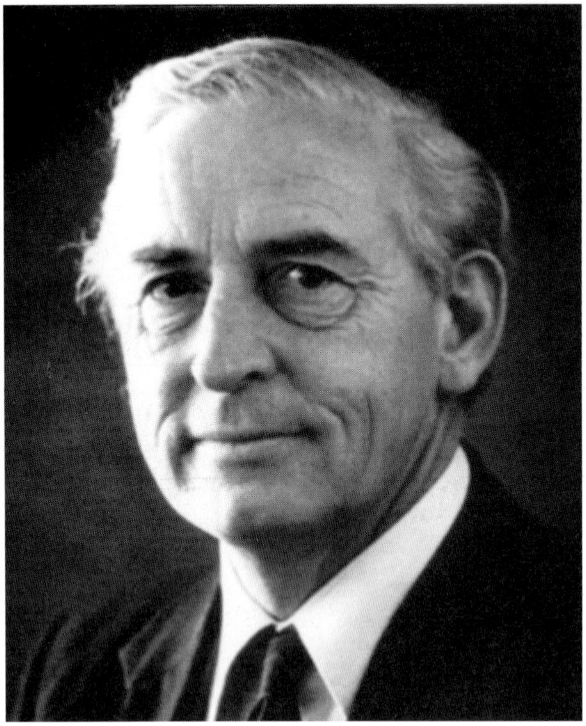

Albert William Liley

Albert William Liley was born in Auckland, New Zealand and received his early education there. He graduated in medicine from the University of Otago in 1954. He received his PhD from the Australian National University in 1957. Liley devoted his professional career to the study of maternal and fetal physiology and, in 1968, was granted a personal chair in perinatal physiology at the Postgraduate School of Obstetrics and Gynaecology of Auckland University. Following his epic work on fetal transfusion Liley was honoured by election, fellow ad eundem, to the Royal College of Obstetricians and Gynaecologists. In 1973 he was knighted by the Queen for services to medicine.

Bill Liley became interested in forestry and had an 80-hectare forest 250 km south of Auckland, where he became a knowledgeable student of silviculture. One of his sons became prominent in this field. Liley had a profound regard for the sanctity of life and in 1970 became a co-founder and president of the Society for the Protection of the Unborn Child. He and his wife had five children and also adopted a two-year-old girl with Down's syndrome.

On June 15 1983, while deeply depressed, Sir William Liley took his own life; he was 54. Liley's breakthrough paved the way for fetal treatment and has led to the normal survival of thousands of otherwise doomed infants. Few men have such an epitaph.

Selected Publications

Liley AW. Liquor amnii analysis in management of pregnancy complicated by rhesus sensitisation. *Am J Obstet Gynecol* 1961; 82: 1359.

Liley AW. Intrauterine transfusion of foetus in haemolytic disease. *BMJ* 1963; 2: 1107–9.

Bibliography References

8, 170, 175, 388, 389, 572, 654, 655, 702, 904, 905, 1690, 1741, 1744, 1748.

Lippes, Jack (b. 1924)

Lippes' Loop

The earliest, serviceable intrauterine contraceptive device (IUCD) was the flexible ring of Ernst Gräfenberg. In the 1950s, Jack Lippes of Buffalo, New York began using the contraceptive ring developed in the 1930s by the Japanese physician, Tenrei Ota (1900–1985). He found removal difficult and added a thread to the device to overcome this problem. This was against the teaching of Gräfenberg, who felt this would increase the risk of infection. Lippes decided to change the design of the device so it would conform to the shape of the uterine cavity and not rotate, pulling the thread up into the uterus:

> *My attention was focused on how to prevent rotation of the IUD with disappearance of the useful removal thread. A departure from the geometry of the ring was essential. Perhaps, if the IUD closely fitted the contours of the uterine cavity, rotation might be prevented or at least minimized.*

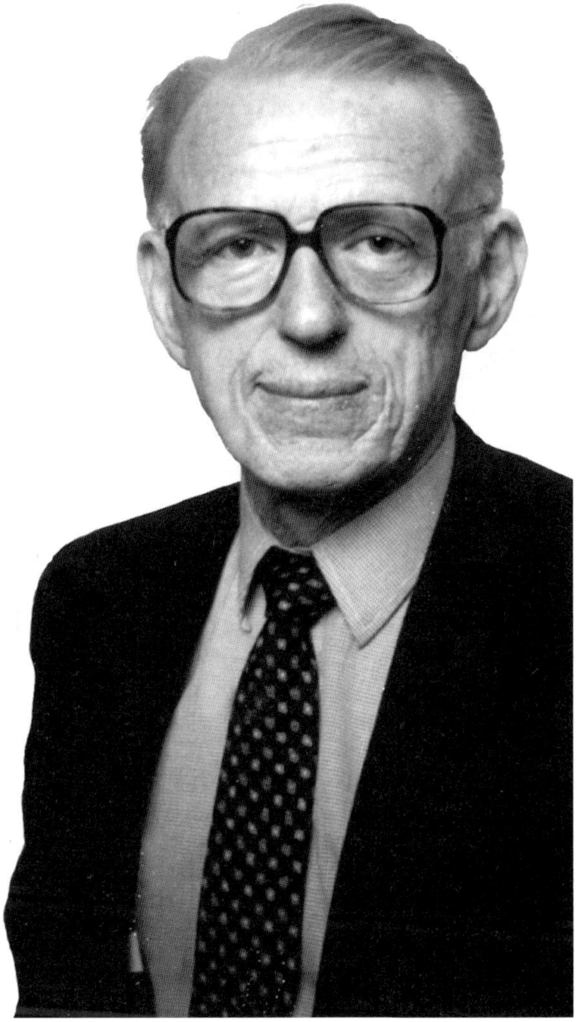

Jack Lippes

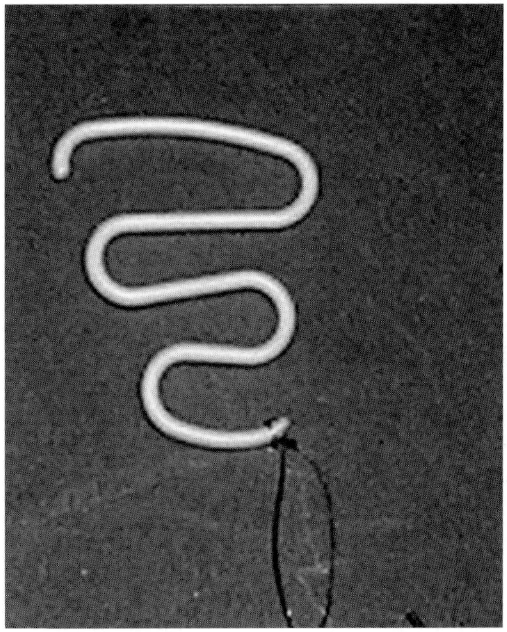

Lippes' loop

He settled on the now familiar double-S shape of the Lippes' loop. With the advent of thermoplastics with 'memory', the device could be straightened to fit into an insertion tube, pushed into the uterine cavity and regain its original shape. He produced his first loop in 1959. It was Lazar Margulies who devised the insertion tube for use with his own IUCD, the Margulies spiral.

Lippes utilised data from Robert Dickinson on measurements of the uterine cavity to produce four different sized loops: A, B, C and D. In a study comparing the smallest loop A with the largest loop D, he found an overall pregnancy rate of 2.2 per hundred women years, 4.8 for the smaller and 1.0 for the larger. As a result, loop D was recommended for parous women and loop A only for the nulliparous. Lippes carried out this work in his private practice and at the Buffalo Planned Parenthood Centre.

In addition to the Ota ring and Margulies spiral, several other eponymous devices were developed – the Zipper ring (Jaime Zipper), the Birnberg bow (Charles Birnberg) and the Majzlin spring (Gregory Majzlin) – as well as the Saf-T-Coil devised by Ralph Robinson.

Jack Lippes was born in Buffalo, New York and received his MD from the State University of New York at Buffalo in 1947. He did his residency in obstetrics and gynaecology at the University of Nebraska Hospital in Omaha. In 1952 he rejoined the faculty of his alma mater in Buffalo, rising to the rank of professor. He was chief of the department of obstetrics and gynaecology at the Deaconess Hospital of Buffalo from 1975 to 1981. He was also involved at the other end of the fertility spectrum and helped establish the first in vitro fertilisation clinic in Buffalo in 1981. He has acted as consultant in family planning to a number of government agencies.

Selected Publications

Lippes J. A study of intra-uterine contraception: development of a plastic loop. In Tietze C, Lewit S (eds) *Proceedings Conference Population Council: Intra-uterine contraceptive devices.* Amsterdam: Excerpta Medica Foundation; 1962: 69–75.

Lippes J. Contraception with intrauterine plastic loops. *Am J Obstet Gynecol* 1965; 93: 1024–30.

Ota T. A study on birth control with an intrauterine instrument. *Jap J Obstet Gynecol* 1934; 17: 210.

Bibliography References

368, 504, 909, 1599, 1600, 1614.

Little, William John (1810–1894)

Little's Disease (Cerebral Palsy)

In the early part of the nineteenth century, cases of cerebral palsy were often attributed to febrile convulsions. In part this was because the clinical manifestations of cerebral palsy may not be apparent until later childhood. William Little first drew attention to the condition in his series of lectures on the *Deformities of the Human Frame*, published in the *Lancet* in 1843. In 1853 he produced a book based on these lectures, which also included a case report describing muscular dystrophy almost 10 years before Guillaume Duchenne. In his first lecture on the subject, Little implied an association among cerebral palsy, prematurity and difficult birth. After 20 years of further reflection and study of these cases, he clearly implicated prematurity, trauma and asphyxia at birth. He presented these revolutionary findings to general disbelief before the Obstetrical Society of London on 2 October 1861. Up to this time it was felt that asphyxia at birth either led to death or survival with complete recovery. Little declared:

> *... abnormal parturition, besides ending in death or recovery, not infrequently had a third termination in other diseases ... a delay of only a few moments in the substitution of pulmonary for the ceased placental respiration would lead to the apprehension that even the want of a few breathings, if not fatal to the economy, may imprint a lasting injury upon it.*

It was only three years after Little's death that Sigmund Freud, a neurologist in his early career, made this observation in his treatise on cerebral palsy:

> *One has to consider that the anomaly of the birth process, rather than being the causal etiological factor, may itself be the consequence of the real prenatal etiology.*

This prescient comment is more in accord with the modern theory that the majority of cases of cerebral palsy are due to antepartum factors.

William John Little was born in the Red Lion Inn in the Aldgate district of London, where his father was the landlord. A sickly child, as a four-year-old he had infantile paralysis (poliomyelitis), which left him with a club foot (talipes equinovarus). He was sent to the country but was left with a permanent limp and nicknamed 'lame duck' at school. He initially attended school in Dover and then a Jesuit school in St Omer, where he became fluent in French. Little returned to London at the age of 16 and became an apothecary's apprentice. After two years he transferred to the London Hospital as a medical student, qualifying in 1831. In 1835 he went to Berlin to complete a two-year university course in order to quality for membership in the Royal College of Physicians. There he studied under Johannes Müller and was a fellow pupil of Jakob Henle and Theodor Schwann.

Little sought a cure for his own club foot and had the new procedure of subcutaneous tenotomy performed by the pioneer of this technique, Louis Stromyer of Hanover (1804–1876). He was delighted with the improvement in his own mobility and adopted and modified the technique, making it the subject of his MD thesis at Berlin. On returning to London, he founded the Hospital for the Cure of Deformities in 1838, later expanded and moved to Hanover Square to become the Royal Orthopaedic Hospital. His personal insight and compassion for those with deformities was revealed in these words from one of his lectures:

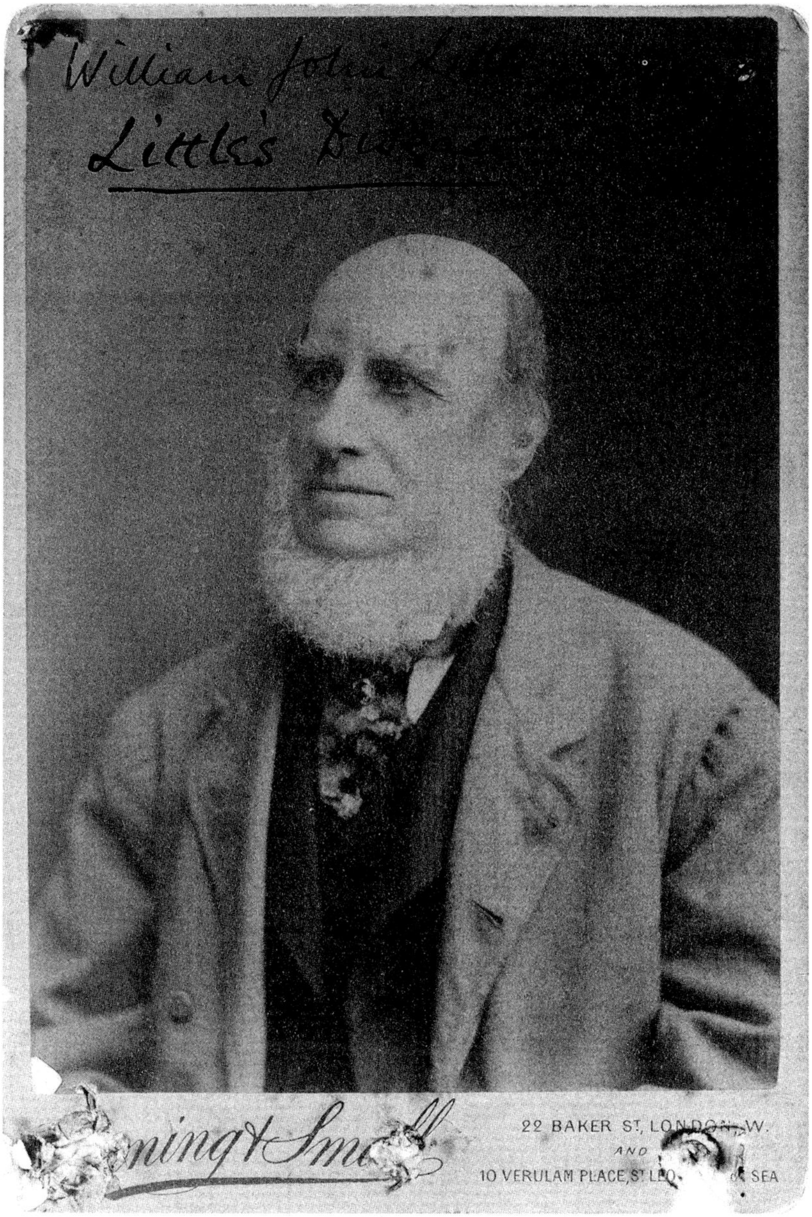

William John Little

Society is responsible for the humiliating position in which the deformed have been placed . . . The evils of deformities are not confined to verbally expressed anguish.

In the discussion following his lecture to the Obstetrical Society of London, Little postulated that the title character in Shakespeare's play *Richard III* was an example of 'one kind of deformity originating at birth'. He based this on Richard's words bemoaning his physical misfortune:

That I am curtailed of this fair proportion, cheated of feature by dissembling nature, deformed, unfinished, sent before my time into this breathing world, scarce half made up - and that so lamely and unfashionable that dogs bark at me as I halt by them.

Little became increasingly deaf, retired from practice in 1884, and moved to Kent. He suffered from an enlarged prostate, chronic cystitis and uraemia, dying at the age of 83. He had seven daughters and four sons. Two of his sons became physicians, one of whom was elected the first president of the British Orthopaedic Association.

Selected Publications

Freud S. *Die infantile Cerebrallähmung.* 1897. (English translation by LA Russin. Coral Gables, FL: University of Miami Press; 1968.)

Little WJ. Course of lectures on the deformities of the human frame. *Lancet* 1843; 1: 318–22.

Little WJ. *On the Nature and Treatment of the Deformities of the Human Frame.* London: Longman, Brown, Greene and Longmans; 1853.

Little WJ. On the influence of abnormal parturition, difficult labours, premature birth, and asphyxia neonatorum, on the mental and physical condition of the child, especially in relation to deformities. *Trans Obstet Soc London* 1861–62; 3: 293–344.

Bibliography References

6, 7, 233, 611, 913, 914, 928, 933, 968, 1101, 1162, 1353, 1721.

Litzmann, Carl Conrad Theodor (1815–1890)

Litzmann's Obliquity (Posterior Asynclitism)

A guiding principle in the dynamics and mechanics of labour is that things anterior are favourable and those posterior are abnormal, with the potential for dystocia. Franz Naegele had previously observed anterior asynclitism as a common occurrence during engagement of the fetal head in the pelvis. Litzmann described the opposite situation, wherein the posterior parietal bone presented at the pelvic inlet-posterior asynclitism. Others had observed this presentation before, but it was Litzmann who described it in detail and received the eponym, 'Litzmann's obliquity'. He observed that this presentation could be the case in labour with normal progression but noted that when it persisted there was an association with prolonged labour and dystocia, saying 'progress in labour is out of the question without a change in the position of the head'.

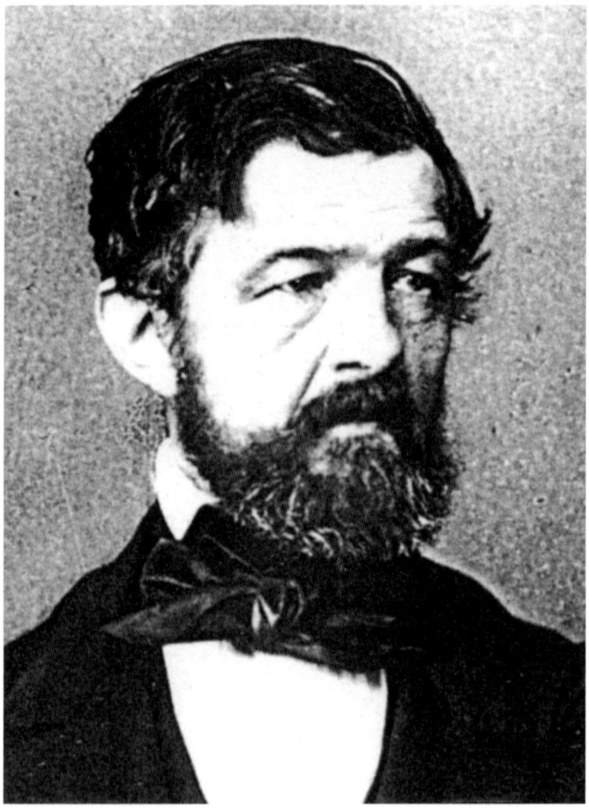

Carl Conrad Theodor Litzmann

Carl Conrad Theodor Litzmann was born in Gadebusch, Germany, the son of a physician. During Litzmann's early education his main focus was literature and poetry, an interest he retained all his life. His father encouraged him to study medicine, but he was reluctant until the death of two of his siblings from typhus stimulated him to enrol in the University of Berlin. Here he was taught by Johannes Müller. Litzmann finished his medical degree at the University of Halle. In 1848 he succeeded Gustav Michaelis and became professor of obstetrics, gynaecology and paediatrics at the University of Kiel, where he remained until he retired aged 70.

Selected Publications

Litzmann CCT. Über die hintere Scheitelbeinstellung, eine nicht seltene Art von fehlerhafter Einstellung des Kopfes unter der Geburt. *Arch Gynäkol* 1871; 2: 433–440.

Bibliography References

548, 553, 648, 1261, 1367, 1480, 1595.

Logothetopoulos, Konstantinos (1878–1961)

Pelvic Pressure Pack

In some cases following hysterectomy, there is persistent oozing from the tissues at the base of the pelvis, despite ligation of all obvious bleeding points. This is often associated with some degree of disseminated intravascular coagulation (DIC), especially after emergency obstetric hysterectomy. Packing is a time-honoured method of dealing with such bleeding until additional definitive steps can be taken, such as major vessel embolisation and transfusion to correct the DIC.

Almost a century ago, Konstantinos Logothetopoulos of Athens described a special type of pack that could provide tamponade over the wide area of the pelvic basin, combined with the ability to remove the pack without having to reopen the abdomen. In Logothetopoulos' original paper, the pack was made with a large piece of flat gauze filled with loose gauze. A mushroom-shaped pack was formed by bringing the four corners and edges of the flat piece of gauze together and pulling them down into a narrow neck that was placed through the open vaginal vault. Traction on the gauze neck from below causes compression and tamponade by the head of the mushroom pack against the oozing tissues of the pelvic basin. When the bleeding has been stopped, the gauze can be slowly withdrawn vaginally. In modern practice, a plastic bag filled with gauze is used to facilitate placement and withdrawal of the pack. This technique has been variously called the mushroom, parachute or umbrella pack, as well as the Logothetopoulos pack. It is now usually described as the pelvic pressure pack. It is effective and can be life-saving.

Konstantinos Logothetopoulos was born in Nafplio, Greece in 1878. He left for Munich in 1896 to study medicine and graduated MD from Munich University in 1903. There he took his postgraduate training in obstetrics and gynaecology and became a lecturer at Munich University Hospital. In 1910 he returned to Greece and established a private clinic in Athens. During the Balkan Wars of 1912 to 1913 he served with distinction as a surgeon with the Greek Army in Thessalonika. He was conscripted again to serve in the Military Hospital at Athens during the Greco-Turkish War.

In 1922 Logothetopoulos was appointed professor of gynaecology at the University of Athens and served as dean of the medical school from 1928 to 1929. His organisational abilities led to considerable enlargement of the university and hospital facilities in Athens. It was at this time he published, in the German literature, his work on the pelvic pressure pack. He was among the most eminent gynaecological teachers and practitioners of his era in Greece.

Logothetopoulos was a Germanophile, a fluent German speaker, his wife was German and his sympathies were with Nazi German aspirations. After Greece capitulated in 1941, Logothetopoulos was appointed vice-president and minister of health and education in the first collaborationist government. He served as prime minister from December 1942 to April 1943 and failed to avert the genocide of the Salonika Jewish community.

When the German occupying forces left Greece in late 1944, Logothetopoulos went with them. He was captured by the US army in 1946 and returned to the Greek Authorities. The Greek Special court found him guilty of treason and sentenced him to life in prison. In 1948 he published a book, *Behold the Truth*, in an attempt to salvage his reputation. However, his distinguished clinical and academic career was nullified by his well-documented Nazi sympathies and collaboration. Because of poor health he was pardoned and released from prison in 1951. He died of cancer on 8 July 1961.

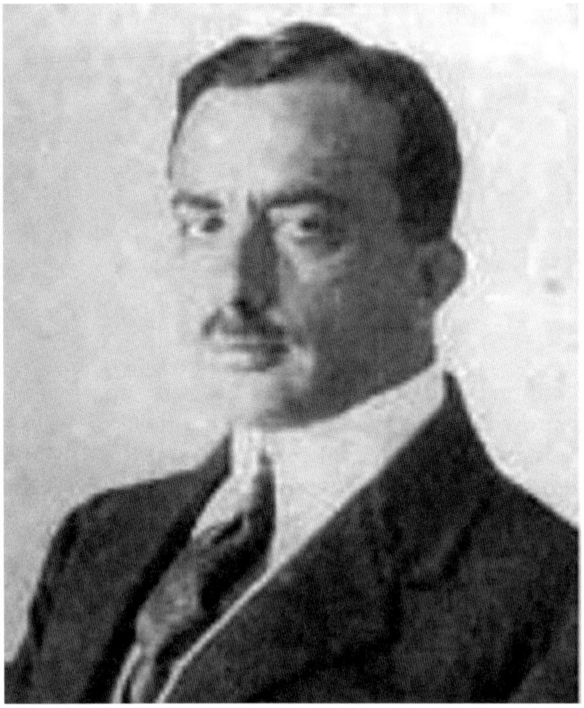

Konstantinos Logothetopoulos

Selected Publications

Logothetopoulos K. Eine absolut sichere blutstillungsmethode bei vaginalen and abdominalen Gynäkologischen operationen. (An absolutely certain method of haemostasis during vaginal and abdominal gynaecological operations). *Zentralbl Gynäkol* 1926; 50: 3202–4.

Bibliography References

99, 102, 398.

Løvset, Jørgen (1896–1981)

Løvset's Manoeuvre

One of the potential dangers associated with vaginal breech delivery is extension of the arms as the trunk delivers. In 1933 Jørgen Løvset, the Norwegian obstetrician from Bergen, devised a technique for dealing with this complication that was so logical, simple and effective that it received worldwide acceptance. In fact, Løvset advised this manoeuvre should be used for the delivery of the shoulders in all cases, but emphasised its particular value in those with extended arms:

> *There are few obstetric operations which offer so many technical difficulties as the troublesome shoulder delivery in breech presentation ...*
>
> *During the last 4 years a trial has been made with a new method of shoulder-arm delivery in breech presentation, at the Women's Hospital in Bergen. The theoretical basis for this procedure is that the posterior shoulder is always the lower one, owing to the pelvic inclination and the direction of the birth axis in the pelvic outlet ... When the body of the foetus is delivered so far that one may see or feel the inferior angle of the anterior scapula, the posterior shoulder is resting under the promontory of the sacrum. The position of the anterior shoulder at that time is behind or over the pubis.*
>
> *If the body of the foetus is turned 180° with its back to the front, the shoulder will appear under the pubis if the body descends sufficiently during the last 90° to 130° of the manoeuvre. To make this possible the posterior shoulder must be below the promontory when the rotation begins, whether spontaneously or by traction ... This method has been practised by ourselves till the present time (1937) and no failures occurred.*

In his book, *Vaginal Operative Delivery*, published in 1968, Løvset described his manoeuvre thus:

> *It consists of making the posterior shoulder the anterior one rotating the body of the baby 180° or a little more.*

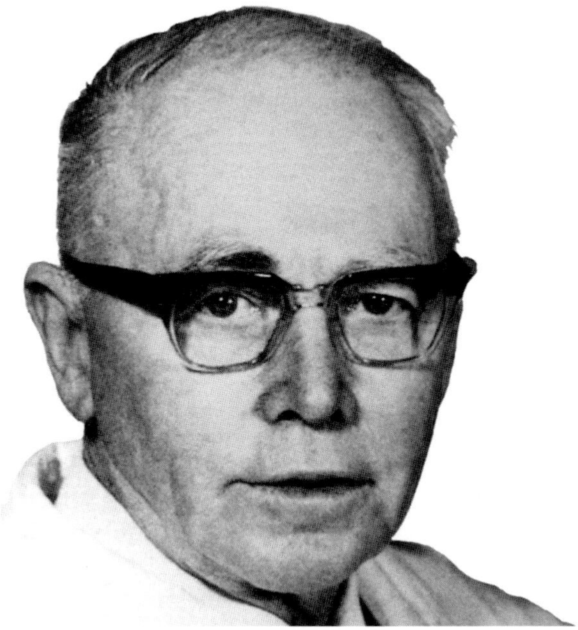

Jørgen Løvset

The rotation should take place in the hollow of the pelvis where all diameters have the same size. The rotation starts as soon as the angle of the scapula has arrived under the pubic arch. The baby's body is kept horizontal and this keeps the posterior shoulder fairly well beyond the linea terminalis. To prevent it gliding above the pelvic inlet, the body should be kept in the horizontal plane during the first 90 of the rotation. If it were kept horizontal during the next 90° of rotation, the shoulder would find its way above the symphysis. Therefore, the body of the baby is lowered as far as possible during that part of rotation. To get hold of the now anterior elbow without breaking the arm, rotation is continued until the elbow has come under the symphysis. As soon as the first shoulder and arm have been delivered, the body is rotated 180°–200° in the opposite direction. The same rule applies for the direction of the body, horizontally the first 90° and lowered during the next 90°–100°.

Løvset's manoeuvre was taught to the midwives of Norway. This graceful procedure has saved many breech deliveries from trauma and brought comfort and a sense of accomplishment to many an accoucheur. The principle of Charles Woods' screw manoeuvre for shoulder dystocia relies on a similar rationale and understanding of feto-pelvic anatomical relationships. Indeed, Løvset proposed a similar technique for shoulder dystocia in 1948.

Løvset also developed a vacuum extractor cup with four traction points and a system of attached cords to allow variation in the axis of traction.

Jørgen Løvset was a 1924 medical graduate of the University of Oslo. His postgraduate training was taken in the Women's Clinic in Bergen, with additional time in Oslo. Most of his professional life was spent in Bergen, and when the University of Bergen was founded in 1947, he became professor of obstetrics and gynaecology. He also served as director of the school of midwifery and was dean of the medical faculty from 1952 to 1957.

Selected Publications

Løvset J. Shoulder delivery by breech presentation. *J Obstet Gynaecol Br Emp* 1937; 44: 696–701.

Løvset J. Skulderlosing ved hodefodsel. *Nord Med.* 1948; 38: 1127.

Løvset J. Modern techniques of vaginal operative delivery in cephalic presentation. *Acta Obstet Gynecol Scand* 1965; 44: 102–6.

Løvset J. *Vaginal Operative Delivery.* Oslo: Scandinavian University Books; 1968.

Bibliography References

648, 942, 943, 1261.

Lugol, Jean Guillaume Auguste (1788–1851)

Lugol's Iodine

Jean Lugol worked at the Hôpital de St Louis in Paris and laboriously studied scrofula, which was the name given to tuberculous lymphadenitis before the etiology was known. Most of his theories about the disease were wrong. He believed it was not contagious but that those who married before the age of 25 or after 40 years of age were likely to give birth to a child that would develop scrofula. He advocated iodine

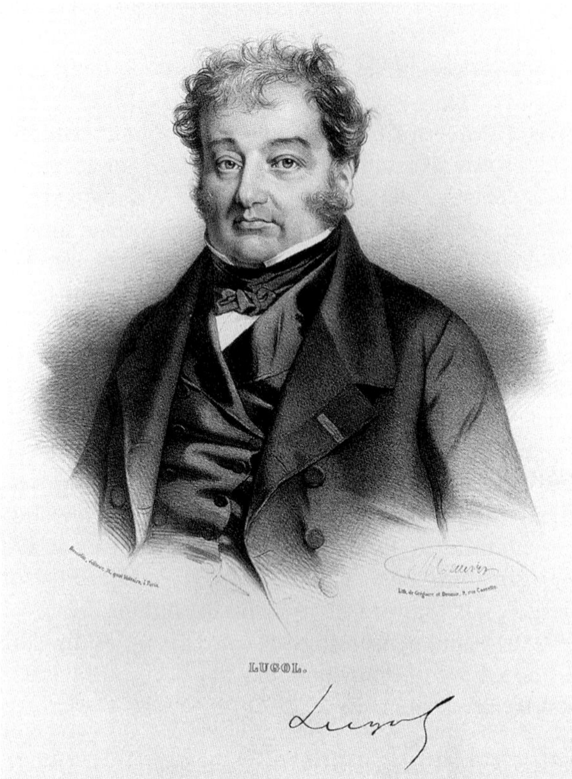

Jean Guillaume Auguste Lugol

treatments by virtually every available route: local application, plasters, general bath and orally. The solution was in various strengths of iodine, potassium iodide and distilled water. Lugol also advocated exercise, fresh air and cold baths. He presented his recommendations to the Royal Academy of Sciences in Paris in 1829.

The current composition of Lugol's iodine solution is iodine 5%, potassium iodide 10% and distilled water 85%. The proportions of both iodine and potassium iodide are higher than in Lugol's original formula.

Jean Guillaume Auguste Lugol was born in Montauban, France. He studied medicine in Paris and received his MD there in 1812. He was appointed to the medical staff of the Hôpital de St Louis in Paris in 1819 and worked there for most of his life. In 1831 he received a prize of 6,000 francs from the Institut de France for his work on behalf of tubercular patients. He died in Geneva on 16 September 1851.

Lugol's solution was used by Walter Schiller as a screening test for the early detection of cervical cancer. It is still used in gynaecology to delineate the margins of normal epithelium in the vagina and cervix.

Selected Publications

Lugol JGA. *Mémoire sur l'émploi de l'iode dans les maladies scrofuleuses.* Paris: Baillière; 1829.

Bibliography References

207, 1031.

M

Macafee, Charles Horner Greer (1898–1978)

Placenta Praevia

In the summer of 1945, within one month of each other, two reports appeared advocating a more conservative approach to the initial management of placenta praevia, one from Houston, Texas by Herman Johnson and the other by Charles Macafee from Belfast, Northern Ireland. At this time the conventional management of antepartum haemorrhage involved vaginal examination and, if placenta praevia was confirmed, early delivery of the fetus. If viable, caesarean section might be performed and if not vaginal delivery, often using the fetus for tamponade with either John Willett's scalp forceps or Braxton Hicks' bipolar version. The rationale behind this early recourse to delivery was the prevailing view that the first bleed associated with placenta praevia could be fatal to the mother. Both Johnson and Macafee, working independently, showed this was almost never the case provided no attempt at interference or delivery was made. Johnson advocated vaginal examination to confirm the diagnosis and then no further interference until induction or spontaneous labour ensued.

The most comprehensive report was that of Macafee, involving an eight-year review of 174 cases of placenta praevia. During this time all cases of antepartum haemorrhage admitted to the Royal Maternity Hospital, Belfast were assigned to Macafee and managed under his direction. He noted:

> *One of the main causes of foetal mortality in placenta praevia is prematurity. This mortality can be reduced only by carrying the pregnancy to as near term as possible ... placenta praevia is not an obstetrical emergency which must necessarily be dealt with at the first haemorrhage, and a vaginal examination must not be made until the appropriate subsequent treatment can be carried out.*

His principles of management involved withholding early digital pelvic examination, expectant hospital management until labour or fetal viability, and then pelvic examination in the operating theatre prepared for caesarean section or amniotomy depending on the presence and degree of placenta praevia.

Most other reports of this era quoted maternal death rates of 6–7% and fetal mortality of 50–60%. Macafee lost one mother of the 174, and the fetal mortality was 23%. In the last three years of his study, the fetal loss was 6%, a remarkable achievement at that time. This work revolutionised the approach to antepartum haemorrhage in general and placenta praevia in particular, resulting in considerable improvement in both maternal and fetal mortality rates. With modifications due to the availability of ultrasound, Macafee's principles of management remain intact.

Charles Horner Greer Macafee, a son of the manse, was born in Omagh, Northern Ireland. In 1921 he graduated in medicine from the Queen's University of Belfast with first-class honours, a rare achievement. He was appointed to the chair of midwifery and gynaecology at Queen's in 1945 and held this position until his retirement in 1963.

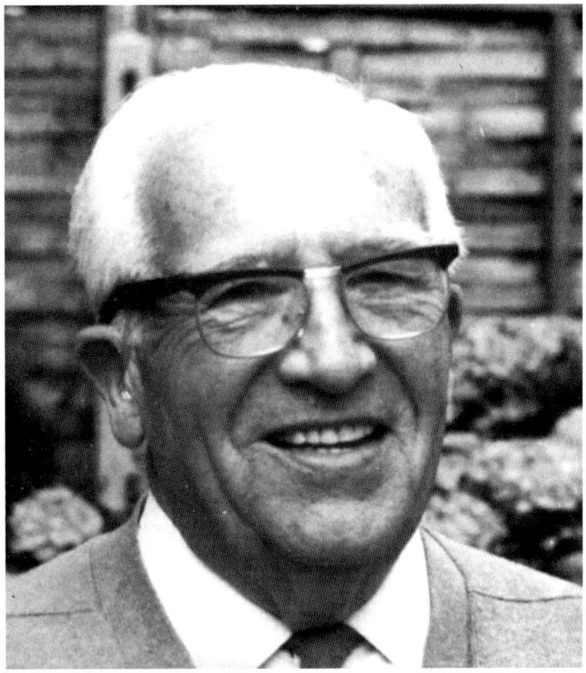

Charles Horner Greer Macafee

He was an accomplished obstetrician, gynaecological surgeon and teacher who attracted many overseas postgraduate students to his department. He was a foundation fellow of the Royal College of Obstetricians and Gynaecologists, serving as vice-president from 1961 to 1964. In 1961 he was appointed a Commander of the Order of the British Empire by the Queen. His guiding philosophy was summed up in his words: 'While medicine is undoubtedly a science, it is a science in which the scientist is dealing with people and not things'. He died on 16 August 1978 at his home in Donaghadee, Northern Ireland.

Selected Publications

Macafee CHG. Placenta praevia: a study of 174 cases. *J Obstet Gynaecol Br Emp* 1945; 52: 313–24.

Johnson HW. The conservative management of some varieties of placenta previa. *Am J Obstet Gynecol* 1945; 50: 248–54.

Bibliography References

88, 952, 983, 1561.

Mackenrodt, Alwin Karl (1859–1925)

Mackenrodt's Ligaments

The understanding of the supporting structures of the pelvic floor and the treatment of prolapse was imperfect in the nineteenth century. Alvin Mackenrodt, in his study of an eight-month-old fetus, pointed out the major role of the transverse cervical ligaments, also known as the cardinal or Mackenrodt's ligaments. He wrote:

> *The idea persists that the inner genitalis, especially the uterus, close the genital opening like a sort of obturator. This assumption does not correspond at all with the facts ... If, in the pelvis of the newborn, one exposes this part of the pelvic fascia, which is readily accessible because it lies in large part directly under the pelvic peritoneum, then firm, bandlike, fibrous processes can be isolated, which attach directly to the uterine cervix, vagina, rectum and bladder ... These masses of fibres extending from the pelvic fascia to the side of the cervix assume an important and independent position ... The purely connective tissue and muscular transverse cervical ligament is the principal means of support of the uterus, and in its upper edge it conducts the principal blood vessel of the uterus, the uterine artery.*

Alvin Mackenrodt was born in Nordhausen, Germany. At his father's urging, he followed his two elder brothers in the study of theology at Jena University. He found this not to his liking and soon transferred to medicine. After four years in general practice in Strassfurt he studied gynaecology in Berlin as an unpaid volunteer. He later established his own gynaecology clinic in Berlin and in 1904 attained the rank of professor at Berlin University. Mackenrodt became one of the dominant gynaecological surgeons in Germany, making many original contributions to prolapse, fistula and cancer surgery. He died of pneumonia.

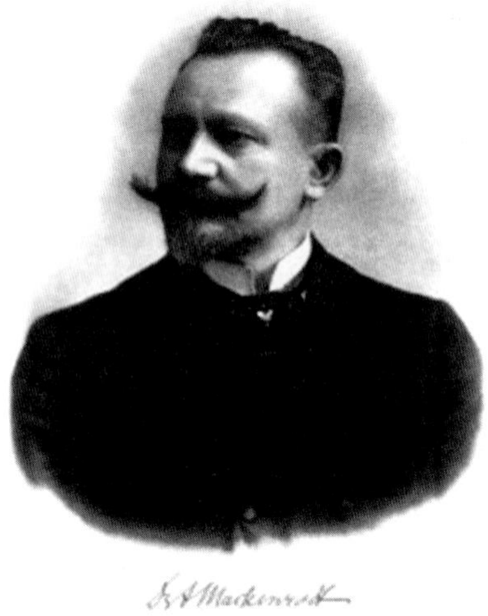

Alwin Karl Mackenrodt

Selected Publications

Mackenrodt A. Über die Ursachen der normalen und pathologischen Lagen des Uterus. *Arch Gynäkol* 1895; 48: 394–421.

Bibliography References

406, 501, 524, 553, 648, 960, 1261, 1291.

Madlener, Max (1868–1951)

Madlener Tubal Ligation

In the early part of the twentieth century, surgical sterilisation of women became acceptable and feasible. One of the more popular procedures was described by Max Madlener. In essence this involved elevating a loop of tube at its most mobile point, crushing the base of the loop with a clamp, removing the clamp and tying a ligature around the crushed area. No portion of the tube was excised:

> *With a pickup forceps, the operator grasps the tube where most mobile, thus not near the uterus, but rather at or distal to its midportion. The tube is elevated to an angle of 90°. With the other hand, one applies the crushing clamp to the tube just under the tip of the forceps. The part of the tube running to and from the forceps is then encountered obliquely, and at the same time a small knuckle of the mesosalpinx is crushed with it . . . One now applies the jaws of the crushing forceps, which are compressed by closing the fist tightly so that the tissue is surely crushed paper thin. After the clamp is removed and while the tube is still held in the forceps, a thin thread ligature is placed in the groove.*

In Madlener's report of 89 cases there were no failures, although he did recognise the possibility of tubal recanalisation. With further experience the failure rate was unacceptably high, and Madlener's technique was abandoned in favour of others.

Max Madlener was born in Memmingen, Germany. His medical studies were taken in Munich, Berlin and Kiel. He practised both surgery and gynaecology in Kempten, where he became medical director of the regional hospital. He died of a stroke.

Selected Publications

Madlener M. Über sterilisierende Operationen an den Tuben. *Zentralbl Gynäkol* 1919; 43: 380–4.

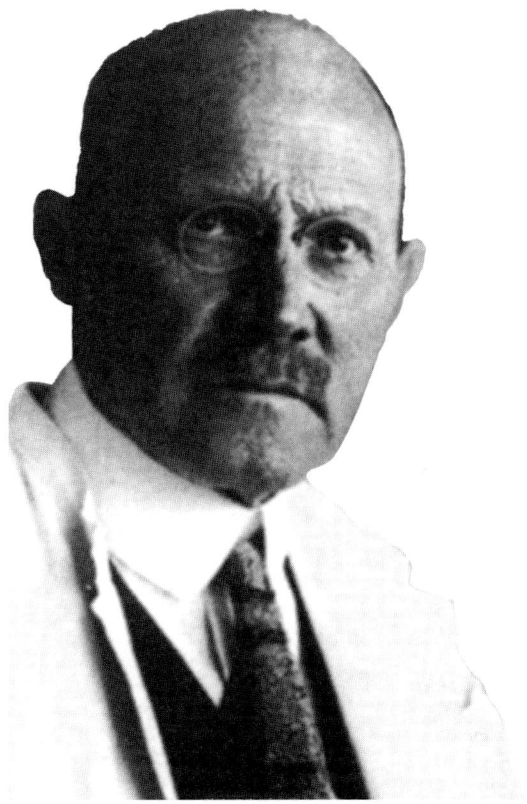

Max Madlener

Bibliography References

168, 645, 891, 1355, 1480.

Mahfouz, Naguib (1882–1974)

Obstetric Fistula

Naguib Mahfouz was born to Coptic Christian parents on 5 January 1882 in Mansoura, Egypt. He began his studies at the Kasr El-Aini Medical School in 1898 at the age of 16. In his final year as a medical student there was an outbreak of cholera in Upper Egypt, and Mahfouz went to the village of Mousha to help. Using the same principles as John Snow some 50 years before, he traced the source of the cholera to an infected well in a farmer's house. Within a week the Mousha cholera epidemic had come to an end.

Mahfouz qualified in medicine at the head of his class in 1902. After two years working as a general practitioner in Suez he took an appointment as anaesthetist at the Kasr El-Aini Hospital. At that time there was no department of obstetrics and gynaecology at the hospital, so Mahfouz started these clinics on the side. They became so popular that the hospital created a department of obstetrics and gynaecology, the first in Egypt. For almost 20 years Mahfouz provided his services as an obstetric consultant to medical officers who delivered women in their homes. They knew they could call on Mahfouz for help in difficult cases, and he acquired enormous clinical experience during this time. One of the children he delivered, in 1911, was named after him and later won the Nobel Prize in Literature: the novelist Naguib Mahfouz.

In 1929 Naguib Mahfouz was appointed professor of obstetrics and gynaecology at Kasr El-Aini Medical School, and he remained in this position until 1947. Mahfouz was also the senior gynaecologist to the Coptic and Lord Kitchener's Memorial Hospitals. He was appointed obstetrician and gynaecologist to the Egyptian Royal Family. Mahfouz established a school of midwifery from which selected graduates went on to provide domiciliary midwifery services in Cairo.

The oldest recorded vesicovaginal fistula was found in the mummy of Henhenit, a woman at the royal court in Cairo c.2050 BC. It was therefore fitting that one of the modern pioneers in the surgical management of obstetric fistula should be Naguib Mahfouz from Egypt. He first began operating on fistulae in 1907, and by 1919, 'I devoted a ward of 10 beds to urinary and faecal fistulae and the beds were always full'. By 1957, when he delivered the Shaw Memorial Lecture to the Royal College of Obstetricians and Gynaecologists, he was able to report on almost 1,000 personal cases: '758 besides 210 of which I kept no record'.

In addition to his pioneering work on fistulae he wrote widely on other aspects of obstetrics and gynaecology. His personal collection of more than 3,000 rare specimens in obstetrics and gynaecology he donated to the Kasr El-Aini Medical School. They created the Naguib Mahfouz Museum of Obstetrics and Gynaecology, which still exists at that institution. He published a three-volume atlas of the specimens in the museum.

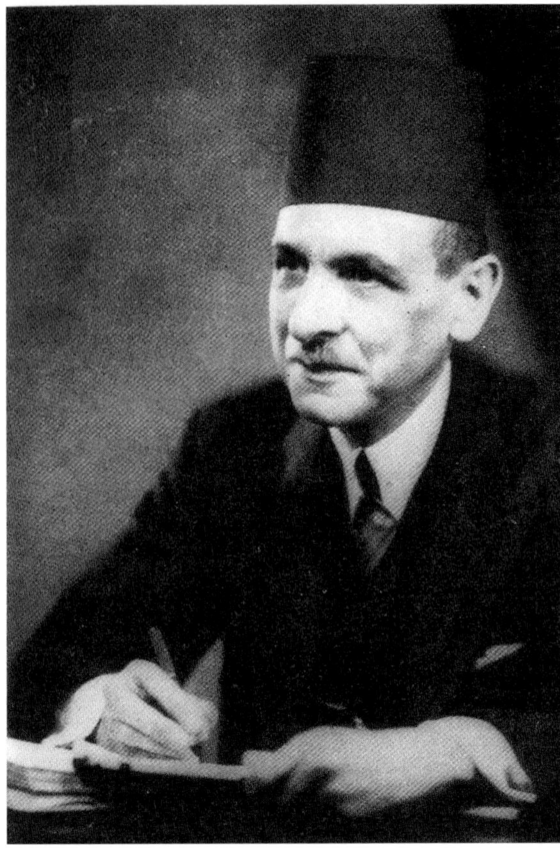
Naguib Mahfouz

Mahfouz was regarded as the father of obstetrics and gynaecology in Egypt and greatly honoured in his time. He was awarded the Order of the Nile and, in 1937, the title of Pasha, the highest civilian honour in Egypt. He was elected honorary fellow of the Royal College of Obstetricians and Gynaecologists and, in 1943, was made an Honorary Fellow of the Royal College of Surgeons of England at the same time as Winston Churchill. Naguib Mahfouz Pasha died at the age of 92 on 25 July 1974.

Selected Publications

Mahfouz, N. Urinary and recto-vaginal fistulae in women. *J Obstet Gynaecol Br Emp* 1929; 37: 581–9.

Mahfouz N. Urinary fistulae in women. *J Obstet Gynaecol Br Emp* 1957; 64: 23–34.

Bibliography References

384, 686, 687, 725, 970, 1739, 1740.

Malmström, Tage (1911–1995)

Vacuum Extractor

The first recorded attempt to deliver an infant by vacuum extraction was in 1706 by James Yonge (1646–1721) of Plymouth, England. He described a failed attempt to deliver a woman 'four days in labour' by 'a cupping glass fixed to the scalp with an air pump'. In 1829, the English surgeon, Neill Arnott (1788–1874), suggested that a 'pneumatic tractor' could act 'as a substitute for the steel forceps in the hands of men who are deficient in manual dexterity, whether from inexperience or natural ineptitude'. It seems Arnott never actually produced or used such a device.

James Young Simpson of Edinburgh developed the first practical instrument, which consisted of a round metal speculum with a leather cuff attached to a piston to create the vacuum. Although he used it several times with success, its value was limited and Simpson soon concentrated on his modification of the obstetric forceps.

Over the next century, many became involved in the development of the vacuum extractor, including in America, Herbert Stillman (1875), Peter McCahey (1890) and Richard Torpin (1938); in France, Soubhy Saleh (1857) and Yves Couzigou (1947); D Kuntzsch (1912) and Korber (1952) of Germany; O Koller (1950) of Norway; T Hasegawa and R Shiojima (1951) in Japan; and Vicktor Finderle (1952) in Yugoslavia.

The most successful of all vacuum extractors was designed by Tage Malmström of Gothenburg, Sweden, in 1953. One of the key elements in the Malmström device was the rounded incurved margin of the cup so that the periphery of the cup underlies the outside diameter of the 'chignon', thereby reducing the risk of cup detachment during traction. Malmström refined his instrument between 1953 and 1957, with a final modification in 1967.

Originally Malmström used the instrument in the first stage of labour to improve uterine action by pulling the head down onto the cervix:

> *In the first stage of labour and also initially in the second stage the vacuum extractor can be used in cases of uterine inertia to stimulate the contractions by pressing the foetal head against the cervix. In such cases one must, of course, make a thorough investigation so that one has full information as to the cephalo-pelvic relation ... In cases of uterine inertia where the foetal head is almost or completely engaged, the situation may be such, that one can not draw out the labour but is compelled to make a direct extraction. At this point the vacuum extractor takes the place of a high or a midhigh forceps, or it can make the situation much easier for a subsequent forceps delivery by bringing the head into a better position.*

As the role of the vacuum extractor developed, it came to be used mainly as an alternative to forceps delivery. It is incorrectly felt by some to be safer than forceps, especially in the hands of the less experienced – to some degree as Arnott had predicted 150 years before.

In 1969, Geoffrey Bird of Australia modified the instrument by placing the vacuum tubing eccentrically on the cup, with the traction cord separately at the centre. This further reduced the chance of detachment due to loss of the vacuum.

Tage Malmström was born in Malmö, Sweden. He studied medicine at the University of Lund, qualifying

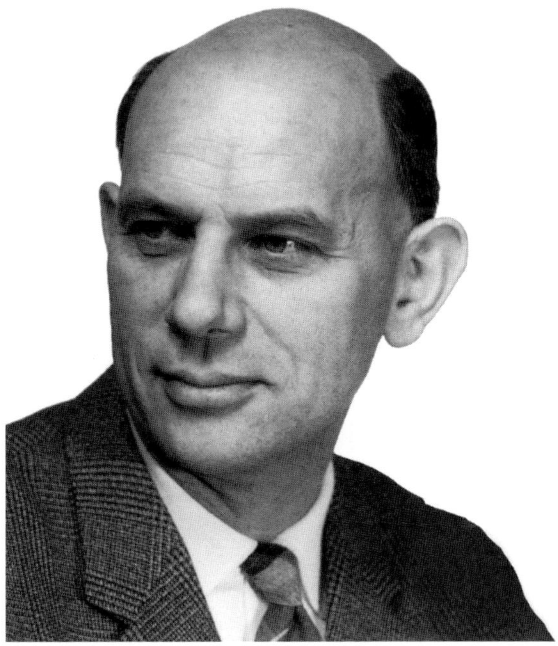

Tage Malmström

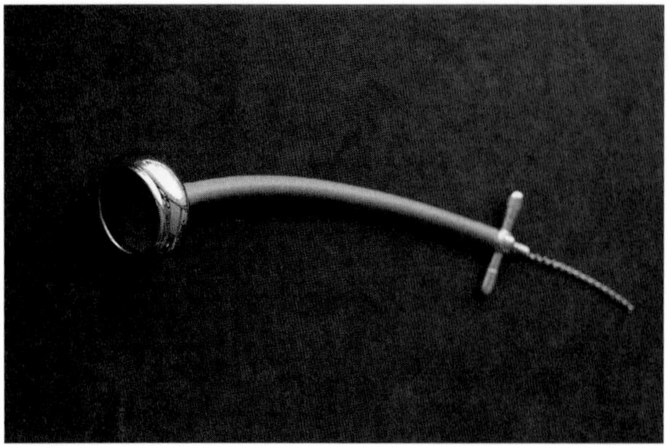

Malmström vacuum cup

in 1940. He initially worked as a surgeon and then specialised in obstetrics and gynaecology. In 1949 he moved to the Women's Clinic in Sahlgrenska Hospital, Gothenburg, where he developed his vacuum extractor. He became docent and professor at the University of Gothenburg.

Malmström's vacuum extractor received acceptance throughout the world, virtually replacing forceps in many areas. He became ill with Menière's disease in 1965, the symptoms of which became so troublesome that he retired in 1969. At the FIGO conference in Montreal in September 1994, Tage Malmström was awarded a special certificate of recognition. He died on 19 January 1995.

Selected Publications

Arnott N. Pneumatics. In: *Elements of Physics or Natural Philosophy (Vol. 1)* 1829; 1: 650.

Bird GC. Modification of Malmström's vacuum extractor. *BMJ* 1969; 3: 526.

Malmström T. Sugklocke-en ersattre for galeatang. *Nord Med* 1953; 50: 1311.

Malmström T. Vacuum extractor: an obstetrical instrument. *Acta Obstet Gynecol Scand* 1954; 33 (Suppl 4): 1–31.

Simpson JY. The air tractor as a substitute for the forceps in tedious labours. *Proc Edinb Obstet Soc* 1848; 124.

Yonge J. An account of balls of hair taken from the uterus and ovaria of several women. *Phil Trans* 1706–7; 25–26: 2387–92.

Bibliography References

92, 99, 260, 532, 1133, 1694.

Malpighi, Marcello (1628–1694)

Embryology

One of the earliest and greatest microscopists of the seventeenth century, Marcello Malpighi made numerous discoveries in anatomy and pioneering observations in embryology. However, in his first embryological foray of 1673 he was misled. Believing he was observing unfertilised chicken eggs, he saw early embryos which he interpreted as miniature chicks. This observation was subsequently used to support the theory of preformation. Two years later he made the most advanced embryological observations of his era in an incubated egg, describing the aortic arches, neural folds and tube, and the cerebral and otic vesicles. Among his many anatomical observations was the capillary anastomosis between arteries and veins, and the red blood cells, which he described as 'fat globules looking like a rosary of red coral'.

Marcello Malpighi was born at Crevacuore, near Bologna, Italy. He graduated in philosophy and medicine from the University of Bologna in 1653. He held chairs in medicine at the universities of Pisa, Messina and Bologna. In 1864 a fire at his home destroyed many of his personal manuscripts. In 1691 Malpighi moved to Rome when Pope Innocent XII persuaded him to become his personal physician. He died in the papal apartments on 29 November 1694.

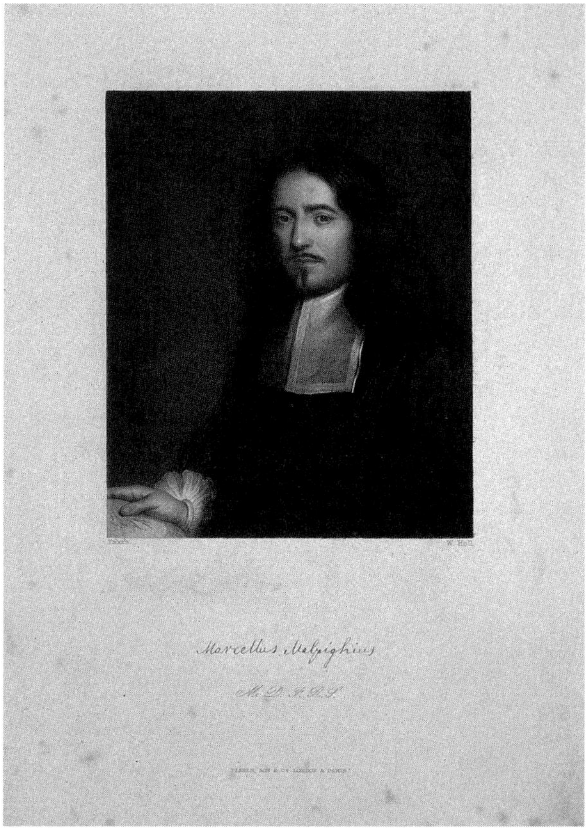
Marcello Malpighi

Selected Publications

Malpighi M. *Dissertio epistolica de formatione pulli in ovo.* London: J. Martyn; 1673.

Malpighi M. *De ovo incubato observationes.* London: J. Martyn; 1675.

Bibliography References

182, 648, 954, 969, 1031, 1230.

Malthus, Thomas Robert (1766–1834)

Malthusian Principle

In his *Essay on the Principle of Population*, Thomas Malthus put forward this maxim:

> *Population, when unchecked, increases in a geometrical ratio. Subsistence increases only in arithmetical ratio. A slight acquaintance with numbers will show the immensity of the first power in comparison of the second. By the law of our nature which makes food necessary to the life of man, the effects of these two unequal powers must be kept equal.*

He argued that populations will naturally tend to increase faster than the means to sustain them and advocated 'moral restraint' and checks on population increase. These ideas had previously been advanced by Plato, Aristotle and Benjamin Franklin but are remembered eponymously as the Malthusian principle. A controversial figure in his time, his writings influenced Charles Darwin, Karl Marx and John Maynard Keynes. He published his work first anonymously in 1798 and then in a much expanded, signed work in 1803. In all, the book went through six editions in his lifetime.

Robert Malthus, as he was generally called, was born in Dorking, Surrey, England, and educated at Jesus College, Cambridge. He became curate of Albury and later professor of political economy at Haileybury College, where he was a popular teacher.

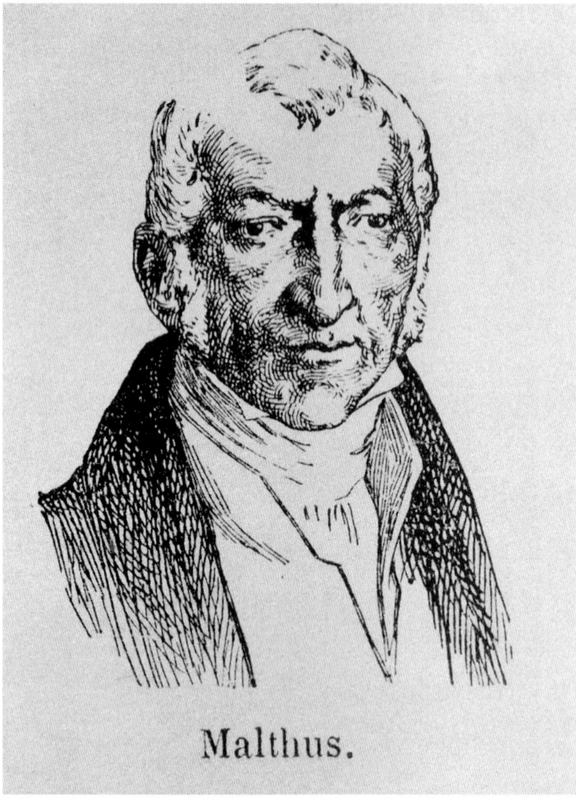

Thomas Robert Malthus

Malthus, who had a cleft palate, married and raised three children. He is buried in Bath Abbey and just inside the entrance on the left is a memorial tablet in his honour.

Selected Publications

Malthus TR. *An Essay on the Principle of Population, as it Affects the Future Improvement of Society*. London: J. Johnson; 1798.

Bibliography References

298, 410, 470, 552, 773, 834, 968, 1026, 1199, 1201.

Marker, Russell Earl (1902–1995)

Synthesis of Progesterone

Russell Marker was born in 1902 into a sharecropper family that lived in a one-room log cabin on a farm near Hagerstown, Maryland. His early experience of farm work convinced him to get an education. To attend high school his daily journey required six miles of walking and a train ride. Supported by his mother, he enrolled at the University of Maryland in, for no particular reason, chemical engineering. After a year, despite having had no science education at high school, he changed to chemistry and earned his bachelor's degree in 1923. He followed this in two years with his master's degree and after a further two years completed his PhD thesis, which was acknowledged to be of high calibre. However, the university would not grant him his doctoral degree unless he took an additional course in physical chemistry. Marker refused to take the course, as he thought it was unnecessary and found the subject boring. Thus, Marker left the university without his PhD.

For a short time, he worked in the laboratory of a gasoline corporation in Yonkers, New York, and there developed the gasoline octane rating. Despite his lack of a PhD, his previous graduate research work gained him a position at the Rockefeller Institute in Manhattan in 1928. It was here that Marker began his interest in steroids, known then as sterols. At that time progesterone could only be produced in minute amounts at great expense. Marker felt that it could be produced from plants and proposed this research to his seniors. This was rejected. Once again Marker refused to yield and left the Rockefeller Institute to become a fellow at Pennsylvania State College. Here he was able to carry out his basic research on steroid chemistry and eventually rose to the rank of full professor, with a prolific publication record. Against all advice he was eventually able to develop an efficient method for converting a plant steroid, sapogenin, which occurs naturally in roots, into progesterone. Marker then began a search across America to find the best plant in sufficient quantities to produce large amounts of progesterone. After much investigation he settled on the Mexican black-headed yam, in which he found the steroid diosgenin. He developed the chemical process to convert diosgenin into progesterone. As the only large quantities of this root were in Mexico, Marker set about obtaining financial backing to set up a laboratory in Mexico. The University could not support him, and he tried all of the major pharmaceutical companies without success.

Once gain his impetuous and stubborn nature took over and he resigned from Penn State, took out his savings and moved to Mexico City. Working in a shed with tons of yams he produced three kilograms of progesterone, at that time worth about $250,000. Marker did not patent his process. In 1944, in conjunction with a small Mexican firm, he founded Syntex, the name being a blend of the two words 'synthesis' and 'Mexico'. After two years he fell out with the other founders of Syntex and for a brief time formed another company to produce progesterone, Botanica-Mex. At the age of 49, and after 213 publications in the field, he forsook the world of chemistry and pharmaceuticals forever. By this time the production of progesterone, using his process, was so efficient that the cost of progesterone had dropped from $80 to $2 per gram.

As he later wrote:

> *When I retired from Chemistry in 1949, after 5 years of production and research in Mexico, I felt I had accomplished what I had set out to do. I had found sources for the production of steroidal hormones in quantity at low prices, developed the process for manufacture, and put them into production. I assisted in establishing many competitive companies in order to insure a fair price to the public and without patent protection or royalties from the producers.*

Marker ultimately went into business in Mexico City commissioning Mexican craftsmen to make replicas of antique European silverworks. He turned up again in the United States in the mid-1980s and had done sufficiently well in the silver business to endow

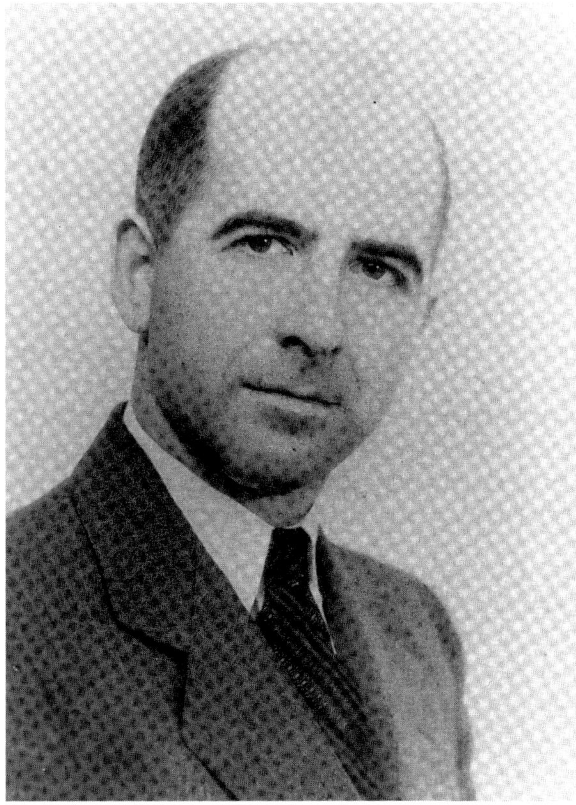

Russell Earl Marker

six annual lectures at Pennsylvania State University. He specified that Carl Djerassi be the first lecturer. He also endowed two annual Russell Marker lectureships at the University of Maryland, which university ultimately awarded him an honorary doctorate, having withheld his PhD for want of a course in physical chemistry some 50 years before. Marker's eccentric independence and tenacity in producing progesterone from the steroid diosgenin was the starting point for hormone synthesis and, ultimately, the contraceptive pill.

Russell Marker died in relative obscurity having lived quietly for many years close to the Penn State University campus.

Selected Publications

Marker RE. Steroidal sapogenins, part 173. *J Am Chem Soc* 1949; 71: 3856.

Bibliography References

31, 82, 101, 304, 401–403, 516, 620, 887, 888, 979, 981, 1309, 1329, 1498.

Marshall, Victor Fray (1913–2001) Marchetti, Andrew Anthony (1901–1970) Krantz, Kermit Edward (1923–2007)

Marshall–Marchetti–Krantz Operation

A co-operative venture between a urologist and two gynaecologists, one with anatomical leanings, led to a suprapubic surgical approach for urinary stress incontinence in females. They started their report, which included the outcome of the operation in 46 female and four male patients, with the confident statement:

> *A procedure for the correction of urinary stress incontinence has been devised which has given results approximately and often surpassing those which follow the commonly used operations . . . the operation is a simple elevation and immobilization of the vesical neck and urethra by suturing them to the pubis and rectus muscles . . . The exact mechanism by which this operation improved urinary control in most of the selected cases is not entirely understood. However, simple elevation and fixation of the vesical outlet and urethra seem to be the only significant change that can result from the technique.*

Of the female patients with stress incontinence, 92 per cent were cured or improved. They also described a preoperative test to assess the likelihood of success:

> *The test was made by filling the bladder with 250 cubic centimetres of saline and observing the patient's urinary control while coughing and straining in the prone and standing positions. After the bladder was refilled to 250 cubic centimetres the same procedures were repeated with the exception that elevation and fixation of the vesical outlet was provided in the following manner: A wheal of novocain which was made in the vaginal wall at a point estimated to be under the interureteric ridge was grasped with an Allis clamp and held firmly upward toward the umbilicus, not permitting downward movement on coughing and straining. If this elevation and fixation provided good urinary control, the test was considered favourable.*

This became known as the 'Marshall test'. A similar manoeuvre was described by Victor Bonney, so it is known by some as the 'Bonney test'. Less credence is put upon this test now, as urodynamic assessment has shown it often works by compressing the urethra. Marshall was also aware of this possibility.

The genesis of this operation arose from Marshall's work at the New York and Memorial Hospitals in the mid-1940s, in which he assessed the problem of urinary incontinence in men following abdomino-perineal resection of the rectum. He found that, by displacing a perineal hernia backwards and upwards with a pad and T-binder, continence was restored: 'In this case lack of support of the bladder and bladder neck seems to be the main factor in the persistent difficulty'. He therefore used a suprapubic surgical approach to suspend the bladder and bladder neck:

> *By means of interrupted chromic catgut sutures, the prostate, bladder neck, and anterior bladder wall were sutured to the periosteum of the symphysis and posterior rectus sheath.*

The operation was a success, and the man remained continent 10 years later. Marshall postulated that the basic mechanism and cure of incontinence would be the same in females, and with this belief he began co-operative work with the gynaecologists.

In the half century since it was first described, the Marshall–Marchetti–Krantz procedure became one of the standard operations for urinary stress incontinence in women.

Victor Fray Marshall was born in Culpepper, Virginia. He received his medical degree from the University of Virginia in Charlottesville. His postgraduate training was in surgery and urology at the New York Hospital and Cornell University. He worked at the New York and Memorial Hospitals. In 1957 he was appointed professor of clinical surgery at the New York Hospital Cornell Center. He retired back to Charlottesville, Virginia and died in 2001.

Andrew Anthony Marchetti, of Italian descent, was born in Richmond, Virginia. His school of medical graduation was Johns Hopkins in 1928. He did

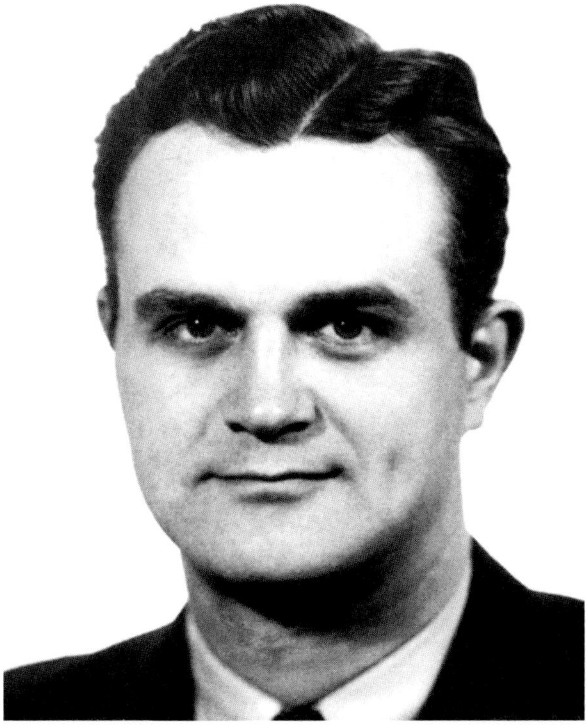

Victor Fray Marshall

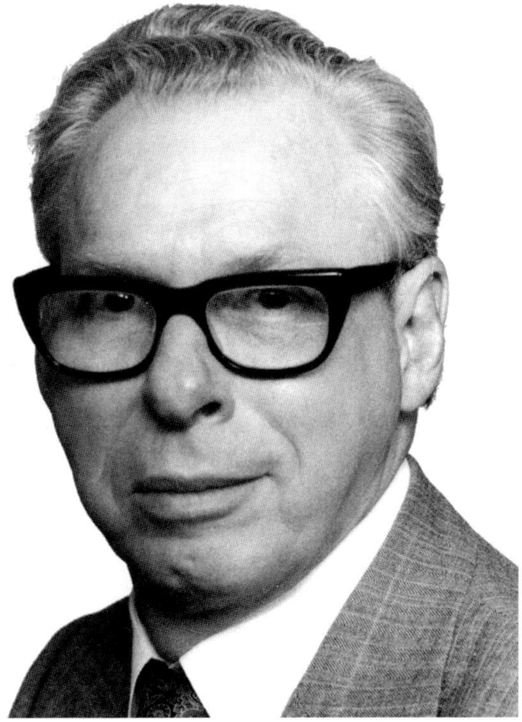

Kermit Edward Krantz

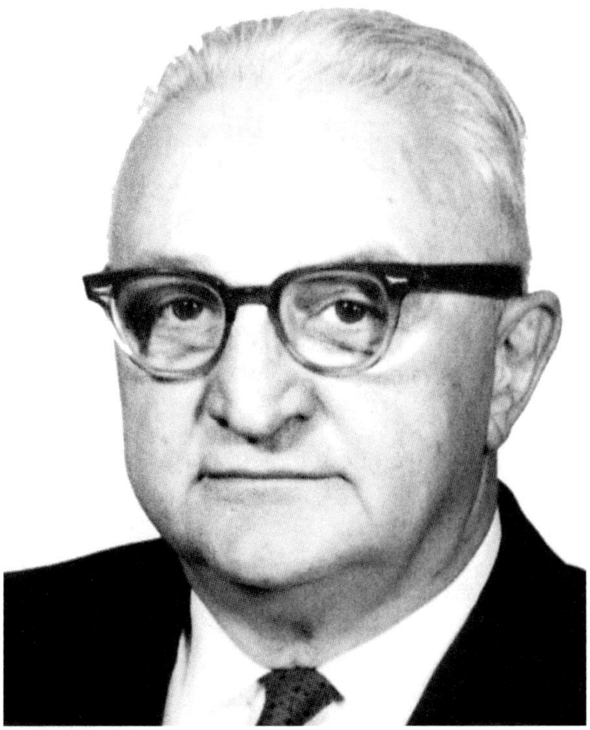

Andrew Anthony Marchetti

postgraduate work at his alma mater, Rochester, New York, Cincinnati General Hospital and the New York Hospital. In 1948 he became professor and chairman of obstetrics and gynaecology at Georgetown University Hospital in Washington DC. Marchetti was also experienced in gynaecological pathology and cytology. He often accompanied George Papanicolaou to medical meetings and assisted with translation. His interests outside medicine included wine, on which he was an expert, and the history of both baseball and medicine. A past president of the American Gynecological Society, he died while attending a meeting of the American Board of Obstetrics and Gynecology.

Kermit Edward Krantz was born in Oak Park, Illinois. He did his undergraduate science degree at Northwestern University, Chicago. There he worked in the zoology department from 1943 to 1947 and was curator of the museum of anatomy from 1944 to 1947. He graduated MD in 1948. It was during his residency from 1948 to 1950 in Cornell Medical College and the New York Lying-in Hospital that he collaborated with Marshall and Marchetti. He was assistant professor of obstetrics and gynaecology at the University of Arkansas from 1955 to 1959. In 1959 he became professor and head of the department of obstetrics and gynaecology at the University of Kansas and after retirement held the title of distinguished professor in that department until his death in 2007. The chair of the department of obstetrics and gynaecology at the University of Kansas is the KE Krantz chair.

Selected Publications

Marshall VF, Pollack RS, Miller C. Observations on urinary dysfunction after excision of the rectum. *J Urol* 1946; 55: 409–16.

Marshall VF, Marchetti AA, Krantz KE. The correction of stress incontinence by simple vesicourethral suspension. *Surg Gynecol Obstet* 1949; 88: 509–18.

Bibliography References

442, 443, 524, 767, 978.

Martius, Heinrich (1885–1965)

Martius Graft

Heinrich Martius was professor of obstetrics and gynaecology at the University of Göttingen. His main interest was gynaecological surgery, and he developed the bulbocavernosus graft, inserted between the bladder and vaginal skin to augment the repair of a vesicovaginal fistula. The aim of this graft was to bring a fresh blood supply into a relatively scarred and ischaemic area and, by keeping the bladder and vaginal wall apart, to reduce the risk of recurrent fistula from adherence between the two healing surfaces. He first described this in 1928 and outlined the technique in his text *Martius' Gynecological Operations*:

> *In this operation a fat muscle flap is formed from one of the labia majora. This is about as thick as a thumb and as long as a finger and is left attached to the pedicle posteriorly. It contains the bulbocavernosus muscle. It is placed around the neck of the bladder and fixed on the other sides with sutures. This is a very simple, safe, and rapid procedure.*

In addition to promoting healing of the fistula, Martius felt that the graft might assist sphincter function of the bladder neck. He later acknowledged that there was little muscle tissue in the graft, and it is generally referred to as the Martius bulbocavernosus fat graft. He advocated use of the graft in all but the smallest and simplest fistulae, saying 'the risk is low, the gain is high'.

Heinrich Martius was born in Berlin, Germany, the son of a professor of medicine. He qualified in medicine in 1910 and worked briefly as a ship's doctor. In the First World War he served as a medical officer with the German cavalry. Martius was one of the most respected gynaecologists in Germany and in

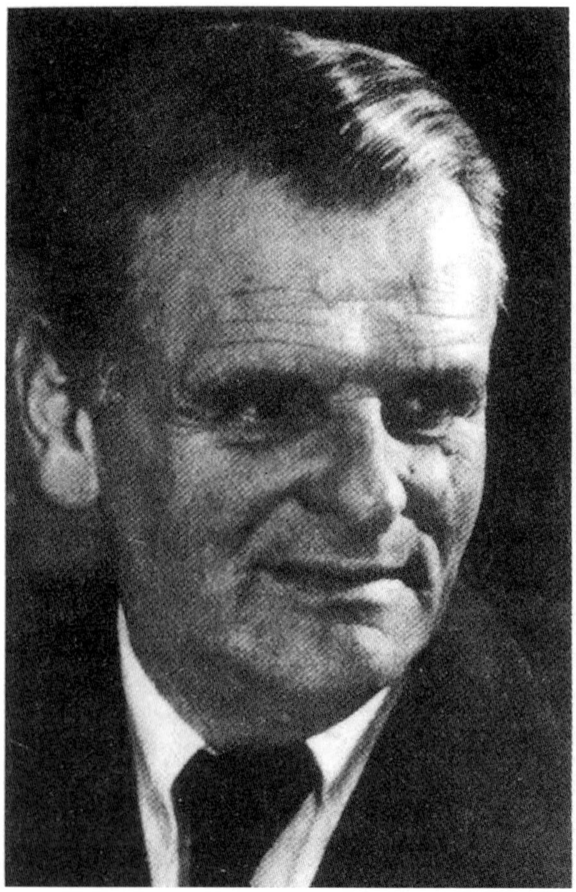

Heinrich Martius

1951 was elected President of the German Society of Gynaecology and Obstetrics. He died in Göttingen on 17 February 1965, two days before his wife's death.

Selected Publications

Martius H. Die operative Wiederherstellung der vollkommen fehlenden Harnröhre und des Schaliessmuskels ders Derslelben. *Zentralbl Gynäkol* 1928; 8: 480–6.

Martius H. *Martius' Gynecological Operations.* (English translation by ML McCall, KA Bolten.) Boston, MA: Little, Brown and Company; 1956, pp. 329–33.

Bibliography References

147, 686, 725, 1248, 1739, 1740.

Mauriceau, François (1637–1709)

Mauriceau–Smellie–Veit Manoeuvre

François Mauriceau was born in Orléans, France, received his training at the Hôtel Dieu and became a member of the company of master surgeons of Paris. Working at the Hôtel Dieu, and through his writings, he became the most famous obstetrician of the seventeenth century. His first work, *Traité des maladies de femmes grosses et de celles qui sont accouchées,* was published in 1668 and went through seven editions. It was translated into English by Hugh Chamberlen, as well as into Latin, Dutch, Flemish, German and Italian. In the preface he wrote:

> *The doctrine of books, which is one of the most wholesome effectual remedies we have to chase away ignorance, is wholly useless to men's wits, when not disposed to receive it.*

It was not until the third edition of this book that Mauriceau's full account of his method for delivering the aftercoming head of the breech was developed. In this he embellished Jacques Guillemeau's method of flexing the head with one or two fingers in the infant's mouth, by also providing traction on the shoulders with the other hand and having an assistant hold the feet:

> *There are nevertheless some infants with a head so large that it remains caught in the passage after the body is completely out . . . the surgeon will disengage the head gradually from the bones of the pelvis. This he will do by gently sliding one or two fingers of his left hand into the infant's mouth, in order to release the chin first, and with his right hand he will grasp the back of the infant's neck, above the shoulders, with the help of one of the fingers of his left hand placed in the infant's mouth, as I have just said, to disengage the chin; for it is chiefly this part that causes, the head to be held up in the pelvis, out of which one cannot extract it until the chin is completely disengaged.*

There are a number of glaring inaccuracies in Mauriceau's work. He maintains that the ovarian ligaments are the conduit between the ovary and uterus by which the 'sperm' of the female and male are joined. He rejects the views of Regnier de Graaf on the ovum: 'This sentiment ought not to be followed by other wise men'.

Most of the treatise, however, is sound clinical sense and dispels a number of myths held at that time. He denied that the bones of the symphysis pubis separate during labour and that the infant born at seven months had a greater chance of survival than one born at eight months. He advocated ambulation in labour:

> *. . . the mother being on her legs, causeth the inward orifice of the womb to dilate sooner than in bed, and her pains to be stronger and frequenter, that her labour be nothing near so long.*

He encouraged women to deliver in the semi-recumbent position in bed rather than on a birth stool:

> *The bed must be so made, that the woman being ready to be delivered, should lie on her back upon it, having her body in a convenient figure, that is her head and breast a little raised so that she be neither lying nor sitting . . .*

Mauriceau was one of the first to advocate suture of perineal tears:

> *But sometimes it happens by an unlucky and deplorable accident, that the perinaeum is rent . . . let it be strongly stitched together with three or four stitches or more, according to the length of the separation, and taking at each stitch good hold of the flesh, that so it may not break out . . .*

His approach to the third stage of labour was rather aggressive, as he advocated early cord traction and manual removal. He favoured early intervention and delivery by internal podalic version and breech extraction in cases of placenta praevia with haemorrhage: 'that a woman in this condition, for the reasons alleged, must necessarily be delivered, that the floodings may be stopt'. In his treatise Mauriceau describes in emotional terms the case of one of his sisters who died from antepartum haemorrhage because of delay in delivery: 'the sad story of one of my sisters, which I shall not again repeat, being too sadly affected with it'.

Mauriceau displays an entertaining and humorous side to his writing. In discussing multiple pregnancy and the possibility of superfetation, he recounts the story of one Monsieur Herbert, whose wife delivered quadruplets. When asked 'whether it were true, that he was so good a fellow as to get his wife with child of those four at one bout', Monsieur Herbert apparently replied 'that he had certainly begot at the same time half a dozen if his foot had not slipt'.

In 1694 Mauriceau published his *Aphorisms*, which was really a synopsis of his larger works and intended for midwives and student physicians. In his time, he helped establish the Hôtel Dieu as the best midwifery training hospital for both midwives and surgeons. He retired to the countryside outside Paris several years before his death on 17 October 1709.

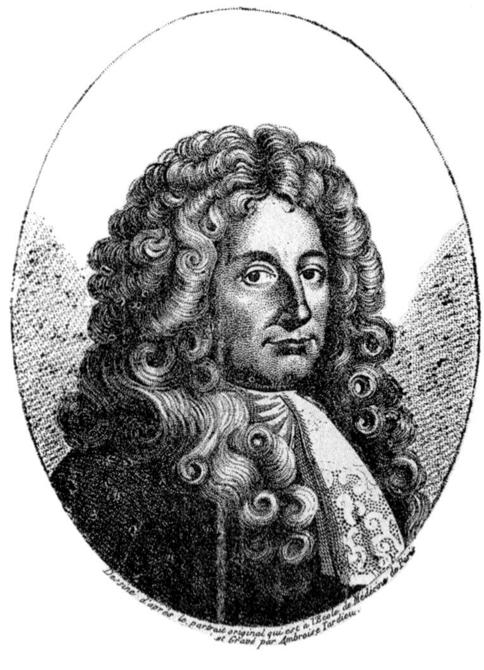

François Mauriceau

Selected Publications

Mauriceau F. *Traité des maladies de femmes grosses et de celles qui sont accouchées.* Paris; 1668.

Mauriceau F. The Diseases of Women with Child, and in Child-bed. (English translation, 2nd edn by Hugh Chamberlen) London: John Darby; 1683. Also published in: The Classics of Obstetrics and Gynecology Library. New York, NY: Gryphon Editions; 1992 (facsimile).

Mauriceau F. *Aphorismes touchant la grossesse, l'accouchément, les maladies et autres dispositions des femmes.* Paris: Laurent D'Houry; 1694.

Bibliography References

88, 113, 268, 298, 320, 347, 359, 448, 461, 648, 925, 983, 1261, 1304, 1408, 1475, 1595.

Maygrier, Jacques Pierre (1771–1835)

Obstetric Atlas

Jacques Pierre Maygrier was born in Angoulême, France, on 11 June 1771. He started his medical career as an army surgeon and later went to Paris as a pupil of Antoine Dubois (1756–1837), the accoucheur of Empress Marie Louise, wife of Napoleon. Maygrier developed an extensive obstetric practice in Paris and published a number of anatomical and obstetric texts. His major work was 'the best and most magnificent obstetrical atlas of the nineteenth century': *Nouvelles demonstrations d'accouchemens.* It was released in 20 parts between 1822 and 1827. The 80 copper plates were made from drawings by the noted Parisian artist,

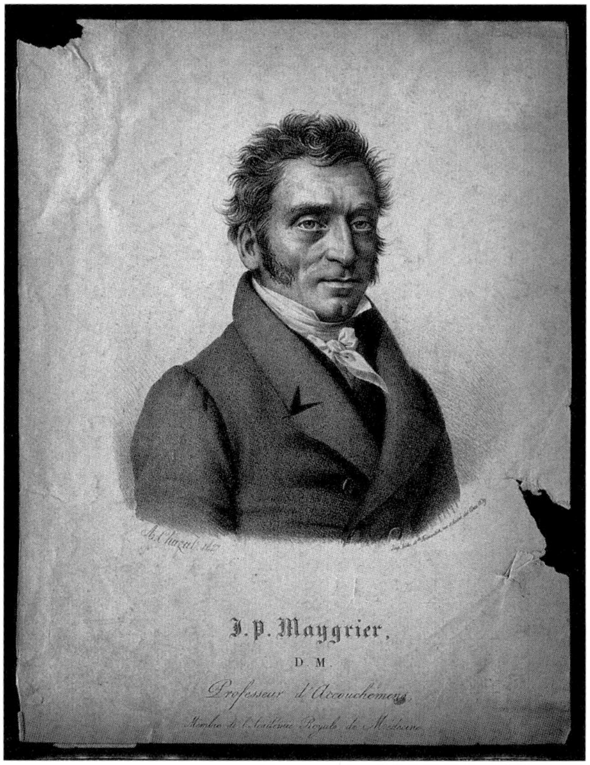

Jacques Pierre Maygrier

Antoine Chazal (1793–1854). The book, which also included a detailed obstetric text, was popular and translated into both Spanish and Dutch. The first of six English editions appeared in 1833, translated by the New York physician, Sidney Doane (1808–1852).

Maygrier also spoke in favour of caesarean section in selected cases, at a time when the operation was almost always fatal:

> *Employed with discernment, and when the female can support its formidable dangers, it may be perfectly successful, and then becomes a brilliant triumph of art over powerless nature.*

He also showed an entertaining turn of phrase with his description of the technique for delivery of the fetus at caesarean section:

> *The operator then introduces one hand within the uterus, seeks for the child's feet, which he grasps and delivers with celerity and prudence.*

Jacques Pierre Maygrier, as professor of obstetrics and gynaecology in the faculty of medicine at Paris, continued to teach and practice at the Hôtel Dieu. He died in Paris in 1835.

Selected Publications

Maygrier JP. *Nouvelles demonstrations d'accouchemens.* Paris: Bechet; 1822–7.

Maygrier JP. *Midwifery Illustrated.* Translated by Sidney Doane. New York, NY: Harper and Brothers; 1833.

Bibliography References

102, 347, 676, 1261, 1291, 1408, 1631, 1734.

Maylard, Alfred Ernest (1854–1947)

Maylard Incision

Ernest Maylard was one of the pioneer abdominal surgeons in Britain during the late nineteenth and early twentieth centuries. At this time most operations were carried out through vertical, usually midline, incisions. Maylard wrote of his conversion to the transverse incision:

> *It was in 1901 that my thoughts were first directed to the possible advantages of the transverse incision through the abdominal parietes. And it came about in this way. When forced to add a transverse incision to a vertical one, in order to obtain the necessary exposure and room for deeper work, I noted that the transverse cut healed quicker, and when healed was firmer than the median vertical one.*

In modern texts the Maylard incision is described as a transverse incision through all layers: skin, rectus sheath and rectus muscles. In fact, Maylard only advocated cutting the muscles on a selective basis:

> *If sufficient room can be obtained by separation of the recti muscles after division of their sheaths, the fibres of these muscles should not be cut; and when division is necessary it should be carried out obliquely, so as, if possible, to leave some of the outer fibres undivided.*

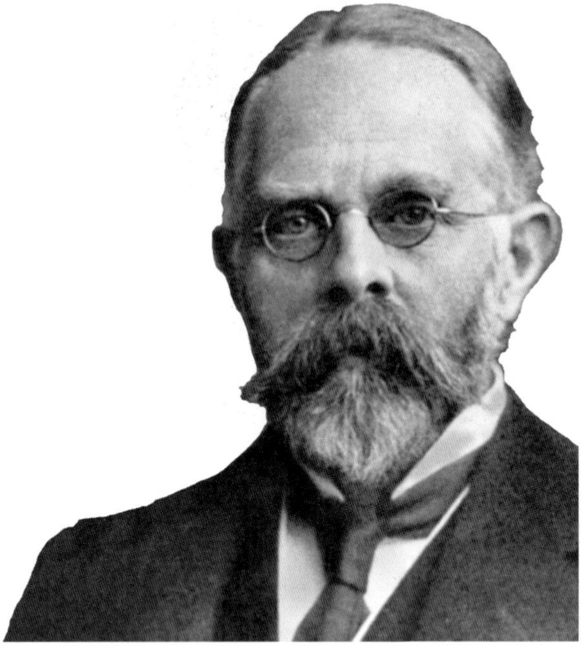

Alfred Ernest Maylard

Thus, in cases without the need to divide the rectus muscles, the incision was similar to that proposed by Hermann Pfannenstiel in 1900. Maylard acknowledged that when speed was essential the vertical, midline incision was required. His advocacy for the transverse incision was based on a greatly reduced incidence of postoperative incisional hernia and that such incisions 'afford more room for the treatment of pelvic diseases'. Maylard's incision is similar to those developed by Bernard Bardenheuer and Alwin Mackenrodt.

Alfred Ernest Maylard graduated from Guy's Hospital medical school, London, in 1879. He spent another year in that school as a house surgeon and demonstrator in anatomy. In 1880 he moved to Glasgow as an assistant surgeon in the Western Infirmary. He visited Vienna and other European clinics to learn the latest techniques in abdominal surgery. When the new Victoria Infirmary of Glasgow was opened in 1890, Maylard was the first surgeon appointed, and he served with distinction until his retirement 30 years later.

He spent his final years in Peebles, Scotland, about which he wrote a book.

Selected Publications

Maylard AE. Direction of abdominal incisions. *BMJ* 1907; 2: 895–901.

Bibliography References

274, 714, 1006, 1432, 1433.

McCall, Milton Lawrence (1911–1963)

McCall Culdeplasty

The development of an enterocoele following vaginal hysterectomy is usually the result of inadequate obliteration of the pouch of Douglas at the time of operation. In 1957 Milton McCall described his posterior culdeplasty to prevent or treat enterocoele formation at the time of vaginal hysterectomy:

> *There has been a tremendous increase recently in the number of vaginal hysterectomies performed in this country. This fact makes the problem of enterocele more significant than ever, since this operation is done frequently without giving adequate support to the cul-de-sac area. In keeping with modern emphasis upon early diagnosis and treatment in medicine, the author believes that it is of great importance to ferret out and treat the early enterocele. It is with this in mind that a new technic is described although large enteroceles have been treated successfully with this method.*

McCall outlined the principles of his technique as follows:

> *This operation is performed from below following vaginal hysterectomy and takes place within the lower portion of the peritoneal cavity. It is a posterior culdeplasty whereby the relaxed cul-de-sac of Douglas is suspended and obliterated between the uterosacral ligaments without dissection of or excision of the hernial sac.*
>
> *The posterior culdeplasty is a simple procedure which obliterates the redundant cul-de-sac of Douglas by a series of continuous sutures so as to suspend it by the uterosacral ligaments, which then are brought together in the midline.*

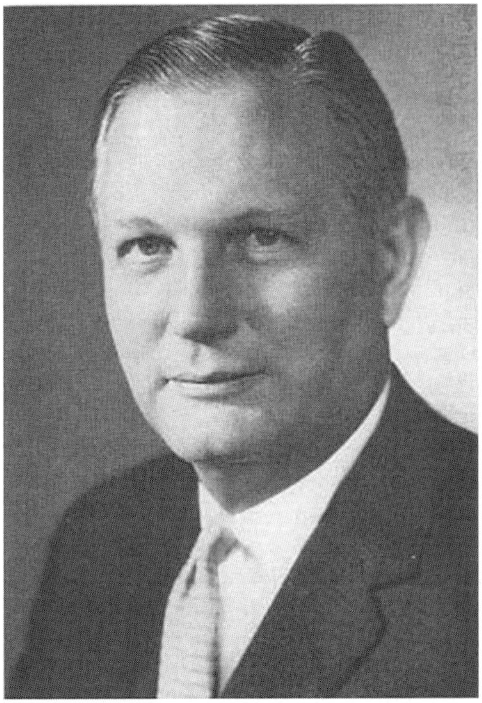

Milton Lawrence McCall

McCall emphasised that, properly performed, his technique did not shorten the vagina. In his 1957 publication he reported that he did the first operation in 1943.

Milton Lawrence McCall was born in Peru, Indiana. He graduated in medicine from Indiana University in 1939. His residency in obstetrics and gynaecology was completed in the Kensington Hospital for Women in Philadelphia. He then entered private practice in the city, changing to the academic stream in 1950 with his appointment as assistant professor at Jefferson Medical College. At this point in his career McCall carried out much original research on eclampsia. He travelled from hospital to hospital at all hours measuring cerebral blood flow in eclamptic patients and the effect of various hypotensive agents on this flow. In 1954 he accepted the position of professor and head of the department of obstetrics and gynaecology at Louisiana State University in New Orleans. It was from this post that he published his work on culdeplasty. In 1959 he moved to the chairmanship of obstetrics and gynaecology at the University of Pittsburgh and Magee Women's Hospital. Widely respected and at the height of his abilities, McCall became ill in the summer of 1963. He had advanced lung cancer and died at home on October 8 1963, in his fifty-third year.

Selected Publications

McCall ML. Posterior culdeplasty: Surgical correction of enterocele during vaginal hysterectomy; a preliminary report. *Obstet Gynecol* 1957; 10: 595–602.

Bibliography References

536, 672, 1086, 1219, 1360, 1485.

McCormick, Katharine Dexter (1875–1967)

Oral Contraception

Katharine McCormick, along with Margaret Sanger, made up the formidable duo that convinced Gregory Pincus to develop the oral contraceptive pill. In the final seven years of its development it was McCormick who provided the financial support and sustained pressure on Pincus to see the pill through to Food and Drug Administration (FDA) approval.

Katharine Dexter was born on 27 August 1875 in Dexter, Michigan, a town near Chicago founded by her grandfather. Her father was a prominent lawyer in Chicago, descended from a charter member of the United States Senate and a long line of Harvard-trained lawyers. Her mother was a school teacher. She was 14 when her father died suddenly from a heart attack, and four years later her older brother succumbed to meningitis. As only the second female student at the Massachusetts Institute of Technology (MIT), she graduated in 1904 with a degree in biology. Shortly after graduation she married Stanley McCormick, the son and heir to the International Harvester Company fortune. Within two years of their marriage Stanley became overtly psychotic and was declared legally insane with schizophrenia. Until his death in 1947, Katharine McCormick organised extensive private treatment for her husband and funding of neuro-psychiatric research, all to no avail.

In 1909, she turned her attention to the American woman's suffrage movement, funding, organising, speaking and marching. She became vice-president and treasurer of the National American Woman Suffrage Association and continued this work until they achieved the vote in 1920.

McCormick and Sanger met in 1917 and thereafter she continued to support Sanger's work and, later, the Planned Parenthood Federation. However, until her husband's death in 1947 she was mainly concerned with his care and the direction of neuro-psychiatric research. Ultimately, McCormick became very wealthy as the sole beneficiary of the family's inheritance and, after a legal battle, the McCormick estate.

Thus, by the early 1950s she was in control of her own considerable fortune and had decided to give her full support to birth control research. She wrote to Margaret Sanger, asking, 'What are the present prospects for birth control research, and by research I mean contraceptive research'. Among other things, Sanger suggested support of Pincus' work at the Worcester Foundation for Experimental Biology. In 1952 McCormick moved from California to Boston and began her single-minded pursuit of the 'perfect contraceptive': 'freezing in Boston for the pill', as she put it.

In June 1952, Sanger and McCormick arrived at the Worcester Foundation to interview Pincus and convince him to direct all of his efforts to developing an effective oral contraceptive. After an initial tour of the facility and observance of pleasantries, it was the 77-year-old McCormick who led the discussion. Could Pincus produce an oral contraceptive pill? Pincus replied that, while he could not guarantee it, he thought it was feasible. Would he be willing to direct all his research efforts to this end and what would it cost for him to commit to this project? Pincus gave an estimate of $125,000 ($1.1 million in 2017 dollars). McCormick wrote a cheque for $40,000 and said the rest would follow shortly. It did, along with a contract outlining the conditions of support, which included a bimonthly written progress report from Pincus.

By this time Sanger had become quite frail after a series of heart attacks, starting in 1949. She had retired to Arizona and, other than correspondence, withdrew from active participation. Thus, it was Katharine McCormick who provided, not only the money, but the sustained pressure and sense of urgency on Pincus and, later, on John Rock. With her background in science she understood the basis of Pincus' research and kept up with the relevant literature. Periodically she would arrive at the Worcester Foundation in her chauffeur-driven Rolls Royce with suggestions and encouragement.

Pincus acknowledged that her support went beyond the financial and was impressed by her grasp of the science involved. He acted on some of her suggestions for improved organisation during the project. As he observed, 'She was tall and carried herself like a ramrod. Little old woman she was not. She was a grenadier'.

She met any reasonable requests for funding, and over the next seven years, until the pill received FDA approval in 1960, her financial support totalled $2 million ($18 million in 2017 dollars). During this time there was no funding from any government agency or pharmaceutical company (mainly because of the restrictive laws against birth control). The laboratory research and clinical trials were funded entirely by Katharine McCormick.

When the pill received FDA approval, she was 85 and, while continuing to fund the Worcester Foundation, she directed her philanthropic attention to improving educational opportunities at her alma mater (MIT), where she financed the construction of two women's dormitories.

Katharine McCormick died on 28 December 1967, age 92. In her will she bequeathed $1 million to the Worcester Foundation, $5 million to the Planned Parent Federation and $5 million to Stanford University to assist female medical students. While she was a forceful presence when fulfilling a project, she kept a low public profile and her death was not recorded with an obituary in any of the major newspapers. However, Pincus dedicated his 1965 autobiography, *The Control of Fertility*, to 'Mrs Stanley McCormick because of her steadfast faith in scientific inquiry and her unswerving encouragement of human dignity'.

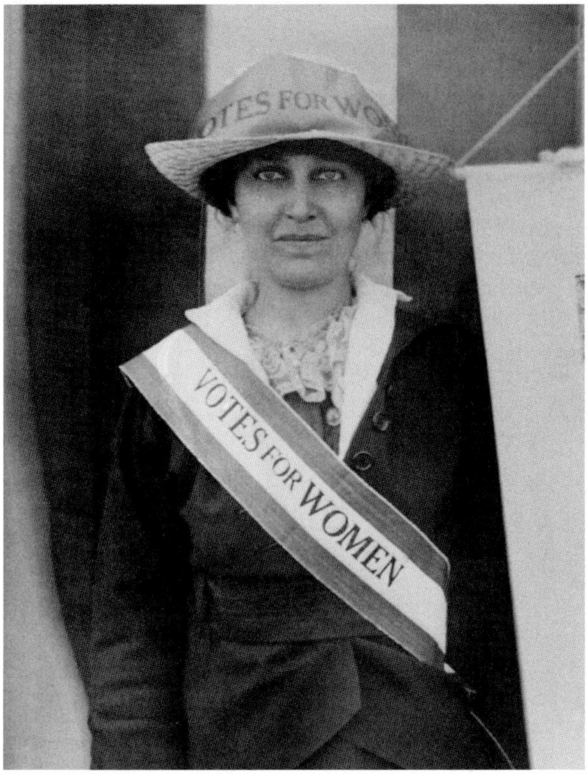

Katharine Dexter McCormick

Selected Publications

Pincus G. *The Control of Fertility*. New York, NY: Academic Press; 1965

Fields A. *Katharine Dexter McCormick: Pioneer for Women's Rights*. Westport, CT: Praeger; 2003.

Bibliography References

31, 101, 267, 402, 433, 516, 817, 866, 981, 1027, 1209, 1297, 1381, 1498.

McDonald, Ian Alexander (1922–1990)

McDonald Cervical Suture

Ian McDonald devised a simple purse-string suture for cervical incompetence in the second trimester of pregnancy. In so doing he simplified the procedure initially developed by Vithal Shirodkar. He first used it during his training at the North Middlesex Hospital, London, in 1952. Following his publication on the procedure in 1957, the simplicity of the method ensured its widespread adoption. He described his technique as follows:

> *A purse-string suture of No. 4 Mersilk on a Mayo needle is inserted around the exo-cervix as high as possible to approximate to the level of the internal os. This is at the junction of the rugose vagina and smooth cervix. Five or six bites with the needle are made, with special attention to the stitches behind the cervix. These are difficult to insert and must be deep. If the ligature pulls out later, it is always from this portion, the silk remaining attached to the anterior lip. The stitch is pulled tight enough to close the internal os, the knot being made in front of the cervix and the ends left long enough to facilitate subsequent division.*

Ian Alexander McDonald was born in Perth, Western Australia, and educated at Geelong College and the University of Melbourne. He completed post-graduate training in obstetrics and gynaecology at the Royal Melbourne Hospital and Queen Charlotte's, Chelsea and North Middlesex hospitals in London. In 1952 he returned to the Royal Melbourne Hospital as assistant gynaecologist and, from 1966 until his retirement in 1982, was gynaecologist-in-chief. In

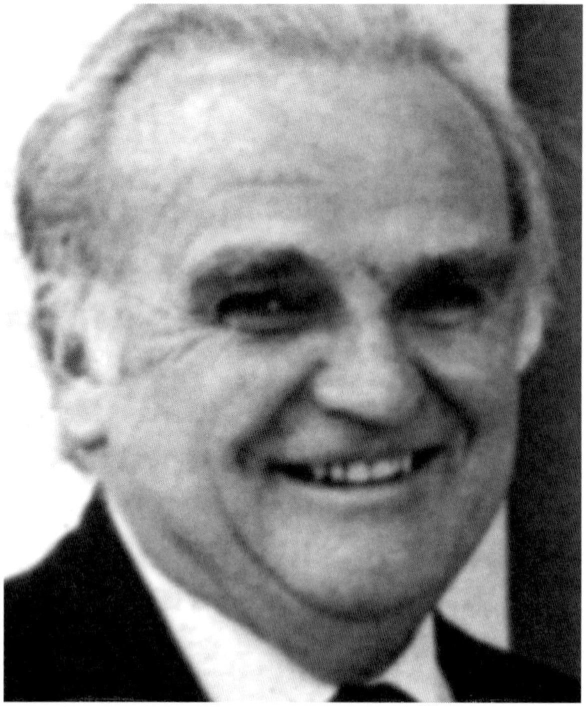

Ian Alexander McDonald

1975 he was elected President of the Royal Australian and New Zealand College of Obstetricians and Gynaecologists. He died on 4 September 1990 after surgery for an abdominal aortic aneurysm.

Selected Publications

McDonald IA. Suture of the cervix for inevitable miscarriage. *J Obstet Gynaecol Br Emp* 1957; 64: 346–50.

McDonald IA. Incompetent cervix as a cause of recurrent abortion. *J Obstet Gynaecol Br Commonw* 1963; 70: 105–8.

Bibliography References

572, 1015, 1240.

McDowell, Ephraim (1771–1830)

Ovariotomy

In the early morning of Christmas Day 1809, Ephraim McDowell, a surgeon with a marked tendency to prayer, was preparing for his and the world's first ovariotomy. He uttered what must have been one of his most ardent pleas for celestial guidance:

> *Direct me, oh! God, in performing this operation, for I am but an instrument in thy hands, and am but thy servant, and if it is thy will, oh! spare this poor afflicted woman.*

The woman in question was 47-year-old Mrs Jane Todd Crawford, suffering much pain from a huge ovarian cyst. McDowell was consulted on 13 December 1809 by two local doctors in Motley's Glen, Kentucky, who thought she was in labour with twins. Having made the diagnosis of an ovarian cyst, McDowell explained that ovariotomy had been proposed in such cases but never performed and that most surgeons thought it would be fatal: 'But notwithstanding this, if she thought herself prepared to die, I would take the lump from her if she would come to Danville'. In her pain and desperation Jane Crawford accepted: 'She appeared willing to undergo an experiment'. Even after her acceptance of this early and brutally frank version of informed consent, Mrs Crawford still had to 'come to Danville'. This was a 60-mile journey by horseback on trails through rough Kentucky terrain. The courageous women 'performed the journey in a few days on horseback', while resting her protuberant abdomen on the pommel of the saddle. The resultant bruising of her abdominal wall caused McDowell to choose a paramedian rather than the midline incision he used in later cases.

After her journey Mrs Crawford rested for six days. McDowell chose to operate the next Sunday, which happened to be Christmas Day, so that the prayers of the church would be with him in full force. He performed the operation in the front room of his house with the assistance of his recently qualified physician nephew, James McDowell:

> *I made an incision . . . continuing the same nine inches in length . . . The tumor then appeared full in view, but was so large that we could not take it away entire. We put a strong ligature around the Fallopian tube near the uterus, and then cut open the tumor, which was the ovarium and fimbrious part of the Fallopian tube very much enlarged. We took out 15 lbs of dirty gelatinous-looking substance, after which we cut through the Fallopian tube and extracted the sac, which weighed 7 lb and one-half . . . we closed the external opening with the interrupted suture, leaving out at the lower end of the incision the ligature which surrounded the Fallopian tube.*

The operation took 25 minutes and in that pre-anaesthetic era the patient apparently 'occupied herself repeating the Psalms', of which no doubt McDowell approved. She recovered uneventfully and later made the trip back to her log cabin in Motley's Glen. In that same year, in another log cabin 35 miles away, Abraham Lincoln was born. He later married Jane Crawford's cousin. In 1932 the road from Motley's Glen to Danville was named the *Jane Todd Crawford Trail* by the Kentucky State Highway Department, in honour of the women who was as much a courageous pioneer as her surgeon. Jane Crawford died at the age of 78, outliving her ovariotomist by 11 years.

McDowell did not report this case for several years. He carried out two more successful ovariotomies in 1813 and 1816, publishing the three cases as one report in 1817.

Ephraim McDowell, the ninth of 11 children, was born near Lexington, Virginia of Ulster-Scots descent. His great-grandfather, also Ephraim, helped close the gates of Londonderry against the Catholic army of King James II in 1688 and later fought at the Battle of the Boyne. At the age of 56 he emigrated to Pennsylvania with his wife and four children. He was reputedly almost seven feet tall, with a 'terrible countenance', and lived to be 100 years old.

The younger Ephraim was initially apprenticed to a surgeon in Kentucky, Dr Alex Humphreys, who was an Edinburgh graduate. In 1793 McDowell went to Edinburgh and was taught by the surgeon John Bell. At that time ovarian cysts were refractory to all medical treatment. Tapping was carried out but could be fatal due to haemorrhage, peritonitis and perforation of adherent bowel. In his lectures Bell suggested that laparotomy and removal of the whole cyst was the only chance for cure, although the potential surgical risks at that time were prohibitive. McDowell did not have the financial means to remain in Edinburgh to complete his medical degree, so he returned to Danville, Kentucky in 1795. He became an able surgeon with experience in herniotomy and lithotomy. In 1812 he performed a successful lithotomy operation on young James Polk who, in 1845, became President of the United States.

McDowell sent a copy of his paper to John Bell in Edinburgh. However, Bell was in Italy, where he became ill and died. His successor in Edinburgh, John Lizars, received the paper and some years later attempted ovariotomy with poor results.

McDowell married the daughter of the first governor of Kentucky, by whom he had eight children. He died at the age of 59 of 'an acute attack of inflammation of the stomach'. Ironically this may have been acute appendicitis, later easily remedied when laparotomy, which he was the first to perform,

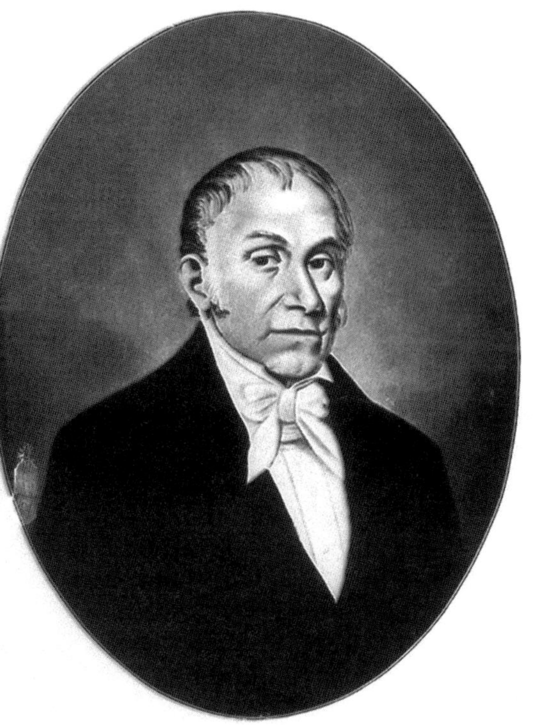

Ephraim McDowell

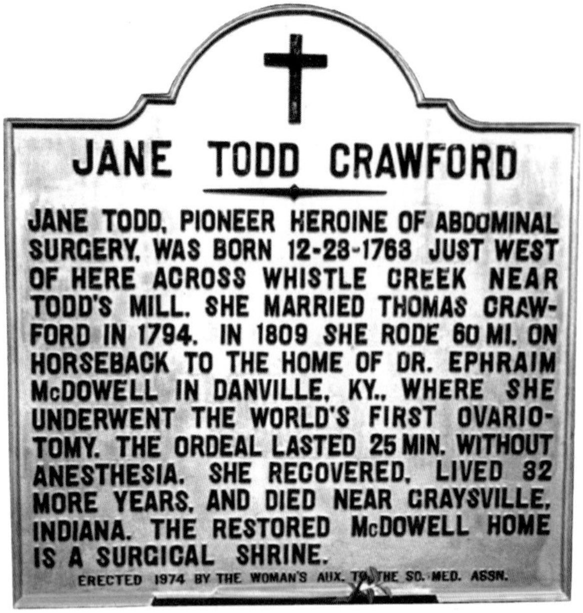

Roadside plaque in Kentucky to commemorate Jane Todd Crawford

became safe. As the gravity of his illness became apparent, his doctors advised him to settle his affairs. In typical fashion, God-fearing to the end, he replied: 'All my earthly affairs are satisfactorily arranged, and, what is of more importance than all else, my peace with God is made'.

McDowell's house, which was built in the 1790s and where the operation took place, has been restored by the Kentucky State Medical Association and, as the McDowell House Museum, is open to the public.

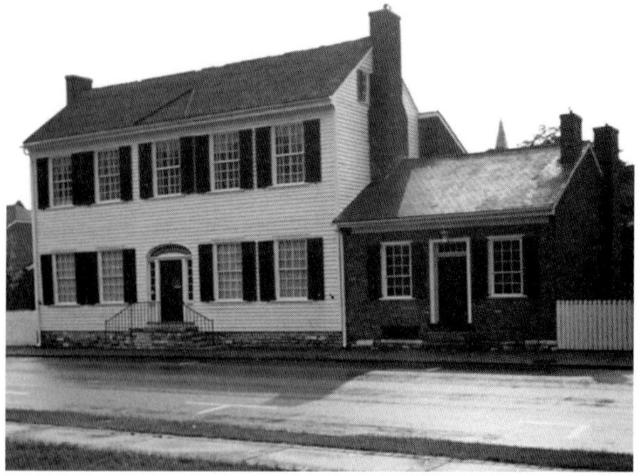

Ephraim McDowell's house

Selected Publications

McDowell E. Three cases of extirpation of diseased ovaria. *Eclect Repertory Analyt Rev Philadelphia* 1817; 7: 242–4.

McDowell E. Observations on diseased ovaria. *Eclect Repertory Analyt Rev Philadelphia* 1819; 9: 546–53.

Bibliography References

346, 356, 496, 518, 519, 599, 651–653, 663, 684, 740, 764, 769, 930, 951, 1018, 1028, 1351, 1419, 1454, 1496, 1497, 1595, 1642, 1746.

McRoberts, William Alexander (1914–2006)

McRoberts' Manoeuvre

The solutions to medical problems have often been forged in desperate circumstances. Thus it was with the development of McRoberts' manoeuvre for the safe delivery of the infant with shoulder dystocia. On Thanksgiving Day 1942, William McRoberts was a junior resident obstetrician alone on duty at the Philadelphia Lying-in Hospital. As he later recounted:

> *A primigravida was admitted in active labour and made rapid progress. When the head was visible with contractions I applied low forceps as we were taught. On removal of the forceps the chin disappeared into the mother's anus. I did not realise then what a problem I had. Forty minutes later, with great difficulty I delivered a dead 12-pound baby. I vowed then that it would never happen to me again.*

Shortly after this, Charles Woods published his screw manoeuvre for managing shoulder dystocia. McRoberts used this with good results for many years. However, in the mid-1950s he encountered a case that was refractory to Woods' manoeuvre. He remembered working with a gynaecologist who insisted on his assistants holding the patient's legs in marked hip flexion, which he claimed gave better surgical access at vaginal hysterectomy. Thus, McRoberts flexed the woman's hips sharply on her abdomen and was gratified to find immediate resolution of the shoulder dystocia. He taught this manoeuvre to generations of residents in training but never published the technique. Upon his retirement from clinical practice in 1982, two of his former residents wrote up the method and named it for McRoberts. The technique was published the following year and since its dissemination in the literature has become the manoeuvre of first choice in shoulder dystocia. Its great advantages are simplicity, effectiveness and absence of neonatal injury. The manoeuvre straightens the lumbo-sacral angulation and sweeps the symphysis cephalad. Although it does not alter the pelvic diameters, it facilitates the descent of the posterior shoulder below the sacral promontory and the rotation and descent of the anterior shoulder.

As always, there is little new under the sun, and a similar manoeuvre had been described by Bonnaire and Bué, of Paris and Lille, respectively, in 1899.

William McRoberts Jr was born on 11 August 1914 to missionary parents, an American father and Canadian mother, in Taichowfu, China. He returned to America at the age of five. He attended Oberlin College in Ohio and medical school at the University of Pittsburgh, graduating in 1940. Residency training in obstetrics and gynaecology followed at the Pennsylvania Hospital, Philadelphia. From 1944 to 1982 he was in the private practice of obstetrics and gynaecology in Houston, Texas. He became chief of obstetrics at the Hermann Hospital and clinical professor at the University of Texas Medical School at Houston.

McRoberts was the first to publish a series of cases with supine hypotensive syndrome in the English literature. He described six cases of what he called 'postural shock in pregnancy'. The term supine hypotensive syndrome was coined two years later.

Outside medicine McRoberts' main interest has been music. He had a well-trained voice as a student, and this talent helped pay some of his university tuition. He was also trained in violin and piano and continued these endeavours in his retirement. William McRoberts died on 18 August 2006.

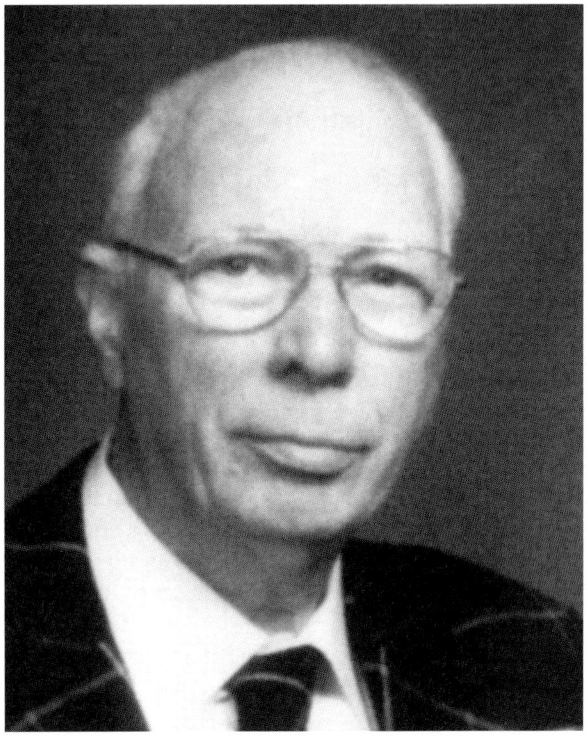

William Alexander McRoberts

Selected Publications

Bonnaire C, Bué E. Influence de la position sur la forme et les dimensions du bassin. *Ann Gynécol Obstet* 1899; 52: 296–310.

Gonik B, Stringer CA, Held B. An alternative maneuver for management of shoulder dystocia. *Am J Obstet Gynecol* 1983; 145: 882–4.

McRoberts WA. Postural shock in pregnancy. *Am J Obstet Gynecol* 1951; 62: 627–32.

Bibliography References

99, 113–116.

Meigs, Joe Vincent (1892–1963)

Meigs' Syndrome

The combination of ovarian fibroma, ascites and pleural effusion was clearly described by at least four other authors – Otto von Spiegelberg, CJ Cullingworth, Albert Demons and Lawson Tait – before Meigs.

Joe Meigs first made reference to the syndrome in 1934, describing three cases in his book *Tumors of the Female Pelvic Organs*. He became aware of the condition when reviewing charts of all patients with pelvic tumours in the Massachusetts General Hospital in preparation for this book. In 1937 Rhoads and Terrell published a case report and suggested the term 'Meigs' syndrome'. Meigs followed this up with six publications on the topic over the next 17 years, securing the eponymous link.

Meigs laid down four criteria for the syndrome:

> *As the first characteristic we must have a fibroma or a fibroma-like tumor (including thecomas, granulosa cell tumors, and Brenner tumors).*
>
> *Second, this tumor must be accompanied by ascites . . . the fluid may be of very great or of small amount, but it must be there.*
>
> *Third, there must be fluid in the chest . . . most often found in the right thoracic cavity but can occur in the left, and even in both sides . . .*
>
> *Fourth, the removal of the benign solid tumor must relieve the patient of her ascites and chest fluid . . .*
>
> *It is not necessary that the fluid always be clear and yellow; it can be bloody or serosanguinous, but this is not common.*

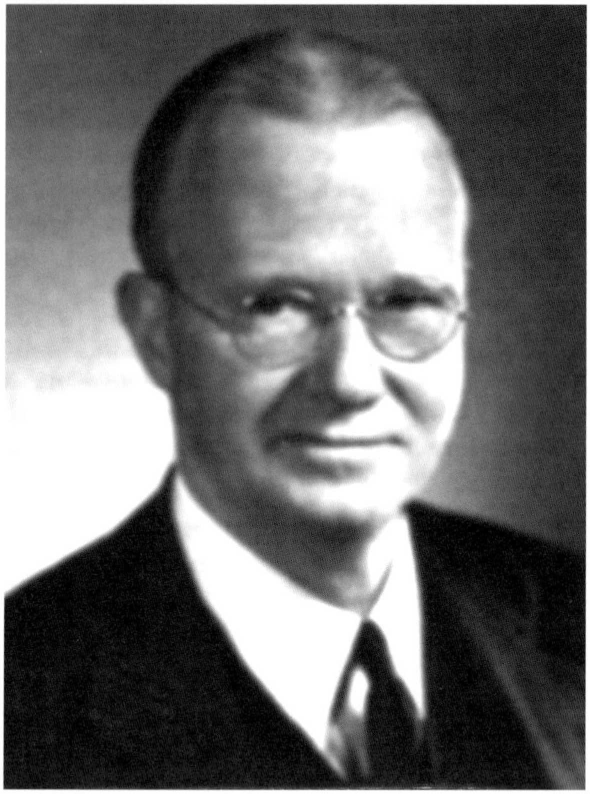

Joe Vincent Meigs

Meigs was born in Lowell, Massachusetts, the son of a physician. He was distantly related to the Charles Meigs of Philadelphia who spoke out so vehemently against the use of anaesthesia in obstetrics and opposed the theory of the contagious nature of puerperal sepsis. Joe Meigs graduated from Princeton in 1915 and attained his MD from Harvard in 1919. His training was mainly surgical, but he became director of gynaecology at the Massachusetts General Hospital and clinical professor of gynaecology at Harvard Medical School. He died on his seventy-first birthday from coronary occlusion while flying home to Boston, having just presented a paper at a meeting in Rochester, New York.

Selected Publications

Cullingworth CJ. Fibroma of both ovaries. *Trans Obstet Soc London* 1879; 21: 276.

Demons A. Épanchements pleurétiques compliquant les kystes de l'ovaire. *Bull Soc Chirug Paris* 1887; 13: 771–6.

Meigs JV. *Tumors of the Female Pelvic Organs*. New York, NY: Macmillan Co; 1934, pp. 262–3.

Meigs JV. Fibroma of the ovary with ascites and hydrothorax: Meig's Syndrome. *Am J Obstet Gynecol* 1954; 67: 962–87.

Rhoads JE, Terrell AW. Ovarian fibroma with ascites and hydrothorax (Meigs' Syndrome): Report of a case. *JAMA* 1937; 109: 1684–7.

Spiegelberg O. Fibrom des Eierstockes von enormer Grosse. *Monatschr Geburtsh Frauenk* 1866; 28: 415–25.

Tait L. On the occurrence of pleural effusion in association with disease of the abdomen. *Med Chir Trans* 1892; 75: 109–18.

Bibliography References

134, 801, 947, 949, 1033, 1480.

Mendelson, Curtis Lester (1913–2002)

Mendelson's Syndrome

At a meeting of the New York Obstetrical Society on 11 December 1945, Curtis Mendelson first presented his study on aspiration of stomach contents associated with general anaesthesia in the pregnant woman. He had reviewed all cases at the New York Lying-in Hospital from 1932 to 1945 and found an incidence of 1.5 per 1,000 deliveries. In doing so, he differentiated between those aspirating liquid as opposed to solid vomitus. He followed his clinical review with experimental studies on rabbits, introducing various substances into their lungs:

> *Following aspiration of liquid containing hydrochloric acid (tenth normal hydrochloric acid or unneutralized liquid vomitus) the animals develop a syndrome similar in many respects to that observed in the human following liquid aspiration ...*
>
> *This study reveals that two entirely different syndromes may follow aspiration. Aspiration of solid food usually produces the well-known picture of laryngeal or bronchial obstruction ...*
>
> *Aspiration of liquid material produces an asthma-like syndrome with distinct clinical, roentgenologic, and pathologic features. Apparently this syndrome has escaped recognition, for to the author's knowledge it has not been previously described ...*
>
> *The animal experiments indicate that hydrochloric acid is responsible for the changes described. The acid produces a bronchiolar spasm and a peri-bronchiolar congestive and exudative reaction interfering with normal intra-pulmonary circulation to the extent that cardiac failure may develop.*

He found a less intense clinical and radiological pulmonary reaction with neutral liquids such as water, normal saline and neutralised liquid vomitus. Mendelson pointed out the dangers of oral intake during labour but foresaw the danger of concentrated hydrochloric acid remaining in the stomach. He thus advocated gastric emptying or giving an oral alkaline solution prior to anaesthesia. This landmark publication helped highlight the dangers of general anaesthesia in obstetrics.

Curtis Lester Mendelson was born on 4 September 1913 in New York City. He did his undergraduate degree at the University of Michigan and took his MD at Cornell University in 1938. His postgraduate training in obstetrics and gynaecology was

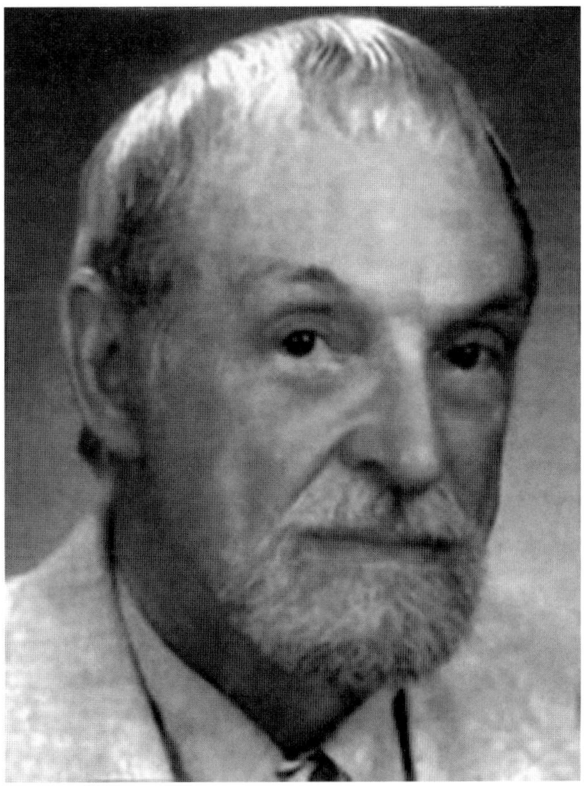

Curtis Lester Mendelson

undertaken at the New York Lying-in and New York Polyclinic hospitals. He later served on the staff of these institutions and became associate professor of obstetrics and gynaecology at Cornell University. From 1950 to 1959 he directed the cardiac clinic at the New York Lying-in Hospital. In 1959, at the age of 46, Mendelson gave up his high-profile clinical and teaching appointments in New York and moved to the Bahamas, where he practised until 1990, when he retired and moved to Florida. Soon after his arrival in the Bahamas, Mendelson set a record by catching a 3.6 metre, 225 kg blue marlin from a three-metre dingy.

Mendelson was a member of the English Channel Swimming Association. He made two attempts to swim the channel from France to England. In the last swim, in 1970, he spent 12 hours in the water and was within sight of the white cliffs of Dover when hypothermia thwarted his attempt to become the oldest person to make the crossing. He attributed this setback to training in the warm Bahamian waters and minimal body fat. Curtis Mendelson died in Florida on 13 October 2002.

Selected Publications

Mendelson CL. The aspiration of stomach contents into the lungs during obstetric anesthesia. *Am J Obstet Gynecol* 1946; 52: 191–205.

Bibliography References

240, 910, 975, 1485.

Menon, Krishna (1908–1988)

Lytic Cocktail for Eclampsia

After a 25-year study of various medical regimes used in the management of eclampsia, Krishna Menon presented his conclusions in a lecture delivered at the University College Hospital, London on 30 May 1960. He spoke from a level of experience gained by few, as his hospital had 12,000 deliveries a year with a 1–2 per cent incidence of eclampsia. Menon presented his results using a 'lytic cocktail' of phenothiazines and pethidine (meperidine). This entailed an intravenous infusion of pethidine in 20% dextrose and intramuscular chlorpromazine and diethazine every four hours. He reported a low maternal mortality of 2.2% in 402 eclamptics. Menon also showed that maternal mortality increased the longer delivery was delayed and advocated the greater use of caesarean section in selected cases:

> *I conclude that the combination of chlorpromazine, diethazine and pethidine constitutes a form of conservative therapy which is reasonably effective in the control of convulsions . . . However, I believe that if within a reasonable time the convulsions cannot be controlled by this treatment LUS caesarean section under local anaesthesia or artificial rupture of membranes in the rest could supplement with advantage the conservative regime.*

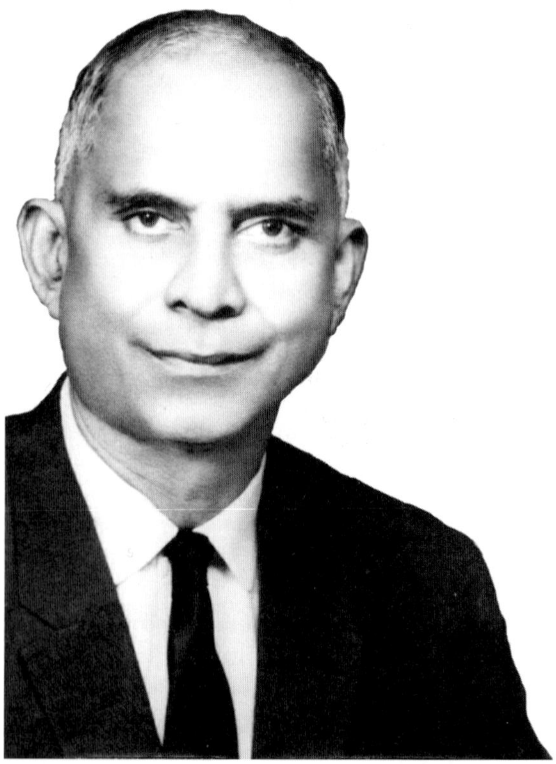

Krishna Menon

Krishna Menon received his medical degree at the Medical College of Madras in 1932. He did postgraduate work in obstetrics and gynaecology in Madras and served in the Indian Medical Service in the Second World War, attaining the rank of lieutenant-colonel. He became professor of obstetrics and gynaecology at the Madras and Stanley Medical Colleges and, in 1957, the director and professor of the Institute of Obstetrics and Gynaecology at the Madras Medical College and Government Hospital for Women and Children. Menon's teaching and writing influenced a generation of Indian obstetricians. He also achieved international recognition, serving on World Health Organization committees and as a visiting professor in Britain and the United States. Menon became president of the Federation of Obstetrical and Gynaecological Societies of India in 1961, an honorary fellow of the Royal College of Obstetricians and Gynaecologists and, in 1973, was awarded the title *'Padma shri'* by the President of India. He was regarded as a cultured, modest and trustworthy man.

Selected Publications

Menon MKK. The evolution of the treatment of eclampsia. *J Obstet Gynaecol Br Cwlth* 1961; 68: 417–26.

Bibliography References

268, 1036, 1037.

Mercier, Louis Auguste (1811–1882)

Mercier's Bar

Gynaecologists who look in the bladder, and there are many who do, will be familiar with the transverse curved ridge joining the two ureteric orifices. This is known as Mercier's bar and represents the posterior border of the trigone. Soon after vulcanised rubber catheters were made, Mercier recommended an elbow bend or *coudé* near the tip to facilitate its insertion.

Louis Auguste Mercier was born in Plessis-Saint-Jean, France. He worked in Paris as a specialist in urogenital surgery and carried out detailed anatomical studies of the bladder and urethra. He died in Paris.

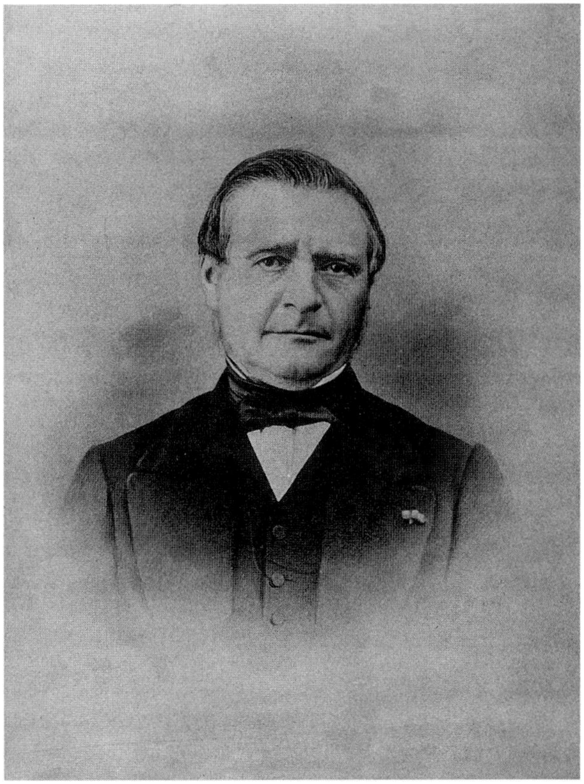

Louis Auguste Mercier

Selected Publications

Mercier LA. *Recherches anatomiques, pathologiques et thérapeutiques sur les valvules du col de la vessie, cause fréquente et peu connue de rétention d'urine, et sur leurs rapports avec les inflammations et les rétrécissements de l'urèthre*. Paris; 1848.

Mercier LA. Memoire sur les sondes elastique et particulièrement sur les sondes coudées et bicoudées. *Gaz Méd Paris* 1863; 18: 365–7.

Bibliography References

266, 716, 843, 1155.

Mettauer, John Peter (1787–1875)

Vesicovaginal Fistula

Although Marion Sims is rightly acknowledged as the most tenacious pioneer in the surgical cure of vesicovaginal fistula, he was not the first. In 1663, Hendrik van Roonhuyse (1622–1672) described a surgical technique to close vesicovaginal fistulae with sharpened swan's quills and waxed threads. About 1675, Johann Fatio (1649–1691) reported a cure using van Roonhuyse's technique. Only one of Fatio's medical texts survives, and that was published anonymously 60 years after his death. The first successful case in Britain was performed by Montague Gosset, a pupil of Astley Cooper, and reported in the *Lancet* of November 1834. Gosset used the knee-chest position, denuded the edges of the fistula and closed it with three sutures 'of gold wire, or, rather silver-gilt wire'. He left an indwelling silver urethral catheter and achieved a cure. However, he did not pursue this endeavour, nor did others take up the technique. In the United States the first surgical cure of vesicovaginal fistula was accomplished in August 1838 by a colourful character called John Peter Mettauer, although he did not report the case until 1840. He used wire sutures of lead and an indwelling silver catheter. By 1855 he reported a total of 27 cures.

In his first report Mettauer wrote, 'I operated in August, 1838. The opening had existed three years and was fully as large as half a dollar'. He described the operation as follows:

> *I was enabled to gain admission to the fistulous opening through a hollow conoidal speculum of proper size and length; through it the operation was executed. The margins at the opening were denuded with curved scissors, using hooks to draw out the portions to be removed. In closing the opening, I employed an instrument similar to the one I constructed for cleft palate, for introducing the ligatures from the vesical surface, and the leaden wire was used as the means of suture. Only one operation was required. Six sutures were introduced; and it was only necessary to tighten them once after the operation. In three weeks the wires were removed, and a firm and perfect union was found to have taken place between the edges of the opening. A short silver tube was kept constantly in the urethra for four weeks. The patient, at the date of this note, is well – nearly two years since the operation was performed.*

A year after Mettauer, George Hayward of Boston also achieved a cure using interrupted sutures of 'thread'. He published his report a year earlier than Mettauer.

John Peter Mettauer was born in Prince Edward County, Virginia. His father was a surgeon with the French army that helped George Washington's forces during the American revolution. Mettauer studied medicine and graduated from the University of Pennsylvania. He served in the war of 1812 and then returned to his birthplace, where he practised medicine until he died of pneumonia at 88 years of age. He had survived four marriages, from which issued six children. His three sons became doctors. In the era of

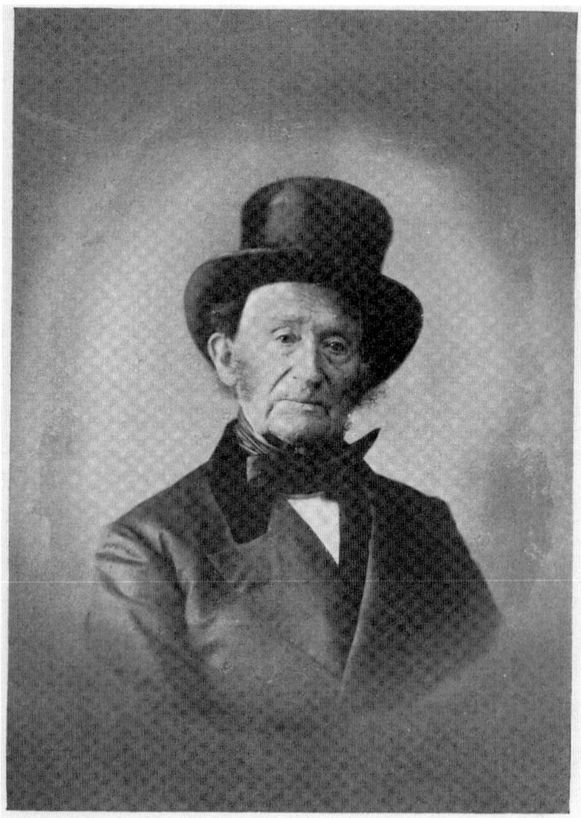

John Peter Mettauer

medical apprenticeship, he grouped his apprentices into a medical school called the Prince Edward Medical Institute. Mettauer was the entire faculty and taught all the courses. He was quite eccentric and always, inside or out, wore a twelve-inch stove-pipe hat. He was buried wearing his hat, accommodated in a custom-made coffin.

Selected Publications

Fatio J. *Helvetisch-Vernünftige Wehe-Mutter (Helvetic Reasonable Midwife)*. Basle: Johann Rudolph Imhof; 1752.

Gosset M. Calculus in the bladder-incontinence of urine: vesicovaginal fistula. Advantages of the gilt-wire suture. *Lancet* 1834; 1: 345–6.

Hayward G. Case of vesico-vaginal fistula, successfully treated by an operation. *Am J Med Sci* 1839; 24: 283–8.

Mettauer JP. Vesico-vaginal fistula. *Boston Med Surg J* 1840; 22: 154–5.

Mettauer JP. On vesico-vaginal fistula. *Am J Med Sci* 1847; 14: 117–21.

Mettauer JP. Contribution to practical surgery (vesico-vaginal fistula). *South Med Surg J* 1855; 11: 417–31.

Roonhuyse H. *Heel-konstige aanmerkkingen betreffende de gebreeken der vrouwen*. Amsterdam: T. Jacobsz; 1663.

Bibliography References

148, 156, 285, 621, 676, 810, 811, 834, 835, 1135, 1136, 1291, 1332, 1334, 1485, 1704, 1739, 1740.

Meyer, Robert Otto (1864–1947)

Endometriosis

Robert Meyer proposed one of the three main theories of pathogenesis of endometriosis, that of coelomic metaplasia. This is based on the rationale that during fetal development the primitive coelomic peritoneum forms the Müllerian ducts and may retain the ability to undergo metaplasia in response to appropriate stimuli. Meyer's theory is sometimes combined with John Sampson's to postulate that retrograde menstruation is the stimulus for peritoneal metaplasia to endometrial cells.

Robert Otto Meyer was born in Hanover, Germany, the third of five children. At 10 years of age he was treated for a traumatic knee infection and during the enforced bedrest learned to play the violin. He was a medical student in Strasburg, where his teachers included Adolf Kussmaul and Friedrich Von Recklinghausen, and among his fellow students were Carl Aschoff, and August von Wassermann. He qualified in 1888 and spent two years at Berlin in hospital jobs to prepare himself for five years as a country doctor in the small town of Dedeleban. Meyer then returned to the University of Berlin and the study of pathology and embryology along with the clinical practice of gynaecology. In 1908 he was given the rank of professor in the Berlin Charité Clinic and became a full-time pathologist. At the age of 66 he published two books totalling 1,700 pages, which he wrote by hand in three drafts.

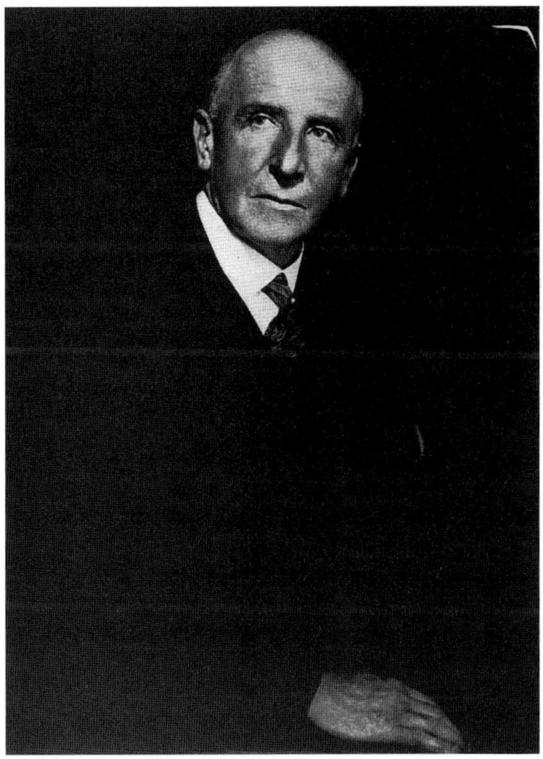

Robert Otto Meyer

Under pressure from the Nazis, he left Germany in 1939 for the United States. He worked at the University of Minnesota as an associate professor until 1946. He died on 12 December 1947 from stomach cancer in Minneapolis. In his final days he wrote to a friend, 'People make such a fuss about dying with cancer, but I don't see how it is any different from dying of some other disease'.

Selected Publications

Meyer R. Über den stand der frage der Adenomyositis und Adenomyome im allgemeinen und insbesondere über Adenomyositis Seroepithelialis und Adenomyometritis Sarcomatosa. *Zentralbl Gynäkol* 1919; 36: 745.

Bibliography References

1024, 1042, 1043, 1116, 1480.

Michaelis, Gustav Adolf (1798–1848)

Michaelis' Rhomboid

Gustav Michaelis was one of the first to demonstrate and write of the inaccuracy of external pelvimetry. It is therefore ironic that his eponymous link is with an external pelvic landmark: the sacrum. His study of the pelvis in a thousand cases led to his conclusion of the clinical uselessness of external pelvimetry. Among his early observations he noted the external features of the sacral surface in an effort to correlate this with internal pelvic dimensions:

> *In normal pelves the sacral surface forms an elongated quadrangle, bounded by the glutei maximi and by two lines, which connect the region of the posterior spines of the ilium with depression over the sacrum; and in the better body conformation this quadrangle approaches a rhomboid. In cases of abnormal body configuration, especially those with rachitic distortion, the upper angle becomes more obtuse at the depression over the sacrum and may even disappear completely, the sacral surface then presenting the appearance of a triangle.*

From his large study Michaelis concluded that only internal pelvic mensuration was valid, although certain marked external deformities could be correlated with pelvic contraction. He observed that pelvic contraction was more common than formerly recognised and advocated dietary restriction during pregnancy, induction of premature labour and, in extreme cases, caesarean section.

Gustav Adolf Michaelis was born in Harburg, Germany. His father and uncle were both obstetricians. His father died when Michaelis was a young boy, and he went to live with his uncle in Kiel. He was educated in Göttingen and Kiel and graduated from the latter city's medical school in 1820. He did further postgraduate work in obstetrics in Paris and returned to work as an assistant to his uncle, who was director of the lying-in hospital at Kiel. Upon the death of his uncle in 1841, Michaelis succeeded him as director. Michaelis was also actively interested in natural history, archaeology and literature. He was one of the first to endorse and adopt Ignac Semmelweis' preventive measures for puerperal sepsis. Using these principles, he succeeded in containing one such

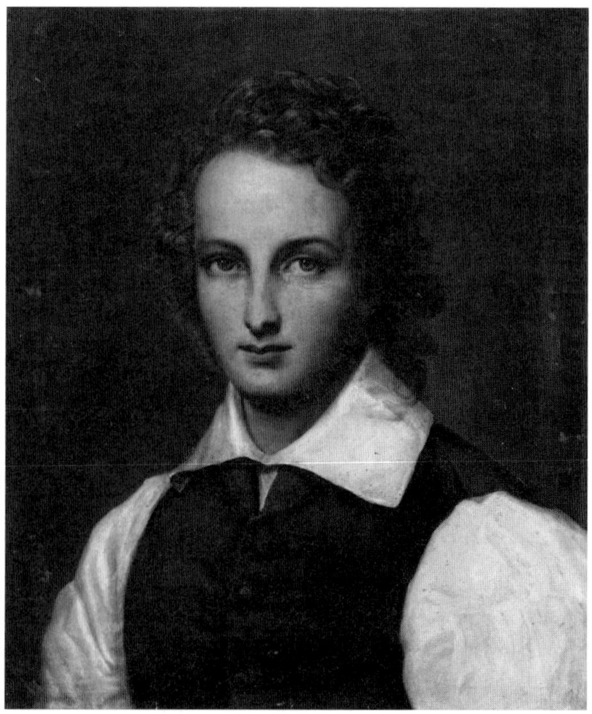

Gustav Adolf Michaelis

epidemic in his hospital. However, sepsis recurred in his wards and caused the death of one of his nieces, whom he had attended. This was too much for his sensitive melancholy nature and, in despair, blaming his own 'dirty hands', he jumped to his death in front of a moving train on 8 August 1848 at the age of 50.

Selected Publications

Michaelis GA. *Das Enge Becken*. Leipzig: Wigand; 1851 (Published posthumously by his associate, Carl Litzmann).

Bibliography References

548, 648, 775, 889, 1018, 1261, 1367, 1368, 1480.

Minnitt, Robert James (1889–1974)

Minnitt Apparatus for Inhalation Analgesia

When chloroform inhalation analgesia was introduced into obstetrics by James Young Simpson in 1847, he rendered the patient unconscious. It was soon realised by John Snow, among others, that full surgical anaesthesia was neither necessary or desirable to provide analgesia in labour. Fatalities associated with chloroform anaesthesia stimulated the use of alternatives in obstetrics, including ether alone and alcohol/chloroform/ether mixtures.

In 1934 Minnitt reported the use of an apparatus designed by himself and Charles King to administer 45% nitrous oxide with 55% air. The method was approved by the Central Midwives Board in 1936 for unsupervised use by midwives. It became the standard technique for inhalation analgesia for domiciliary midwifery in the United Kingdom during the 1940s and 1950s. The drawback was the potential for hypoxia, with the 55% air component providing only 11% oxygen. In 1961 Michael Tunstall (1928–2011) showed that at 2,000 psi, 50% nitrous oxide and 50% oxygen gas mixture could be stored and delivered from one cylinder.

In 1962 the Lucy Baldwin apparatus, named after the wife (1859–1945) of a British prime minister who had been a supporter and benefactor of organised midwifery services, was developed. This provided a varying mixture of oxygen and nitrous oxide, with a minimum of 30% oxygen. In 1963 Michael Tunstall arrived in Aberdeen towards the end of his training in anaesthesia and persuaded the British Oxygen Company to manufacture pre-mixed oxygen and nitrous oxide, marketed as Entonox. With a simple demand valve and pre-mixed 50% and 50% nitrous oxide, Entonox superseded the Minnitt and Lucy Baldwin machines. In many hospitals a blender apparatus is used that produces a 50/50 oxygen/nitrous oxide concentration via hospital gas lines.

Minnitt recognised that his method of pain relief was imperfect and, in the language of the day, wrote:

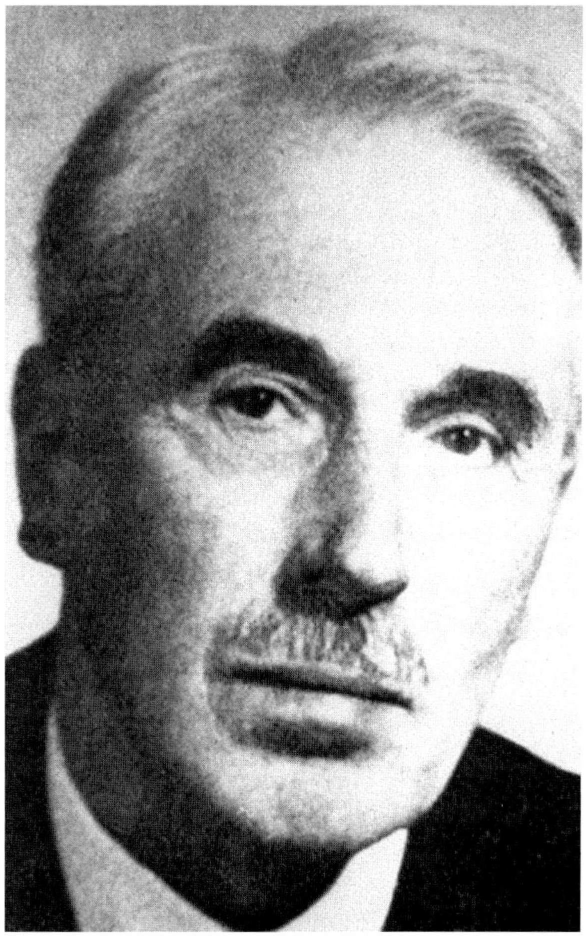
Robert James Minnitt

What has been done is not a terminus. It is a thoroughfare to greater possibilities for painless labour. So may there dawn renewed hope in the hearts of women.

Robert James Minnitt graduated MB from Liverpool University in 1915 and went into general practice. In addition, he held honorary appointments in anaesthesia at the Liverpool Maternity Hospital and Liverpool Royal Infirmary. He also carried out research and was awarded his MD for studies in surgical shock. When the National Health Service was established in 1948, he registered his philosophical opposition by resigning his hospital appointments and continued in private general practice.

For his services to analgesia in labour he was awarded honorary fellowships from the Faculty of Anaesthetists in the Royal College of Surgeons and the Royal College of Obstetricians and Gynaecologists.

Selected Publications

Minnitt RJ. A new technique for the self-administration of gas-air analgesia in labour. *Lancet* 1934; 1: 1278.

Minnitt RJ. Self-administered analgesia for the midwifery of general practice. *Proc R Soc Med* 1934; 27: 1313–5.

Tunstall ME. Obstetric analgesia: the use of a fixed nitrous oxide and oxygen mixture from one cylinder. *Lancet* 1961; 2: 964.

Bibliography References

74, 253, 263, 585, 753, 897, 957, 997, 1051, 1052, 1150, 1438, 1440, 1527, 1584, 1585, 1685.

Moir, John Chassar (1900–1977)

Ergometrine

The discovery of the chemical structure of ergometrine in 1935 made available the first oxytocic compound with a predictable and consistent effect. As such it has been used for more than 80 years in millions of obstetric cases worldwide and reduced the toll from atonic post-partum haemorrhage, one of the commonest causes of maternal death. The drawback to the parent compound, ergot, introduced to conventional medical practice by John Stearns in 1808, was the unpredictable and variable oxytocic effect. Ergot has been described as 'a veritable treasure house of pharmacology'. It contains histamine, tyramine, acetylcholine and a number of alkaloids with oxytocic activity. Two of these, ergotoxine in 1906 and ergotamine in 1918, were isolated in Britain and Switzerland respectively.

Working in the University College Hospital, London, in 1932, Chassar Moir devised a technique of placing a small balloon in the post-partum uterus of a patient in the postnatal ward. He attached this to a device to measure uterine contractions and thus was able to time and quantitate the oxytocic effect of various drugs given to the patient. He was later to describe the setup and economic outlay for this endeavour:

The recording apparatus, save for a revolving-drum kymograph, was all of my own construction. One shilling was used for the lead piping and five shillings were used for the purchase of an alarm clock which, when fitted with electrical contacts and used in conjunction with the mechanism of a worn-out electric bell, enabled me to add minute markings to the kymograph charts. These and other contrivances were all improvised from discarded hospital material. Only the clockwork-moving drum was specially requisitioned, and it was already part of the departmental equipment. Thus, the claim can be made that the discovery of the presence of the new ergot principle, later to be called ergometrine, which I shall presently describe, was accomplished at a total cost of six shillings.

Enough to cause much envy and teeth-grinding from the modern clinical scientist involved with research grant applications.

In a study comparing the oxytocic effects of ergotoxine and ergotamine, Moir found them both to have a slow onset of action. Moir was seeking the rapid onset fraction of ergot – the 'John Stearns effect', as he called it, based on Stearns' words, 'the suddenness of its action will surprise you'. He then tried aqueous extract of ergot and got an almost instantaneous oxytocic response; he had discovered the 'John Stearns effect'.

Harold Dudley, chief research chemist in the National Institute of Medical Research and working under the direction of Sir Henry Dale, was appointed to find the elusive chemical fraction. Each substance he isolated had to be tested by Moir on the post-partum uterus. It was to take three years before Dudley identified the chemical and Moir confirmed its rapid oxytocic action in February 1935:

> *... the isolation of the substance to which ergot owes its long-established reputation as the 'pulvis parturiens'. We propose to name it 'ergometrine'.*

The name was Dale's suggestion. They decided, 'The method of preparation would be published in full. No patent rights or proprietary interests would encumber the new drug; it would be free for any manufacturing firm to produce'. This they did in the 16 March 1935 edition of the *British Medical Journal*, which was published on the same day that Dudley died at the age of 49.

At almost the same time, independent work from Baltimore (M Thompson); Chicago (ME Davis and associates); and Basle (A Stoll and E Burckhardt) isolated the same active principle. It was called ergonovine in the United States and ergobasine in Switzerland, but in the rest of the world it was to be ergometrine. It came into widespread use for the treatment of atonic post-partum haemorrhage. Edward Davis of Chicago was the first to propose its routine use intravenously with the delivery of the anterior shoulder for the prevention of post-partum haemorrhage.

John Chassar Moir was born at Montrose, Scotland, and graduated in medicine from Edinburgh University in 1922. He also travelled to study in Berlin, Vienna and the United States. It was while working as first assistant to Professor FJ Browne at University College Hospital, London that he did his work on ergometrine in the early 1930s. He was appointed the first holder of the Nuffield chair of obstetrics and gynaecology at Oxford University in 1937, which he held for 30 years. During his Oxford era he became expert in the surgical treatment of vesicovaginal fistula and published a small classic text on the subject. He helped Reginald and Catherine Hamlin develop their surgical technique for fistula repair and visited them in Ethiopia on two occasions. He was awarded the CBE in 1961 and received

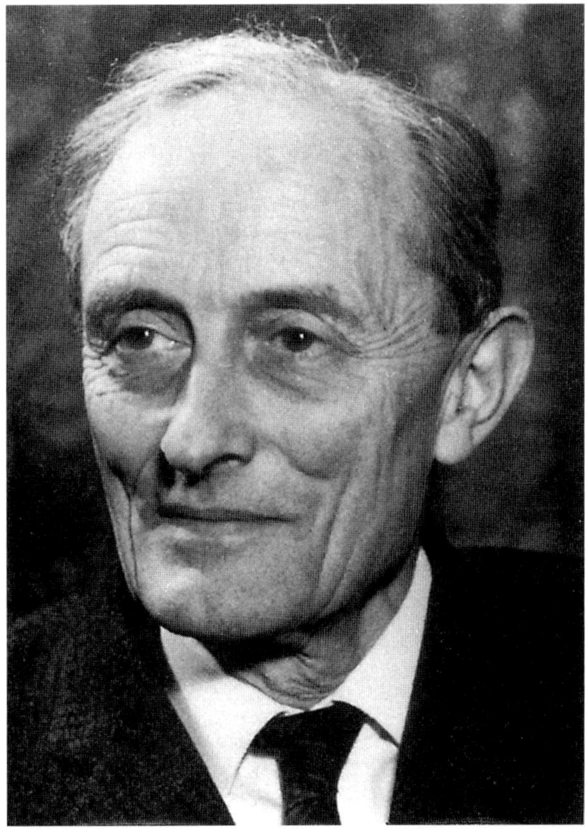

John Chassar Moir

honorary doctorates from the two Queen's Universities: in Belfast, Northern Ireland and Kingston, Ontario. He followed Munro Kerr as the author of the standard text, *Operative Obstetrics*. After vacating the chair at Oxford, he became visiting professor at the Royal Postgraduate Medical School Hammersmith. He died on 14 November 1977.

The worldwide use of ergometrine to prevent and treat post-partum haemorrhage has undoubtedly saved countless lives. Moir was later to say of ergometrine, 'reckoned in the saving of human life, places it among the enduring achievements of medical science' – an achievement in which, it should be added, he played a significant role. He was described by a colleague as 'a gentle gentleman with the face of a poet'.

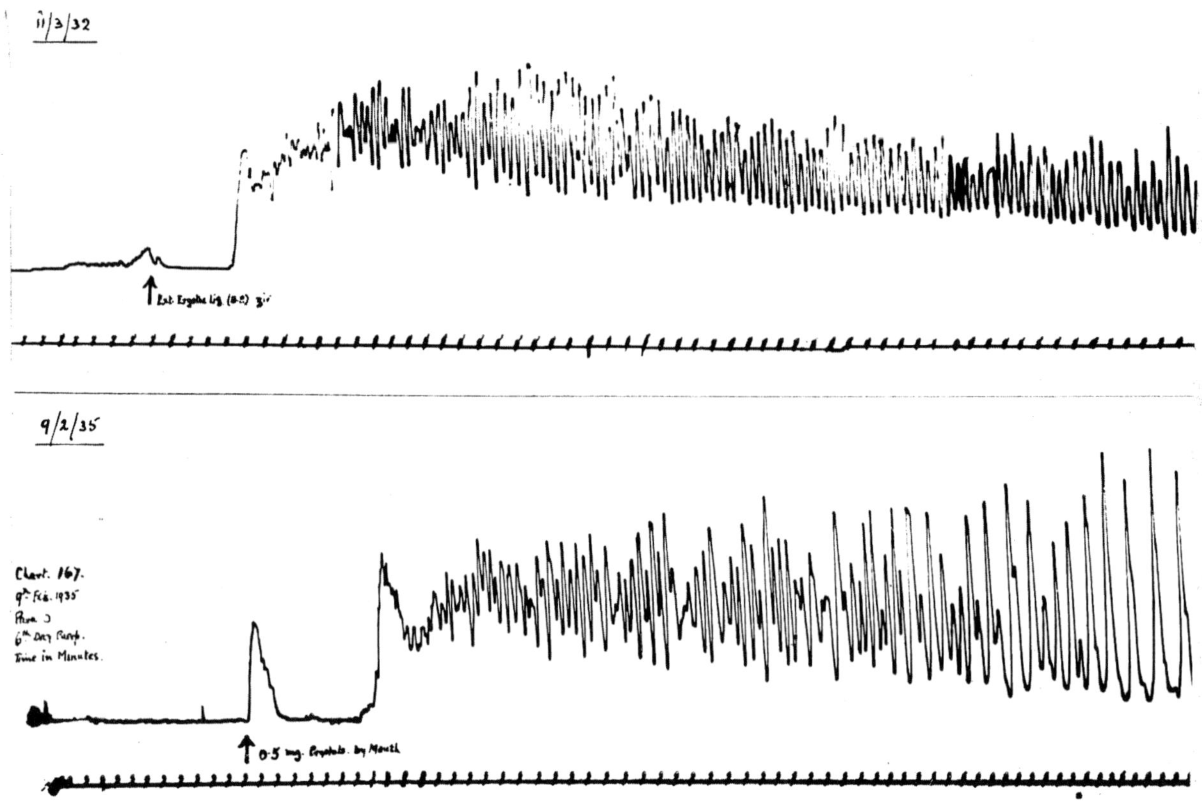

Copies of two of Chassar Moir's kymographic tracings. The upper one shows the 'John Stearns effect' of aqueous extract of ergot. The lower recording is the first demonstration of the oxytocic effect of ergometrine on 9 February 1935.

Selected Publications

Davis ME. Postpartum haemorrhage. *Am J Surg* 1940; 48: 154–63.

Dudley HW, Moir C. The substance responsible for the traditional clinical effect of ergot. *BMJ* 1935; 1: 520–3.

Moir JC. The action of ergot preparations on the puerperal uterus. *BMJ* 1932; 1: 1119–22.

Moir JC. *The Vesicovaginal Fistula*. London: Ballière, Tindall & Cassell; 1967.

Bibliography References

85, 94, 99, 263, 273, 374, 435, 443, 445, 479, 560, 680, 686, 733, 822, 938, 955, 1061, 1063, 1064, 1066–1069, 1130, 1506, 1644.

Monsel, Leon (1816–1878)

Monsel's Solution

Monsel's solution is ferric subsulphate, which he prepared by oxidising ferrous sulphate with nitric acid in the presence of sulphuric acid. He found it worked as 'a powerful haemostatic agent' on bleeding wounds. It acts by causing denaturation and agglutinating proteins, which mechanically seals small blood vessels.

Monsel first used his solution when stationed in Rome with the French army, and he reported this in

October 1852. Monsel later used the solution for haemostasis on otherwise non-life-threatening wounds to stop bleeding during transport from the front lines to the medical stations in the Crimean War.

Leon Monsel was born on 13 March 1816 in Gironde, France. He took his pharmacy training in the military health school of Strasbourg and qualified in 1840. He became a 'pharmacien major' and remained in the French army of Napoléon Bonaparte III until he retired in 1874. He died in Nancy on 15 April 1878.

Monsel's solution remains in widespread use in gynaecology for haemostasis of biopsy sites of the vulva, vagina and cervix. It may also have occasional application in areas of persistent blood oozing in cases of placenta praevia and emergency obstetric hysterectomy.

Selected Publications

Monsel L. *La correspondence scientifique de Roma.* Bull Universale 1852, p. 38.

Monsel L. Proprieté hémostatique du sulfate de peroxyde de fer. *Rec Mem Med Chir Pharm Milit* 1856; 17: 424–5.

Bibliography References

202, 527, 601, 1179, 1247.

Montgomery, William Fetherston (1797–1859)

Montgomery's Tubercles

An Irish obstetrician who graduated from Trinity College Dublin in 1822, Montgomery was appointed the first professor of midwifery in the School of Physic in 1827 and held the position for 30 years. In his book, in the chapter entitled *Mammary Sympathies*, he described and illustrated the small sebaceous glands in the areola surrounding the nipples which become more prominent, elevated and reddened during pregnancy. These became known as 'Montgomery's tubercles'.

While acknowledging the previous description by Johann Georg Roederer (1727–1763) some 84 years earlier, Montgomery wrote:

> *The alteration which takes place in that part of the breast which immediately surrounds the nipple, it is called the areola, appears to me not to have received the degree of notice which its importance merits, as being one of the most certain external indications of pregnancy, arising from the operation of sympathy.*

In a case report he described the changes thus:

> *I therefore examined the state of the breasts which had enlarged a little and were slightly sensitive, the circle of the areola had a faint pinkish hue, with the glandular follicles just beginning to show themselves above the surface of the areola, which exhibited a slight degree of elevation and appeared to be a little more than an inch in diameter, but I did not measure it; the nipple was also beginning to be turgid. These appearances ... induced me to give an opinion in favour of the existence of pregnancy, which the event proved to be correct.*

William Montgomery died on 21 December 1859.

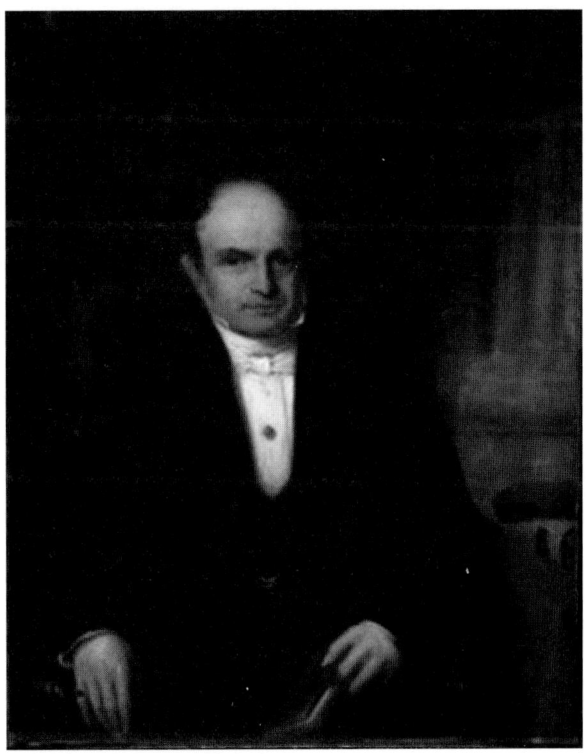

William Fetherston Montgomery

Selected Publications

Montgomery WF. *An Exposition of the Signs and Symptoms of Pregnancy, the Period of Human Gestation and the Signs of Delivery.* London: Sherwood, Gilbert & Piper; 1837.

Roederer JG. *Elementa artis obstetriciae in usum praelectionum academicarum.* Göttingen; 1753, p. 62.

Bibliography References

231, 232, 952, 968, 1073, 1126.

Morgagni, Giovanni Battista (1682–1771)

Hydatid Cyst of Morgagni

Every surgeon operating in the female pelvis is familiar with the small, thin walled, translucent cysts attached by a long slender pedicle near the fimbriated end of the oviduct. These are often bilateral and so common as to be regarded as normal, although on rare occasions they become large enough to cause symptoms. The first description of these cysts was by Giovanni Morgagni.

Morgagni, an only child, was born in Forli, Italy, and educated at the University of Bologna, graduating in philosophy and medicine in 1701. He was a student of Antonio Valsalva (1666–1723). Morgagni was a founder member of a group of young academic staff and senior students in Bologna called *Academia Inquietorum* (The Academy of the Restless) whose mission was to seek proof for old theories rather than accept dogma for its own sake – a forerunner of his own meticulous approach to drawing conclusions only after the facts were established. Appointed to the chair of anatomy in Padua in 1715, he remained there until his death. His first publication was in 1706, but his greatest work he produced 56 years later, in his eightieth year. He revolutionised the study of morbid anatomy by carefully relating his pathological findings to the patient's clinical record:

> *Since in anatomy the morbid state reflects the idea of the healthy, why should not disease indicate the function of an organ especially when experiments cannot assist us . . . those who have dissected or inspected many bodies, have at least learned to doubt; when others, who are ignorant of anatomy and do not take the trouble to attend to it, are in no doubt at all!*

With the advent of percussion and auscultation, symptoms were henceforth seen as 'the cry of the suffering organs', and the era of clinico-pathological correlation was established.

Giovanni Morgagni married a woman from his home town, with whom he had 15 children. He con-

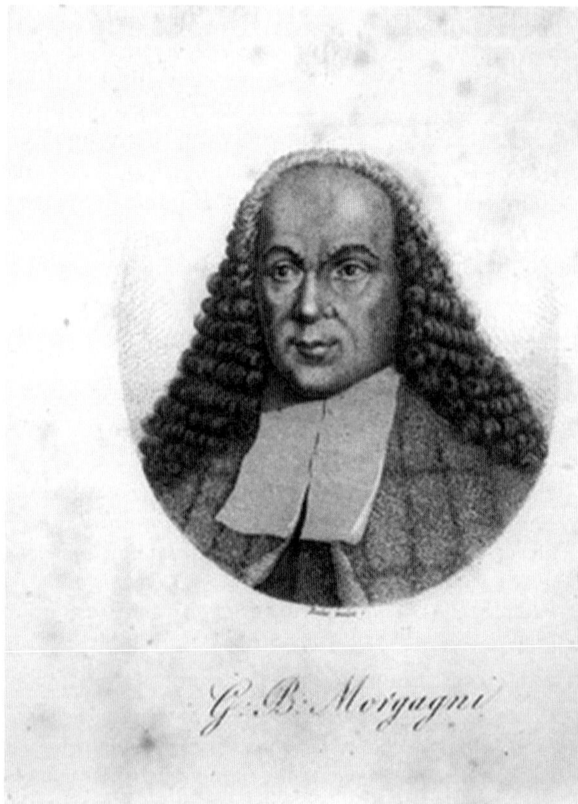

Giovanni Battista Morgagni

tinued to teach until a few weeks before his death in his eighty-ninth year. He died on 6 December 1771, alone except for his servants. His classic text, *De sedibus,* was translated into English in 1769. His manuscript and papers were eventually unearthed in the Laurentian Library of Florence in 1952.

Selected Publications

Morgagni GB. *De sedibus et causis morborum per anatomen indagatis, libri quinque.* Venice; 1761.

Bibliography References

120, 123, 406, 648, 1115, 1121, 1306, 1417, 1461, 1480.

Moro, Ernst (1874–1951)

Moro Reflex

The Moro reflex or response is normally seen in the first six months of life. In response to a loud noise, initial abduction and extension of all extremities is followed by flexion and adduction. The absence of this reflex in a newborn suggests generalised central nervous system damage. Asymmetrical palsies will also become manifest.

Ernst Moro first presented this information to a meeting of the Society of Natural History and Medicine of Heidelberg on 7 May 1918. He finished his presentation by demonstrating the reflex when striking the pillow beside an infant.

Ernst Moro was born in Lalbach, Austria. He received his MD from Graz in 1899 and then worked as an assistant in the Children's Clinic in Vienna for three years. In 1911 Moro became professor of paediatrics and director of the Children's Clinic in Heidelberg.

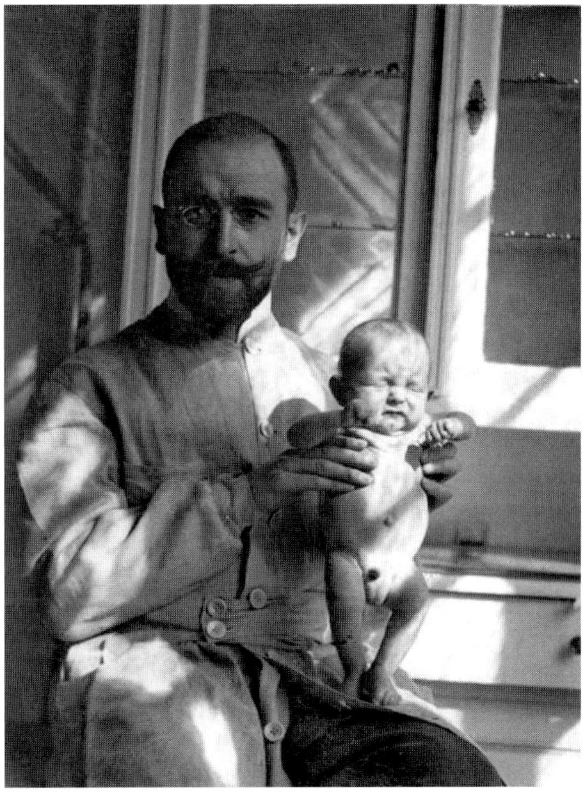

Ernst Moro

Selected Publications

Moro E. Das erste Trimenon. *München Med Wochenschr* 1918; 65: 1147.

Bibliography References

730, 900, 1054.

Moschcowitz, Alexis Victor (1865–1933)

Moschcowitz Procedure

Alexis Moschcowitz presented his detailed studies on prolapse of the rectum to the New York State Medical Society on 16 April 1912. His paper covered extensive anatomical explanations of the pathogenesis of rectal prolapse as a form of sliding hernia:

> *When my studies led me to the conclusion that prolapse of the rectum was in every essential a hernia, I set out to devise an operation in which the principles of an operation for the cure of a hernia could be carried out.*

He went on to describe his operative procedure:

> *. . . silk sutures are passed circularly around the cul de sac of Douglas, and tied. The lowermost suture is placed about one inch above the inferior extremity of the cul de sac; similar sutures, six to eight in number, are passed at intervals, and persisted in as long as the peritoneum comes together until practically the entire pouch of Douglas is obliterated.*
>
> *It is advisable, and I always try to include in my suture the pelvic fascia, particularly that part which covers the levator ani . . .*
>
> *When the sutures reach the region of the supravaginal portion of the cervix and body of the uterus, the sutures are anchored to these structures.*

Moschcowitz pointed out that the ureters and internal iliac vessels were vulnerable in his operation but, happily for him, was able to state, 'neither of the structures have thus far caused me any embarrassment'.

Gynaecologists later appropriated the operation to treat herniation of the pouch of Douglas, with or without enterocoele, particularly at the time of hysterectomy. Classically the procedure is performed abdominally, but the same principles can be applied, to a degree, by the vaginal route.

Alexis Victor Moschcowitz was born in Giralt, Hungary and moved to the United States in 1880, at the age of 15. In 1891 he received his MD from the College of Physicians and Surgeons of Columbia University, New York. When he did his research on prolapse of the rectum, he was associate surgeon at the Mount Sinai Hospital in New York. In addition, he served on the consulting staff of the Bronx Maternity and Women's Hospital. He also improved the surgical technique of femoral hernia repair.

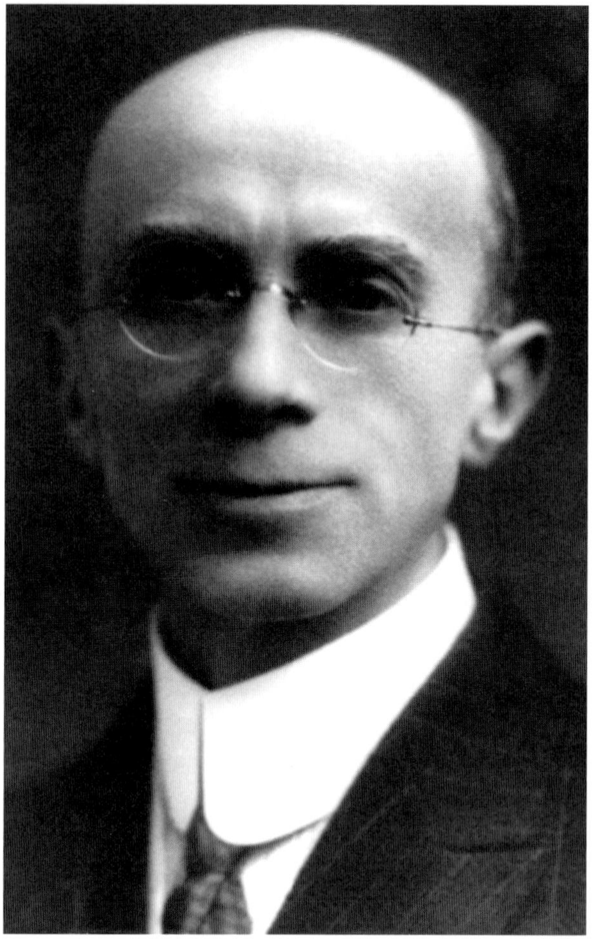

Alexis Victor Moschcowitz

Recognition of his clinical and teaching skills came with his appointment as professor of clinical surgery at his alma mater. He died of a coronary thrombosis on 21 December 1933.

Selected Publications

Moschcowitz AV. The pathogenesis, anatomy and cure of prolapse of the rectum. *Surg Gynecol Obstet* 1912; 15: 7–21.

Bibliography References

30, 112, 1081.

Müller, Johannes Peter (1801–1858)

Müllerian Ducts

The primordial female genital tract is initially paired as the paramesonephric ducts in all vertebrates. Other anatomists, including Johann Meckel and Martin Rathke, contributed to this knowledge, but it was Müller who amalgamated and interpreted the existing facts in his treatise on the embryology of the genitalia. Thus, he received the eponymous recognition.

Johannes Peter Müller was born in Coblenz, Germany, the eldest son of a shoemaker. His forebears were winegrowers in the Moselle Valley. He vacillated between study for the priesthood and medicine and was said to have been influenced toward the latter by the writings of Goethe. He graduated MD from the University of Bonn in 1822. He undertook further study in Berlin but returned to Bonn in 1824 and rose to the rank of professor in 1830. In 1833 he proposed himself as the suitable candidate for the vacant chair of anatomy, physiology and pathology at Berlin. This unorthodox self-promotion proved successful. His academic output was enormous and included 20 books and more than 250 scientific papers; during his professional life he produced an average of one scientific publication every seven weeks. He inspired many illustrious students, including Theodor Schwann, Jakob Henle and Rudolph Virchow. In his early academic career, he was very competitive and it was only later in life that he remarked, 'Envy within me is changed into admiration, but that is a height only gradually attained'.

In 1855, returning from holiday in Norway, his ship was sunk in a collision. Müller was rescued, but his assistant drowned. For many years he had been plagued with insomnia and depression and following this catastrophe his health failed badly. On 28 April 1858 he was found dead in bed. He had forbidden an autopsy. The cause of his death was unknown, but suicide was suspected by those close to him.

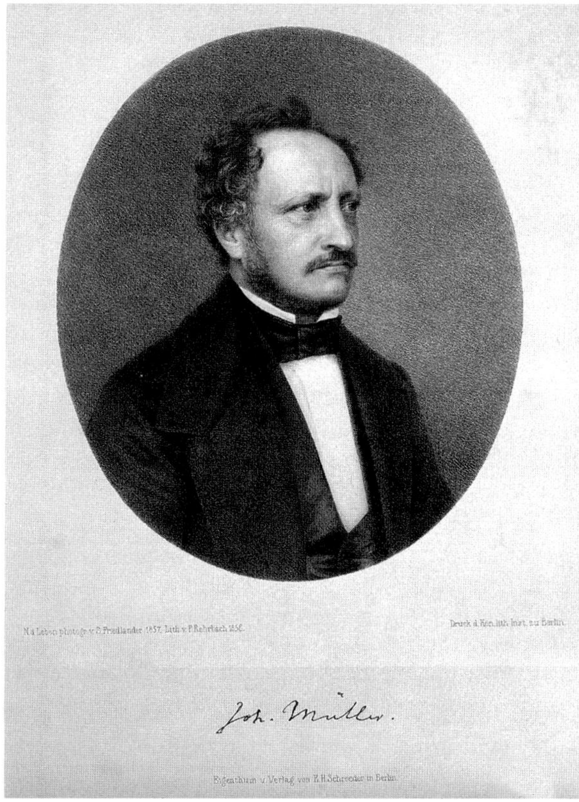

Johannes Peter Müller

Selected Publications

Müller JP. *Bildungsgeschicte der Genitalien.* Düsseldorf; 1830.

Bibliography References

552, 590, 615, 648, 689, 703, 968, 969, 1087, 1223, 1330, 1417, 1517, 1534, 1611, 1651.

Murray, Robert Milne (1855–1904)

Milne Murray Forceps

In 1891, Robert Milne Murray read a paper before the Edinburgh Obstetrical Society and summarised the ideals of forceps delivery thus:

> *To draw the foetal head through the pelvic canal with the least expenditure of force. Any force expended above that needed to overcome the resistance of the birth canal is likely to cause injury.*

Milne Murray applied his considerable mathematical talents to the geometry of forceps application and the axis of traction required to fulfil the ideals he espoused. He therefore designed his own forceps with traction rods attached to the middle of the fenestra and curved backwards to the handles. In addition to his obstetric talents, he was a noted electrophysiologist. In his own laboratory he investigated the action of hot water on smooth muscle in an attempt to establish some scientific basis for hot water douches in the treatment of atonic post-partum haemorrhage.

Robert Milne Murray, the son of a schoolmaster, was born in the small Scottish village of Fettercairn. He initially read arts in St Andrew's University, moving to Edinburgh for the study of medicine and graduating with first-class honours. He was appointed to the staff of the Royal Infirmary and Royal Maternity Hospital.

His health was poor, and he developed pneumonia after attending his father's funeral. He never fully recovered, developed chronic lung infections, and died a few days after an operation to remove some ribs and obliterate the pleural cavity. He was highly regarded as a trusted and generous colleague.

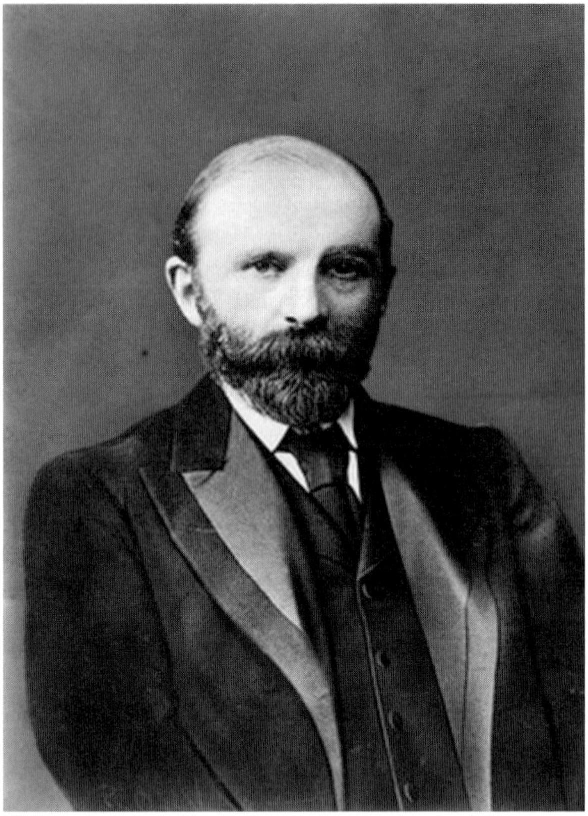

Robert Milne Murray

Selected Publications

Murray RM. The axis-traction forceps: their mechanical principles, construction and scope. *Trans Edinb Obstet Soc* 1891; 16: 58–89.

Murray RM. A discussion on the relative advantages of forceps and version as a means of extraction in cases of moderate pelvic deformity. *BMJ* 1896; 2: 1281–3.

Bibliography References

305, 361, 399, 648, 718, 721, 822, 956, 1065, 1092, 1285, 1420.

N

Naboth, Martin (1675–1721)

Nabothian Cyst

Mucous retention cysts of the cervix are so common as to be considered a variant of normal. They were first described in 1681 by the French surgeon Guillaume Desnoues (1650–1735), subsequently appointed professor of anatomy in Genoa. He felt they represented a reservoir for a spermatic substance. Martin Naboth acknowledged the earlier work of Desnoues but interpreted their function differently in his treatise on sterility in women published in 1707. Naboth felt the cysts represented a repository for ova; he called them 'ovarium novum' and described them as follows:

> *The vesicles vary somewhat in size as well as number; while some are as large as a pea, others are smaller, some being the size of a hemp seed, a greater number, though equal in size, resembling a grain of millet. In younger subjects a greater or lesser number of vesicles may be seen, in older subjects their number is greater and they develop more rapidly, but in the aged they are fewer.*

Martin Naboth was born in Kalau, Saxony. He received his medical degree in 1703 having studied in Leipzig and Halle. While working in general medical practice he pursued anatomical studies. In 1707 he was appointed professor of chemistry in Leipzig.

Selected Publications

Naboth M. *De sterilitate mulierum*. Leipzig: A. Zeidler; 1707.

Bibliography References

406, 1463, 1480.

Naegele, Franz Carl (1778–1851)

Naegele's Rule/Naegele's Obliquity/Naegele's Pelvis

Franz Carl Naegele is remembered eponymously for three things: a rare type of pelvic deformity, a common presentation in labour and a rule for calculating gestational age that he did not invent. The most commonly used clinical formula for calculating the expected date of confinement is to add seven days to the first day of the last menstrual period and count forward nine months. Although commonly known as 'Naegele's rule', it was not formulated by Naegele, nor did he lay claim to it. In his publication of 1812 he clearly attributed it to, and quoted from, Herman Boerhaave (1668–1738):

> *Women are usually impregnated after the end of their menstrual flow . . . 99 out of 100 births occur in the ninth month after the last menstruation, adding a week after the last menses and counting nine months of gestation.*

Having acknowledged the primacy of Boerhaave's work, Naegele wrote,

> *The usual calculation of the duration of pregnancy, namely starting from the last menstruation is correct in most instances; and conception within the last third of the cycle or in the second half between two periods is unusual and an exception to the rule.*

It should be noted that neither Boerhaave or Naegele were specific about calculating from the first or the last day of menstruation, merely 'after the last menses' and 'starting from the last menstruation'. Later clinicians interpreted the calculation as being

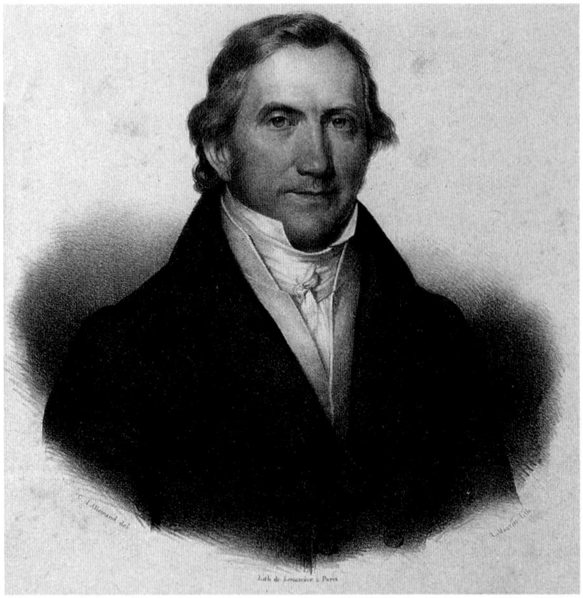

Franz Carl Naegele

from the first day of the last menstrual period and attributed the rule to Naegele.

In his 1819 monograph, *Mechanism of Birth*, Naegele described the tendency in normal labour for the anterior parietal bone to present as the head engages. He emphasised that this anterior asynclitism, or so-called 'Naegele's obliquity', was normal. In describing the circumstances in a left occipito-anterior presentation, he wrote:

The head assumes an oblique rather than a vertical position at the pelvic inlet, so that neither the vertex nor the sagittal suture, but rather the right parietal bone, is the presenting part. The sagittal suture is much closer to the sacral promontory than to the pubis . . .

Naegele was also the first to describe the rare obliquely contracted pelvis that bears his name. He encountered his first case in 1803 and assiduously set about collecting more. He first published his observations in 1834. His expanded treatise on these cases and other causes of contracted pelvis was published in 1839. The Naegele pelvis is obliquely contracted, with the sacral ala on one side missing or deficient so that the sacral body is fused with the iliac bone. The outcome for infant and mother in the 35 cases described was uniformly bad, with lethal destructive operations required for delivery. As he wrote:

Moreover the contraction of our pelves may be so great that caesarean section may be indicated in the case of a normal sized foetus. The cases described above speak only too loudly for this alternative.

Franz Carl Naegele was born in Düsseldorf, Germany, the son of a military surgeon. He studied medicine at the universities of Freiburg, Strasburg and Bamberg. After service as a medical officer to the town of Elberfeld-Barmen he was appointed professor at the University of Heidelberg in 1807. Three years later he was also appointed director of the lying-in hospital, succeeding his father-in-law in this position. Naegele exclusively practised obstetrics and over 40 years in Heidelberg gained international renown for his studies of the mechanism of labour and the contracted pelvis. His son, Franz Joseph, followed in his footsteps.

Selected Publications

Boerhaave H. *Praelectiones academicae in proprias institutiones rei medicae* (Vol. 5). In: Von Haller A (ed.) Göttingen: Vandenhoeck; 1744: 437.

Naegele FC. *Erfahrungen und Abhandlungen aus dem Gebiethe der Krantheiten des Weiblichen Geschlechtes. Nebst Grundzügen einer Methodenlehre der Geburtshülfe.* Mannheim: Loeffler; 1812, pp. 280–1.

Naegele FC. Veber den Mechanismus der Geburt. *Deutsche Arch Physiol* 1819; 5: 483–531.

Naegele FC. *Das schräg berengte Becken nebst einem Anhange über die wichtigsten Fehler des weiblichen Beckens überhaupt.* Mainz: Von Zabern; 1839.

Naegele FC. *The Obliquely Contracted Pelvis Containing Also an Appendix of the Most Important Defects of the Female Pelvis.* (Centennial Edition. Newly Translated from the Original German). New York, NY; 1939. Also published in: The Classics of Obstetrics and Gynecology Library. Birmingham: Gryphon Editions; 1991 (facsimile).

Bibliography References

86, 347, 522, 548, 648, 676, 775, 920, 1349, 1480.

Neisser, Albert Ludwig Siegmund (1855–1916)

Neisseria Gonorrhoeae

At the age of 24, two years after receiving his medical degree, Albert Neisser described the micro-organism responsible for gonorrhoea:

> *If gonorrhoeal pus is spread in as thin a layer as possible, allowed to dry, stained by simply pouring an aqueous solution of methyl violet over it . . . a number of more or less concentrated masses of micrococci are seen at first glance. These have a quite characteristic, typical form, immediately recognizable . . . These characteristic micrococci thus appear to be a constant work of all gonorrhoeal affections . . . which has repeatedly allowed me to diagnose the specific gonorrhoeal nature of pus.*

Albert Ludwig Siegmund Neisser was born in Schweidnitz, Germany, the son of a prominent physician. He studied medicine in Erlangen and Breslau and upon qualification in 1877 was appointed assistant to the dermatology clinic at the latter university. He studied leprosy and identified the leprosy bacillus, previously discovered by the Norwegian Gerhard Hansen, as the causative organism of the disease. In 1882 he was appointed extraordinarius professor of dermatology and venereal diseases at Breslau. Neisser carried out clinical and pathological studies of venereal diseases and for years attempted to find an antiserum against syphilis. In his animal experiments he went so far as to build a house for 200 monkeys in his garden. He worked with Paul Ehrlich on the use of arsenicals in the treatment of syphilis and collaborated with August von Wassermann in the development of his serological test.

In his later years his health deteriorated, and he died from septicaemia shortly after removal of a bladder stone in July 1916.

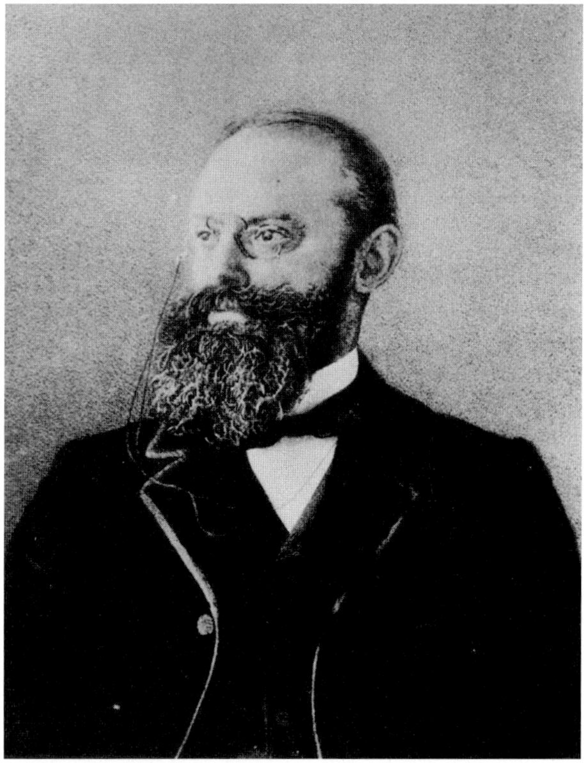

Albert Ludwig Siegmund Neisser

Selected Publications

Neisser A. Über eine der Gonorrhoe eigentümliche Micrococcusform. *Zentralbl med Wiss* 1879; 17: 497–500.

Bibliography References

553, 648, 1103, 1104, 1145, 1146, 1352, 1480.

Nihell, Elizabeth (b. 1723)

Midwife

Elizabeth Nihell was the most prominent English midwife of her era; not because of her competence, but because of the ferocity of her attacks on man-midwives and forceps. She became incensed at the intrusion of men into midwifery and devoted much of her time to vitriolic attacks against them and, in particular, their use of forceps. Much of this was articulated in her 1760 publication, *A Treatise on the Art of Midwifery*. In the preface she clearly laid down the gauntlet:

> *The truth is, that my very natural and strong attachment to the profession, which I have long exercised and actually do exercise, created in me an unsuppressible indignation at the errors and pernicious innovations introduced into it, and every day gaining ground, under the protection of fashion, sillily fostering a preference of men to women in the practice of midwifery.*

Nihell considered women who employed man-midwives to have 'sunk to so low a degree of cheapness ... a sort of prostitution'. Many of her strongest attacks were directed at William Smellie who, through his classes for both male and female midwives, had increasing influence. She belittled his physique, alluding to his large hands, 'the delicate fist of a great-horse-godmother of a he-midwife'.

At this time most midwives were poorly trained, if trained at all. Nihell's public attacks served to bring the whole area of care during labour into general debate, which did not always serve her cause. Indeed, around this time the first lying-in hospitals were established in London and the dominance of medical men in midwifery began. Nihell acknowledged that the standard of some female midwives was poor: 'I own however there are but too few midwives who are sufficiently mistresses in their profession'. She managed only the most reluctant recognition of the male midwife:

> *I will also, with the same candour, own that there are some not entirely incapable men-midwives: but they are so very rare, and must for ever necessarily be so, and even, at the best, so inferior to good midwives ...*

She reserved her most dramatic prose for the condemnation of the instruments used by the man-midwife:

> *... till at length, not infrequently, some infernal instrument is produced, like the dagger, in the fifth act of a tragedy, and forms the catastrophe of mother, of child, or of both? ... Art should aim at imitating Nature: now Nature proceeds leisurely, instead of which the forceps goes too quick to work.*

Elizabeth Nihell was born in London. She trained at the Hôtel Dieu in Paris as an apprentice-midwife, 'which I accomplished with great difficulty on account of being born a subject of England, and consequently a foreigner there ...'. At that time there were about 500 deliveries a month at the Hôtel Dieu.

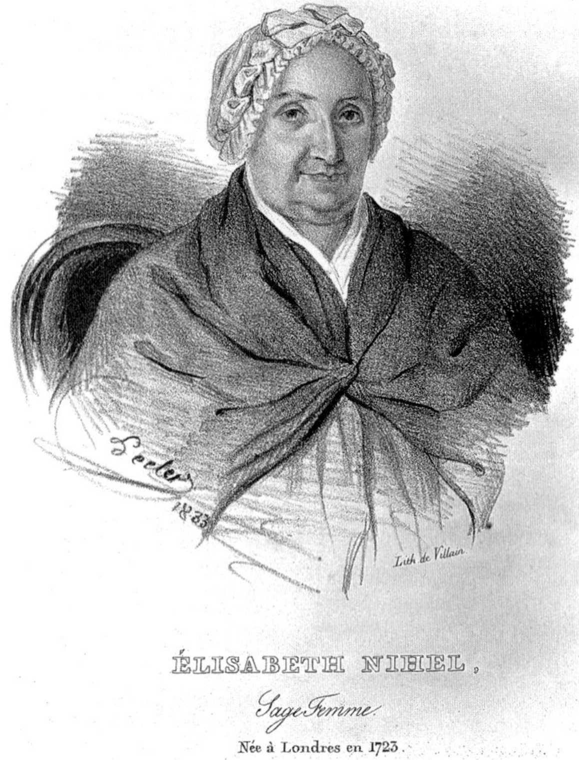

Elizabeth Nihell

Her husband was a surgeon-apothecary, and they practised in the Haymarket district of London. Few other details of her are known, although she presumably had children: 'I am myself a mother'. She was known to be in practice as late as 1772, but the exact date of her death is unknown.

Selected Publications

Nihell E. *A Treatise on the Art of Midwifery. Setting Forth Various Abuses Therin, Especially as to the Practice with Instruments: the Whole Serving to Put all Rational Inquirers in a Fair Way of Very Safely Forming Their Own Judgement upon the Question; Which Is It Best To Employ, In Cases of Pregnancy and Lying-In, A Man-Midwife Or A Midwife*. London: A. Morley; 1760. Also published in: The Classics of Obstetrics and Gynecology Library. New York, NY: Gryphon Editions; 1994 (facsimile).

Bibliography References

43, 46, 298, 419, 534, 568, 610, 648, 982, 1261, 1386, 1495.

Noeggerath, Emil Oscar Jacob Bruno (1827–1895)

Latent Gonorrhoea

At the inaugural meeting of the American Gynecological Society in 1876, Emil Noeggerath, as a founding member, read his paper on *Latent Gonorrhoea, Especially with Regard to its Influence on Fertility in Women*. He concluded that gonorrhoeal infection could remain latent in both the male and female for life and that the wives of men who had ever had gonorrhoea were usually sterile:

> *I have chosen the term latent gonorrhea instead of chronic gonorrhea . . . better to define the truly imperceptible manner by which the disease works its slow progress in the organs affected up to the first more or less severe attack, when it passes from the latent into the active state; and secondly because the disease in the female, although she be discharged, cured to all appearances, after an attack, say of gonorrheal ovaritis, keeps within her, at least up to the time of menopause, the germ of similar more or less severe relapses . . .*
>
> *About ninety per cent of sterile women are married to husbands who have suffered from gonorrhea either previous to, or during married life.*

Most of the discussants of this paper expressed disbelief and even outrage at Noeggerath's views. At the end Noeggerath replied, 'After the gentlemen have given five years or more of careful study to this question, I shall expect to hear more approval than I have done today'. In fact, Noeggerath had published these findings four years earlier in a German monograph. It was to be three years later, in 1879, that Albert Neisser isolated the causative organism for gonorrhoea.

Emil Noeggerath was born in Bonn, Germany. He graduated in medicine from the University of Bonn in 1852, following which he worked as an assistant in the Bonn Gynaecological Clinic. He emigrated to New York in 1856 and later became professor of obstetrics and diseases of women in the New York Medical College. In 1868, along with Abraham Jacobi (1830–1919), he founded, and for five years edited, the *American Journal of Obstetrics and Diseases of Women and Children*, which was published until 1919 and resurfaced in 1921 as the *American Journal of Obstetrics and Gynecology*.

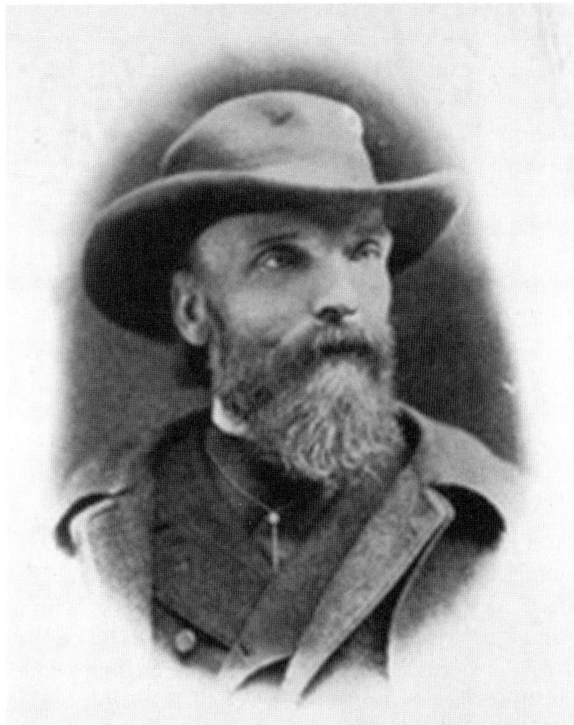

Emil Oscar Jacob Bruno Noeggerath

In 1885 he returned to his homeland and worked in Wiesbaden, where he died on 3 May 1895.

Selected Publications

Noeggerath E. *Die latente Gonorrhoea im weiblichen Geschlecht*. Bonn: Max Cohen & Sohn; 1872.

Noeggerath E. Latent gonorrhea, especially with regard to its influence on fertility in women. *Trans Am Gynecol Soc* 1877; 1: 268–300.

Bibliography References

602, 638, 801, 1146, 1276, 1480, 1485, 1595, 1747.

Novak, Emil (1884–1957)

Novak Curette

Like many clinical gynaecologists of his era at Johns Hopkins Hospital, Emil Novak was steeped in gynaecological pathology. Succeeding Thomas Cullen as head of the gynaecological pathology laboratory, he developed a special interest in the endometrium and designed a curette to facilitate outpatient biopsy. In differentiating endometrial biopsy from therapeutic curettage, he wrote:

> *In other cases it is necessary only to secure smaller amounts of endometrium, as in the differentiation of the physiologic responses of the mucosa to one type or another of hormone stimulation. In this respect the endometrium is the registering board of ovarian endocrine activity, and its microscopic study often yields much more useful information than blood or urine hormone studies.*

Novak originally used his hollow curette attached to an electric motor to create suction, with an intervening bottle to collect the aspirated endometrial tissue. Later the curette was used alone or with a syringe to create the aspiration vacuum. The curette is still in occasional use for endometrial biopsy but has been largely replaced by small bore disposable aspiration cannulae.

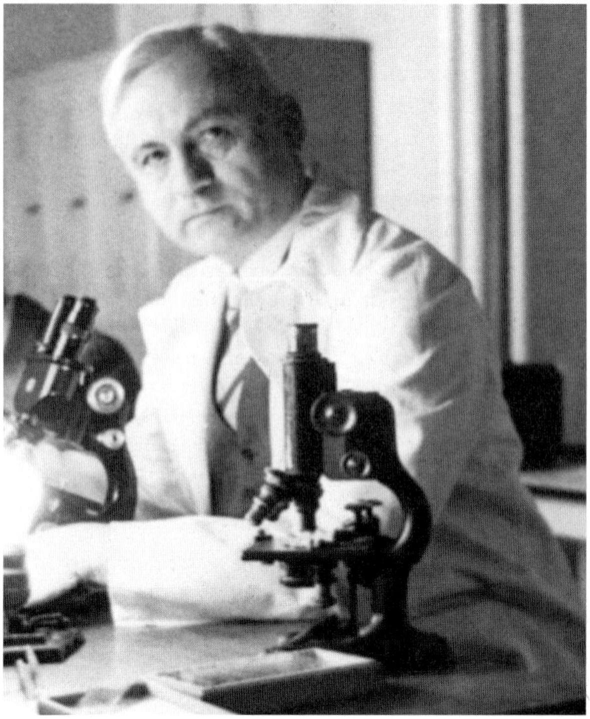

Emil Novak

Emil Novak was born in Baltimore to immigrant parents from Bohemia. His father had a small tailor's shop. He studied at Loyola College and received his medical degree from Baltimore Medical College in 1904, at the age of 20. He did his postgraduate training at the Maryland General Hospital. In 1915 he began his association with the gynaecological pathology laboratory at Johns Hopkins. He became a prolific contributor to the literature, with more than 160 original articles and two textbooks, *Gynecological and Obstetrical Pathology* and *Textbook of Gynecology*. These ran to several editions and were subsequently edited by his son Edmund. He became the inaugural chairman of the American registries of Chorionepithelioma and Rare Ovarian Tumors. In 1948 he was elected president of the American Gynecological Society.

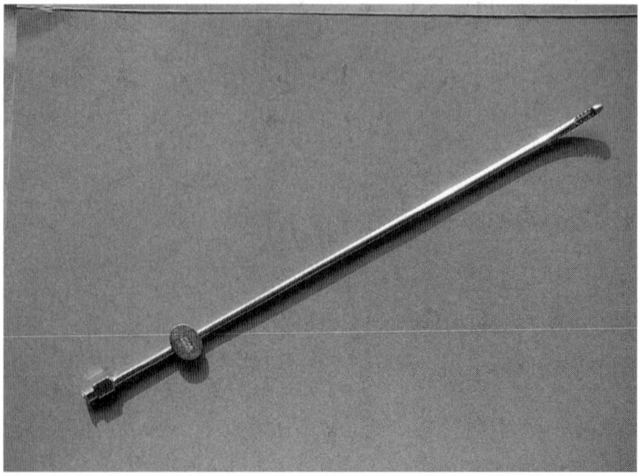

Novak curette

Novak received considerable international recognition, with honorary fellowships from medical societies in Britain, Ireland, Brazil, France, Mexico, Bolivia, Hungary and Greece. In 1949 he was made an honorary fellow of the Royal College of Obstetricians and Gynaecologists. Novak responded by presenting the college with a gavel carved from wood of the attic of Ephraim McDowell's house. He died suddenly from ischaemic heart disease at his home in Baltimore on 3 February 1957.

Selected Publications

Novak E. A suction-curet apparatus for endometrial biopsy. *JAMA* 1935; 104: 1497–8.

Bibliography References

132, 617, 801, 1117, 1480, 1485, 1490.

Nuck, Anton (1650–1692)

Canal of Nuck

Anton Nuck was born in Harderwyck, Holland and obtained his MD from Leyden in 1677. He was a reader in anatomy and surgery at The Hague and later professor at Leyden. Nuck described the prolongation of the peritoneum – *processus vaginalis peritonei* – into the inguinal canal in the female. Known as the canal of Nuck, this pouch of peritoneum is normally obliterated but may remain patent and form the sac of an oblique inguinal hernia. On rare occasions fluid may accumulate and distend a portion of this rudimentary structure presenting as a swelling in the forepart of the labium majus: hydrocoele of the canal of Nuck.

Selected Publications

Nuck A. *Adenographia curiosa et uteri foeminei anatome nova*. Leyden: Jordan Luchtmans; 1691, pp. 130–8.

Bibliography References

406, 676, 917, 1480.

O

O'Driscoll, Kieran (1920–2007)

Active Management of Labour

When Kieran O'Driscoll became Master of the National Maternity Hospital in Dublin, Ireland for the statutory seven-year period, 1963–1969, he directed his attention to the problem of prolonged labour. During his years as master, when he was responsible to the board of governors for all clinical care, teaching and administration within the hospital, O'Driscoll defined the problems of prolonged labour and enunciated the principle of active management in the course of four daily rounds on the labour ward, during which each woman's care and progress in labour was reviewed. O'Driscoll summarised the problem of prolonged labour in the following terms:

> *Prolonged labour presents a picture of mental anguish and physical morbidity which often leads to surgical intervention and may produce a permanent revulsion to childbirth, expressed by the mother as voluntary infertility; it constitutes a danger to the survival and subsequent neurological development in the infant. The harrowing experience is shared by relatives and by doctors and nurses to the extent that few complications so tarnish the image of obstetrics.*

O'Driscoll's mastership culminated in the publication of his classic paper in the *British Medical Journal* in May 1969. A prospective study of 1,000 consecutive primigravid deliveries showed that active management in labour ensured that every woman was delivered within 24 hours. Five years later, a second prospective study of 1,000 cases led to the statement, 'Active management of labour has been developed to the extent that an assurance is given to every woman who attends this hospital that her first baby will be born within 12 hours'. O'Driscoll continued this work in collaboration with his successor, Declan Meagher, and the two of them were to publish the first edition of the book *Active Management of Labour* in 1980. In this book, particular emphasis was laid on the importance of differentiating between first and subsequent labours and the potential detrimental effect upon the woman and her family of a bad experience in the first labour. As they wrote:

> *There are fundamental differences between a first and a later birth. These differences are so great that they warrant the statement that primigravidae and multigravidae behave as different biological species ... The birth of a first child, however, is almost surely the most profound emotional experience, for good or ill, in a lifetime ... A woman who has had an unhappy first experience is likely to be terrified at the prospect of a repeat performance. These fears can have serious consequences outside the narrow confines of obstetrics; they can haunt a woman for the rest of her life and affect her attitude towards her husband and possibly to her child.*

Thus, in clear prose, uncluttered by jargon, they captured the essence of the potential psychological impact of this seminal event in a woman's life.

In addition to an emphasis on the unique nature of the first labour, the principles of active management involved antenatal education of the pregnant woman, a clear diagnosis of labour, one-to-one nursing care during labour, and early correction by amniotomy and oxytocin of slow progress as detected by partographic analysis. Using these principles O'Driscoll abolished prolonged labour in nulliparous women, such that all were promised delivery within 12 hours of the onset of labour. In addition, the operative intervention rates of caesarean section and forceps delivery were low. Contrary to the belief of many, the latter point was never the rationale for active management of labour; rather, it was the prevention of prolonged labour and its deleterious effect on the woman's physical and emotional well-being. O'Driscoll emphasised that the word 'active' referred to more involvement of the obstetrician during labour, as opposed to more active surgical intervention. Some trials of active management of labour in other hospitals were unable to show a reduction in operative delivery, often because the whole philosophy of education and of patient and staff involvement that O'Driscoll imbued in his unit could not be replicated. Many concentrated on the more physical aspects of the package – amniotomy and oxytocin – and found this approach wanting.

Kieran O'Driscoll, the son of a family doctor, was born in 1920 in Kildare, which is located close to the Curragh, a leading centre for thoroughbred horses. His love of thoroughbred horse racing and rugby were two of his main interests outside his family and his work. He was also a great admirer of the poetry of William Butler Yeats, whom he regarded as the finest poet in the English language of the late nineteenth and early twentieth centuries. He was educated at Clongowes Wood College and University College Dublin, graduating in medicine with first-class honours in 1943. His postgraduate training in obstetrics and gynaecology was in Dublin, Liverpool and London. He returned to the National Maternity Hospital as a senior registrar and maintained his attachment there until his retirement in 1986. He was appointed the first clinical professor of obstetrics and gynaecology at University College Dublin, based at the National Maternity Hospital, in 1971. During his time as master, O'Driscoll established the first family planning clinic in the country in April 1963. He also abolished any hospital differences between private and public patients.

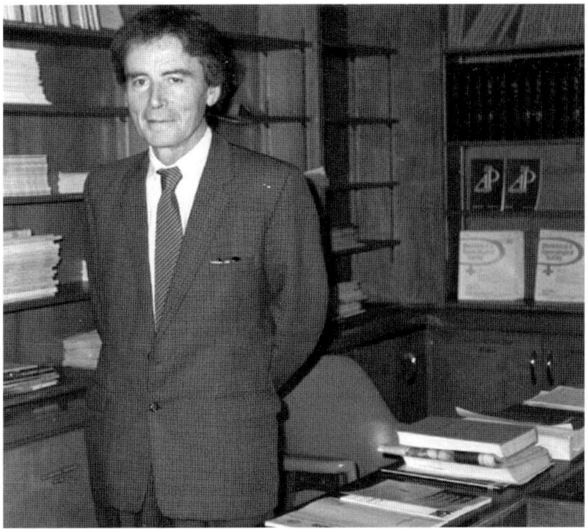

Kieran O'Driscoll

O'Driscoll was a shy and complex man with an exceptional level of integrity and honesty. He was quiet-spoken but could be quite formidable, and occasionally dismissive, as he defended the logic of his clinical programme. His position, as outlined in the first edition of his book, was based on the experience of two masters of a maternity hospital in which they were directly responsible for 100,000 births. By the time the fourth edition of *Active Management of Labour* was published in 2004, the experience was based on 300,000 births.

Caesarean section rates have risen in the National Maternity Hospital, as they have elsewhere in the world, mostly in relation to a change in the maternal demographics of age, parity, body habitus and co-morbidities. However, the humane elements and principles of active management of labour remain intact and relevant. O'Driscoll's contribution in helping to make the harrowing event of prolonged labour obsolete represented one of the most significant Irish contributions to obstetrics in the second half of the twentieth century. Kieran O'Driscoll died suddenly at his home on 17 January 2007, some four months after the death of his wife. Irish obstetrics had lost one of the greats.

Selected Publications

O'Driscoll K, Jackson RJA, Gallagher JT. Prevention of prolonged labour. *BMJ* 1969; 24: 447–80

O'Driscoll K, Stronge JM, Minogue M. Active management of labour. *BMJ* 1973; 3: 135–7.

O'Driscoll K, Meagher D. *Active Management of Labour.* London: W.B. Saunders Company Limited; 1980.

O'Driscoll K, Meagher D, Robson M. *Active Management of Labour.* 4th edn. London: Mosby; 2004.

Bibliography References

99, 100, 102.

O'Sullivan, James Vincent (1899–1976)

Acute Uterine Inversion

On 15 February 1945 Vincent O'Sullivan was trying to reduce an inverted uterus under ether anaesthesia some three hours and three pints of transfused blood after delivery. Before attempted manual replacement, he administered an antiseptic douche. He described the events that followed:

> *In carrying out the douche the tip of the nozzle, guarded by my fingers, was passed towards the posterior fornix: my forearm happened to block the vaginal orifice and the vagina ballooned out, and to my surprise and pleasure the uterus promptly returned to its correct position. The signs of shock rapidly disappeared, and the patient made an uninterrupted recovery.*

Thus, serendipitously, O'Sullivan's method of hydrostatic replacement of acute inversion was discovered. This technique represented an enormous breakthrough in the management of a condition which at that time had a mortality up to 80 per cent.

James Vincent O'Sullivan was born in Wales, the son of an Irish general practitioner, and grew up in

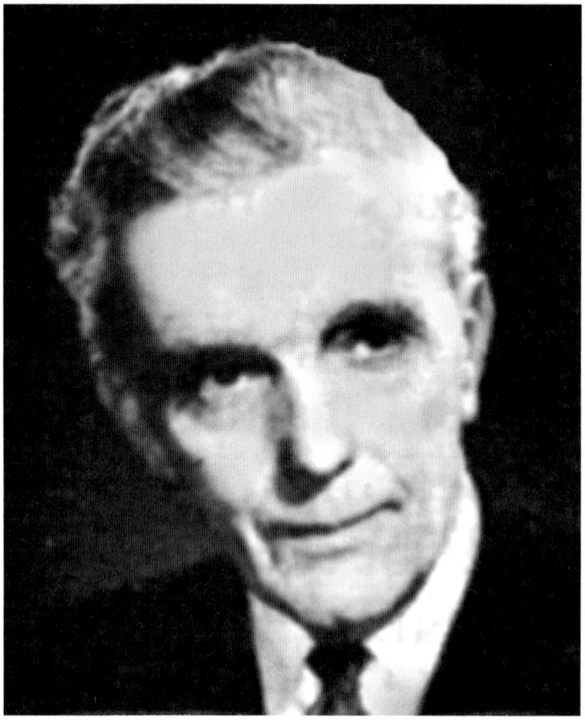

James Vincent O'Sullivan

County Cork. He received his medical education at the University of Galway and the London Hospital Medical College, graduating MB with first-class honours in 1924. He became consultant obstetrician to the City of London Maternity Hospital and St Theresa's Hospital, Wimbledon. He conceived the idea of an international hospital where leading specialists from around the world would spend time developing the highest standards and techniques and train others to maintain them. Despite some early success in planning this vision, practical difficulties prevented it from being realised.

In his youth he was a good rugby player, and later in life he excelled at skiing, shooting and fishing. He was also a considerable raconteur. He had four children, all of whom became doctors.

Selected Publications

O'Sullivan JV. Acute inversion of the uterus. *BMJ* 1945; 2: 282–3.

Bibliography References

79, 99, 822, 1151, 1152.

Ould, Fielding (1710–1789)

Mechanism of Labour/Episiotomy

Fielding Ould was the first to recognise that during labour the fetal head could not remain with its long axis at right angles to that of the shoulders and traverse the pelvic brim:

> *So that supposing the woman on her back, the head coming into the world, is a kind of ellipsis in a vertical position; and the shoulders of the same form in a horizontal position; thirdly that the pelvis is of an elliptical form, from one to the other hip . . . it must of necessity, from what has been said above, acquire another form for the admission of the shoulders . . . it is evident that when the child is turned, so as to have the chin on one shoulder, all the above objections are removed; for the head and shoulders are on a parallel line, in respect of their shape, and at the same time, both answer the form of the passage from the pelvis.*

In reasoning that the fetal head rotated towards one shoulder to traverse the pelvic brim, Ould wrote:

> *It is to be hoped that this opinion, being founded on theory, and confirmed by experience, will meet with few opponents; and without doubt, the due application of it will be of infinite use.*

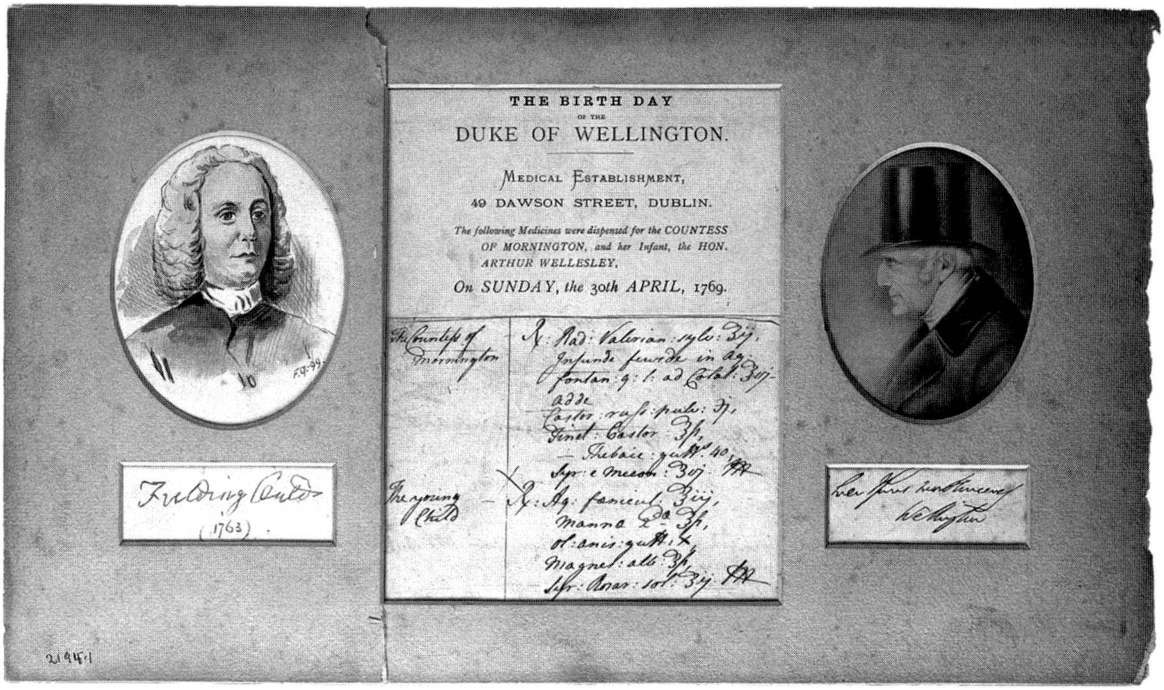

Post-partum medication orders for the Countess of Mornington and her infant son, the future Duke of Wellington, delivered by Fielding Ould

Fielding Ould was born in Galway, Ireland into an English military family. His grandfather commanded the Royal Regiment of Welch Fusiliers at the Battle of the Boyne in 1690. In his early childhood, Fielding Ould lived in London, until his father was 'assassinated at night in the streets of London'. Ould's mother returned with her children to Galway when Fielding was five. From the age of 19 Ould spent five years as a prosector in the anatomy department of Trinity College Medical School in Dublin. For unknown reasons he did not take his medical degree but went to Paris to study midwifery under Grégoire. He returned to Dublin, becoming a licentiate in midwifery of the College of Physicians in Ireland in 1738. His single publication, *A Treatise of Midwifery*, was published in 1742 and became influential in British obstetrics. He was one of the first to advocate delivery in the left lateral position and the selected use of episiotomy and its suture:

It sometimes happens that the head of the child . . . cannot however come forward, by reason of the extraordinary construction of the external orifice of the vagina . . . wherefore it must be dilated if possible by the fingers . . . if this cannot be accomplished, there must be an incision made towards the anus with a pair of crooked probe-scissors, introducing one blade between the head and vagina, as far as shall be thought necessary for the present purpose, and the businesses done at one pinch, by which the whole body will easily come forth . . . After the delivery, the wound must be united by a stitch.

Along with others, he taught a more conservative attitude to delivery of the placenta, in contrast to the common practice of immediate manual removal. At a time when few mothers survived caesarean section, Ould registered his disapproval in strong terms: 'Repugnant, not only to all rules of theory or practice, but even to humanity . . . this detestable, barbarous, illegal piece of inhumanity'.

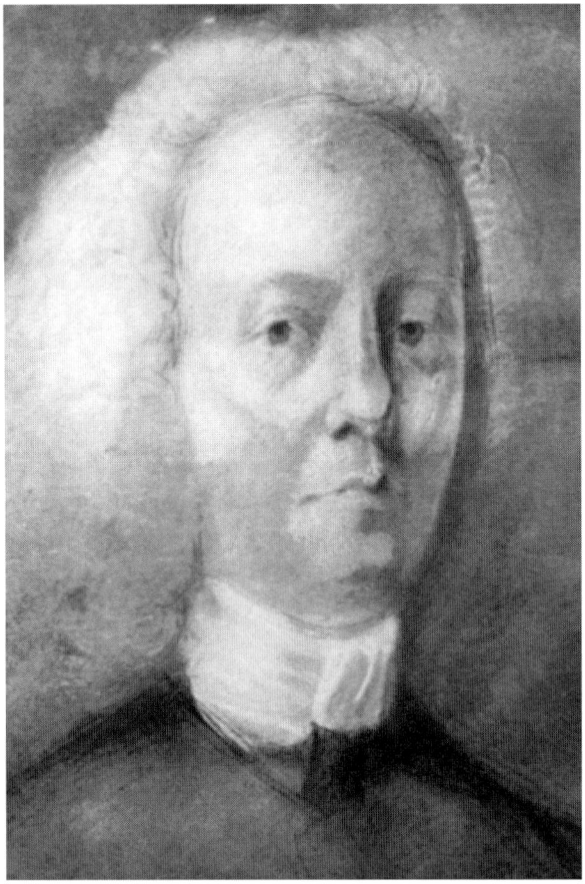

Fielding Ould

In 1759 Ould was knighted and appointed Master of the Rotunda Lying-in Hospital to succeed the founding master, Bartholomew Mosse. Some idea of the low status of midwifery within the medical profession at the time is shown by the attitude of the College of Physicians to the request by Dublin University to examine Fielding Ould for its medical degree. The college refused, on the grounds that man-midwives should not be eligible for a full medical degree. The university went ahead, examined Ould, and granted him the MB in 1761. The dispute smouldered between the two institutions for years thereafter.

Ould had an extensive practice among the upper classes in Dublin and delivered the Countess of Mornington of her sixth child, a son, Arthur, destined to become the Duke of Wellington.

Sir Fielding Ould died suddenly from a stroke, shortly after delivering a patient.

Selected Publications

Ould F. *A Treatise of Midwifery in Three Parts.* Dublin: Nelson and Connor; 1742. Also published in: The Classics of Obstetrics and Gynecology Library. Birmingham: Gryphon Editions; 1990 (facsimile).

Bibliography References

99, 195, 293, 929, 1011, 1126, 1261, 1595.

P

Paget, James (1814–1899)

Paget's Disease of the Vulva

Paget's disease of the breast is characterised by an eczematous looking change in the skin of the nipple associated with underlying ductal carcinoma. Paget first drew attention to this in 1874:

I believe it has not yet been published that certain chronic affections in the skin of the nipple and areola are very often succeeded by the formation of scirrhous cancer in the mammary gland . . . In the majority it had the appearance of a florid, intensely red, raw surface, very finely granular . . . like the surface of very acute diffuse eczema . . . But it has happened that in every case which I have been able to watch, cancer of the mammary gland has followed within at the most two years, and usually within one year.

Paget realised that such an association may occur in other areas of the body: 'I believe that a nearly similar sequence of events may be observed in other parts'. Indeed, this turned out to be the case, and such lesions came to be known as extramammary Paget's disease.

The first case of Paget's disease of the vulva was described by William Dubreuilh, professor of dermatology at the University of Bordeaux. He reported this to the British Medical Association meeting in 1903. In discussing extramammary Paget's disease, he said, 'no case has been observed in which the vulva was affected, and no histological examination of Paget's disease of a mucous surface has been published'. Dubreuilh went on to describe such a case in a 51-year-old woman, 'little addicted to habits of cleanliness'. He described the typical Paget cells found in both the breast and extramammary types of the disease: 'Some of them were very large, with a clear protoplasm and a dark nucleus in process of karyokinetic division'.

James Paget was born in Great Yarmouth, England, the youngest of nine surviving children of a brewer. At the age of 16 he was apprenticed to a local surgeon, moving on to St Bartholomew's Hospital in

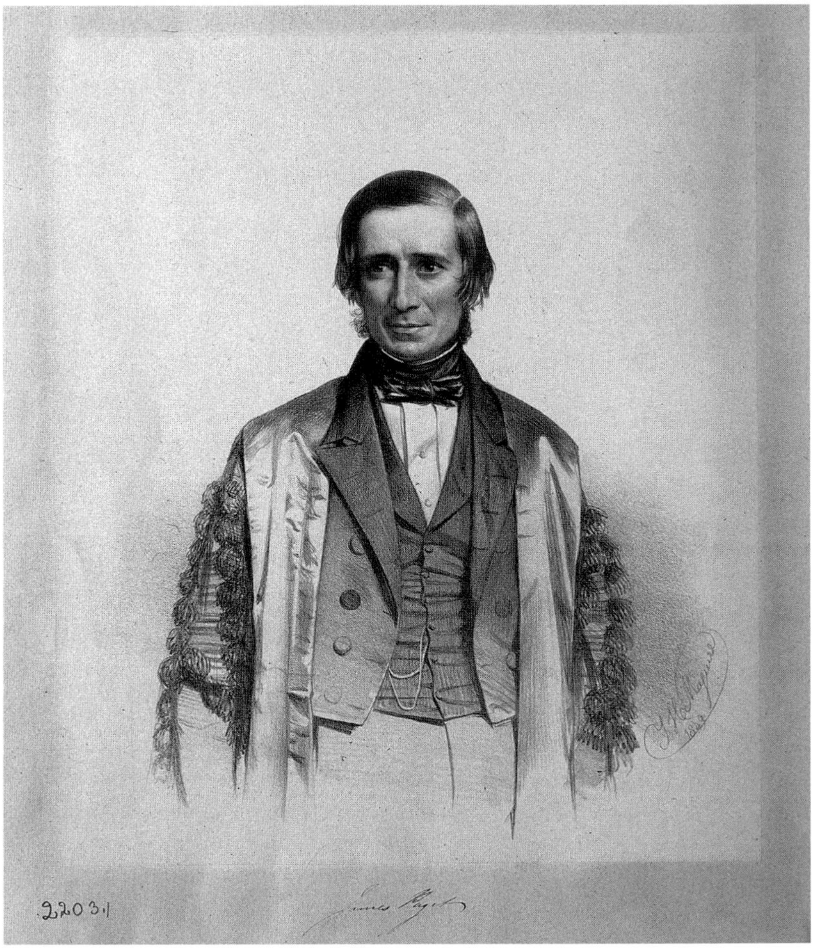

James Paget

London as a medical student four years later. He qualified in 1836 and became curator of the anatomy museum and demonstrator in anatomy at St Bartholomew's Hospital. In 1844 he was appointed surgeon to the hospital. He was a prodigious worker, and despite a huge private practice he continued to write and lecture extensively. He was an adherent to the Paget family motto, *Labor ipse voluptas* (work itself is a pleasure). Paget also campaigned for the abolition of slavery and for education of the poor. He pursued these objectives through a lay organisation, the Society for the Diffusion of Useful Knowledge. He described Paget's disease of bone, osteitis deformans, in 1877. Acknowledged as an extraordinary surgical leader in his lifetime he was appointed sergeant-surgeon extraordinary to Queen Victoria in 1858 and knighted in 1871. He liked music, walking and whist, but disliked sports. He died on 30 December 1899.

Selected Publications

Dubreuilh W. Paget's disease of the vulva. *Br J Dermatol* 1901; 13: 407–13.

Paget J. On disease of the mammary areola preceding cancer of the mammary gland. *St Bartholomew Hosp Rep* 1874; 10: 87–9.

Bibliography References

684, 854, 867, 962, 963, 1157, 1308, 1322, 1387, 1588.

Pajot, Charles (1816–1896)

Pajot's Manoeuvre

Traction during forceps delivery should follow the curve of the pelvis. Using standard obstetric forceps with straight shanks, this may be achieved using Pajot's manoeuvre, in which traction by one hand on the handles of the forceps is associated with downward pressure on the shanks by the other. This was first described by the Danish obstetrician, Matthias Saxtorph in 1772 and is often called the Saxtorph–Pajot manoeuvre. It was also taught by Friedrich Osiander (1759–1822).

Charles Pajot was born in Paris and graduated from that university in 1842. He became professor of obstetrics and gynaecology in 1863 and a dominant figure in French obstetrics in the second half of the nineteenth century. He was a conservative obstetrician, with a pithy turn of phrase and well known for his aphorisms. With regard to the application of forceps, he declared, 'Left blade, from the left hand, to the left and the first: everything must be 'gauche' – except the accoucheur'. Like many of his generation he designed his own forceps. He spoke against analgesia in labour and caesarean section: 'To prepare for a caesarean section is to prepare for a scientific assassination'. Pajot devised a hook for fetal decapitation, achieved by the sawing movements of a wire string in a groove in the hook. However, he lectured his students against fetal destructive procedures, saying,

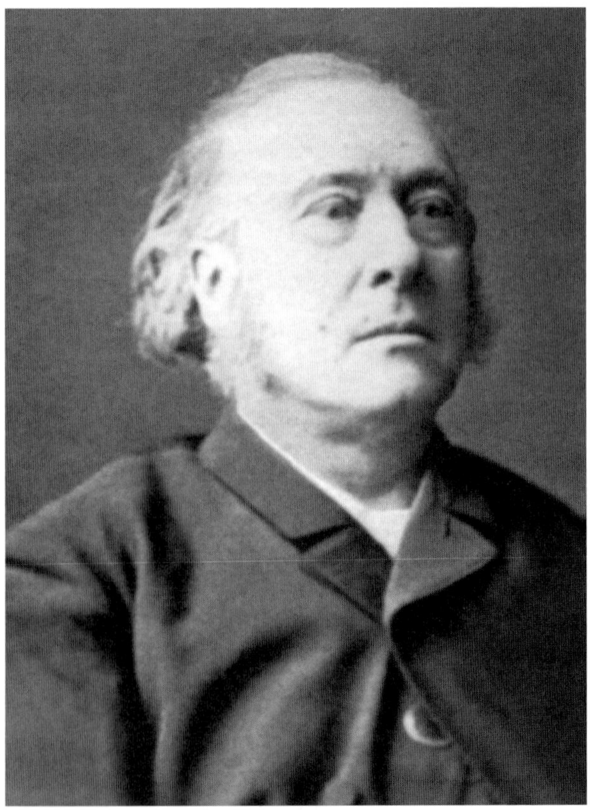

Charles Pajot

'Remember gentlemen, that this hook and this perforator have been put here to remind you never to use them'.

Pajot was a keen angler and habitually fished the River Seine. He frequently spent his nights in a boat under the Pont Marie, which was often used as a jumping site for would-be suicides. Over the years he is said to have rescued no fewer than 16 of these despairing souls, probably only marginally less than his level of piscatorial success. This talent was noted by his colleagues, who nicknamed him 'the Newfoundland dog' of the faculty. He was described by Adolphe Pinard, at that time one of his assistants, as having 'a casual air – a superb presence – an astonishing mimic'.

Selected Publications

Osiander EB. *Lehrbuch der Hebaummenkunst* Göttingen: JG Rosenbusch; 1796.

Pajot C. La seconde sur le forceps à aiguille. *Ann de Gynéc (Paris)* 1877; 7: 21–31.

Saxtorph M. *Theoria de diverso partu*. Copenhagen: AH Godiche; 1772

Bibliography References

99, 399, 451, 548, 604, 721, 1158, 1261.

Palfyn, Jan (1650–1730)

Obstetric Forceps

Jan Palfyn was an anatomist and surgeon, but as such he was also familiar with obstetrics and the destructive operations used on the fetus in obstructed labour. As he wrote in his treatise on surgical anatomy:

> *The doctor is often the cause of death of the child by inflicting a head wound, demonstrated in a case which I witnessed not long ago, where the fetus, apparently dead, was with the aid of a hook inserted in the occiput, extracted. It was alive but lived only one day. But what shall I say? There are many difficulties in medicine which cannot be overcome by the wisest physicians.*

He conceived the idea of an instrument gripping the fetal head like a pair of hands. He called them *mains de fer* and showed them before the Royal Academy of Sciences in Paris in 1720. The blades were made of metal with a cephalic curve and a slight pelvic curve. André Levret was familiar with Palfyn's forceps and it may have been from these that he got the idea for his long forceps with their pelvic curve. The handles of Palfyn's forceps were wooden, with no overlap or locking mechanism. Each blade was inserted and held separately, rather in the manner of salad spoons – indeed, the French described them as Palfyn's *cuillières*. As a result, the blades allowed little or no traction before slipping off the fetal head. Others tied the handles together with more success. The Chamberlen forceps had been in use, albeit in secret, for over a century when Palfyn presented his relatively unserviceable forceps. However, Palfyn openly shared his idea and sought no profit from it. He never mentioned or described his forceps in any of his publications, which were all written before his invention.

Jan Palfyn was born in Courtrai, Belgium, the son of a barber-surgeon, which at that time was a profession in the lower ranks of society. Having learned what he could from his father, he decided that a good knowledge of anatomy was essential to the improved practice of surgery:

> *I have always loved the science of anatomy beyond measure: I have applied myself to it with an insatiable passion; having in view the aim to be able to practice surgery with the greatest security.*

To further his anatomical education he dissected cadavers which, due to residual plague in Flanders, were relatively plentiful at that time. However, this practice was frowned upon in Courtrai, and when he was discovered opening a grave he had to leave town

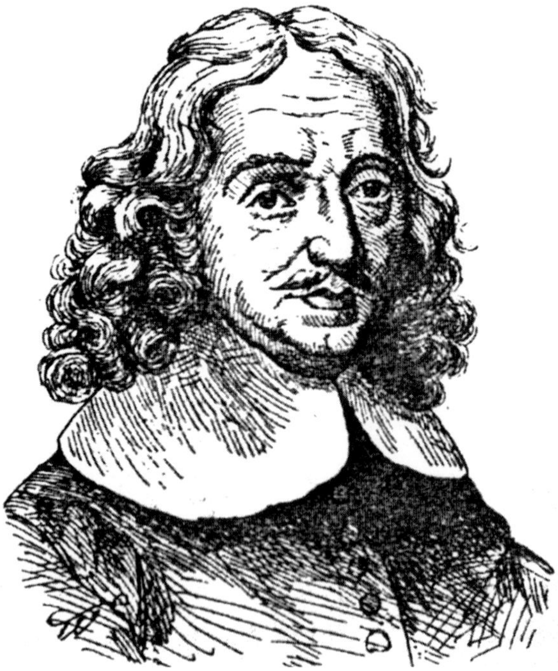

Jan Palfyn

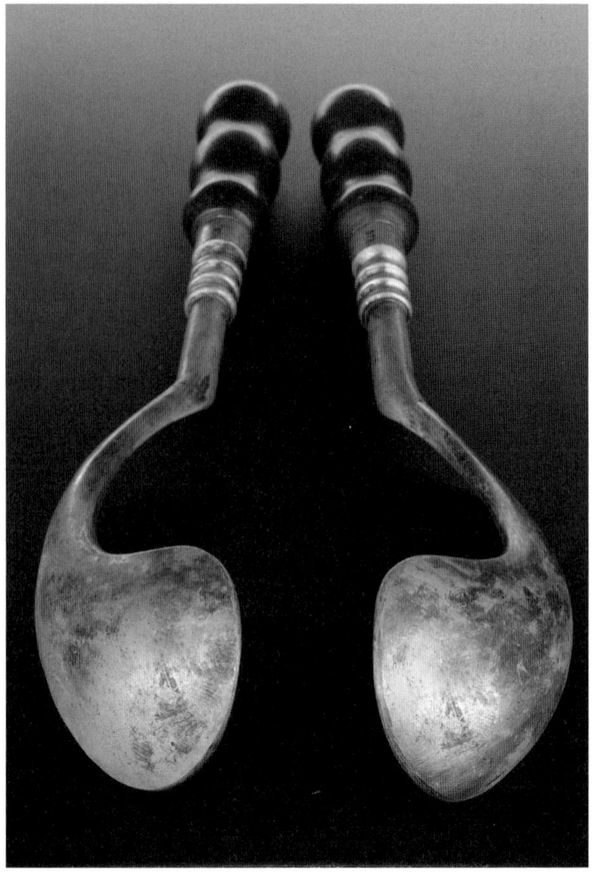

Palfyn 'mains de fer'

in some haste to escape the wrath of the law. He went to Ghent, was apprenticed to a surgeon and attended lectures at the medical school. In 1674 he moved to Paris and established his reputation as an anatomist and surgeon. Having been pardoned for his previous anatomical indiscretions, he returned to his home city of Courtrai, intending to devote himself to teaching and writing. His continued anatomical inquisitiveness again brought him into conflict with the establishment, and he was fined by the Royal College of Medicine at Courtrai for 'inobedience in refusing to explain satisfactorily a skeleton found in his possession'. As a result, he left for Ypres in 1687. He visited schools of medicine in England, France, Germany and Holland in his quest for the latest anatomical and surgical knowledge. In 1695 he moved back to Ghent, where he was later appointed professor of anatomy and surgery. In his time, he did much to promote the knowledge of surgical anatomy and wrote a number of treatises on the subject between 1701 and 1714. He died in Ghent on 21 April 1730.

Selected Publications

Palfyn J. *Heelkonstige antleding des Menschelyk lichaems.* Leyden; 1710.

Palfyn J. *Traité d'anatomie chirurgicale.* Paris; 1726.

Bibliography References

347, 361, 399, 451, 548, 648, 676, 721, 1261, 1285, 1511.

Palmer, Raoul (1905–1985)

Laparoscopy

Raoul Palmer was largely responsible for the application of laparoscopy to gynaecology. He started using this technique in 1943, at a time when it was mainly used to visualise the upper abdomen by surgeons. Over the years he was instrumental in developing the procedure, using the Trendelenburg position and a uterine cannula to improve the view of the pelvic organs. He delineated its role in both infertility and birth control, pioneering laparoscopic tubal ligation with electrocoagulation. Later in his career he was to write:

> *It is my privilege, as a senior laparoscopist, to state that laparoscopy is an innocuous, rapid and elegant procedure in the hands of well-trained specialists. It can also be a source of errors and accidents if it is put in the hands of every gynecologist without the proper training and the proper spirit of continuous attention to all the technical details, indispensable for total safety.*

He is remembered eponymously for his laparoscopy forceps and 'Palmer's point', the area in the left hypochondrium least likely to have adhesions in patients with previous extensive surgery: 'In case of previous laparotomy, I still use an entry 3 cm below the middle of the left costal border'.

Palmer was also one of the earliest colposcopists in France. As a young gynaecologist he assisted Vivian Green-Armytage when the latter visited Paris in 1938 at the invitation of the French Gynaecological Society to demonstrate his technique of vaginal hysterectomy. Palmer later did the pen and ink drawings for Green-Armytage's paper on the subject in the *Journal of Obstetrics and Gynaecology of the British Empire* of 1939.

He played a leading role in the fight for contraception and termination of pregnancy in France in the 1960s, often at odds with the medical establishment. Among those who came to learn the technique of laparoscopy was Patrick Steptoe in 1958.

Raoul Palmer was born in Paris to Swedish parents. He became head of the Gynaecological Clinic at the Broca hospital in Paris. In addition to his laparoscopic skills, he was a noted tubal and vaginal surgeon. He was a renowned international teacher and in 1974 was elected fellow ad eundum of the Royal College of Obstetricians and Gynaecologists.

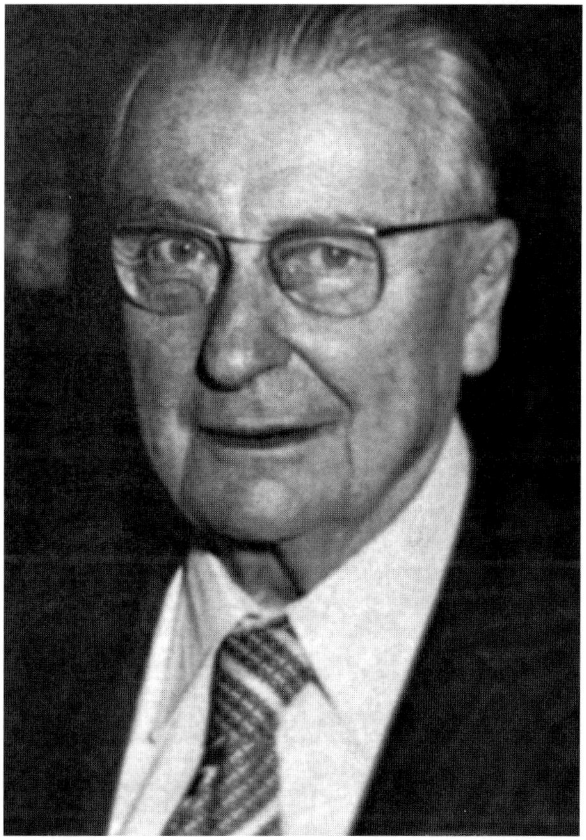

Raoul Palmer

Selected Publications

Palmer R. La coelioscopie gynécologique. *Acad de Chir* 1946; 72: 363–8.

Palmer R. Technique et instrumentation de la coelioscopie gynécologique. *Gynécol Obstét (Paris)* 1947; 46: 420.

Palmer R. Essais de stérilisation tubaire coelioscopique per electrocoagulation isthmique. *Bull Fed Soc Gynécol Obstét* 1962; 14: 298–302.

Palmer R. Safety in laparoscopy. *J Reprod Med* 1974; 13: 1–5.

Bibliography References

128, 168, 580, 670, 1084, 1160, 1161, 1315, 1512.

Pantaleoni, D Commander (c. 1869)

Hysteroscopy

After the initial endoscopic efforts of Philipp Bozzini in 1805, a practical endoscope was developed by Antonin Jean Desormeaux of the Hôpital Necker in Paris. Desormeaux used the instrument to study the urethra and bladder. In 1865, Francis Cruise (1834–1912) of Dublin improved the illumination of Desormeaux's instrument with a modified paraffin lamp light source.

The first reported use of the endoscope to diagnose and treat an intrauterine lesion was by D. Commander Pantaleoni, MD in the *Medical Press and Circular* of 1869. In this article he acknowledges the help of Francis Cruise:

> *It is always the instrument of Dr Cruise that I have employed in my practice, and I am so well satisfied with it, that I owe a public testimony of thankfulness to its inventor, for the kindness with which he treated me in Dublin, and his willingness to show to me the employment of this instrument on several cases.*

He wrote that three years later he examined a 60-year-old woman with postmenopausal bleeding and, finding nothing abnormal in the vagina or cervix, prepared her for hysteroscopy by insertion of a laminaria tent, 'sponge tent', for 24 hours. At that time this technique was used to dilate the cervix and allow diagnostic digital exploration of the uterine cavity. Pantaleoni then described precautions for reasons that would appal the modern endoscopist, spoiled by the cold light source:

> *The next day I proceeded to the removal of the sponge tent. I had the lady lying on her left side, as is usual in England in specular examinations or confinements, and I took the only precaution, that the lady should be as near and as much as possible on the borders of the bed, as otherwise the lamp of Dr Cruise's instrument might set fire to the curtains and at all events the endoscope be not so easily managed.*

He then inserted a 20 cm long cylindrical tube through the cervix 'with the greatest ease', and through it passed the endoscope:

> *Having in such a way applied the endoscope I could see most clearly in the inside of the cavity of the womb, and inspect the condition of the internal membrane.*
> *A polypous vegetation was easily discovered at the bottom of the cavity and towards the posterior part of the fundus uteri in my case. It was a vivid red colour, unequal like a sponge, and of the largeness of a small strawberry. It was striking the difference with the pale yellowish colour of the rest of the membrane. I withdrew the endoscope fixing the tube however, upon the vegetation, and I introduced the caustic through the tube itself, being therefore quite sure of the impossibility of touching anything but the vegetation itself, and then each time, I looked in again with the endoscope to certify the effect of the cauterisation before removing the tube. I was obliged to return six or seven times to the use of the caustic. I employed the nitrate of silver, the chromic acid, which I have experienced particularly useful ...*

The polyp must have been benign, as the result 'proved to be one of the most perfect success, and with no return of illness'. Pantaleoni finished his paper in speculative mode:

> *Those considerations decided me to put under the judgement of the profession this system, in the hope to open a door to some future progress of our knowledge in gynecology.*

It was to be more than a century before diagnostic and operative hysteroscopy would become common gynaecological practice. It seems from this article that Pantaleoni visited Dublin and learned the use of the endoscope from Cruise. However, where he practised and whence he came is not known.

Selected Publications

Cruise FR. The utility of the endoscope as an aid in the diagnosis and treatment of disease. *Dublin Quart J Med Sci* 1865; 39: 329–63.

Desormeaux AJ. *De l'endoscope et de ses applications au diagnostic et au traitement des affections de l'urètre et de la vessie.* Paris: Baillière; 1865.

Pantaleoni DC. On endoscopic examination of the cavity of the womb. *Med Press Circ* 1869; 8: 26–7.

Bibliography References

908.

Papanicolaou, George Nicholas (1883–1962)

Papanicolaou Smear

George Nicholas Papanicolaou was born in Kyme on the Greek island of Euboea. His father was a doctor and the mayor of Kyme. Young George was sent to school in Athens at the age of 11. He entered medical school at 15 and was awarded his MD from the University of Athens in 1904. He served two years in the medical corps of the Greek Army and returned to practise in his home town. Within a year he became dissatisfied and left to study philosophy and natural sciences in Germany. He received his PhD in zoology from the University of Munich in 1910. After working for a time in the Oceanographic Institute of Monaco, he was called up to serve as a medical officer in the Greek Army during the Balkan War. He met several volunteers from the United States and in 1913 emigrated to New York. When Papanicolaou and his wife arrived in New York, they had little money and no medical contacts. For several months they both worked at Gimbels Department Store. Papanicolaou then got a part-time job in the pathology laboratory of the New York Hospital and the following year was appointed a research biologist in the department of anatomy at Cornell Medical College. He remained working at these two institutions until 1961.

In his early years in New York, Papanicolaou studied sex differentiation in guinea pig ova. Needing to determine the time of ovulation, he took serial vaginal smears from the guinea pig using a nasal speculum. Ultimately, he was able to correlate the vaginal cytological changes with ovulation. He later applied this to the human and devised a staining technique using alcohol as a counter stain with the dyes, giving greater transparency and better cell type differentiation. While studying vaginal smears at the New York Hospital, he identified tumour cells by chance in a woman with cervical cancer. He gave a preliminary report on this finding at the Third Race Betterment Conference in Battle Creek, Michigan, in January 1928:

> *It is not an exaggeration to say that certain cases of cancer of the cervix may be diagnosed by the presence of only one of these cells.*

The conference was not geared to this information, and the published proceedings were of poor quality and thus made no impact. The pathology establishment still felt that accurate histological diagnosis required a viable tissue sample rather than exfoliated 'dead' cells. Furthermore, Papanicolaou was not trained as a pathologist. Papanicolaou remained convinced of the potential value of exfoliative cytology in the diagnosis of cancer of the female genital tract. In the late 1930s he teamed up with Dr Herbert Trout in the department of gynaecology at the New York Lying-in Hospital. This collaboration resulted in the landmark publication in 1941. In the concluding paragraph they wrote:

> *In presenting this method of diagnosis at this time we hope that it may prove to be a dependable means whereby the principle malignant diseases of the uterus can be recognised; and further that because of its simplicity, it may eventually be applied widely so that the incipient phases of the disease may come more promptly within the range of our modern modes of treatment which have proved highly effective in early carcinoma.*

Few medical prophesies have been so comprehensively vindicated. Papanicolaou and Trout used a

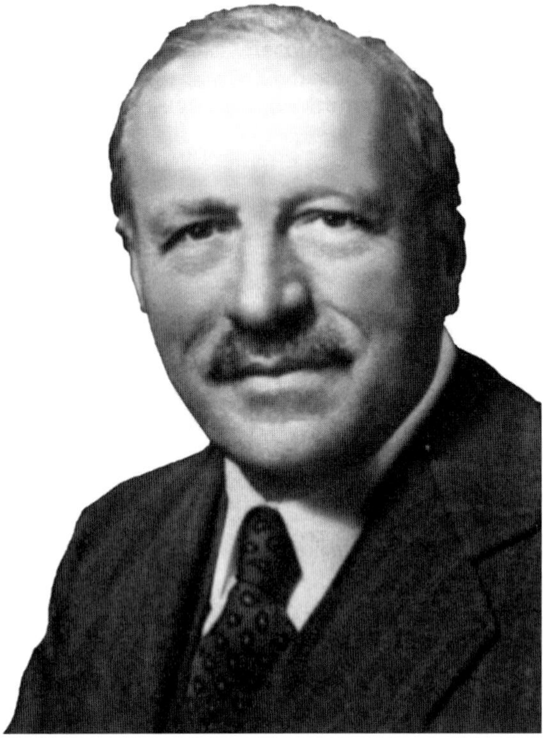

George Nicholas Papanicolaou

curved glass pipette with a rubber bulb to produce suction and aspirate cells from the posterior vaginal fornix. Later, in 1947, James Ayre simplified cell collection with a wooden spatula that continues in use to this day.

Papanicolaou left New York in 1961 and moved to Miami Beach, Florida. He was named director of the Miami Cancer Institute. On the morning of 19 February 1962, he awoke with chest pain and died a few hours later from myocardial infarction.

Selected Publications

Papanicolaou GN. New cancer diagnosis. In: *Proceedings of the Third Race Betterment Conference*. Battle Creek, MI: Race Betterment Foundation; 1928: 528–34.

Papanicolaou GN, Trout HF. The diagnostic value of vaginal smears in carcinoma of the uterus. *Am J Obstet Gynecol* 1941; 42: 193–206.

Papanicolaou GN, Trout HF. *Diagnosis of Cancer by Vaginal Smears*. New York, NY: Commonwealth Fund; 1943.

Bibliography References

137, 241, 383, 387, 665, 853, 854, 1044, 1099, 1100, 1377, 1389, 1650.

Paré, Ambroise (1510–1590)

Internal Podalic Version

Ambroise Paré was born in Laval to a Huguenot family. When he was 15 years old he became an apprentice to a barber-surgeon in Angers. He continued his apprenticeship at the Hôtel Dieu in Paris and worked there for three years from 1533–6.

In 1541 he qualified as a master barber-surgeon. He spent most of his life as a military surgeon, serving through the reigns of six kings. His keen powers of observation and logical approach revolutionised the surgical management of wounds. Paré was one of the first to publish a medical book in a colloquial language, instead of the customary scholarly Latin. For this he was reproached by his colleagues in the faculty of medicine at Paris. However, he was subsequently vindicated, as his extensive writings in French were translated into several other European languages and had a profound effect on surgical practice for at least a century.

His obstetrical experience was gained in the Hôtel Dieu. He reintroduced internal podalic version and breech extraction into the medical literature. In his writing on the subject he says he learned podalic version from two master barber-surgeons in Paris: Thierry de Héry and Nicole Lambert. Paré taught this method to deal with transverse lie and shoulder presentation. He also used it to hasten delivery in cases of antepartum haemorrhage. It was by using this technique that one of his pupils, Jacques Guillemeau, subsequently saved the life of Paré's daughter.

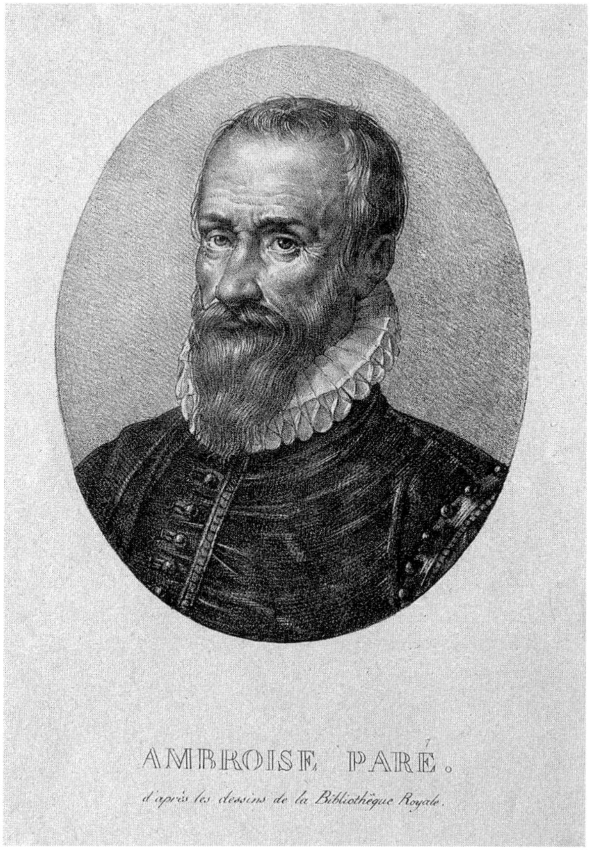

Ambroise Paré

Excerpts from the translation of Paré's description of internal podalic version and breech extraction follow:

> *. . . and then let him put his hand gently into the mouth of the womb, having first made it gentle and slippery with much oil; and when his hand is in let him find out the form and situation of the child . . . and so turn him that his feet may come forwards . . . and when he hath them both out, let him join them both together, and so by little and little let him draw the whole body from the womb.*

Paré was aware of the risk of the uterus trapping the aftercoming head of the breech during extraction and advocated leaving one arm alongside the head:

> *Neither is it meet that he should come out with his arms along by his sides, or be drawn out on that sort, but one of his arms must be stretched out above his head, and the other down by his side; for otherwise the orifice of the womb . . . would so shrink and draw itself when the body should come unto the neck . . . that it would strangle and kill the infant.*

Paré advocated repair of the perineum following traumatic childbirth: 'We should by means of some stitches unite the parts unnaturally separated and treat the wound according to art'.

In 1562 Paré was appointed premier surgeon to King Charles IX, who thought so highly of him that he hid him in his own rooms during the St Bartholomew's Day massacre of Huguenots, saying, 'It is not right for a man so useful to the world to perish in such a manner'.

In this profile, only his obstetrical contribution is outlined, but Paré's work and influence helped elevate surgery from its barbarous roots to an organised profession. He outlined his surgical principles as follows:

> *Five things are proper to the duty of a surgeon: to take away that which is superfluous; to restore to their places such things as are displaced; to separate those things which are joined together; to join those things which are separated; and to supply the defects of nature. Thou shalt far more easily and happily attain to the knowledge of these things by long use and much exercise, than by much reading of books or daily hearing of teachers.*

Between military campaigns, Paré lived and practised in Paris. When he was 64 his wife died; he remarried and had six more children. He died in Paris on 20 December 1590.

Selected Publications

Paré A. *Briefe collection de l'administration anatomique.* Paris; 1549.

The Works of Ambroise Paré. Translated by TH Johnston. London: Clark; 1678.

Bibliography References

32, 74, 88, 95, 99, 102, 320, 339, 408, 420, 519, 548, 648, 682, 827, 973, 983, 1057, 1121, 1283, 1372, 1375, 1589, 1698.

Pawlik, Karl (1849–1914)

Pawlik's Grip/Pawlik's Triangle

Karl Pawlik was born in Klattau, Bohemia and received his MD from the University of Vienna in 1873. He became director of the Bohemia obstetrics and gynaecology clinic in Prague and later professor of the Bohemia medical faculty at Prague University. Pawlik was amazingly multilingual, being fluent in German, English, French, Italian, Spanish, Portuguese, Polish and Russian. He contributed to the knowledge of urological disease in women and was the first to catheterise the ureters using reflected light via a urethral speculum. In 1889 Pawlik performed the first successful total cystectomy for cancer in a female and implanted the ureters into the vagina – although with a ureterovaginal fistula, the woman must have regarded this as a pyrrhic victory

He is remembered eponymously for 'Pawlik's grip', when the fetal head is grasped one-handed abdominally like a ball to assess the degree of mobility and relationship to the pelvic brim. The area of the anterior vaginal wall in contact with the trigone of the bladder, identifiable by the absence of vaginal rugae, is known as 'Pawlik's triangle'.

He was elected an honorary fellow of the American Gynecological Society in 1901. He retired in November 1913 and died on 7 September 1914

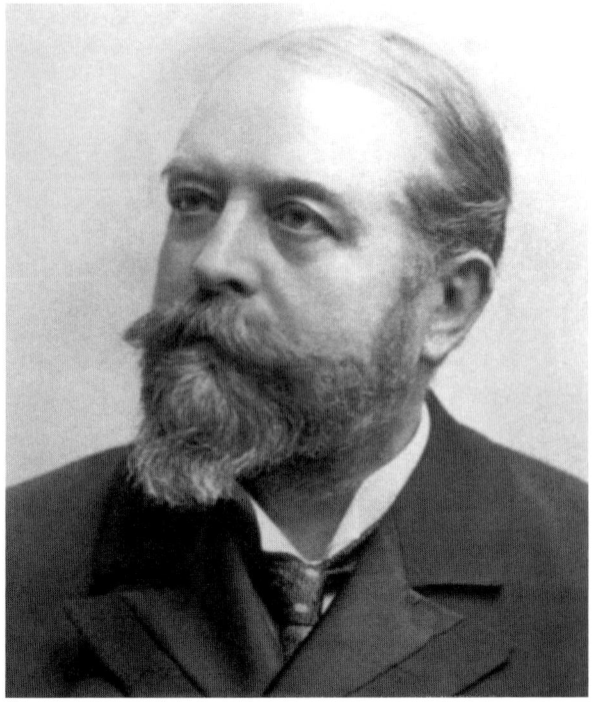

Karl Pawlik

Selected Publications

Pawlik K. *Über die Sondirung der Ureteren der weiblichen Blase. Arch Gynäkol* 1881; 18: 491–5.

Pawlik, K Über Blasenextirpation. *Wein Med Wochenschr* 1891; 41: 1816–7.

Bibliography References

889, 1174, 1175, 1291.

Pearl, Raymond (1879–1940)

Pearl Index

The Pearl index is the oldest and most commonly used measure of contraceptive efficacy. It is defined as the number of failures per 100 woman-years of exposure. The numerator is the number of unintended pregnancies, and the denominator is the total months or cycles of exposure from the start of the contraceptive method until the study ends, the method is discontinued or unintended pregnancy occurs. The quotient is multiplied by 1,200 if the denominator is months or by 1,300 if the

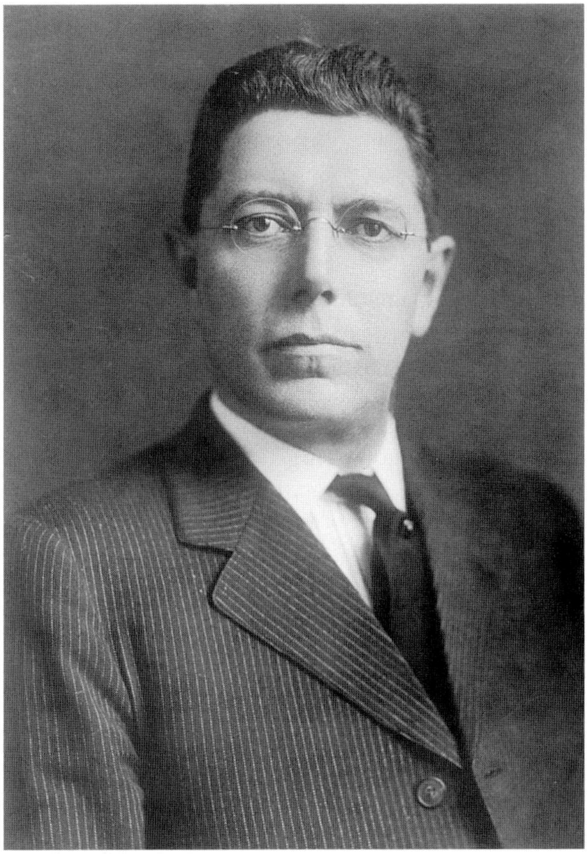

Raymond Pearl

denominator is cycles. The limitation of the Pearl index is that it does not compare variable durations of exposure and the fact that failure rates of most methods of contraception decline with prolonged use. This can be overcome by using life table analysis.

Raymond Pearl did his undergraduate degree in biology at Dartmouth College and his PhD, on the behaviour of flatworms, at the University of Michigan. In 1907 he joined the department of zoology at Johns Hopkins University and in 1918 was appointed the first professor of biometry and vital statistics in the school of hygiene and public health at the same university. Pearl approached biology from a broad but statistical perspective, studying the implications of life, fertility, population growth, eugenics, genetics, disease and death. He defined biostatistics as the 'biology of groups' and applied both statistical analysis and experimental methods to these groups. He sought to define the influence of genetics and environment on disease and longevity. He was an early advocate of birth control.

Outside his work Pearl enjoyed food, drink, music and the company of a circle of friends in Baltimore with similar tastes, including the journalist HL Mencken (1880–1956). They formed the Saturday Night Club, which met during prohibition in Mencken's basement to debate, play music and drink beer brewed in the cellar. On one occasion the group sat down to play the first eight Beethoven symphonies in a row, Pearl contributing a rather mediocre French horn. They reached the fifth symphony before fatigue supervened. During prohibition Pearl defiantly carried out a study showing that moderate alcohol intake did not shorten life. Pearl was a large man who put his views forcefully and dismissed his critics with disdain. However, his enemies fought back to deny him a much-wanted appointment at Harvard in 1929. He remained at Johns Hopkins until his death.

Selected Publications

Pearl R. Contraception and fertility in 2000 women. *Hum Biol* 1932; 4: 363–407.

Pearl R. *The Natural History of Population*. New York, NY: Oxford University Press; 1939.

Bibliography References

840, 1525.

Penrose, Charles Bingham (1862–1925)

Penrose Drain

Drainage of surgical wounds with rigid, hollow pipes was carried out in the Hippocratic era as 'an outlet for any humour collecting within'. This principle was lost to medicine until the nineteenth century, when it was reintroduced for certain cases of abdominal surgery: sepsis, incomplete haemostasis and repair of bowel

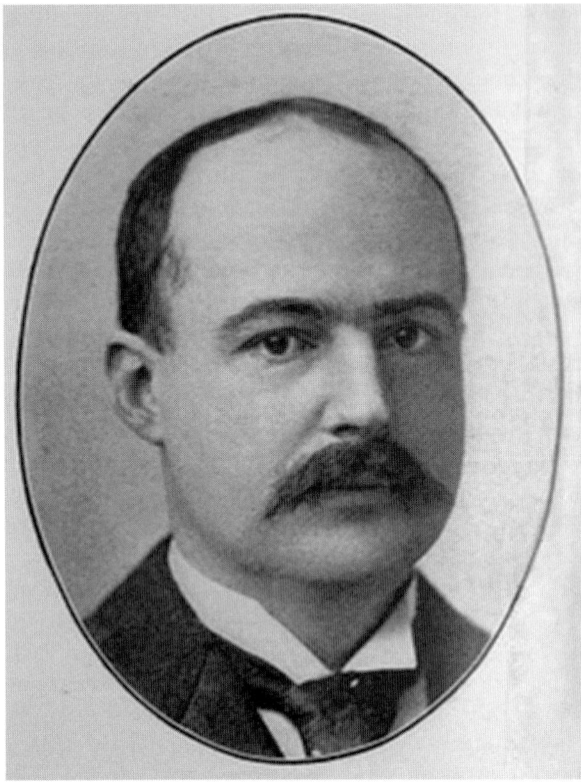

Charles Bingham Penrose

injury. Surgeons fell into two camps, frequent and infrequent drainers.

Charles Penrose was of the frequent drainage camp: 'When in doubt, drain'. Common methods of drainage in the late nineteenth century included gauze or perforated glass tubes. In both types there could be damaging adherence of bowel or omentum to the drain. As Penrose put it:

> *One objection to the gauze drain is the difficulty of removal. Lymph processes and granulations penetrate the interstices of the gauze and often render its removal very difficult. The surgeon fears to use too much force in attempts at withdrawal, because an adherent loop of intestine or omentum may be pulled out of place or damaged, or the lymph wall of the drainage tract may become open and expose the general peritoneum to infection. To avoid this difficulty, the writer has for some time used a drain made by surrounding the gauze bag with an ordinary rubber condom, the end of which has been cut open. With this arrangement, the surgeon may feel certain that there are no adhesions except at the end of the drain.*

The Penrose type of rubber tube drain was widely used in the twentieth century and became standard, until polyethylene drains attached to negative pressure, sealed containers became available.

Charles Bingham Penrose was born in Philadelphia on 1 February 1862 to a distinguished family. His grandfather was Pennsylvania state senator, his father was professor of obstetrics and gynaecology at the University of Pennsylvania and one of his brothers became a United States senator.

In 1884 he received both his PhD in physics from Harvard University and his MD from the University of Pennsylvania. He did resident training in Philadelphia hospitals from 1885 to 1887 and acquired a reputation as a good surgeon. In 1888 he was cofounder of the Gynecean Hospital in Philadelphia, 'for the medical and surgical treatment of diseases of women'. This, the first women's hospital in Philadelphia, started as two rooms in a private house and developed into a 40-bed hospital with operating theatres and a laboratory.

In 1891 he developed pulmonary tuberculosis. A college friend, who was now the governor of Wyoming, advised him to come to the favourable western climate. Penrose, who was quite athletic, embarked upon a regimen of digging ditches for the town of Cheyenne, Wyoming. He recovered, but before returning east agreed to serve as surgeon to a group of cattlemen who decided to eliminate settlers they believed were cattle rustlers. The conflict became known as the Johnson County War. Penrose was captured, jailed and only escaped lynching due to the intervention of the governor.

On another occasion, while on a hunting trip to Montana, he showed poor judgement in shooting and killing a grizzly bear cub, which predictably precipitated an attack on him by the cub's large mother. In the ensuing tussle he shot the mother bear but sustained a compound dislocation of his wrist – which he treated himself.

Quickly rediscovering his love of the east, Penrose returned to his hospital practice and was appointed professor of gynaecology at the University of Pennsylvania in 1893. He had married well and was able to retire from medical practice in 1899.

In retirement he established the Penrose Research Laboratory at the Philadelphia Zoo. He also helped create the Pennsylvania Department of Health. Charles Penrose died of a heart attack on 28 February 1925 while returning home on a train.

Selected Publications

Penrose CB. Drainage in abdominal surgery. *JAMA* 1890; 14: 264–8.

Penrose CB. *A Textbook of Diseases of Women.* Philadelphia, PA: WB Saunders; 1897.

Bibliography References

3, 973, 1239, 1324, 1485.

Pereyra, Armand Joseph (1904–1988)

Needle Suspension Operation

In 1959, Armand Pereyra, chief medical officer and gynaecologist to the California Institution for Women, reported a new surgical approach in the treatment of stress urinary incontinence. Until then the standard operation to elevate the urethrovesical junction was the anterior vaginal repair or the more extensive abdominal operation of Marshall–Marchetti–Krantz. Working with the prison population, Pereyra found a significant number with troublesome stress incontinence and decided to try a less invasive surgical approach. He devised a ligature carrier that was inserted through a small suprapubic stab incision and used this to pass wire sutures into the paraurethral tissue and vagina with no additional dissection. These sutures were tightened to elevate the urethrovesical junction to the appropriate level and were then anchored to the rectus fascia. His report on 31 patients showed a 90 per cent cure rate and, as the women were mostly in prison, his follow-up to 14 months was 100 per cent. Pereyra outlined his rationale as follows:

> *The purpose of this paper is to present a simplified surgical procedure whereby such support and angulation of the urethra on the bladder is obtained by sutures placed in the paraurethral tissues and anchored to the abdominal fascia near its junction with the symphysis. A special cannula was devised to permit the insertion of these sutures without resorting to wide opening of the abdominal wall, so that what is commonly a major procedure is converted to a minor operation.*

A number of others modified this procedure, including Benson Harer of San Bernadino, California, Shlomo Raz of Los Angeles and Thomas Stamey (1928–2015) of Stanford University. Pereyra himself continued to refine and modify his technique over the next 20 years. These refinements included the use of various sutures – absorbable, non-absorbable and helical – and vaginal dissection of the paraurethral tissues. The short-term results were good but long-term failures were common. By

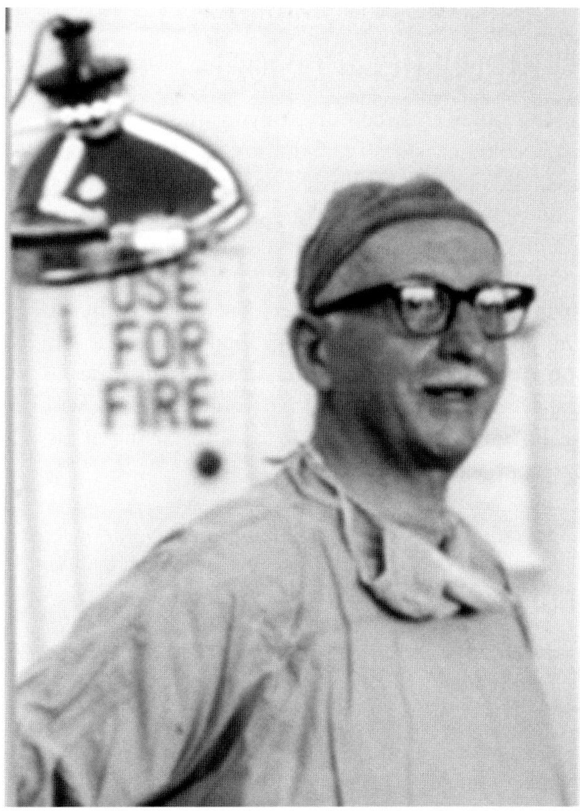

Armand Joseph Pereyra

the twenty-first century, many gynaecologists turned to sling procedures.

Armand Pereyra was born on 14 January 1904 in Mazatlán, Mexico. As a teenager he invented a successful tortilla-making machine. He graduated MD from the University of California, Berkeley, School of Medicine in 1930. He joined the United States Navy and served for the next 26 years, during which he carried out his postgraduate training in obstetrics and gynaecology. He was with the navy at Pearl Harbour during the Japanese attack in December 1941. From 1956 to 1972 he was chief medical officer and medical director of the hospital at the California Institution for Women. At the same time, he carried on a private practice in Ontario, California, and continued this until 1982. Armand Pereyra died on 11 October 1988 of a pulmonary embolus after a hip fracture.

Selected Publications

Pereyra, AJ. A simplified surgical procedure for the correction of stress incontinence in women. *West J Surg Obstet Gynecol* 1959; 67: 223–6.

Harer WB, Gunther RE. Simplified urethrovesical suspension and urethroplasty. *Am J Obstet Gynecol* 1965; 91: 1017–21.

Pereyra AJ, Lebherz TB, Growdon WA, Powers JA. Pubourethral supports in perspective: modified Pereyra procedure for urinary incontinence. *Obstet Gynecol* 1982; 59: 643–8.

Bibliography References

311, 312, 1241.

Pfannenstiel, Hermann Johann (1862–1909)

Pfannenstiel Incision

In the nineteenth century, during the early years of gynaecological surgery, abdominal access to the pelvis was via the longitudinal, usually midline, incision. This was associated with a significant risk of subsequent incisional hernia. At the turn of the century some gynaecologists, including Otto Küstner, began to incise the skin transversely but still cut the fascia and peritoneum in the longitudinal plane. The crucial contribution of Pfannenstiel was to incise the fascia transversely, feeling that this would improve wound healing and strength. In 1900, after using it in 51 cases, he wrote:

> *It appears to give absolutely certain protection against hernias . . . as we know that hernia occurs in the defective healing of the fascia . . . I therefore cut through not only the skin (transversely) but also the entire fascial layer, and only then, after separating the fascia towards the umbilicus, did I divide the muscle layer and peritoneum longitudinally . . . My expectation was confirmed, namely to thus obtain an absolutely firm scar.*

The incision provided good exposure for most gynaecological surgery, although Pfannenstiel acknowledged that the longitudinal incision was still necessary for large pelvic masses and cancer. He said, 'an ultimate verdict will only be possible after years'

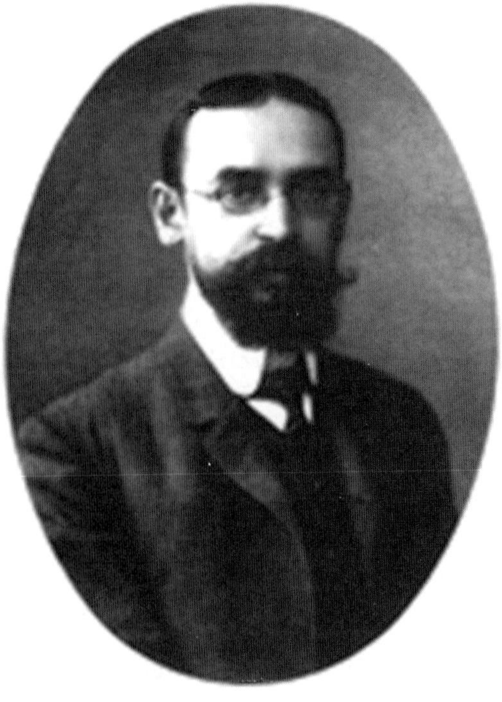

Hermann Johann Pfannenstiel

but was convinced that the long-term superiority and integrity of the incision would be confirmed; and so it proved to be.

Herman Johann Pfannenstiel was born in Berlin and received his medical degree from the University of Berlin in 1885. He was later appointed assistant gynaecologist to the Breslau Frauenklinik. In 1902 he became professor and chairman of the department of obstetrics and gynaecology in the University of Giessen and, in 1907, assumed a similar position in Kiel. Pfannenstiel was an accomplished gynaecological surgeon whose main research interest, on which he published widely, was ovarian tumours. It was ironic that he should die just after his forty-seventh birthday, from sepsis following a needle-stick injury in the middle finger of his left hand sustained at the removal of a tubo-ovarian abscess.

Selected Publications

Pfannenstiel J. Über die vortheile des suprasymphysären Fascienquerschnitts für die Gynäkologischen Köliotomein zugleich ein Beitrag zu der Indikationsstellung der Operationswerge. *Samml Klin Vortr Leipzig* 1900; 268: 1735–56.

Bibliography References

274, 499, 553, 647, 648, 1200, 1291, 1292, 1376, 1480.

Philpott, Robert Hugh (b. 1927)

Partographic Analysis of Labour

In the early 1970s Hugh Philpott, Professor of Obstetrics and Gynaecology at the University of Rhodesia in Salisbury, Rhodesia (now Harare, Zimbabwe) was faced with the problem of early diagnosis of cephalopelvic disproportion in women in rural areas. As he wrote:

> *Cephalopelvic disproportion and inefficient uterine action are two of the biggest obstetrical problems in the African primigravidae ... Our difficulty is not only that of evaluating the degree of disproportion in the individual but also that of teaching the midwives how best to assess these patients in the rural areas. All primigravidae are managed with a trial of labour and a simple, efficient method of conducting such a trial, we have found, is the analysis of a cervicographic record of progress as first propounded by Friedman. This is based on the recognition that cephalopelvic disproportion in the primigravidae is accompanied by inefficient uterine action and that this will be the most evident in the cervicograph.*

In Philpott's cervicograph, zero time started when the patient arrived at hospital with a dilatation of at least 3 cm. He then added a single straight Alert Line presenting four hours from zero time at a rate of 1 cm per hour. If, on assessment four hours after admission, the patient crossed the Alert Line, midwives in the rural area transferred the woman to the central hospital, where more

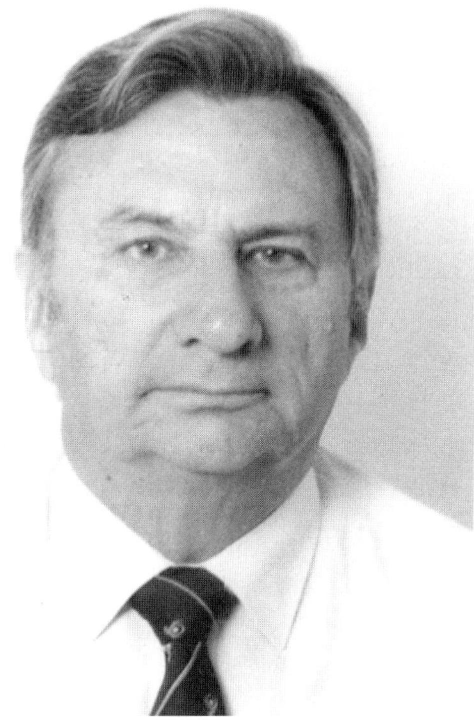

Robert Hugh Philpott

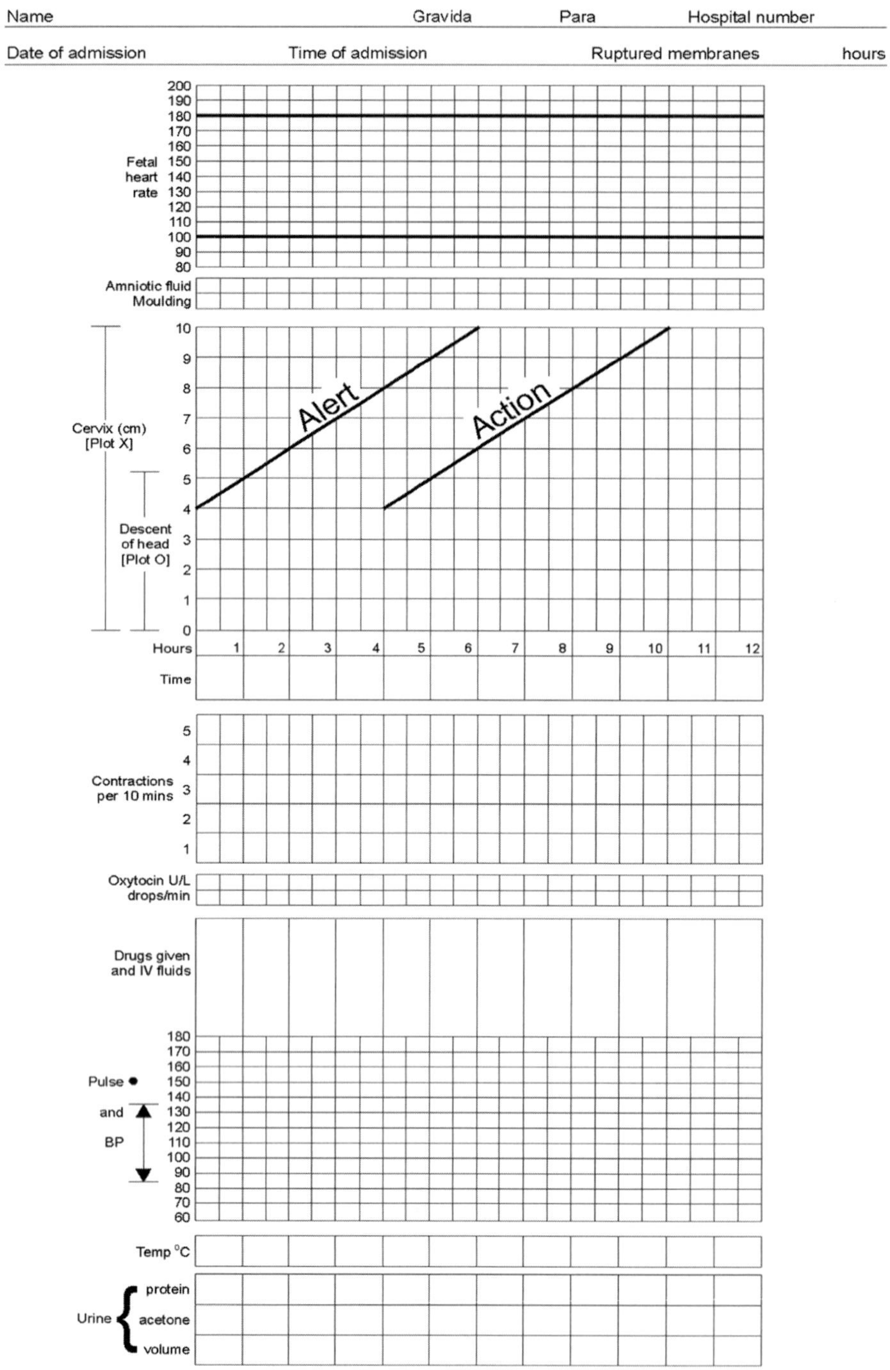

Modified WHO partogram incorporating Philpott's principles

advanced management, including oxytocin augmentation and caesarean section, was available. He then added an Action Line parallel to and four hours to the right of the Alert Line. They found, 'in our practice the cervicographs of 22% of African primigravidae crossed the Alert Line. Half of these patients delivered normally in the next four hours and the other half required oxytocin augmentation of labour and of these 80% ultimately delivered vaginally and 20% by caesarean section'. At the conclusion of their study of 624 consecutive primigravidae women, they were able to show that 'the regime outlined in this paper has reduced the caesarean section rate, the incidence of prolonged labour and the perinatal mortality rate'. This was an achievement unequalled in hospitals using partographic analysis of labour at that time.

The full Philpott partogram included a record of the fetal condition and maternal condition as well as the graphic representation of the progress of labour. In 1988 the World Health Organization (WHO) adopted the main elements of Philpott's partogram. The WHO workshop that produced the partogram did not include Philpott, as he was not invited during the apartheid era, despite his demonstrated opposition to the apartheid government. Apparently, the committee would phone him at night for comments on their deliberations.

A review of Hugh Philpott's life brings to mind the saying, 'they don't make them like this anymore'. He was born on 9 April 1927 in Honiton, Devon, when his father, a student minister, was on study leave from South Africa. The following year the family returned to South Africa. His birth in the United Kingdom enabled him to get a British passport and allowed him to travel overseas during the apartheid years. Upon graduation from high school, Philpott jointed the 6th South African Armored Division and saw action in Italy as a tank driver. After the war he returned to South Africa and graduated in medicine from the University of Cape Town in 1952. After two years of junior hospital positions in Port Elizabeth and Durban, Philpott spent seven years as a medical missionary in Nigeria. During this time, he was director of leprosy services and organised reconstructive surgery programmes. He also developed a post-polio service after a polio epidemic and organised community obstetrical services with the University of Ibidan. In 1962 he returned to South Africa and undertook his postgraduate training in obstetrics and gynaecology at the King Edward VIII Hospital and the University of Natal.

In 1966 he was appointed professor and head of the department of obstetrics and gynaecology in the new medical school in Salisbury, Rhodesia. It was here that he developed his work on the partogram, which formed the basis of his MD thesis. In 1974 he was appointed professor and head of the department of obstetrics and gynaecology at the University of Natal, Durban. Using the same principles, he had established in Rhodesia, he decentralised maternity services to health centres and clinics in the townships, cutting in half the number of deliveries that took place in the central city hospital. He initiated a flying doctor service to rural hospitals and a training programme for advanced midwives. In 1985 he was appointed dean of student services in the University of Kwazulu, Natal, with the mandate to develop programmes to increase access to university for disadvantaged students.

After retiring from the chair of obstetrics and gynaecology in 1992, he was appointed director of the Centre for Rural Health at the University of Natal, a position he held until 2001. Since then he has been a part-time consultant in the centre.

Selected Publications

Philpott RH, Castle WM. Cervicographs in the management of labour in primigravidae I. The Alert Line for detecting the abnormal labour. *J Obstet Gynaecol Br Commonw* 1972; 79: 592–8.

Philpott RH, Castle WM. Cervicographs in the management of labour in primigravidae II. The Action Line and treatment of abnormal labour. *J Obstet Gynaecol Br Commonw* 1972; 79: 599–602.

Bibliography References

99, 102.

Pinard, Adolphe (1844–1934)

Obstetric Palpation

It was Adolphe Pinard who helped establish the value of a logical and systematic approach to abdominal palpation in pregnancy. In outlining his rationale for a consistent technique, he wrote, 'every time I have made students palpate without giving them other rules, I have seen them misled and make false diagnosis'. He laid down clear guidelines for abdominal palpation of the fetus, in particular seeking the presenting part at the pelvic brim, or 'pelvic excavation' as he called it:

> *For that purpose, placing the hands about five or six centimetres to the right and left of the median line, the extremities of the fingers being in relation with the anterior curve of the pelvis, he depresses the abdominal wall from above downwards and from before backwards, just grazing over the horizontal rami of the pubes.*
>
> *When properly palpating, only two sensations may be perceived, viz: the fingers experiencing a sensation of resistance, resulting from contact with a hard round and voluminous body which fills the excavation, can not penetrate deeper; or, on the contrary, they only meet with the resistance offered by the soft parts, and can therefore sink more or less deeply into the excavation.*

Pinard helped lay the foundations of antenatal care by emphasising the need for examination of women in the later weeks of pregnancy with a view to version for the correction of breech and other malpresentations. His description of the manoeuvres necessary for external cephalic version remains clinically pertinent:

> *... apply one hand over the foetal head, and the other over the breech, and by gentle and sustained pressure exerted inversely over one and the other extremity, turn the two poles of the foetus...the pressure made over the breech is more efficient than that made over the head, in as much as it is more directly transmitted to the trunk.*

Pinard also described a technique to bring down the extended leg of the frank breech for extraction. The fore and middle fingers are applied to the thigh flexing and pressing it back against the trunk. This helps flex the knee and bring the foot into reach. It is known as 'Pinard's manoeuvre'.

Adolphe Pinard was born in Méry-sur-Seine in the Champagne region of France. He was the eldest of five sons born to a family of humble means. As a medical student he served in the Franco-Prussian War and was destined to lose his own son in the First World War. He worked as assistant to Charles Pajot and Étienne Tarnier at the Paris Maternité Hospital. Pinard became a great clinical teacher and worked hard to reduce the mainly theoretical teaching philosophy of that time. In 1881, he wrote, 'A number of students have become doctors without ever examining a woman or attending a birth. That is monstrous, but a fact'. In 1890 he became chairman of clinical obstetrics in the faculty of medicine. The change from a theoretical to a clinical chair was at his request. Pinard was among the first to promote antenatal care and rest in the later weeks of pregnancy. He showed that the infants were larger and in better health at birth as a result of this attention. He coined the term 'intrauterine paediatric care'. He established shelters and nurseries for poor women and their infants.

In his time, Pinard also served as mayor of Méry-sur-Seine and in his later years held a seat in the parliament at the Palais Bourbon. He is also remembered eponymously for the Pinard fetal stethoscope.

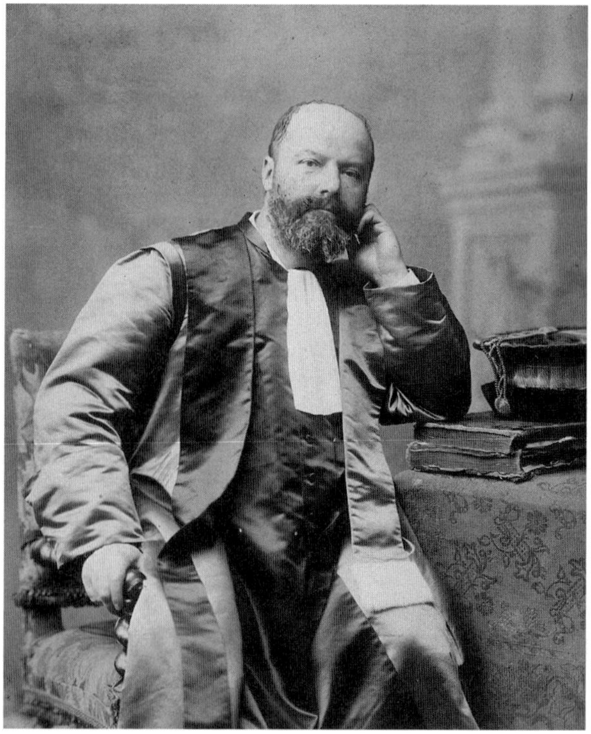

Adolphe Pinard

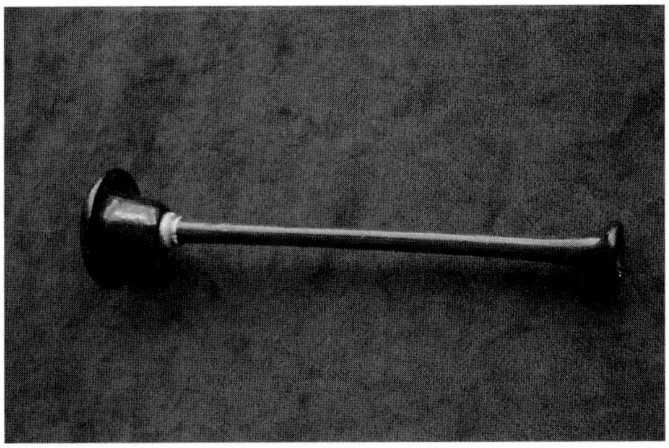

Pinard stethoscope

Selected Publications

Pinard A. *Traité du palper abdominal au point de vue obstétrical.* Paris: H. Lauwereyns, 1878. English translation by LE Neale. A Treatise on Abdominal Palpation as Applied to Obstetrics and Version by External Manipulations. New York, NY: JH Vail & Co; 1885. Also published in: The Classics of Obstetrics and Gynecology Library. New York, NY: Gryphon Editions; 1995 (facsimile).

Bibliography References

41, 648, 1261, 1435, 1478, 1558, 1595.

Pincus, Gregory Goodwin (1903–1967) Rock, John Charles (1890–1984)

Oral Contraception

It is to some extent inappropriate to link only two people to the discovery of the oral contraceptive pill, as the development and testing involved so many individuals. Often overlooked was the early realisation by two Austrian physicians, working independently, that such a development was feasible.

Ludwig Haberlandt (1885–1932) was professor of physiology at the University of Innsbruck, and in 1919 he showed that the transplanted ovaries from pregnant rabbits to fertile does rendered them infertile. In 1921 Otfried Otto Fellner (b. 1873), a gynaecologist in Vienna, used oestrogenic ovarian extracts to create infertility in guinea pigs. By 1931, continued studies on animals convinced Haberlandt that hormonal contraception was feasible:

> *Of all the methods available, hormonal sterilisation, based on a biological principle, if it can be applied unobjectionably in the human, is the ideal method for practical medicine and its future task of birth control.*

Haberlandt's prophetic words were forgotten. However, research into the identification and action of ovarian hormones continued. During the 1920s, evidence of the hormone-secreting activity of the ovary accumulated, and assays for oestrogen and progesterone activity were developed. Oestrogen was isolated in 1929 and progesterone soon after. The main problem was that these steroids were not active when taken by mouth. Pharmaceutical companies expended much effort to find synthetic, orally active compounds. In 1938 the addition of an ethinyl group to estradiol produced the orally active ethinylestradiol. Although this was used for many gynaecological conditions, including dysmenorrhoea in which the pain was reduced by inhibiting ovulation, the potential for contraception was not pursued.

In 1943, Russell Marker, an eccentric organic chemist, left Pennsylvania State University for Mexico. His earlier plant work with the Mexican black-headed yam had revealed a steroid, diosgenin. He was able to chemically degrade diosgenin and produce progesterone, which previously could only be obtained in minute quantities from animal ovaries.

Thus, progesterone could now be produced cheaply in bulk, but it was still not active when taken by mouth. Carl Djerassi (1923–2015), whose Bulgarian father and Austrian mother were both doctors, left Vienna for the United States at the age of 16 when the Nazis annexed Austria. In 1951 he worked at the

Syntex laboratory and synthesised the potent, orally active progestational compound norethindrone. Of all the protagonists who contributed to the development of the pill, only Djerassi gained financial success – through the allotment of shares from the Syntex company. In 1952, Frank Coulton (1923–2003), working with the GD Searle company, synthesised norethynodrel, which was the progestin chosen for the first iteration of the pill.

The tools were now available, and it was Gregory Pincus at the Worcester Foundation for Experimental Biology in Massachusetts who took up the challenge. He was encouraged to do so by Margaret Sanger and Katharine McCormick, who helped organise research funds. In 1953 he and his research scientist Min Cheuh Chang (1908–1991) published their study on the effect of progesterone and other progestational agents on ovulation in rabbits. They found that:

> *The effectiveness of progesterone as an inhibitor of ovulation is reaffirmed by our data. Furthermore, certain active progestins, namely ethinyl testosterone and 17-methyl progesterone are also effective. Since 17-hydroxyprogesterone is also effective, it is suggested that substitutions at carbon 17 in the progesterone molecule do not notably interfere with the ovulation-inhibiting capacity.*

In 1954 Pincus enlisted the help of John Rock, a respected Boston gynaecologist with a special interest in infertility. By giving orally active progestins to women from day 5 to 25 of the menstrual cycle, ovulation was inhibited but menstruation occurred normally. Rock gave this to patients at his infertility clinic for one to three cycles, hoping to achieve 'rebound' fertility upon stopping the progestin.

In view of the legal and social attitudes towards contraception, trials of birth control efficacy were not feasible in the United States in the 1950s. Thus, large-scale trials were set up in Puerto Rico with the guidance of Celso-Ramón Garcia (1922–2004), a gynaecologist training with Rock, who had previously worked at the Puerto Rico medical school. The local clinical co-ordinator was Edris Rice-Wray (1904–1990), an American doctor from Detroit and the director of the Puerto Rico Family Planning Association. Further trials were carried out in Haiti and Los Angeles. The progestins used were found to be impure and contain significant amounts of an oestrogen, later identified as mestranol. This helped to reduce the amount of irregular breakthrough bleeding found with pure progestins.

The first oral contraceptive was approved by the United States Food and Drug Administration on 9 May 1960. It was produced by GD Searle and Company and called Enovid. It contained almost 10 mg of progesterone as norethynodrel and 150 μg of mestranol.

Gregory Goodwin Pincus, known as Goody, was born in Woodbine, New Jersey to Russian immigrant parents. He took his undergraduate science degree from Cornell University in 1924 and his master's and doctorate degrees from Harvard University. From 1929 to 1930 he studied in England and Germany. He was appointed assistant professor at Harvard in 1931. Among his prodigious research output was the creation of a rabbit embryo by fertilising a rabbit ovum and sperm in a petri dish – the forerunner of in vitro fertilisation. Denied tenure at Harvard in 1944, he established the Worcester Foundation for Experimental Biology in Worcester, Massachusetts as a centre for research in mammalian reproduction. He was appointed professor at Tufts Medical School, Boston in 1945 and at Boston University in 1951. He died in Boston from myeloid leukaemia. Pincus received no royalties from the pill.

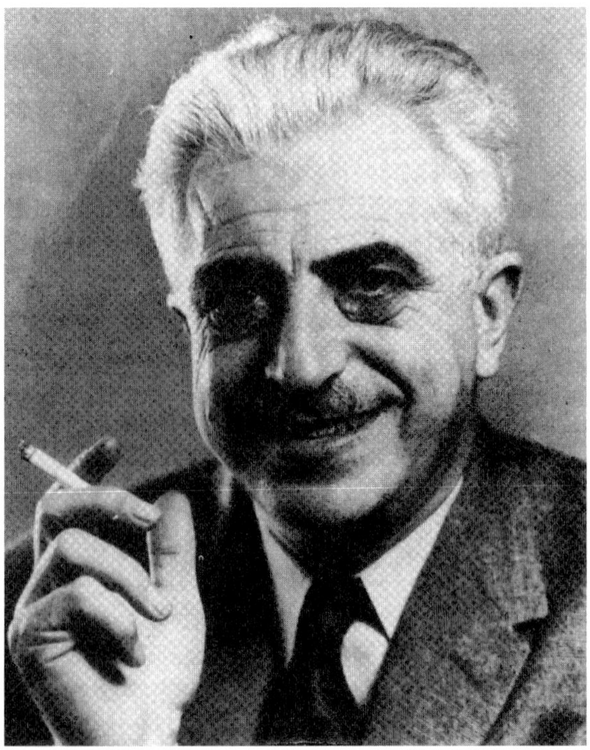

Gregory Goodwin Pincus

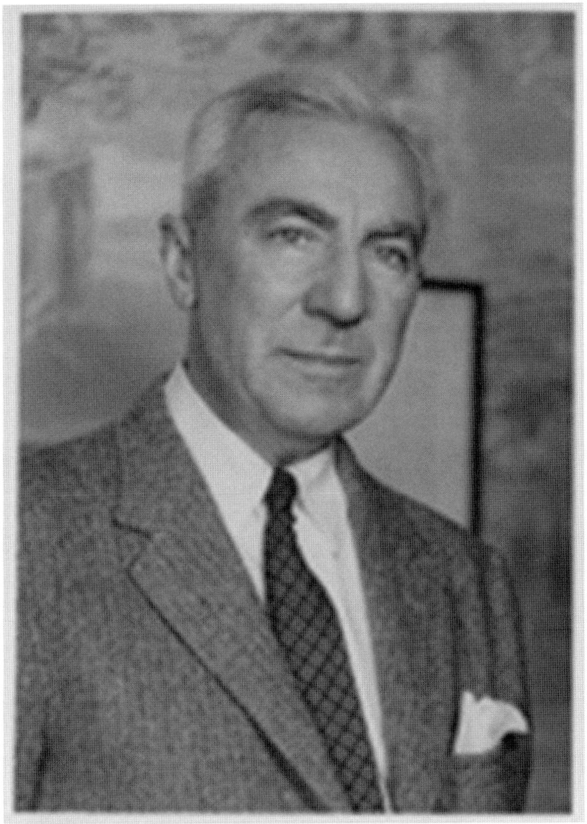

John Charles Rock

John Rock, a twin, was born in Marlborough, Massachusetts. His grandfather came from Armagh, Northern Ireland and emigrated to Boston at the time of the potato famine. He attended the High School of Commerce in Boston, which led to his first job managing a banana firm in Guatemala for the United Fruit Company. He did not enjoy the commerce of bananas, returned to Boston and, with a dramatic change of course, graduated from the Harvard Medical School in 1918. He took his postgraduate training in Boston in surgery, obstetrics and gynaecology and was appointed clinical professor of gynaecology at Harvard in 1947. He carried out much research related to infertility and detailed the histological changes of the endometrial cycle. Working with Arthur Hertig (1904–1990), he helped develop the classic collection of very early embryo implantation.

By the 1950s Rock, a staunch Roman Catholic, had begun to realise that safe, effective birth control was a worldwide imperative. During his years at Harvard he was an imposing but controversial figure as he spoke out against the strict birth control laws of Massachusetts, where even birth control information was against the law. He reached the mandatory retirement age of 65 in 1955 but continued his clinical and research work on the pill in a privately funded clinic building on the grounds of the Free Hospital for Women in Boston. Rock felt that the oral contraceptive pill worked in a physiological manner that should be acceptable to Catholics. Indeed, the papal birth control commission of the mid-1960s reported as much. However, on 29 July 1968, Pope Paul VI released his restrictive encyclical on birth control, *Humanae vitae*, which ultimately undermined the credibility and authority of the church in the lives of many couples. About this time Rock was evicted from his clinic by the university department. He ultimately retired, with a modest income, to a secluded farmhouse in Temple, New Hampshire and died there at the age of 94 on 4 December 1984.

Selected Publications

Fellner OO. Über die Tätigkeit des ovarium in der Schwangerschaft (interstitielle Zellen). *Mschr Geburtsh Gynäkol* 1921; 54: 88–94.

Haberlandt L. Über hormonale Sterilisierung des weiblichen Tierkoerpers. *Münich Med Wochenschr* 1921; 68: 1577–8.

Pincus G, Chang MC. The effects of progesterone and related compounds on ovulation and early development in the rabbit. *Acta Physiol Lat Amer* 1953; 3: 177–83.

Pincus G, Rock J, Garcia CR, Rice-Way E, Paniaagua M, Rodriguez I. Fertility control with oral medication. *Am J Obstet Gynecol* 1958; 75: 1333–46.

Rock J, Pincus G, Garcia CR. Effects of certain 19-norsteroids upon reproductive processes. *Ann NY Acad Sci* 1958; 71: 677–90.

Rock J. *The Time Has Come: A Catholic Doctor's Proposals to End the Battle Over Birth Control.* New York, NY: Knoff; 1963.

Bibliography References

31, 82, 101, 136, 197, 264, 288, 304, 401–403, 447, 516, 528, 586, 598, 620, 630, 667, 792, 888, 972, 979, 981, 1026, 1027, 1031, 1154, 1209, 1309, 1316, 1329, 1379, 1381, 1414, 1416, 1686, 1716.

Piper, Edmund Brown (1891–1935)

Piper's Forceps

The first description of forceps for use in delivering the aftercoming head of the breech was by William Smellie in his *Sett of Anatomical Tables* published in 1754. In modern obstetrics, forceps to the aftercoming head of the breech are used to aid flexion and protection of the fetal head from sudden decompression at delivery. Many different obstetric forceps have been used for this purpose. In 1929 Piper reported five years' experience with forceps that he designed specifically for assisted delivery of the aftercoming head of the breech. On the rare occasions that vaginal breech delivery is undertaken, these forceps have retained their popularity for this purpose, mainly in the United States. In their original paper on the subject Piper and Bachman described the three characteristics of the forceps:

> *1. A blade having a somewhat flattened pelvic curve for high applications, as in the Tarnier forceps; 2. A lengthened shank, which permits an unusual degree of 'spring' between the blades and thus prevents compression of the head; 3. Depressed handles for greater ease of application and manipulation in the presence of the delivered fetal body.*

Piper stressed that the fetal trunk should be held horizontally so that there would not be excessive extension of the fetal neck. He emphasised, 'The chief function of the instrument is that of flexion and not of traction'.

Edmund Brown Piper was born in Williamsport, Pennsylvania. He graduated in sciences from Princeton and initially worked for the Williamsport Water Company. He studied medicine at the University of Pennsylvania, graduating in 1911. During the First World War he served with the American Expeditionary Forces in France, commanding camp hospitals. He returned to practice, specialising in obstetrics and gynaecology, and ultimately became professor at the University of Pennsylvania.

Apparently the first use of Piper's forceps was by Dr Clifford Hull at the Philadelphia Lying-in Hospital to deliver Dr Piper's daughter of her first child.

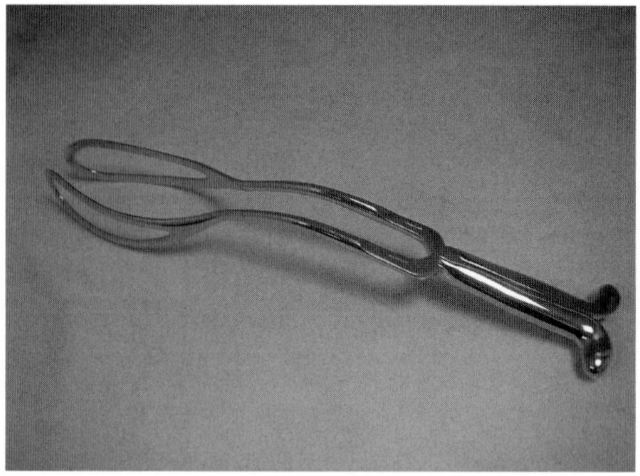

Piper's forceps

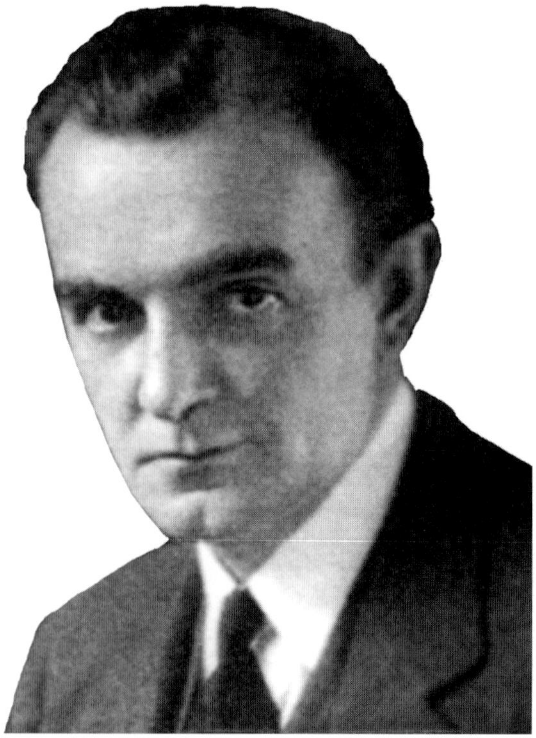

Edmund Brown Piper

Selected Publications

Piper EB. Bachman C. The prevention of fetal injuries in breech delivery. *JAMA* 1929; 92: 217–21.

Bibliography References

399, 728, 801, 1468, 1480.

Piskaçek, Ludwig (1854–1932)

Piskaçek's Sign

In early pregnancy the uterus may appear to be asymmetrical, as the implantation site can enlarge one cornu before the other. This was described by Ludwig Piskaçek of Vienna in 1899. It had been previously noted by Robert Dickinson of New York in 1892 but is usually known as Piskaçek's sign. Carl von Fernwald Braun described a similar sign, emphasising the palpable furrow between the enlarged side of the uterus and the other.

Ludwig Piskaçek was born on 16 November 1854 in Karcag, Hungary. He trained in Vienna and proceeded to MD in 1882. He became lecturer in obstetrics and gynaecology at the University of Vienna. In 1890 he took up the position of director of obstetrics in the School for Midwives in Linz, and in 1901 moved to the same post in Vienna. He died in Vienna on 19 September 1932.

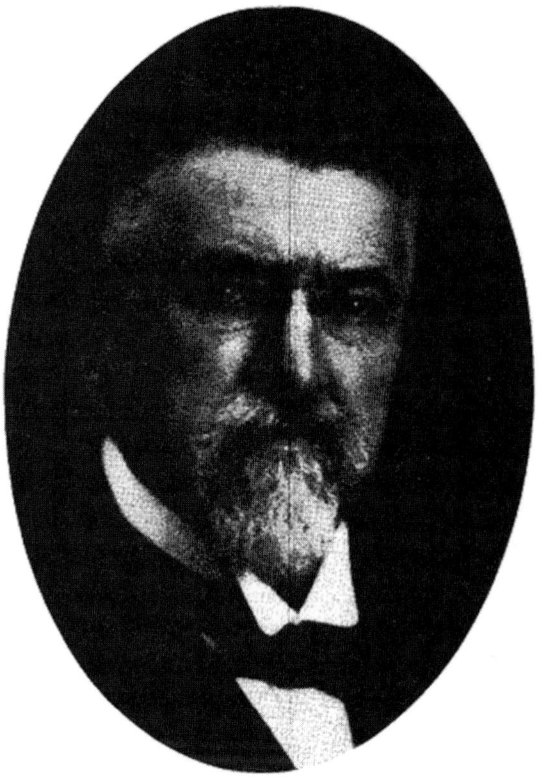

Ludwig Piskaçek

Selected Publications

Braun-Fernwald, CR von. *Wien Klin Wochenschr* 1899; 10: 12.

Dickinson RL. The diagnosis of pregnancy between the second and seventh weeks by bimanual examination. *NY J Gynecol Obstet* 1892; 10: 544–55.

Piskaçek L. *Über Ausladungen umschriebener Gerbärmutterabschnitte* Vienna: W. Braumueller; 1899.

Bibliography References

889, 896, 968, 1014, 1216.

Pollitzer, Sigmund (1859–1937)

Acanthosis Nigricans

Acanthosis nigricans is a dark, raised hyperpigmentation of the skin, usually found on the nape of the neck and axilla. It is most often manifest in hyperandrogenic women with polycystic ovarian syndrome, especially those cases associated with insulin resistance and obesity. It was first described by Sigmund Pollitzer in 1889 when he was working with the renowned German dermatologist, Dr PG Unna, in his clinic for skin diseases in Hamburg, Germany. With Dr Unna's permission, Pollitzer studied and published this first description of the condition as follows:

> *The skin of the hands is in general of a dirty brownish colour; on the dorsum manus there are patches of a bluish-grey, somewhat deeper in colour along the course of the veins. The normal areas of the cuticle are very prominent, standing out somewhat convex and with a glassy shimmer ... The natural furrows are deeply marked, the skin of the entire hand looking as if it were too large for them ... On the dorsal surface of the forearms the discolouration is especially marked over and along the course of a vein ... The neck appears as if encircled by a dirty greyish band which sends irregular offshoots downwards towards the sternum, clavicles, shoulders and scapulae, and upwards towards the face. The skin here shows the changes described as existing on the hands but in a much more marked degree. Some of the cuticular areas project above the general area almost like papillae, others are flatter; the whole running together to run a diffused, discoloured warty surface. Similar changes are seen in both axillae and under both breasts, only here the colouration is a rather greyish-white. On the abdomen there are a few horizontal streaky indications of a similar condition. The crurogenital folds of the large labia show the skin changes in a marked degree.*

Sigmund Pollitzer was born on Staten Island, New York on 1 November 1859. His initial degree, granted by the College of the City of New York, was in physics, astronomy and mathematics. His first publication was a manual of algorithmic computation, which was apparently very successful with those interested in that topic. He changed course, entered Columbia University to study medicine and graduated MD in 1884. He followed this with study in Heidelberg and Berlin, Germany. While he was there in 1885, war broke out between Serbia and Bulgaria. Pollitzer volunteered for service with the Serbians and organised two of the base hospitals until the end of the war a year later. He returned to the United States and practised general medicine for three years. He decided to specialise in dermatology and returned to Germany to study with Dr Unna in Hamburg. Returning to the United States in 1890, he was appointed professor of dermatology at the New York Postgraduate Medical School and Hospital, in which position he remained until 1915. He was one of the first to use arsphenamine in the treatment of syphilis. At meetings he was apparently a lively discussant and critic and it was said, 'His insistence on regular parliamentary procedures often involved him in polemics from which he emerged more frequently in defeat than victory'. Sigmund Pollitzer died in New York in 1937.

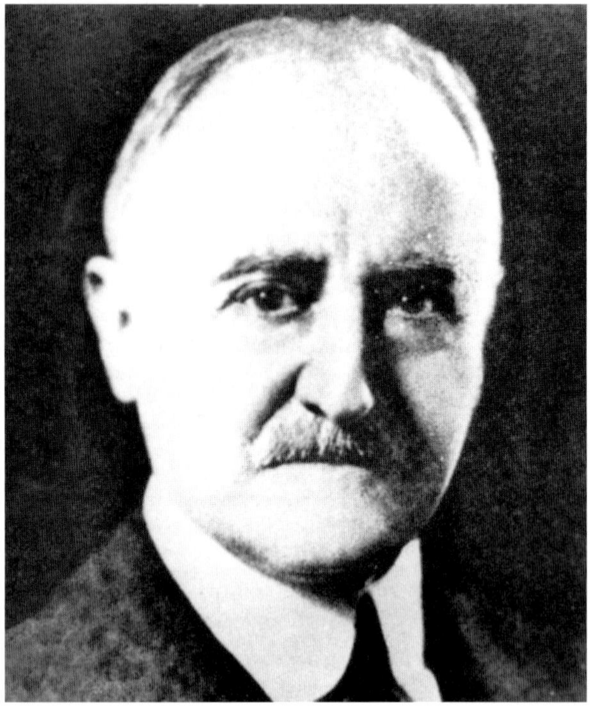

Sigmund Pollitzer

Selected Publications

International Atlas of Rare Skin Diseases. Part X. Hamburg: Leopold Voss; 1891.

Bibliography References

968, 1226, 1398.

Pomeroy, Ralph Hayward (1867–1925)

Pomeroy Tubal Ligation

Ralph Pomeroy developed his simple procedure for tubal ligation but never presented or published the technique. Four years after his death, two of his colleagues, Drs Eliot Bishop and WF Nelms, presented Pomeroy's technique and reported on 100 cases to the New York State Medical Society on 6 June 1929. They noted:

> *Its simplicity lies in the fact that it is nothing more or less than that a loop in the loose, middle portion of the tube is ligated with absorbable suture material and resected.*

Ralph Pomeroy was born in New York and was a medical graduate of Long Island College Hospital in 1889. He practised obstetrics and gynaecology in Brooklyn. In 1912 he was appointed associate professor in his alma mater.

As a youth a hip disorder kept him bed-bound for several months and left him permanently lame. After his early training he started general practice in hard times and earned $290 in his first year.

Pomeroy was an early and strong advocate of adequate analgesia in labour, saying the aim was 'to convert primiparae into undamaged, unterrified and competent multiparae'. He was also known for his procedure to correct occipito-posterior position in labour by manipulation of the fetal shoulder in concert with manual rotation of the fetal head.

Pomeroy was twice elected president of the New York Obstetrical Society. He was known to his close friends as 'Pom'.

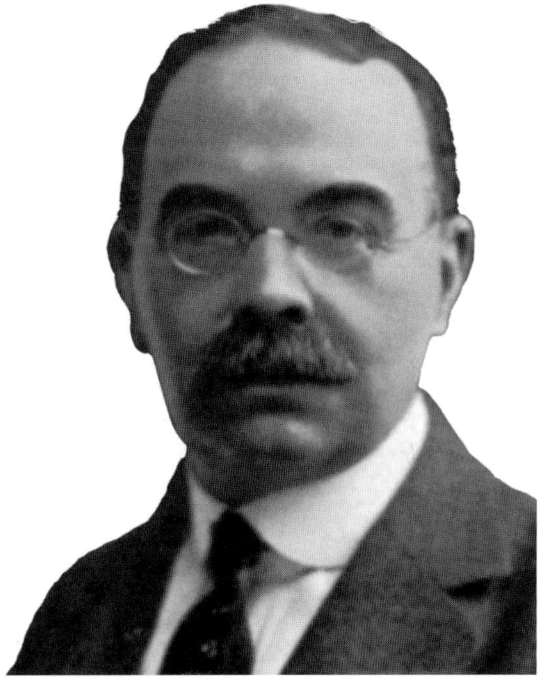

Ralph Hayward Pomeroy

Selected Publications

Bishop E, Nelms WF. A simple method of tubal sterilisation. *NY State J Med* 1930; 30: 214–6.

Pomeroy RH. The treatment of occipito-posterior positions. *Am J Obstet Dis Women Child* 1914; 69: 354–6.

Bibliography References

152, 168, 801, 852, 1410, 1480.

Porro, Edoardo (1842–1902)

Caesarean Hysterectomy

Up to the nineteenth century, almost all women subjected to caesarean section died from shock, haemorrhage or sepsis. Even in the early 1800s Friedrich Osiander (1759–1822) wrote, 'Before undertaking this procedure, one should allow the patient to draw up her will and grant her time to prepare herself for death' – a rather extreme early example of informed consent. By the latter part of the nineteenth century, despite the advent of anaesthesia and antisepsis, the threat of fatal haemorrhage and infection remained high in caesarean section. A thoughtful Italian obstetrician, Edoardo Porro, offered a radical, albeit partial solution to this problem. He decided to remove the uterus as a potential source of haemorrhage and sepsis. After careful review of his own cases of contracted pelvis and experimental work on the removal of the uterus in pregnant rabbits and cadavers, Porro felt ready to perform his operation. The opportunity came on 21 May 1876 when he was presented with a rachitic primigravida with a true conjugate of 4 cm. Porro delivered the infant by caesarean section and then amputated the tubes, ovaries and body of the uterus, fixing the cervical stump to the abdominal incision. Thus, he diverted the potentially septic contents of the cervix and vagina away from the peritoneal cavity. The woman was the first to survive caesarean section at that clinic and left hospital with her infant after six weeks. Porro published the case later that year and for a time it found favour, until Ferdinand Kehrer and Max Sänger showed that careful suture of the uterus allowed its conservation.

Edoardo Porro was born at Padua. He received his MD from the University of Pavia in 1865, despite what was described as 'considerable embarrassment owing to want of pecuniary means'. For a year after graduation he served as a soldier under Garibaldi in the 1866 campaign for Italian unity. In 1867 he became an assistant in obstetrics at Milan and by dint of honest industry and teaching ability became the professor of obstetrics at the University of Pavia. He resigned from this position in 1882 and returned to Milan as the director of the maternity hospital. He spent most of his later years on hospital administration.

Selected Publications

Porro E. Della amputazione utero-ovarica come complemento di taglio cesareo. *Ann Univ Med Chir (Milan)* 1876; 237: 289–350.

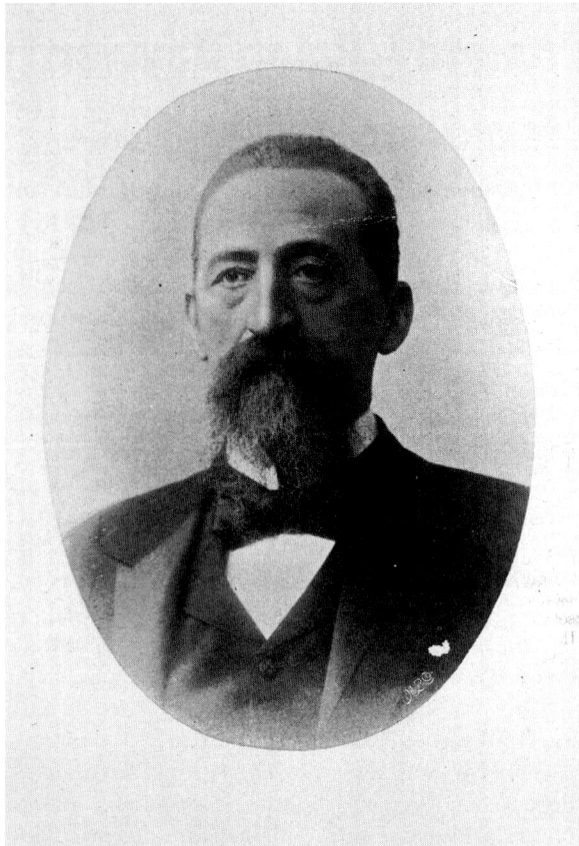

Edoardo Porro

Bibliography References

25, 97, 102, 225, 276, 323, 492, 648, 950, 987, 1093, 1205, 1227, 1291, 1333, 1483, 1618, 1620, 1631, 1646, 1734.

Portal, Paul (1630–1703)

Placenta Praevia

Paul Portal started his surgical studies in his birthplace, Montpellier, but completed his medical education in Paris. There he attended the lectures of François Mauriceau and studied at the Hotel Dieu. In 1657 he was appointed companion surgeon to the Hôtel Dieu and confined his practice to obstetrics. He was the first to point out that in cases of placenta praevia the placenta was attached to the lower uterine segment. Before this, it was thought the placenta had fallen down from its fundal attachment. In his book Portal asserts:

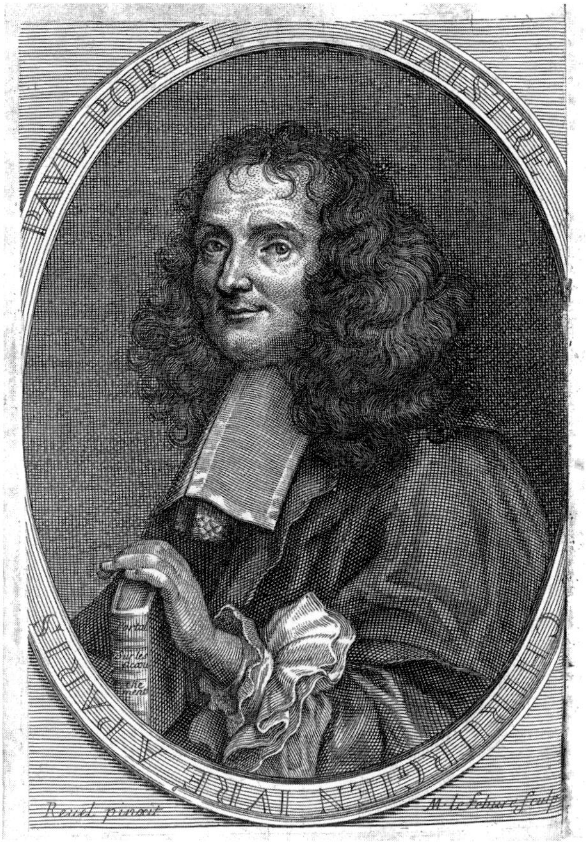

Paul Portal

... the placenta does not always attach itself at the bottom (fundus) *of the womb, sometimes it can fasten itself to the neighbourhood of the neck.*

He confirmed this in one of his case descriptions:

I put my fingers into the orifice and felt the afterbirth which covered the orifice of the matrix from all sides and adhered in all its parts with the exception of the middle.

In his text Portal describes the case of a woman with placenta praevia who bled repeatedly for 19 days and died after refusing any intervention:

Wherefore, in such cases as this the delivery ought to be dispatched with all possible speed, without which the woman must expect nothing but present death.

In describing one case of a women with 'a most violent flux of blood' in which he was consulted, he revealed a high degree of self-esteem:

No less than four of the most noted physicians of Paris ... required her to take all the Sacraments, which being done, they desired me to endeavour her delivery, as the only means (next to God) to save the woman's life.

Portal also pointed out that face presentations could be left to deliver normally, whereas the practice of that era was to advocate manual conversion to a normal vertex or destructive instrumental delivery.

He showed an understanding of the risks incurred with footling breech presentation, combined with an ecclesiastical twist, when he wrote, 'If the feet of the child come foremost, you must take care to baptise them immediately'.

Selected Publications

Portal P. *La pratique des accouchemens soutenue d'un grand nombre d'observations.* Paris: G. Martin; 1685.

Portal P. *The Compleat Practice of Men and Women Midwives: Or, the True Manner of Assisting a Woman in Child-Bearing.* (English translation from the original 1685). London: J. Johnson; 1763.

Bibliography References

73, 88, 99, 102, 340, 359, 485, 648, 676, 983, 1112, 1408.

Potter, Edith Louise (1901–1993)

Potter's Syndrome/Potter's Facies

Potter's syndrome consists of renal agenesis, hypoplastic lungs, characteristic facies and variable sequelae from the associated oligohydramnios – usually limb deformities. The infants are commonly male and usually die within hours from respiratory distress before uraemia supervenes. Potter's first report in 1946 concentrated on the facial characteristics, 'Potter's facies':

Bilateral renal agenesis is associated with a type of facies so characteristic that the absence of kidneys can be

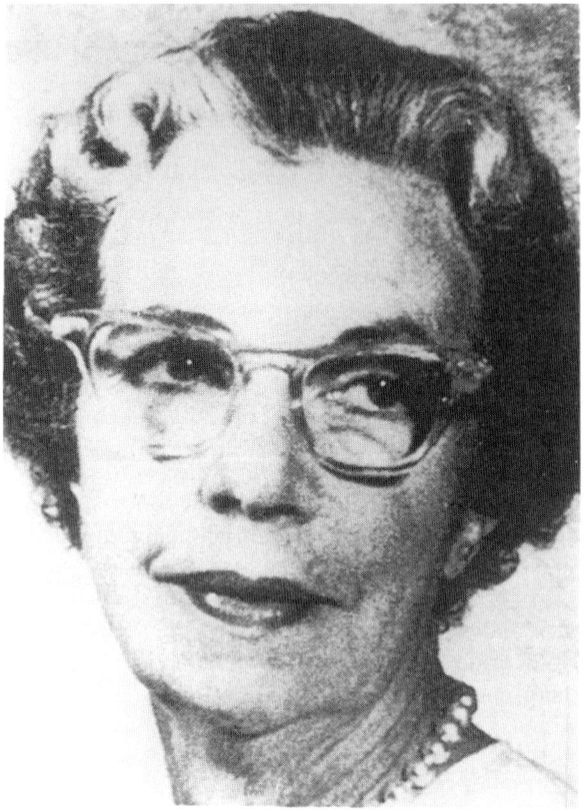

Edith Louise Potter

diagnosed in most instances on this finding alone. The principal change consists of a mild increase in width between the eyes, a very prominent fold of skin arising at the inner canthus, a flattening of the nose, mild retraction of the lower jaw, and large, low-lying ears with incomplete cartilaginous development.

Edith Potter was born in Clinton, Iowa. She qualified in medicine from the University of Minnesota in 1925 and entered clinical practice for five years. She then undertook additional training in pathology, obtaining her PhD in 1934. Potter was appointed to the department of obstetrics and gynaecology at the University of Chicago in 1934 and became professor of pathology and pathologist to the Chicago Lying-in Hospital. She retired to Fort Myers, Florida in 1967. She received the Distinguished Service Award from the American College of Obstetricians and Gynecologists in 1975. The college has also established the Edith Potter Memorial Lecture to be given at the annual clinical meeting.

Selected Publications

Potter EL. Facial characteristics of infants with bilateral renal agenesis. *Am J Obstet Gynecol* 1946; 51: 885–8.

Potter EL. Bilateral renal agenesis. *J Pediatr* 1946; 29: 68–76

Bibliography References

616, 731, 1221, 1485, 1752.

Potter, Irving White (1868–1956)

Internal Podalic Version

Irving Potter of Buffalo, New York, became so skilled in the performance of internal podalic version and breech extraction that by the end of his career he was delivering more than 90 per cent of all infants in his practice by this technique. At the height of his career he was delivering more than 1,000 infants per year. In his monograph, *The Place of Version in Obstetrics*, first published in 1922, he wrote:

During an obstetric practice extending over many years, in which I have personally delivered over fourteen thousand women, I early realized the value of internal podalic version as a maneuvre enabling one to overcome many difficult situations, and as my knowledge of aseptic and antiseptic surgery increased, together with my ability to operate with confidence, I gradually extended its sphere of usefulness as the years passed on.

Potter's technique was to induce surgical anaesthesia with chloroform once the woman reached full dilatation. He spent several minutes 'ironing out' the vagina and then pushed the fetal head up, brought both feet down together, and proceeded with breech extraction. He rarely performed episiotomy and did not use any abdominal pressure, 'realizing that this was unnecessary as well as being responsible for the arms of the child coming up over the head and other difficulties'. Potter advocated this technique for all normal vertex presentations at full dilatation:

> *The second stage of labor has been eliminated; the women have not suffered any of the pain usually consequent upon this stage; the vagina and perineum have not been subjected to long hours of stretching, which resulted in quick retraction so that relaxed and gaping outlets with protruding and falling bladders and rectocele did not occur in my patients. Finally, I have been enabled to complete the delivery within an hour and still be fresh and ready for my other work. The more women I delivered, the more satisfied was I with their condition during the whole puerperium, and I found less morbidity and suffering, as the weeks and months went by. I gradually increased the indications and enlarged the field of the version operation and now, I can say that at least ninety percent of my cases are delivered by version and my last 938 cases had no maternal mortality and fetal mortality of 2.3 percent ...*

Potter's presentations of his results were met with surprise and condemnation. It was generally acknowledged that his results were good, but it was felt that if others tried to emulate his achievements the results for the infants would be disastrous. Potter was unmoved by this criticism and continued his practice and publications. By 1942 he had delivered more than 25,000 infants.

Potter's approach had previously been advocated by Edward Garland Figg (1815–1902), an obstetrician from Glasgow. Soon after the introduction of chloroform anaesthesia, Figg began to perform internal podalic version and breech extraction as an alternative to high forceps. He found this so satisfactory that he started to use the technique for normal cases. He published a series of 55 of 58 infants in vertex presentation delivered by internal podalic version and breech extraction. For this he was soundly condemned by his medical colleagues.

Irving White Potter was born into a prosperous medical family with three generations of physicians. He received his schooling at home and then graduated from the Buffalo Medical School in 1891. For seven years he carried out a general medical practice and

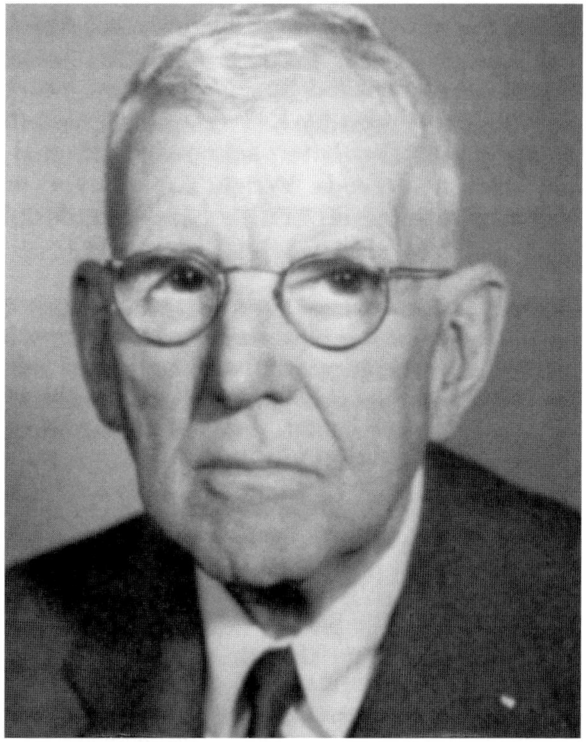
Irving White Potter

then limited his work to obstetrics. He received no formal postgraduate training and was to a large extent self-taught and did not travel outside Buffalo. He had one son, who followed him into obstetrical practice. Irving Potter delivered his three grandsons by internal podalic version and breech extraction, all of whom became obstetricians. Potter was a workaholic who did not take holidays and delivered his patients in six different hospitals in Buffalo. He was receptive to observers at his deliveries, but he insisted upon one rule: 'I'll show you how to do an internal version operation if we do not discuss the indications'. Irving Potter practised well into his eighties despite failing eyesight, the latter presumably being a minor handicap as the majority of his work relied on touch alone. It could be said that he raised the art of obstetric braille to its illogical conclusion.

Selected Publications

Figg EG. On delivery of the child by turning as a general rule in labour. *Med Times Gaz* 1858; 17: 493–5.

Potter IW. Version, with a report of 200 additional cases since September 1916. *Am J Obstet* 1918; 77: 215–20.

Potter IW. Version. *Am J Obstet Gynecol* 1921; 1560–73.

Potter IW. *The Place of Version in Obstetrics*. St Louis, MO: CV Mosby Co; 1922.

Bibliography References

349, 801, 1269, 1485, 1561.

Poupart, François (1661–1709)

Poupart's (Inguinal) Ligament

The inguinal ligament was briefly described by Gabriel Fallopius in 1561. François Poupart gave a full description and outline of its function in a presentation to the French Royal Academy in 1705, as reported in the minutes:

> *They are attached at one end on the crest of the ilium and at the other end on the crest of the os pubis, and the middle section has no attachment. They perform the function of bone in this area, because they support the three great muscles of the abdomen . . .they can sustain in part, and break the thrust which severe coughing, violent strains, etc, give to the intestines . . . Inasmuch as these ligaments take the place of bones which nature might have created in their place, the abdomen has the liberty of distending, especially in pregnancy.*

François Poupart was born in Le Mans, France. He studied natural sciences in Le Mans and Paris and wrote extensively on entomology and comparative anatomy. In 1685 he studied human anatomy and surgery at the Hôtel Dieu in Paris and received his MD from the University of Rheims. He published an outline of surgery in 1695. Poupart lived in relative obscurity and poverty. One of his biographers, Delauney, said, 'Poupart hid his life as a sage under a cloak of mediocrity'.

Selected Publications

Poupart F. *Suspenseurs de l'abdomen. Hist Acad Roy Sci.* Paris; 1705, p. 64.

Bibliography References

378, 406, 732, 831.

Pratt, Edwin Hartley (1849–1930)

Pratt's Cervical Dilators

Edwin Hartley Pratt graduated MD from Hahnemann Medical College of Chicago in 1873. He became a homeopathic general practitioner and surgeon. In 1883 he became professor of surgery at the Chicago Homeopathic Medical College and later founded a Society of Orificial Surgery, which he claimed was successful in the treatment of chronic diseases. It is not clear exactly what is meant by 'orificial surgery', but the phrase does not have a comforting ring to it. Presumably one of the orifices involved was the cervix, because Pratt designed and produced a tapered cervical dilator in 1887. The tapered nature of the dilator allowed for gradual dilatation of the cervix with less trauma.

Edwin Pratt was born in Towanda, Pennsylvania, and although he had a yen to practise law, he followed his father's wishes and footsteps into medicine. He was extremely successful in the world of homeopathic

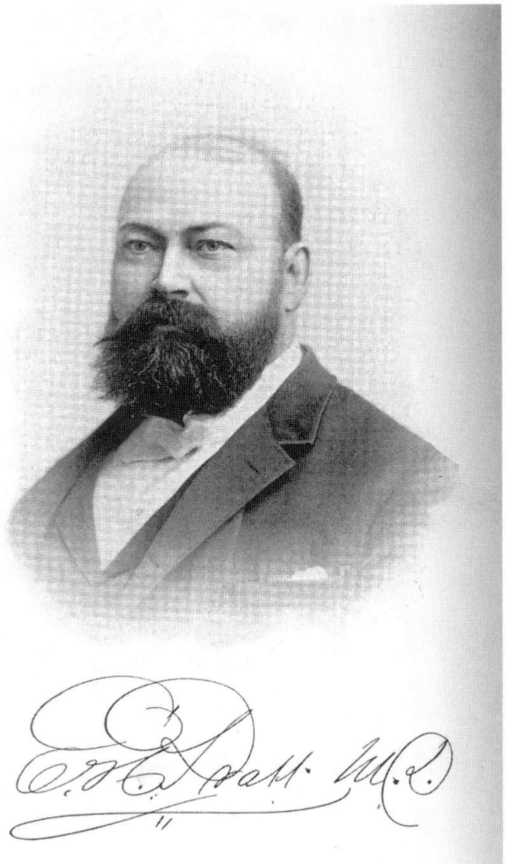

Edwin Hartley Pratt

medicine and built his own private hospital, the Lincoln Park Sanitarium in Chicago. He retired at the age of 70 and died 10 years later at Galva, Illinois. Pratt's cervical dilators continued to be widely used throughout North America.

Selected Publications

Pratt EH. *Orificial Surgery and its Application to the Treatment of Chronic Diseases*. Chicago, IL: WT Keener; 1887.

Bibliography References

1291, 1485.

Pugh, Benjamin (1715–1798)

Obstetric Forceps/Neonatal Resuscitation

Benjamin Pugh, one of 10 children, was born in Bishop's Castle, Shropshire in 1715. His uncle was a surgeon and probably supervised his early training. He spent some time in London and then set up practice in Chelmsford, Essex in 1738 as an apothecary and surgeon. Pugh devised forceps with a pelvic curve but did not publish his invention until 1754. He claimed to have invented the pelvic curve in 1740, which would have given him priority over William Smellie and André Levret, who independently published their descriptions of the pelvic curve in 1751. Apparently, Pugh's manuscript was ready for publication in 1750, but as the subscription to publish was not filled it was delayed until 1754. The book chronicles the meticulous observation and ingenuity of an experienced country practitioner. In the preface to his book he extolled the virtues of his forceps:

> *I have succeeded in deliveries, without opening one child's head for these fourteen years past . . . The curved forceps I invented upwards of fourteen years ago, made me by a*

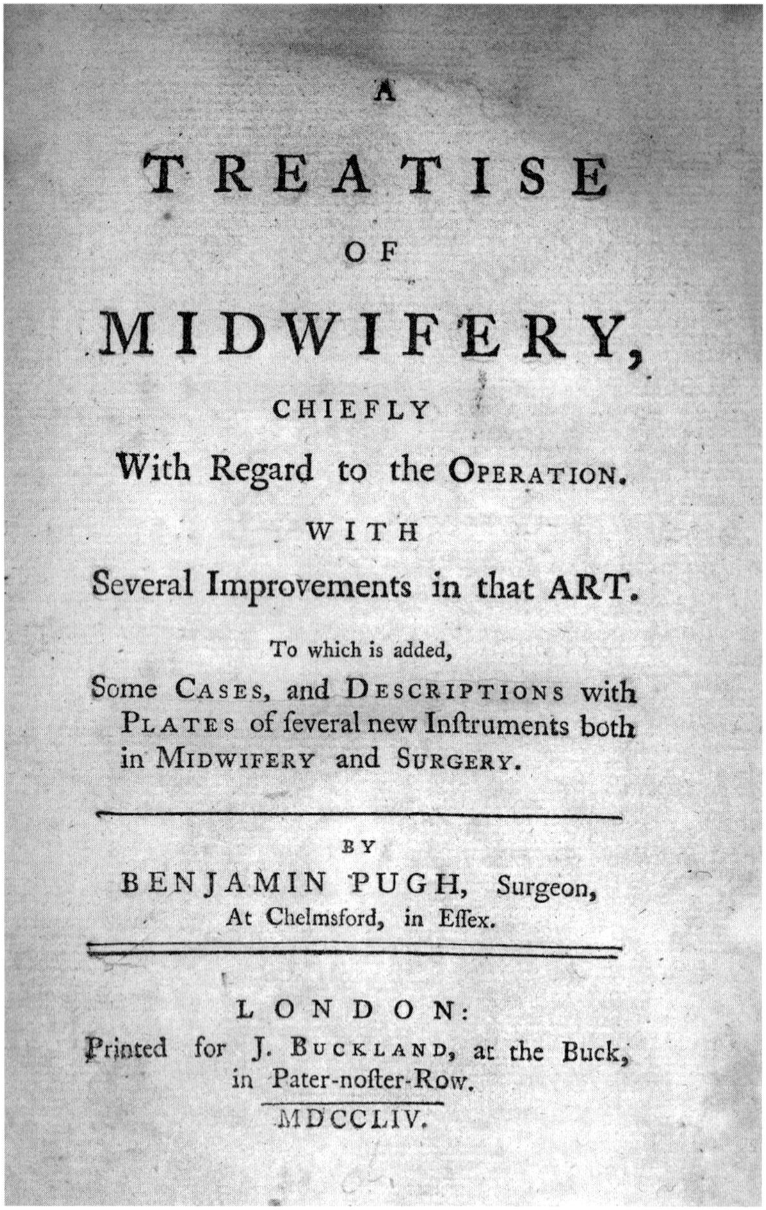

A

TREATISE

OF

MIDWIFERY,

CHIEFLY

With Regard to the OPERATION.

WITH

Several Improvements in that ART.

To which is added,

Some CASES, and DESCRIPTIONS with PLATES of ſeveral new Inſtruments both in MIDWIFERY and SURGERY.

BY

BENJAMIN PUGH, Surgeon,
At Chelmsford, in Eſſex.

LONDON:
Printed for J. BUCKLAND, at the Buck, in Pater-noſter-Row.
MDCCLIV.

Title page of Pugh's *Treatise on Midwifery*

man of Mr Archers, Cutler, now living in Chelmsford. The preference between them and the common straight forceps in every respect is great.

Some support for Pugh's claim is found in an advertisement in the 16 April 1748 edition of the *Ipswich Journal*, offering the treatise and forceps for sale at half a guinea each. Pugh wrote of the use of forceps with some feeling:

The operation is often one of the most difficult in all surgery, and the art depends upon as nice a foundation as any, and some cases you will find will make you sweat plentifully in the coldest day in winter.

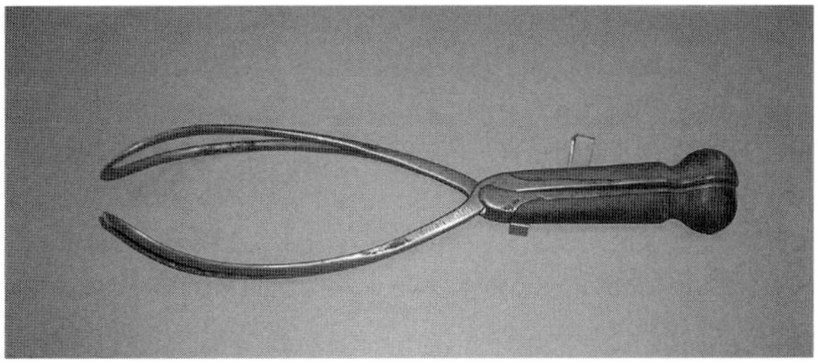

Pugh's forceps

He also gave a remarkable description of neonatal mouth-to-mouth ventilation, that has changed little in the intervening 250 years:

> *If the child does not breath immediately upon delivery, which sometimes it will not, especially if it has taken air in the womb; wipe its mouth, and press your mouth to the child's at the same time pinching the nose with your thumb and finger, to prevent the air escaping; inflate the lungs, rubbing it before the fire: by which method I have saved many.*

In addition, he devised an 'air-pipe' of leather wrapped around a wire spring for use in the infant's mouth to prevent suffocation during breech extraction.

Pugh retired from practice in 1779 and lived in a small estate outside Bath. He died on 14 February 1798 and was buried at St Peter's Church, Freshford. Inside and above the entrance to the church there is a memorial plaque that reads in part, 'He was a sincere friend and a punctual honest man. Requiem in pace'.

Selected Publications

Pugh B. *A Treatise on Midwifery, Chiefly with Regard to the Operation: with Several Improvements in That Art.* London: Buckland; 1754.

Bibliography References

44, 74, 83, 99, 399, 419, 423, 451, 548, 648, 721, 1128, 1265, 1287, 1420, 1519, 1695.

R

Ramsey, Elizabeth Maplesden (1906–1993)

Utero-Placental-Fetal Circulation

In 1933 Elizabeth Ramsey was a junior resident in pathology at Yale University when she made the unexpected discovery of a 14-day embryo during a routine autopsy. The earliest known human embryo at that time, it was donated, as the 'Yale embryo', to the Carnegie Institution of Washington, situated in Baltimore. This discovery ensured Ramsey's part-time appointment to the Carnegie Institution, an association that would last until her retirement in 1971. Here, as part of George Corner's group, she participated in the study of the institution's 600 embryos. She moved on with her own studies of blastocyst implantation and, using a colony of rhesus monkeys, began her detailed work on the utero-placental circulation.

Ramsey used meticulous cineradiographic techniques, with a slow injection of radio contrast material to avoid disruption of the circulation under study. She showed that the maternal blood entered the basal plate under pressure via the spiral arteries, bathed the chorionic villi within the intervillous space and exited passively through the basal plate into the maternal uterine veins. This work established the principle of the utero-placental-fetal interface and was relevant to those investigating the pathogenesis of pre-eclampsia and abruptio placentae. It was also applicable to the understanding of fetal oxygenation during labour. Ramsey studied the circulation during uterine contractions and showed that both the inflow and outflow of blood to the intervillous space ceased but that the

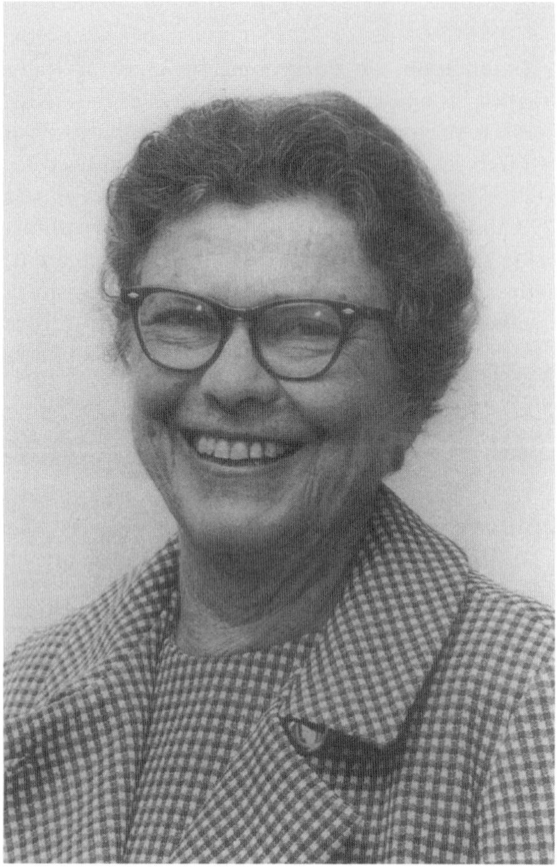

Elizabeth Maplesden Ramsey

volume of blood within the space was not expelled, allowing continued, albeit reduced gaseous exchange.

Elizabeth Ramsey was born in New York City on 17 February 1906 but grew up in California. In 1928 she took her undergraduate BA at Mills College in Oakland, California. As one of two women in her class, she graduated in medicine from Yale University in 1932. In addition to her work at the Carnegie Institution, she was lecturer and associate pathologist at George Washington University in Washington DC.

She married in 1934 and lived in Washington DC with her lawyer husband. During the Second World War she was assistant chief for the Office of Medical Information at the National Research Council. Apart from this interregnum, she devoted her entire professional life to research into the embryo, implantation and placentation.

Outside work, she was knowledgeable in art and music and served on the board of the National Symphony Orchestra. She died on 2 July 1993, 12 days after her husband.

Selected Publications

Ramsey EM. Circulation in the intervillous space of the primate placenta. *Am J Obstet Gynecol* 1962; 84: 1649–63.

Ramsey EM, Corner GW, Donner MW. Serial and cineradioangiographic visualization of maternal circulation in the primate (hemochorial) placenta. *Am J Obstet Gynecol* 1963; 86: 213–25.

Bibliography References

698, 932, 1733.

Read, Grantly Dick (1890–1959)

Natural Childbirth

It is not uncommon in medicine, as in other facets of life, for opposition to develop against established practice. In this case, the so-called natural childbirth movement was a reaction to heavy sedation in the twilight sleep era of the early twentieth century. In the forefront of this movement was the English obstetrician, Grantly Dick Read. He wrote:

> *It is not generally recognised that in childbirth there is an 'emotional labour' which is as definite and important as its physical counterpart. This must be understood if parturition is to be conducted as a physiological performance.*

As a student Read was very impressed by the attitude of a young woman he attended at a home delivery. During the late stages of labour, he offered her chloroform analgesia. However, she refused and after delivery said, 'It didn't hurt doctor; it wasn't meant to hurt, was it?' Read posed the question:

Is a woman pained and frightened because her labour is difficult, or is her labour difficult and painful because she is frightened?

He hypothesised that 'Fear is in some way the chief pain-producing agent in otherwise normal labour', which led to what he called the 'pain-fear-tension syndrome of labour':

Pain is the mental interpretation of harmful stimulus, and fear the intensifier of stimulus-interpretation. The biological purpose of each is protective. The physiological reaction to each is tension.

He argued that the resultant tension stimulated the sympathetic nerve supply of the cervix and lower uterine segment, causing a relative obstruction to progressive labour. He said, 'if fear is eliminated very few physiological labours are so distressing that women will demand relief from pain'. Read advocated a series of antenatal classes and exercises to engender confidence and promote relaxation. He was not a zealot and recognised that some women required and should be given conventional analgesia, but he emphasised that this could be kept to a minimum by breaking the pain-fear-tension cycle:

I do not wish to disagree with the advocates of applied anaesthesia, whether it is caudal, inhalation or parenteral, for pain must be prevented and relieved. Every effort to make childbirth a painless function should be carefully considered.

Read published his influential book, *Natural Childbirth*, in 1933. It was later produced under the title *Childbirth Without Fear*. Others were to follow and modify Read's approach, including I Velvovski in Russia and Fernand Lamaze and Frederick Leboyer in France.

Grantly Dick Read was one of seven children born in Norfolk, England. He studied medicine at St John's College, Cambridge and the London Hospital, qualifying in 1914. He was an accomplished athlete, excelling in boxing, cricket and soccer. He served in the medical corps in the First World War in France and Gallipoli, where he was badly wounded. After the war he returned to the London Hospital for one year as a resident in obstetrics, during which he worked among the poor of the Whitechapel and Bethnal Green districts. He then went into general practice in Woking, Surrey, with an emphasis on obstetrics. It was here that he crystallised his views on childbirth. As his reputation grew, he established his own clinic and worked exclusively in obstetrics. In 1948, unenamoured with the new National Health Service, he moved to South Africa and practised in Johannesburg for five years. He returned to England after a long journey back through Africa, during which he studied childbirth practices in many regions. This confirmed his previous views on the need to regard the process as physiological. He had a charismatic presence and speaking style, and his lectures and writings gained him an international reputation. He lectured widely in the United States, and Herbert Thoms adopted his principles at Yale. Like most who challenge the medical establishment he was, with some exceptions, not honoured by his peers during his lifetime. His surname is sometimes written Dick-Read. He was born Read but added the hyphen one year before his death. He died in Norfolk on 11 June 1959.

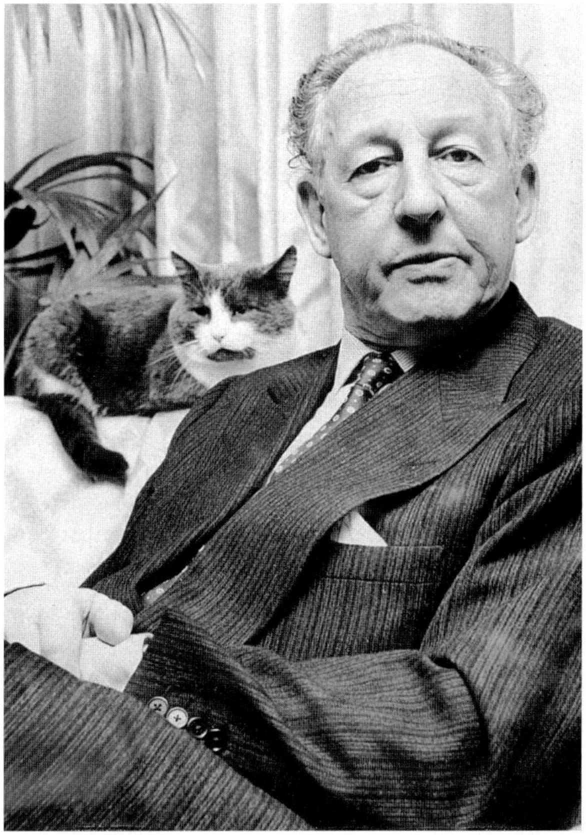

Grantly Dick Read

Selected Publications

Read GD. *Natural Childbirth*. London: Heinemann; 1933.

Read GD. *Childbirth without Fear*. New York, NY: Harper; 1944.

Read GD. Correlation of physical and emotional phenomena of natural labour. *J Obstet Gynaecol Br Emp* 1946; 53: 55–61.

Read GD. The discomforts of childbirth. *BMJ* 1949; 1: 651–4.

Bibliography References

253, 273, 467, 822, 879, 1055, 1272, 1578.

Récamier, Joseph Claude Anthelme (1774–1852)

Vaginal Speculum

Joseph Récamier was a French gynaecologist and surgeon who, in 1801, reintroduced the systematic use of the vaginal speculum to inspect and treat ulcers and infections of the vagina and cervix. Before this, Soranus had used a vaginal speculum and recognisable specula were discovered, preserved in the ashes of

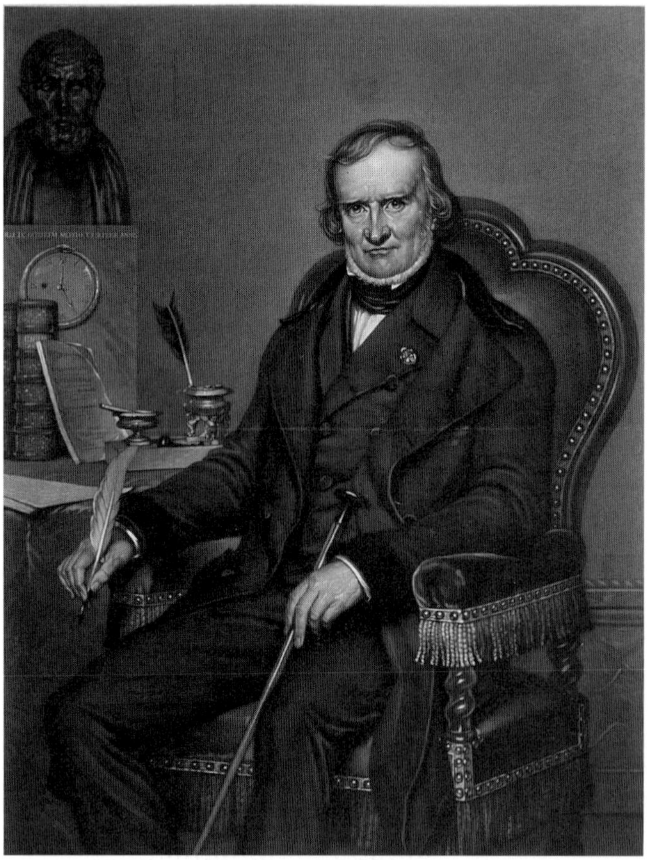

Joseph Claude Anthelme Récamier

Pompeii. Récamier used a thin tin tube, 12 cm long. Later he increased the diameter to improve the field of vision. He was one of the first to perform vaginal hysterectomy for cancer of the cervix, on 26 July 1829. In his book on cancer he gives one of the earliest references to metastasis – 'metastase'. He also reintroduced the curette into gynaecological practice in 1846.

Récamier grew up near Lyon, France, and began a medical apprenticeship with his uncle. He initially served as a military surgeon and then studied medicine at the Hôtel Dieu in Lyon and later at the Hôtel Dieu in Paris. He later became physician and professor of clinical medicine at the Hôtel Dieu in Paris. In 1827 he succeeded René Laennec as professor at the Collège de France. Récamier remained faithful to the Bourbons and resigned these positions rather than take the oath of the new government.

Selected Publications

Récamier JCA. *Recherches sur le traitement du cancer par la compression méthodique simple ou combinée et sur l'histoire général de la même maladie.* Paris: Gabon; 1829

Récamier JCA. Invention du spéculum plein et brisé. *Bull Acad Med (Paris)* 1842–3; 8: 661–8.

Bibliography References

243, 353, 648, 674, 1140, 1141, 1143, 1144, 1278, 1588.

Reinke, Friedrich Berthold (1862–1919)

Crystalloids of Reinke

The ovoid cells in the hilum of the ovary lie adjacent to the mesovarium and may be homologues of the interstitial or Leydig cells of the testis. Within these cells may be seen rectangular hyaline inclusion bodies: the crystalloids of Reinke. They may also be observed in the rare hilus cell or Leydig cell ovarian tumour, in which their presence usually represents androgenic steroid production.

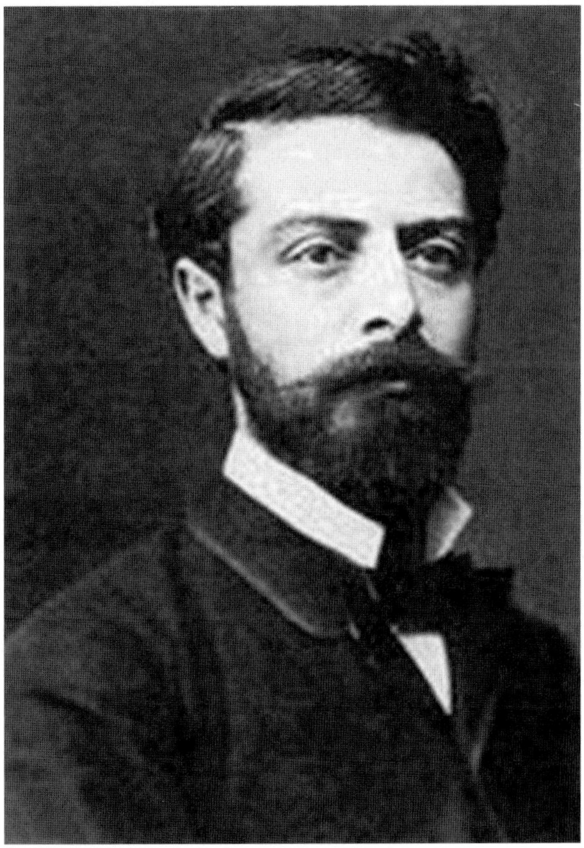

Friedrich Berthold Reinke

Friedrich Reinke was the ninth of 10 children born to a Lutheran Pastor in Ziethen, Germany. He studied medicine at Göttingen and Kiel. He worked successively in the anatomy departments of Kiel, Zurich, Rostock and Wiesbaden. Reinke's main area of research was in cell division and tumour formation. He also described the boundaries of the vocal fold, which bears his name as Reinke's space. While at Rostock, he obtained the testes of a 25-year-old criminal shortly after his execution. In his study of these and other testicular tissue, he described the crystalloids and only found them in testes undergoing spermatogenesis.

Reinke could be impetuous and was described by colleagues as coarse and reckless. He clashed with his department head at Rostock and ended his professional career in Wiesbaden. He died of stomach cancer on 12 May 1919 in a charity hospital in Wiesbaden, which suggests that he was impoverished.

Selected Publications

Reinke F. Beiträge zur Histologie des Menschen. *Arch mikrosk Anat* 1896; 47: 34–44.

Bibliography References

406, 1125, 1369, 1480.

Retzius, Anders Adolf (1796–1860)

Cave of Retzius

Anders Adolph Retzius, anatomist and anthropologist, was born in Lund, Sweden. His father was professor of natural history in the University of Lund. He graduated in medicine in 1819 from his home university. He became professor of anatomy at the Karolinska Institute of Medicine and Surgery in Stockholm, having previously served as the professor of veterinary science at the Veterinary Institute. In addition to many other anatomical contributions, he described the retropubic or pre-vesical space, known as the cave of Retzius. Via this space, surgical access to the bladder is gained without entering the peritoneal cavity – the 'blasporten' (door of the bladder) as Retzius called it. Many of the urethrovesical suspension operations for stress incontinence are performed via this surgical portal. His son, Magnus Gustav, succeeded him in the chair of anatomy.

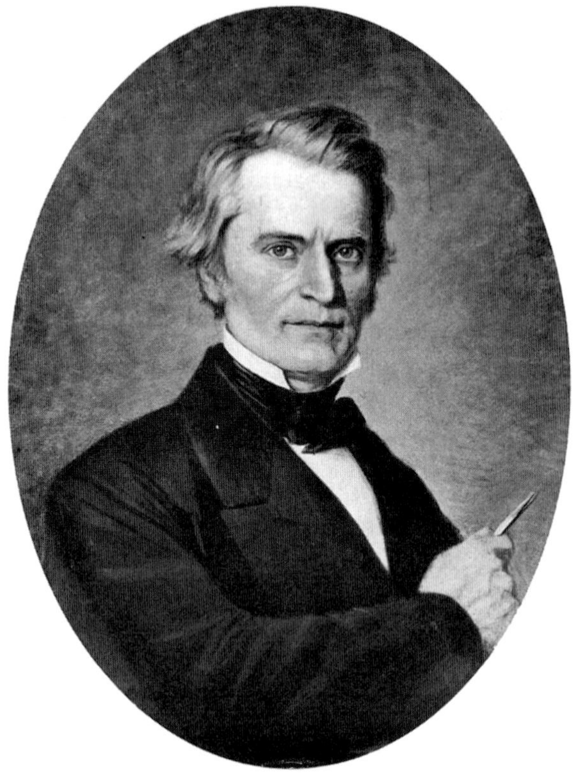

Anders Adolf Retzius

Selected Publications

Retzius AA. Über das Ligamentum pelvoprostaticum oder den Apparat, durch welchen die Harnblase, die Prostata und die Harnröhre an den untren Beckenöffnung befestigt sind. *Müller's Arch Anat Physiol Wiss Med* 1849: 182–96.

Bibliography References

406, 676, 875, 1261, 1281, 1480.

Rigby, Edward (1747–1821)

Antepartum Haemorrhage

Edward Rigby was a general medical practitioner in Norwich, England, who was the first to clearly differentiate between the two main causes of antepartum haemorrhage: one 'unavoidable', due to placenta praevia, and the other 'accidental', due to premature separation of the normally situated placenta – abruptio placentae. He came to his conclusions after carefully observing and writing up the cases in his own practice. He published his first set of results in 1775 in his *Essay on the Uterine Haemorrhage*, which he started by saying:

> *No circumstance that attends parturition, exposes women to so much danger, as profuse Haemorrhages from the Uterus, towards the latter end of pregnancy, and in the time of labour; the art of midwifery is likewise, in no instance, more at a loss in the use of means for the relief of the patient; an inquiry into the causes of them, and an attempt to improve the practice in such cases, cannot, therefore, be useless.*

At this time the general method of managing all cases of significant antepartum bleeding was to forcibly dilate the cervix and empty the uterus by internal version and breech extraction – *accouchement forcé*. By demonstrating the difference between the two causes of haemorrhage, Rigby showed that for cases of placenta praevia this was appropriate, but for abruptio placentae, amniotomy and allowing labour to proceed was effective and safer:

> *From what has been said it appears, then, that the placenta is fixed to the os uteri much more frequently than has hitherto been supposed; that when it is so situated, nothing but turning the child will put a stop to the flooding; that when it is not so situated, nature will, for the most part, expel it safely herself . . .*

Rigby continued to collect cases and his book went into six editions. In the sixth edition his experience with 106 cases is recorded. There were 64 cases of abruptio placentae with no maternal death and 42 cases of placenta praevia with 26 per cent maternal mortality. Rigby's powers of observation and humanity are evident in the individual case histories:

> *Her countenance was pale, her eyes sunk and her whole appearance exhibited a miserable spectacle of poverty, famine, disease and approaching death . . . The pain which a surgeon ever feels when an important operation terminates unfortunately, was in this instance much aggravated by the reflection, that this poor woman would, probably have been saved, had she been in any other than the wretched situation in which her extreme poverty had placed her.*

Rigby's book is one of the genuine landmark publications in obstetrics. In addition to the six English editions it was published in the United States and translated into French, German and Russian.

Edward Rigby was born in Chowbent, near Manchester, England. In 1762 he was apprenticed to a skilled Norwich surgeon, Mr David Martineau. He then studied in London and attended lectures by the Hunter brothers. He became a member of the Corporation of Surgeons in 1769. In that year he returned to Norwich, where he was to remain. In some aspects of his life Rigby was a late bloomer. He only took his MD degree when he was 67 years old. He served as alderman, magistrate, sheriff and, in 1805, as mayor of Norwich. He introduced smallpox vaccination to Norwich. After his first wife died he remarried in 1803 and had 12 children. He fathered twins when he was 57 and quadruplets when he was 70. One of the twins, Edward Rigby junior (1804–1861), became a prominent obstetrician in London and lecturer in midwifery at St Thomas' Hospital.

Rigby also found time, in 1815, to write an article on 'Suggestions for an improved and extended cultivation of the Mangel Wurzel'. He wrote the preface to the sixth edition of his book on his deathbed, dated 21 October 1821, and died six days later.

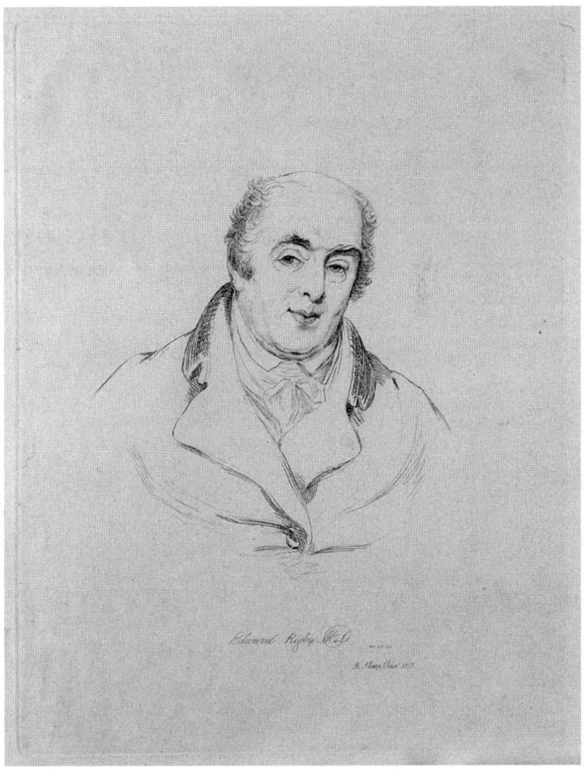

Edward Rigby

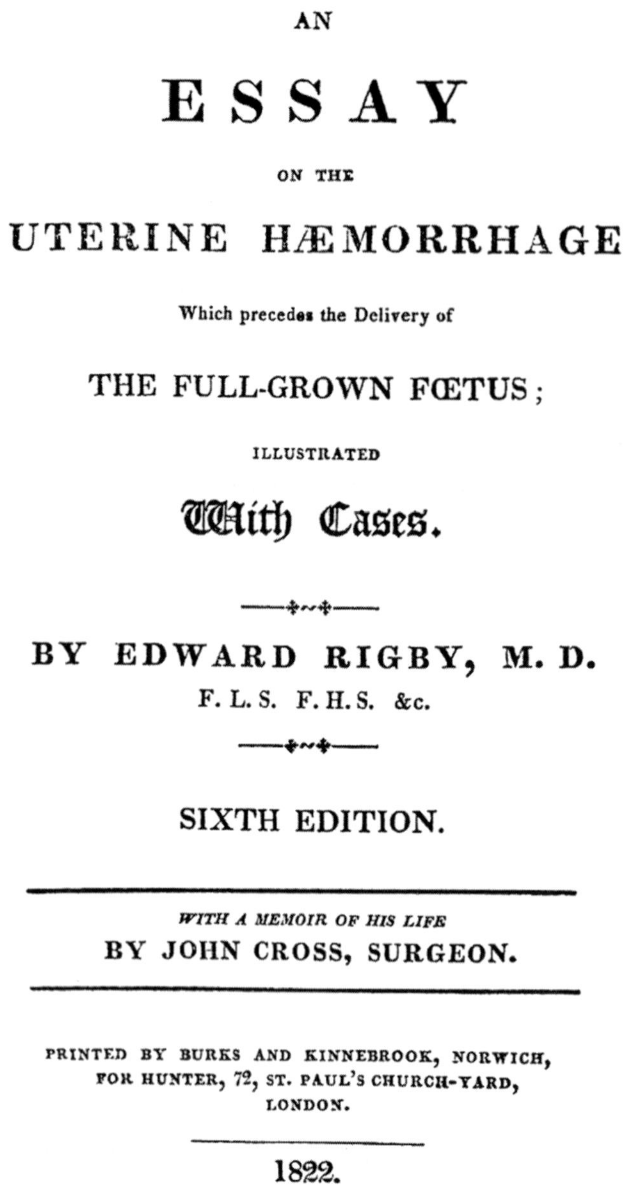

AN

ESSAY

ON THE

UTERINE HÆMORRHAGE

Which precedes the Delivery of

THE FULL-GROWN FŒTUS;

ILLUSTRATED

With Cases.

BY EDWARD RIGBY, M. D.

F. L. S. F. H. S. &c.

SIXTH EDITION.

WITH A MEMOIR OF HIS LIFE

BY JOHN CROSS, SURGEON.

PRINTED BY BURKS AND KINNEBROOK, NORWICH,
FOR HUNTER, 72, ST. PAUL'S CHURCH-YARD,
LONDON.

1822.

Title page of Edward Rigby's sixth and final edition of his text on antepartum haemorrhage

Selected Publications

Rigby E. *An Essay on the Uterine Haemorrhage, Which Precedes the Delivery of the Full Grown Foetus; Illustrated With Cases*. London: J. Johnson; 1775. Sixth edn. London: Hunter; 1822.

Bibliography References

88, 90, 99, 328, 475, 548, 752, 822, 983, 1112, 1261, 1298, 1387, 1595.

Ritgen, Ferdinand August Maria Franz von (1787–1867)

Ritgen's Manoeuvre

From time immemorial, advice has been issued to safeguard the perineum during delivery and, to some extent, this has been the hallmark of the skilful accoucheur. The manoeuvre, or modification thereof, most commonly used is that devised by Ferdinand von Ritgen, although similar techniques were advised by William Giffard and John Harvie in the previous century. Ritgen first described his manoeuvre in 1826 and modified it through the years, publishing his final words on the subject in 1855. He emphasised that this technique was often unnecessary: 'If that passage can proceed without risk of a perineal tear, then head and perineum should *not be touched at all*'. However, he advocated his manoeuvre in selected cases: 'Holding back the head is the more necessary the wider, tighter, thinner and smoother the perineum is'.

In essence Ritgen's manoeuvre provides controlled delivery of the head, as the fingers of one hand press gently on the occiput, while the palmar surface of the other hand is placed on the perineum just in front of the coccyx. Between contractions one gently extends the head with pressure on the fetal chin from the perineal hand and eases it over the perineum. Ritgen described it thus:

> *Pressure is applied in such a way that the three fingers holding the head back are placed at the back of the head, not to be removed until it is delivered. The tips of the four fingers of the other hand are placed outside at the posterior perineum, behind the opening of the anus, next to the tip of the coccyx and a little to the side of the median raphe; between pains preferably immediately after a pain, pressure is exerted inward and forward, usually encountering the baby's chin and causing it to slide forward; at the same time the three fingers on the back of head follow its forward motion, causing it to advance slowly around the fulcrum formed by the nape near the lower edge of the symphysis. From the time that a contraction resumes, both hands remain motionless until it ceases. Immediately thereafter pressure upon the chin is resumed. To the extent that the chin gradually moves forward, the external pressure upon it must also be directed forward from the posterior perineum, until the chin passed over the transverse perineal band. The external pressure must therefore be exerted somewhat to the side of the median raphe, in order that one parietal boss may pass through the vaginal orifice before the other; in this way the vaginal outlet is better protected from rupture than if both bosses were to pass through it simultaneously.*

On rarer occasions Ritgen advocated a technique of 'scarification' of the perineum with several (up to 14) very shallow incisions, which he found allowed the more unyielding perineum to stretch intact. In 1855 he reported a series of 757 deliveries using his manoeuvre, aided by scarification in 11 per cent, with 'not one single tear of the perineum, not even a small one'.

After many years using and teaching his technique Ritgen felt emboldened to write:

> *May every teacher of midwives study most carefully the success of these two manoeuvres and then ask himself in full conscience whether it is not his sacred duty to instruct his students in them and to prevent the graduation of any who do not have sufficient experience in them.*

He introduced his final paragraph with this parting salvo:

> *These pages have not been written for those who lay them aside saying or thinking, 'Much ado about a perineal tear!' They will have to come to terms with their own consciences.*

Ferdinand von Ritgen was born in Wulfen, Germany. He took his medical training in Münster. At the early age of 27 he was appointed professor of surgery and obstetrics in Giessen, where he remained for 53 years until his death. Although his main interest was in obstetrics, his other activities were legion. In 1816 he established a school for midwives in Giessen. In addition to his obstetrical duties he also served at different times as head of psychiatry, dean of the medical faculty and rector of the University of

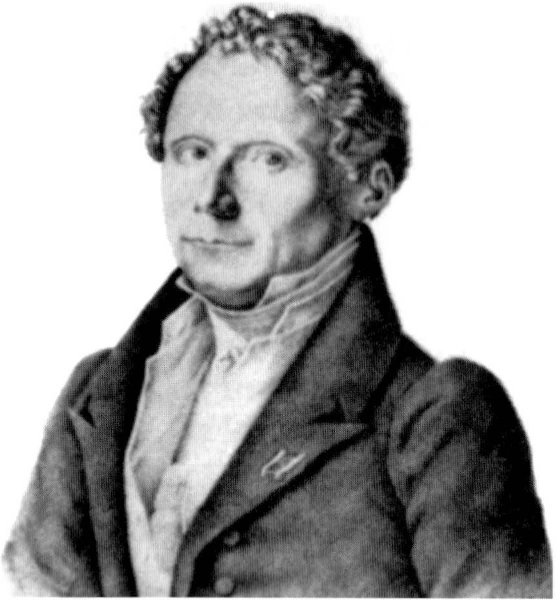

Ferdinand August Maria Franz von Ritgen

Giessen. He published extensively, not only on medical topics but also on astronomy, botany, chemistry, physics, philosophy and the history of obstetrics. On 21 October 1821 he was the first to conceive and attempt extraperitoneal caesarean section. Like many of his era he invented a number of instruments, including obstetric forceps. He was much honoured during his lifetime and received a gold medal from the King of Prussia and was ennobled by Grand Duke Ludwig II in 1840.

Selected Publications

Ritgen F von. Geburtshülfliche Erfahrungen und Bernerkungen. *Geimen Dth Ztschr Geburtsk* 1828; 3: 147–69.

Ritgen F von. Concerning his method for protection of the perineum. *Monatschr Geburtsk Frauenk* 1855; 6: 21. English Translation by Wynn RM. *Am J Obstet Gynecol* 1965; 93: 421–33.

Bibliography References

99, 102, 361, 548, 553, 636, 648, 673, 1261, 1301.

Robert, Heinrich Ludwig Ferdinand (1814–1878)

Robert Pelvis

One of the rarest of all pelvic deformities was first described in 1842 by Ferdinand Robert. He was able to study the pelvis in detail as the woman died following a caesarean section for obstructed labour due to 'such transverse narrowing of the pelvis that there was not enough room for two fingers alongside each other'. Her death on the fifth postoperative day was pithily ascribed: 'the patient committed an error of diet'.

Robert performed the post-mortem examination and found the absence of both sacral alae with the body of the sacrum fused to both ilia. In this so-called 'double Naegele' pelvis, the resultant transverse narrowing is so marked that vaginal delivery is impossible. The cause is unknown and only a handful of cases have been reported.

Heinrich Ludwig Ferdinand Robert was born in Marburg, Germany. He studied medicine at Berlin,

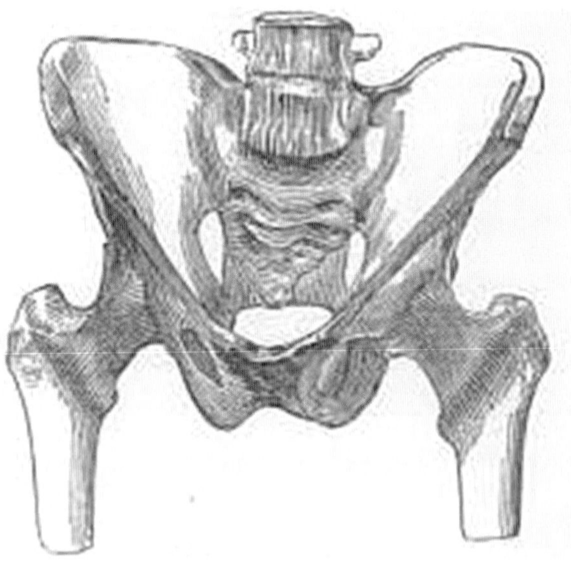

Robert pelvis showing bilateral absence of sacral alae

Göttingen and Würzburg, qualifying in 1838. He practised medicine in his home town and lectured at the University of Marburg. He later practised in Coblenz and Wiesbaden.

Selected Publications

Robert F. *Beschreibung eines im höchsten Grade Querverengten Beckens, bedingt durch Mangelhafte Entwickelung der Flügel des Kreuzbeins und Synostosis Congenialis beider Kreuzdarmbeinfügen*. Carlsruhe and Freiburg: Herder; 1842.

Bibliography References

553, 648, 775, 1261, 1480.

Roberts, James Boyd (1907–1980)

Roberts' Sign

In modern obstetrical practice, suspected intrauterine death is easily confirmed or denied within minutes by ultrasound. Before the reliability of real-time ultrasound was established, radiological signs depended on the post-mortem changes of decreased muscle tone, softening of supporting ligaments and liquefaction; for example, the 'halo' sign due to scalp oedema elevating the dermis from the skull, or 'Spalding's sign' due to overriding and separation of the fetal skull bones.

In April 1943, Boyd Roberts evaluated an X-ray of the fetus of a diabetic woman in whom fetal movements had been absent for 66 hours and fetal death was suspected. None of the then-accepted radiological signs of fetal death were present, but he noticed radiolucent areas, which he interpreted as evidence of gas in the fetal circulatory system. He postulated that this confirmed fetal death. The fetus was delivered three days later and immediate X-ray of the stillborn fetus showed that:

> *these radiotranslucent areas appeared to demonstrate portions of the fetal circulatory system and the following structures were identified: both umbilical arteries and portions of the umbilical vein; the common iliac arteries; external iliac arteries; the femoral arteries; the abdominal aorta; blood vessels of the liver and mesentery; the chambers of the heart; pulmonary vessels; carotid, facial, and intracranial vessels.*

Within an hour of delivery, an autopsy was performed. The heart was opened under water, and gas was noted to escape from both right and left ventricles. A similar escape of gas occurred when the liver and umbilical cord were opened under water. Roberts reported this case in the *American Journal of Roentgenology* in May 1944.

'Roberts' sign', as it became known, was the earliest radiological change, developing within 24 to 72 hours of fetal death. It was, however, transient, remaining for up to 14 days. Although Roberts' sign was frequently absent, it was, when present, the only absolutely reliable sign of fetal death, and there were no false positive results. The type of gas is unknown and has been variously attributed to oxygen, carbon dioxide, carbon monoxide or nitrogen. The origin of the gas is also unknown. Some of the postulated sources include the liberation of gas from the post-mortem breakdown of fetal haemoglobin or passive transfer from the maternal circulation via the placenta.

James Boyd Roberts was born on 2 May 1907, on a farm in Lanark County near Ottawa, Ontario. He was of Irish-Scots descent and one of seven children. He received his education in Lanark, after which he taught school for several years before entering the Queen's University School of Medicine in Kingston, graduating in 1935. He undertook residency training in radiology at the Victoria Hospital in London, Ontario. In November, 1937, he was appointed associate radiologist at the Royal Jubilee Hospital in

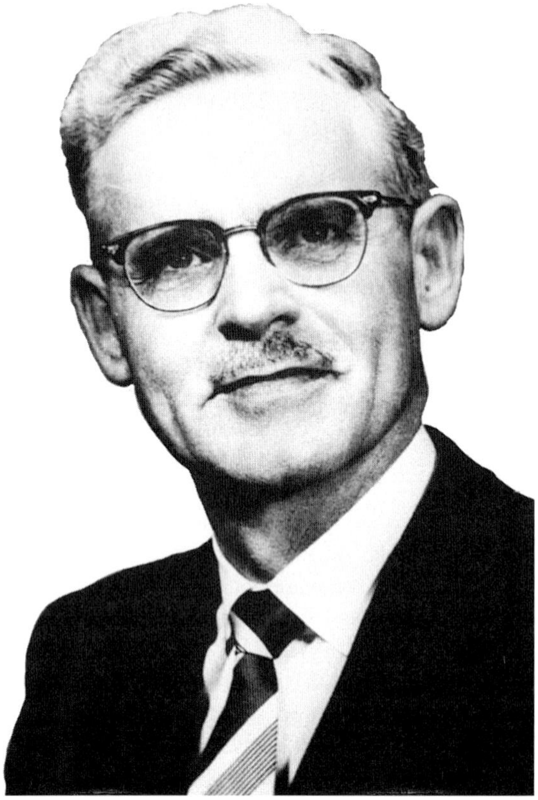

James Boyd Roberts

Victoria, British Columbia. Three months later he developed active pulmonary tuberculosis and spent four months in the tuberculosis ward of the hospital undergoing artificial pneumothorax therapy. He recovered sufficiently to return to work in October 1938, although recurrent pleural effusions continued to plague him intermittently for the rest of his life. He retired from active practice in 1969 and died on 10 May 1980.

Selected Publications

Roberts JB. Gas in the fetal circulatory system as a sign of intrauterine fetal death. *Am J Roentgenol* 1944; 51: 631–4.

Bibliography References

78, 91.

Robin, Pierre (1867–1950)

Pierre Robin Syndrome

Although it is rare (1 in 30,000 births), the Pierre Robin syndrome is known to all obstetricians because of the possibility of acute airway obstruction in the first minutes of life. The cardinal features are micrognathia and glossoptosis, with the posteriorly placed tongue liable to cause respiratory obstruction and difficulty with swallowing. This anomaly is frequently associated with cleft palate. In addition, there may be associated congenital heart defects, strabismus and glaucoma. Robin noted the very poor prognosis for severe cases:

> *I have never seen a child live more than 16 to 18 months who presented hypoplasia such that the lower maxilla was pushed more than 1 cm behind the upper.*

The Pierre Robin syndrome is now known as the Robin sequence, as it does not have a single cause.

Pierre Robin was a dental surgeon and professor of stomatology in Paris and editor of the journal *Stomatologie*. The syndrome was previously reported but has been ascribed to Robin following his full description published in 1923. He went on to write 17 articles on the subject. Pierre Robin died in Paris on 16 January 1950.

Selected Publications

Robin P. La glossoptose: son diagnostic, ses conséquences, son traitement. *J Méd Paris* 1923; 43: 235–7.

Bibliography References

382, 1270, 1310.

Robson, Michael Stephen (b. 1957)

Robson 10-Group Classification System of Caesarean Section

When Michael Robson moved to Pembury Hospital, Tunbridge Wells in 1989, he had just finished a one-year appointment as registrar (resident) at the National Maternity Hospital in Dublin. As such, he was steeped in the clinical principles and philosophy of Active Management of Labour established at that hospital by Kieran O'Driscoll. At that time, in Europe and North America, there was considerable debate about the application and effectiveness of active management of labour in the proportion of the obstetric population represented by the nulliparous woman in spontaneous labour with a single, cephalic fetus at term, this group being the biggest contributor to primary caesarean section.

Robson recognised that in the debate about caesarean delivery rates it was essential to know the profile of the obstetric population under consideration. Furthermore, the obstetric population of any given hospital or region would have varying proportions of women with different obstetric characteristics, based on parity, gestation, malpresentations, multiple pregnancy, previous caesarean section and the proportion of women that labour spontaneously, are induced or are delivered by pre-labour caesarean section. From these obstetric characteristics, 10 groups were identified as a starting point for further analysis. The women within these different categories or groups would have very different caesarean delivery rates. Thus, the proportion of these different groups in any hospital would be the main influencing factor in the overall caesarean section rate.

Robson started by concentrating on the nulliparous group in Pembury Hospital but, in the early 1990s, after his appointment as consultant to the Wycombe General Hospital, he expanded his appraisal to the entire obstetric population. He published his 10-group classification system and its rationale in 2001:

> *The background to the development of this method of classification arose from the aim to identify prospective, clinically relevant groups of women in which there were differences in their caesarean section rates. The purpose of the classification was to make possible comparisons over time in one unit and between different units. This would then allow changes to be made that would improve perinatal care. The groups needed to be well defined, mutually exclusive but totally inclusive, prospective and clinically relevant. Lastly they needed to be simple to understand and organise. It was thought that these different groups of women could be used to give an insight into the makeup of a caesarean section rate.*

Robson published his analysis of one year's deliveries at the Wycombe General Hospital and emphasised the universal applicability of this classification system which, at its heart, allowed any hospital, region or country to identify the contribution of each obstetric group to their caesarean delivery rate:

> *The important issue is that, internationally, it is possible with the minimum of resources, for every obstetric unit to classify their caesarean sections in this manner without the need for specialised information technology.*

The ten groups selected were as follows:

1. nulliparous, singleton, cephalic, ≥ 37 weeks, spontaneous labour
2. nulliparous, singleton, cephalic, ≥ 37 weeks, induced labour or CS before labour

3. multiparous, singleton, cephalic, $\geq$ 37 weeks, no previous CS, spontaneous labour
4. multiparous, singleton, cephalic, $\geq$ 37 weeks, no uterine scar, induced labour or CS before labour
5. multiparous, singleton, cephalic, $\geq$ 37 weeks, with a previous CS
6. nulliparous, singleton, breech
7. multiparous, singleton, breech, including previous CS
8. multiple pregnancy (twins or high-order multiples), including previous CS
9. singleton, transverse or oblique lie, including previous CS
10. singleton, cephalic, $<$ 37 weeks, including previous CS

After initial analysis, groups 2, 4 and 5–10 can be subdivided into those who had labour induced and those delivered by pre-labour caesarean section.

This classification system allows each hospital, region or country to monitor the caesarean rate in each of the 10 groups and to calculate the size of each group as a proportion of their total obstetric population, and therefore the contribution that each group makes to the overall caesarean section rate. It facilitates the analysis and comparison of caesarean rates within and across the groups and provides a reliable and consistent method for comparison of rates over time within and between hospitals or regions. Furthermore, seemingly high or low rates within any group could then be analysed in more detail, with a view to change in management and subsequent audit to assess the effect of that change.

Over the years, many hospitals and regions have applied the 10-group classification system and found it to be useable and relevant to clinical audit and practice. It has been applied in more than 50 countries. As a result, the World Health Organization endorsed its use in 2017: 'WHO proposes the Robson Classification system as a global standard for assessing, monitoring and comparing caesarean section rates within health care facilities over time, and between facilities'.

Robson emphasised that this classification system should be used as the foundation of clinical audit of intrapartum care, into which other aspects of maternal and perinatal outcome should be incorporated:

> *It is important to remember that, although we are talking about an analysis of caesarean sections, we should not interpret the results in isolation from other parameters of perinatal care. This should include perinatal and maternal morbidity and mortality as well as an assessment of maternal satisfaction. It should also include allowances for the case-mix of the population as well as the available resources to provide the care.*

Michael Robson was born on New Year's Eve 1957. He grew up in Norway until the age of 13. A fluent Norwegian speaker, he embraced life in Norway and became proficient in cross-country skiing and other winter sports. In 1971 he moved to England and continued his education at Judd School in Tonbridge, Kent. He qualified in medicine from St Thomas' Hospital, London in 1982 and undertook postgraduate training in general surgery and obstetrics and gynaecology in and around London. From 1991 to 1994 he was assistant master at the National Maternity Hospital in Dublin. In 1994 he was appointed consultant in obstetrics and gynaecology at Wycombe General Hospital, where he developed and refined the 10-group classification.

From 2005 to 2011 he served as Master of the National Maternity Hospital, the first non-Irish master to be appointed in the more than hundred-year history of that Dublin institution. Since 2012 he has remained as a consultant at the National

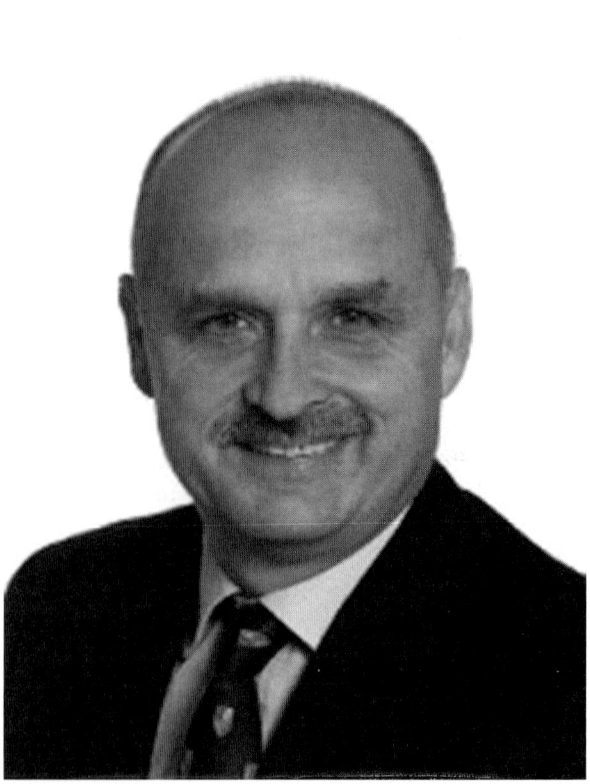

Michael Stephen Robson

Maternity Hospital, where, in addition to the clinical practice of both obstetrics and gynaecology, he maintains an active role in audit. In particular, he is the clinical director of the national electronic patient record for the Maternal and Neonatal Clinical Management System (MNCMS) for Ireland. This aims to improve clinical care as well as enhance clinical audit, governance and quality assurance.

Selected Publications

Robson MS, Scudamore IW, Walsh SM. Using the medical audit cycle to reduce cesarean section rates. *Am J Obstet Gynecol* 1996; 174: 199–205.

Robson MS. Classification of caesarean sections. *Fetal Matern Med Rev* 2001; 12: 23–39.

World Health Organization. *Robson Classification Implementation Manual*. Geneva: World Health Organization; 2017.

Bibliography References

99, 102, 1313, 1652, 1691, 1692.

Rodeck, Charles Henry (b. 1944)

Intravascular Fetal Transfusion

Charles Rodeck was born in Bohemia (then Czechoslovakia) on 23 August 1944. In 1946 he was expelled from the country, along with his parents and 3 million others of the German speaking population. After spending time in various refugee camps, and following his father's death from pulmonary tuberculosis, he and his mother came to England in 1949. He grew up in Banstead, Surrey and graduated from medical school at University College London in 1969. After training posts in London, he was appointed lecturer in obstetrics and gynaecology at King's College Hospital, London in 1976. It was here that he started his work in the fledgling specialty of fetal medicine to which he was to contribute so much over a 40-year career.

His first endeavour was to explore the role of fetoscopy in fetal diagnosis. In the early 1970s advances in fibre-optic technology produced a 2.2 mm diameter fetoscope that allowed visual assessment of dysmorphic features in the fetus with genetic disease. John Hobbins of Yale University had used the fetoscope to puncture small fetal vessels on the chorionic plate, but this did not yield pure samples of fetal blood. Rodeck went for the large fetal vessels at the site of the cord insertion into the placenta and obtained the first sample of pure fetal blood on 16 August 1977. Using a 26-gauge needle, he went on to perfect this technique between 18 and 22 weeks gestation for rapid karyotyping and the diagnosis of many genetic conditions, including haemophilia and muscular dystrophy. He also pioneered biopsies of fetal skin, liver and muscle.

Rodeck realised that direct intravascular access would allow fetal treatment as well as diagnosis. He therefore turned his attention to the problem of severe rhesus isoimmunisation. Since the initial work by William Liley in 1963, the standard method of diagnosis was by amniotic fluid analysis of bilirubin levels and treatment was by fetal intraperitoneal transfusion (IPT). Rodeck felt that fetal intravascular transfusion (IVT) should be feasible via the fetosope: 'Since pure blood can be removed from the fetal circulation by fetoscopy, we thought it should also be possible to transfuse it'. In addition, direct fetal blood sampling before and after transfusion would allow more accurate estimation of the severity of the anaemia and the adequacy of the corrective transfusion. The potential benefit of IVT was highest in severe cases with fetal hydrops, in which the success rate of IPT was low ($<$ 10 per cent) because of poor absorption of red cells from the peritoneal cavity. Rodeck did the first intravascular transfusion on 7 February 1980 on a 23-week hydropic fetus, with a second IVT at 25 weeks. Subsequent IPT at 26 and 28 weeks was followed by caesarean delivery and infant survival. In his 1981 report of the first two cases of IVT Rodeck wrote:

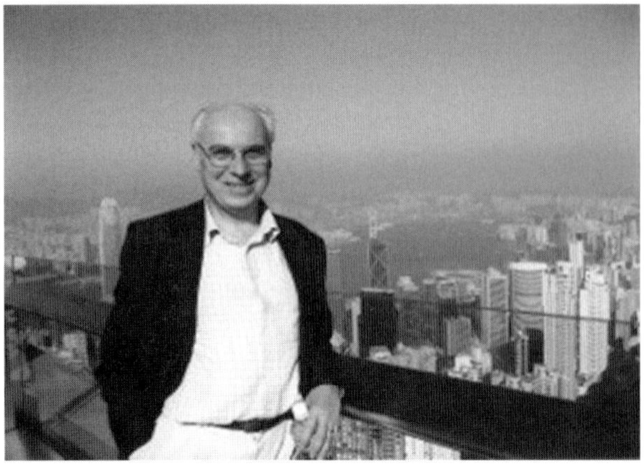

Charles Henry Rodeck

> *The fetus can receive an IVT at an earlier stage of gestation than IPT (optimum time for fetoscopy is 18–20 weeks), and hence hydrops fetalis and congestive cardiac failure may be ameliorated, delayed or even prevented. Absorption of intraperitoneal blood is poor in hydrops fetalis, and IVT is likely to be more effective.*

By 1984 Rodeck and his group reported 19 cases of severe rhesus isoimmunisation treated by fetoscopic IVT with an unprecedented 84 per cent survival rate. After technical improvements to ultrasound resolution in the 1980s, Fernand Daffos of Paris refined and simplified an ultrasound guided technique for needling the umbilical cord (cordocentesis) with a larger bore, 20-gauge needle, although he used this only for blood sampling and not for transfusion. Fetoscopic IVT was technically very difficult, and the simpler ultrasound guided technique of cordocentesis allowed the expansion of IVT to more perinatal units. However, the principles of IVT laid down by Rodeck remained intact.

Rodeck made many original contributions to fetal medicine, including development of the double pig tail catheter as a shunt for obstructive uropathy and fetal hydrothorax, often called the Rodeck shunt. He left King's College Hospital in 1986 to become professor and head of obstetrics and gynaecology at the Royal Postgraduate Medical School in Queen Charlotte's Hospital and ultimately, in 1990, head of department at his alma mater, University College London. In each of these posts he established fetal medicine units; the first in the United Kingdom was the Harris Birthright Research Centre at King's College in 1983. His academic output was prodigious, and he trained many British and international fellows, through whom his influence on fetal medicine has been worldwide.

Charles Rodeck retired in 2007 and in 2010 received the Eardley Holland medal from the Royal College of Obstetricians and Gynaecologists – its highest award. In retirement he strokes cats, supports Tottenham Hotspur Football Club and looks out of aeroplane windows en route to the great opera houses of Europe.

Selected Publications

Rodeck CH, Campbell S. Sampling pure fetal blood by fetoscopy in second trimester of pregnancy. *BMJ* 1978; 11: 728–30.

Rodeck CH, Kemp JR, Holman CA, Whitmore DN, Kernicki J, Austin NA. Direct intravascular fetal blood transfusion by fetoscopy in severe rhesus isoimmunisation. *Lancet* 1981; 1: 625–7.

Rodeck CH, Nicolaides KH, Warsof SL, Fysh WJ, Gamsu HR, Kemp JR. The management of severe rhesus isoimmunisation by fetoscopic intravascular transfusion. *Am J Obstet Gynecol* 1984; 150: 769–74.

Bibliography References

128, 175, 388, 1690, 1741.

Rösslin, Eucharius (d. 1526)

First Midwifery Text

In the early 1500s the training of midwives was virtually non-existent. In England the regulation and licensing of midwives was church-based with emphasis placed on the need to baptise babies that

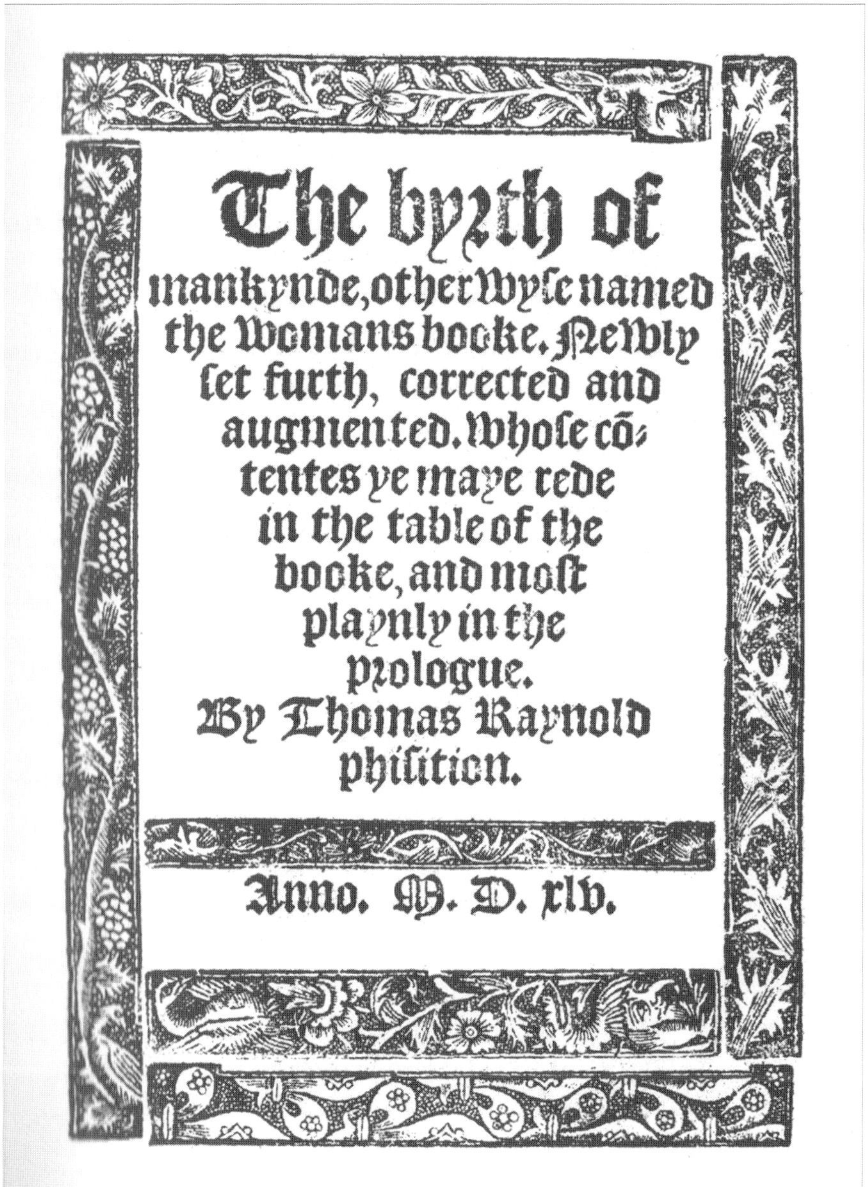
The byrth of
mankynde, otherwyse named
the Womans booke. Newly
set furth, corrected and
augmented. Whose co̅-
tentes ye maye rede
in the table of the
booke, and most
playnly in the
prologue.
By Thomas Raynold
phisition.

Anno. M. D. xlv.

1545 English translation of Rösslin's midwifery text

might not survive. The level of instruction can be gleaned from a sixteenth century oath taken by a midwife for a licence granted by the Archbishop of Canterbury: 'I will faithfully and diligently exercise the said office according to such cunning and knowledge as God hath given me'.

In France, practical experience could be acquired at the Hôtel Dieu in Paris, but the first midwifery text in French, by Louyse Bourgeois, was not available until 1609.

Eucharius Rösslin, whose date of birth is unknown, was an apothecary in Freiburg, Germany, from 1493 to 1498. He served as physician to the cities of Worms and Frankfurt. Part of his job was supervision of the city's midwives, which led him to conclude that much of the infant mortality was due to substandard care. Whether he practised obstetrics himself is unclear, but he produced the first book on midwifery in German, for 'unlatined' midwives. The book was published in 1513 as *Der Swangern Frauen und Hebammen Rosengarten* (A Rose Garden for Pregnant Women and Midwives). The reason for Rose Garden in the title is unclear, but speculation includes the Greek form of the name Rösslin as Rhodion (little rose) and that the city of Worms had a famous rose garden.

At the time of its publication Rösslin worked in the service of the court of Katherine, Duchess of Brunswick and Lüneburg, to whom he dedicated the book. In the prologue he criticised midwives for their ignorance and their reliance on superstition. The text was largely a summary of the obstetrical teachings of the ancients, particularly that of Soranus. It included woodcut illustrations, with some of the more fanciful poses of the fetus in utero. There was also a section on care and rearing of the infant.

The book became a bestseller, was translated into most European languages and remained popular for the next 150 years. Rösslin's son, also named Eucharius, who succeeded his father as physician to the city of Frankfurt, produced a Latin version in 1532 with the title *De partu hominis*. It was from this edition that most of the foreign language editions were produced.

In 1540 the first English translation came from the work of Richard Jonas:

> *. . . a certain studious and diligent clerk, at the request, and desire of diverse honest and sad matrons, being of his acquaintance, did translate out of Latin into English, a great part of this book . . . De Partu Hominis that is to say the Byrth of Mankynde, which we now do name The Woman's Booke.*

The first English edition of *The Byrth of Mankynde* was printed by Thomas Raynold of St Paul's Churchyard, London. The second to fourth editions, in 1545, 1552 and 1560, were under the authorship of 'Thomas Raynold, Phisition'. It seems the two Thomas Raynolds were separate, probably related individuals – publisher and physician, respectively.

In the prologue to the second (1545) English edition, the controversial nature of providing a translation in the mother or vulgar tongue was acknowledged:

> *Some alleging that it is shame . . . and not fitting such matters to be intreated of so plainly in our mother and vulgar language, to the dishonour (as they say) of womanhood, and the derision of their own secrets, by detection and discovering whereof, men its reading or hearing shall be moved thereby the more to abhor and loathe the company of women.*

Multiple other English editions followed up to the late 1600s. Of note, and in keeping with the need for heretic baptism, instructions were included for post-mortem caesarean section:

> *If it chance that the woman in her labour die, and the child having life in it, then shall it be need to keep open the woman's mouth, and also the nether places, so that the child may by that means both receive and also expel air and breath, which otherwise might be stopped to the destruction of the child. And then to turn her on the left side, and there to cut her open, and so to take out the child.*

In 1517 Rösslin returned to Frankfurt where he died in 1526.

Selected Publications

Rösslin E. *The Byrth of Mankynde*. London: Thomas Raynold; 1545. Also published in the Classics of Obstetrics and Gynaecology Library. New York, NY: Gryphon Editions, 1994 (facsimile).

Bibliography References

43, 46, 102, 199, 441, 676, 762, 1130, 1261, 1480, 1486.

Rousset, François (c. 1530–1603)

First Text on Caesarean Section

In 1581, François Rousset was the first physician to advocate caesarean section on a living woman and had the audacity to do so in a text devoted solely to that subject: *Traitté nouveau de l'hysterotomotokie, ou enfantement caesarien* (A New Treatise on Hysterotomotokie or Caesarean Childbirth). The subtitle of the book outlined the essence of the text:

> *The extraction of a child through a lateral incision of the abdomen and uterus of a pregnant woman who cannot deliver by other means. And this without compromising the life of either or preventing subsequent pregnancy.*

François Rousset was born in Pithiviers, France. After study in Paris and Montpellier he graduated in medicine from the latter university. On the title page of his book Rousset identified himself as a physician, *Médecin*, rather than as a surgeon. The distinction was important: physicians were well educated and acted as consultants and diagnosticians but did not do surgical procedures. In contrast, surgeons were usually barbers who also performed the limited surgical procedures of that era: drain abscesses, cut for bladder stone, limb amputation and, at the request of a physician or midwife, carry out caesarean section.

In the 1500s, caesarean delivery was almost exclusively carried out post mortem, mostly to conform to religious edicts and in a usually vain attempt to salvage a live baby. There were isolated cases of caesarean section on living women, but these were mostly anecdotal and unsubstantiated.

Into this environment Rousset launched his text advocating a much more liberal approach to caesarean delivery in the living woman. Furthermore, he published it in French, rather than Latin, which was the working language of academics, including physicians. As most surgeons did not understand Latin, Rousset chose to publish in the vernacular French in order to reach his intended audience:

> *To please the many French surgeons with little or no command of Latin who have been urging me to share this information with them, I have included in this abbreviated French version most of the principal points of the original – not wanting to delay the life-saving and urgent help that women reduced to this last resort may require (as happens when all other solutions have failed.)*

Rousset included 10 case histories: four from 'reliable observers' and six 'that I can vouch for personally'. Two women died when a surgeon could not be found to carry out a repeat caesarean section; the other eight women survived, as did seven of the infants. He advised caesarean section if the woman 'cannot be delivered using easier or more common methods, and it becomes apparent that the mother will otherwise die undelivered'. Surprisingly, five of the ten cases had vaginal delivery in a subsequent pregnancy, suggesting that contracted pelvis was not the reason for the primary caesarean delivery.

Rousset also emphasised the need to perform the caesarean section before the woman was 'exhausted and beyond hope'. On this point he was far ahead of his time, as the high mortality of caesarean delivery in the nineteenth century was found to be due to delay in performing caesarean section until the woman was moribund and in *articulo mortis*.

Although Rousset did not perform the operation, his description of the surgical technique is detailed and plausible, suggesting that he was familiar with the procedure. At this time the rare cases of caesarean section in living women were virtually 100 per cent mortal. Thus, the optimistic results reported by Rousset were not believed and, based on the results of that era, understandably so. It seems that Rousset only reported cases with favourable outcome and that he exaggerated the safety and simplicity of the operation. Indeed, he emphasised this in one case report with a successful outcome in which the surgeon was drunk, saying, 'If the operation succeeded with him drunk, what may he not expect who performs it when sober, according to the justest rules of his art'.

The medical and surgical establishment of the day were virtually all opposed to his opinion. Many questioned the veracity of his reports as 'fable and imposture', and one referred to him as a 'decrepit old man': an uncompromising and frank example of peer review.

During his career Rousset gained a considerable reputation and served a number of ancient and noble families, including appointment as physician to the king, Henry IV. His date of death is unknown, and there are no known portraits of him.

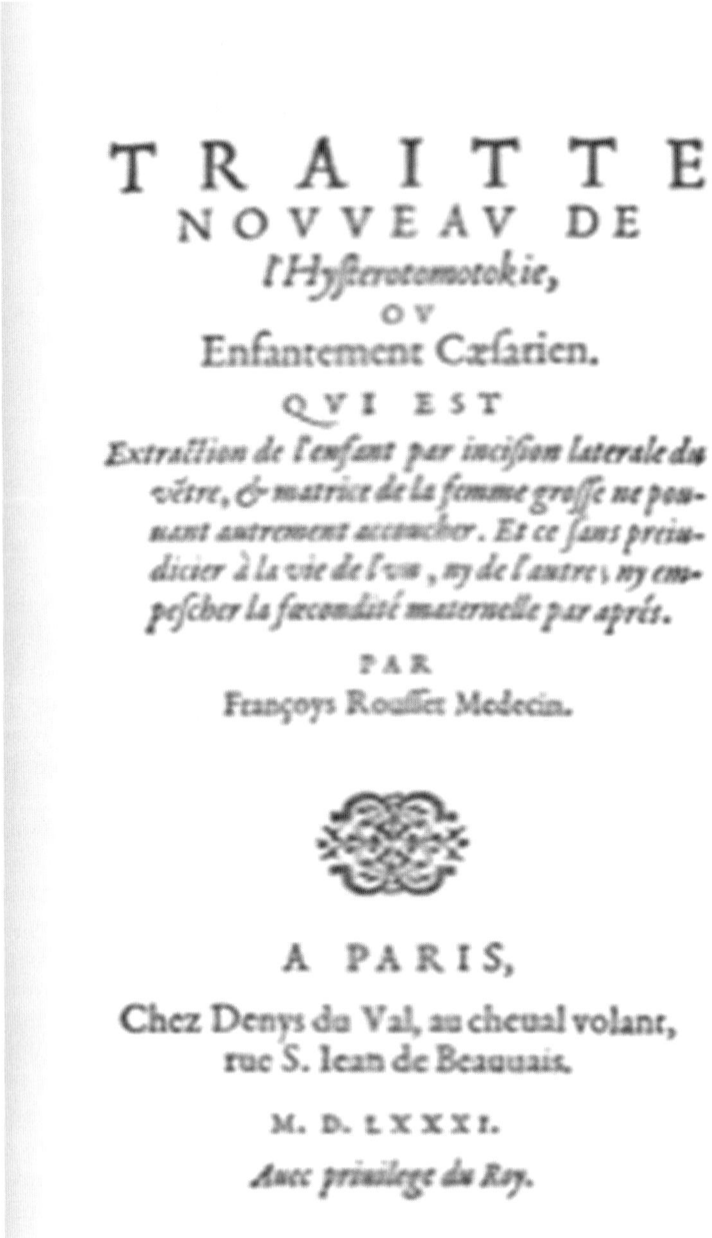

TRAITTE
NOVVEAV DE
l'Hysterotomotokie,
OV
Enfantement Cæsarien.
QVI EST
Extraction de l'enfant par incision laterale du vêtre, & matrice de la femme grosse ne pouuant autrement accoucher. Et ce sans preiudicier à la vie de l'vn, ny de l'autre, ny empescher la fœcondité maternelle par après.
PAR
Françoys Rousset Medecin.

A PARIS,
Chez Denys du Val, au cheual volant, rue S. Iean de Beauuais.
M. D. LXXXI.
Auec priuilege du Roy.

Title page of François Rousset's 1581 text on caesarean delivery

Selected Publications

Rousset F. *Traitté nouveau de l'hysterotomotokie ou enfantement caesarien*. Paris: Denys duVal; 1581.

Sebezius M. *German translation of Rousset's Hysterotomotokie*. Strasbourg: B. Jobin;1583.

Bauhin G. Francisci Rousseti. De partu caesaro tractatus. In: *Gynaeciorum sive de mulierum affectibus commentarii*. Basle: Conrad Vualdkirch; 1586.

Rousset F. *Caesarei partus assertio historiolog*. Paris: Denys duVal; 1590.

Cyr RM, Baskett TF. *Caesarean Birth: the Work of François Rousset in Renaissance France*. Cambridge: Cambridge University Press; 2010.

Bibliography References

99, 102, 159, 351, 548, 604, 1038, 1205, 1233, 1256, 1291, 1631, 1636, 1734.

Rubin, Alan (1923–2011)

Rubin's Manoeuvre

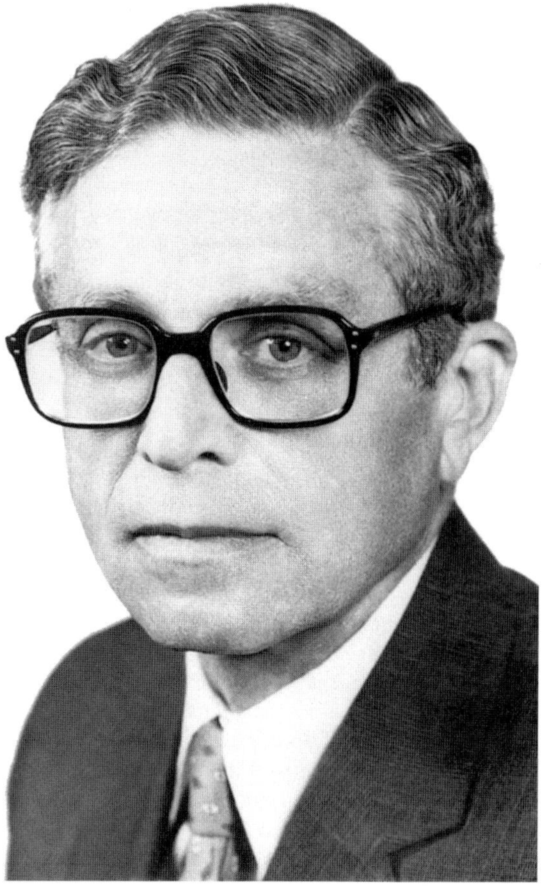

Alan Rubin

Stimulated by a study of neonatal trauma in his own hospital, Alan Rubin sought ways to improve the management of shoulder dystocia. Measuring 25 newborn infants, he found that the transverse diameter of their shoulders was about 2 cm less when adducted as opposed to straight or abducted. He therefore proposed placing the fingers on the scapula and pushing the fetal shoulder towards its chest, thereby adducting and reducing the diameter of the shoulders. In so doing he was, to some extent, modifying Woods' manoeuvre, in which the fetal shoulders are rotated by pressure on the anterior aspect of the shoulder, causing abduction. Rubin reported using this manipulation with good results in cases of shoulder dystocia, and it came to be called 'Rubin's manoeuvre'. He also advocated suprapubic pressure to rock the fetal shoulders from side to side and help disimpaction.

Alan Rubin graduated from the University of Pennsylvania medical school in 1947 and did his residency training in obstetrics and gynaecology at the same university. He became clinical professor of obstetrics and gynaecology at Temple University School of Medicine and chief of the department at the Graduate Hospital in Philadelphia. In 1943 he held the university strength record for servicemen's physical fitness tests. Rubin retired in 1989 and died in Philadelphia on 6 May 2011.

Selected Publications

Rubin A. Management of shoulder dystocia. *JAMA* 1964; 189: 835–7.

Bibliography References

99, 113, 115, 117.

Rubin, Isidor Clinton (1883–1958)

Rubin's Test

Isidor Rubin was born in Friedrichshof, Germany and migrated to the United States as a young boy. His medical degree was granted in 1905 by the College of Physicians and Surgeons of Columbia University. He worked successively at the Beth Israel and Mount Sinai hospitals in New York. He was president of the American Gynecological Society in 1955 to 1956.

Rubin made many contributions to the investigation of infertility and is remembered for his test of fallopian tube patency involving transcervical, uterotubal insufflation. The first test was performed on 3 November 1919, at Mount Sinai Hospital, New York, using oxygen. Rubin later wrote:

> *Theoretically we expected to see the abdominal wall rise in case the oxygen gas succeeded in gaining access through open tubes into the abdominal cavity. The actual rise of the abdominal wall was corroborated by everyone present. This constituted first-hand proof that the oxygen actually passed through the tubes and into the peritoneal cavity.*

The presence of oxygen in the abdominal cavity was confirmed by X-ray, and the women had shoulder tip pain from the sub-diaphragmatic gas for three days. Rubin subsequently modified his technique using the more rapidly resorbed carbon dioxide and a kymograph attachment to evaluate the patency of the fallopian tubes:

> *As carbon-dioxide was found to be more rapidly resorbed than oxygen in equal quantities and thereby also minimizing the shoulder pains and epigastric discomfort, it was early adopted as the gas of choice for uterotubal insufflation. The danger of gas embolism was also eliminated by carbon-dioxide insufflation … The apparatus was shortly thereafter improved by a kymograph thus providing a method of precision in determining tubal patency and nonpatency and at the same time increasing its safety. By means of this apparatus it became possible to demonstrate graphically the functional status of patent Fallopian tubes and in cases with impaired patency the varying degrees of tubal strictures and adhesion.*

Up to the 1960s Rubin's test was widely used in the clinical assessment of infertility. Rubin was one of the first to recognise the potential value of hysteroscopy for infertility investigation. He helped pioneer the use of carbon dioxide as the distension medium using a modified cystoscope. Rubin was also trained in gynaecological pathology, having spent a year of postgraduate study in Vienna. Here he was one of the first to recognise and describe what he later called carcinoma in situ of the cervix. His first publication was on this topic and he referred to 'the microscopic diagnosis of exceedingly young cancer of the cervix'.

He died suddenly while visiting London on 10 July 1958.

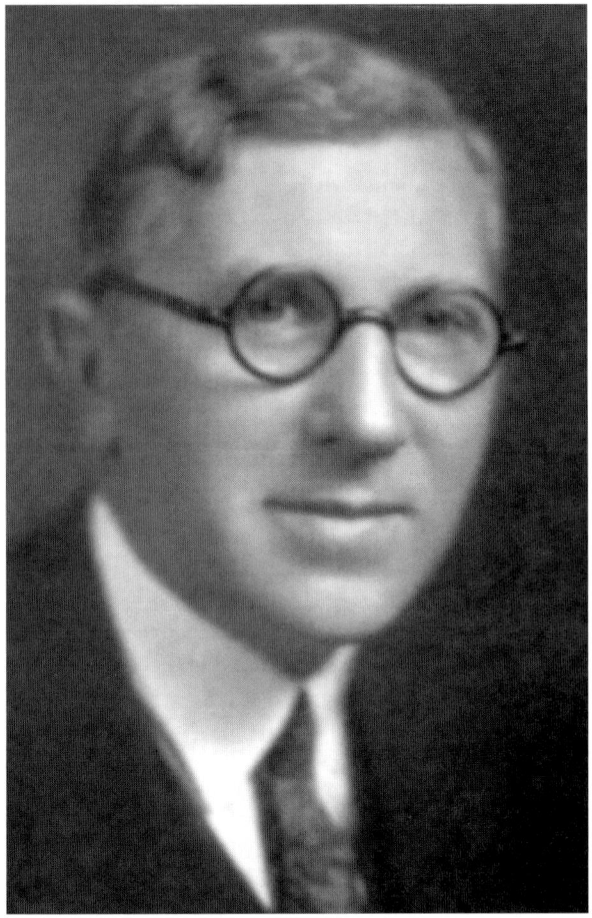

Isidor Clinton Rubin

Selected Publications

Rubin IC. The pathological diagnosis of incipient carcinoma of the uterus. *Am J Obstet Dis Women Child* 1910; 62: 668–73.

Rubin IC. Non-operative determination of patency of fallopian tubes in sterility. Intra-uterine inflation with oxygen and production of an artificial pneumoperitoneum. Preliminary report. *JAMA* 1920; 74: 1017.

Rubin IC. Uterine endoscopy, endometroscopy with the aid of uterine insufflation. *Am J Obstet Gynecol* 1925; 10: 313–6.

Rubin IC. The beginnings of uterotubal insufflation. *J Mt Sinai Hosp* 1943; 10: 231–7.

Bibliography References

133, 793, 801, 1075, 1331, 1409, 1480, 1481, 1485, 1492.

Rueff, Jacob (1500–1558)

Birth Stool/Paravaginal Haematoma

Jacob Rueff was appointed city physician of Zurich and as such was responsible for the instruction and regulation of public midwives. In 1554 he published his text on midwifery aimed primarily at midwives but also for physicians and educated pregnant women. It was published in both German, under the title *Ein Schön Lustig Trostbüchle (A Very Cheerful Booklet of Encouragement)* and in Latin as *De conceptu et generatione hominis*. In 1637 an English translation was produced, *The Expert Midwife*. The last edition of Rueff's text was printed in Amsterdam in 1670. Thus, Rueff's book, which placed emphasis on anatomical knowledge in obstetrics, was influential for more than a century. He described his motive for writing the text:

> *I bequeath to all grave, modest and discreet women, as also to such by profession, practising either physicke or*

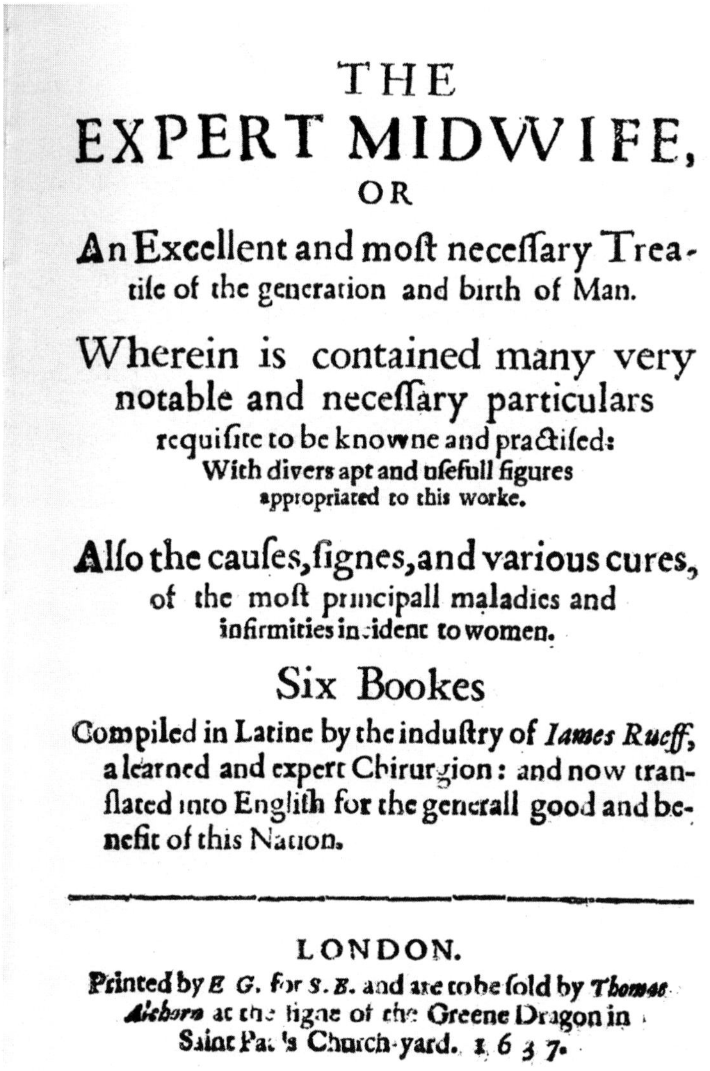
THE
EXPERT MIDWIFE,
OR
An Excellent and moſt neceſſary Treatiſe of the generation and birth of Man.
Wherein is contained many very notable and neceſſary particulars requiſite to be knowne and practiſed: With divers apt and uſefull figures appropriated to this worke.
Alſo the cauſes, ſignes, and various cures, of the moſt principall maladies and infirmities incident to women.
Six Bookes
Compiled in Latine by the induſtry of *James Rueff*, a learned and expert Chirurgion: and now tranſlated into Engliſh for the generall good and benefit of this Nation.

LONDON.
Printed by E. G. for S. B. and are to be ſold by *Thomas Alchorn* at the ſigne of the Greene Dragon in Saint Pauls Church-yard. 1637.

Title page of the English translation of Jacob Rueff's *The Expert Midwife*, published in 1637

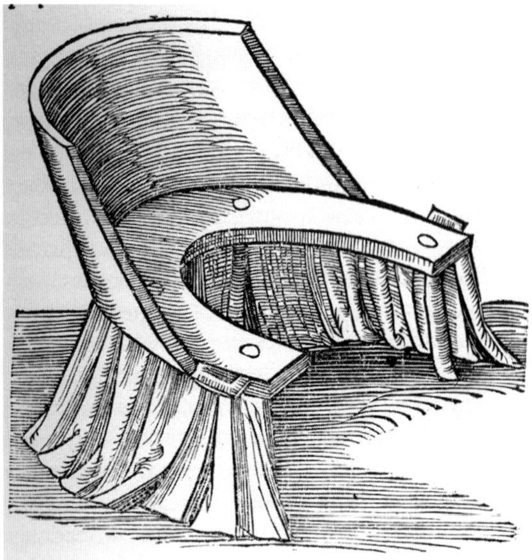

Illustration of Rueff's birth stool

chirurgery. And whose helpe upon occasion of extreme necessity may be useful and good both for mother, child and midwife.

He provided a wood cut illustration of a birth stool and described its use as follows:

Let the stoole be made compassewise, underpropped with foure feet, the stay of it behind bending backeward, hollow in the midst, covered with a blacke cloth underneath, hanging downe to the ground, by that meanes that the labouring woman may be covered . . . And after the labouring woman shall be set in her chaire about to be delivered, the midwife shall place one woman behind her back which may gently hold the labouring woman, taking her by both the armes, and if need be, the pains waxing grievous, and the woman labouring, may stroke and press downe the womb and may somewhat drive and depresse the infant downward . . . This being done, let the midwive her selfe sit stooping forward before the labouring-woman . . . and encourage the party to her labour, to abide her paines with patience and then gently apply her hands to the work as she ought, by feeling and searching with her fingers how the child lieth, and by relaxing and opening the way and passage conveniently for him, while the mother is in pain . . .

Thus, Rueff clearly described fundal pressure, the Kristeller manoevure, applied by the assistant standing behind the labouring woman.

Rueff was the first to describe paravaginal haematoma:

But if it shall happen that some swelling, or congealed blood doe appeare in the fore-skins of the matrix under the skinne, arising from the pains and difficulty of the birth, the veines or fibres being broken because of overmuch distension, opening and enlargement, as it falleth out: or some inward swelling or tumour of blood shall be bred . . . let the midwife make incision of that tumour, and open it with a cleane knife, when the matter shall be perceived to be digested and ripe, whether it shall appear before or after the birth, let her squeeze out the clotted blood, and let her press downe the swelling, wipe and clean those things which are defiled . . .

Rueff also illustrates four instruments: a vaginal speculum, a vaginal dilator, a duckbill pincer with teeth and a locked pincer with smooth ends shaped like small spoons. Some writers have interpreted the latter instrument as obstetric forceps. However, Rueff was a surgeon and lithotomist, and these are probably lithotomy forceps adapted to extract portions of a dead fetus. This instrument is illustrated in the chapter which is entitled 'How, and with what instruments children sticking in the wombe, and being dead are to be brought forth'.

Not a great deal is known about Rueff's early life although, as well as being a physician and surgeon, he was a poet and composer of folk songs. He followed the teaching of Martin Luther and served with the troops of Zurich against the Catholic cantons in defence of religious freedom. He died in Zurich in 1558.

Selected Publications

Rueff, J. *Ein schön lustig Trostbüchle.* Zürich: Christoffel Froschouer; 1554.

Rueff J. *De conceptu et generatione hominis.* Tiguri: Christophorous Froschouerus; 1554.

Rueff J. *The Expert Midwife.* London: T Wykes; 1637.

Bibliography References

18, 199, 347, 477, 503, 548, 648, 685, 1261, 1588.

Rymsdyk, Jan van (c.1750)

Medical Illustration

Two of the great obstetrical atlases of the eighteenth century were produced by William Smellie and William Hunter. At that time authors were responsible for all aspects of the published book; they employed the artists and engravers, supplied the text and often paid for or at least contributed towards the cost of printing. Both Smellie and Hunter had the good sense to employ the superb Dutch artist Jan van Rymsdyk. Working in mezzotint and coloured crayon, his drawings of the anatomical specimens prepared by Smellie and Hunter used perspective and shading to attain an almost three-dimensional quality. Smellie's atlas was published in 1754 and contained 39 plates, of which 26 were made by Rymsdyk. The rest were drawn by Pieter Camper and Smellie himself. In an advertisement for his atlas, Smellie noted that he had 'with great care and expense employed Mr Riemsdyk to draw anatomical figures as large as humans themselves, for the use of those who attend his lectures and in order to illustrate his theory and practice of midwifery'. In the preface to the atlas he also explained that 'delicacy and elegance however was not so much consulted as to have them done in a strong and distinct manner'. Rymsdyk's original coloured drawings for Smellie's atlas were later purchased by Hunter and bequeathed to the University of Glasgow. In 1971 the University of Auckland Postgraduate School of Obstetrics and Gynaecology issued a facsimile reprint of Smellie's atlas.

William Hunter worked on his atlas for some 30 years before its publication in 1774. He employed Rymsdyk off and on between 1750 and 1772. In addition, he employed up to 20 engravers to produce the copper plates. The atlas consisted of 34 plates, of which Rymsdyk made 31. The quality of Rymsdyk's work was even greater in the Hunter atlas than in that of Smellie, with more depth and anatomical detail: 'Every part is represented just as it is found, not so much as one joint of a finger has been moved'. In the preface to his atlas, Hunter said:

> *The art of engraving supplies us, upon many occasions, with what has been the great desideratum of the lovers of science, an universal language. Nay, it conveys clearer ideas of most natural objects, than words can express; makes stronger impressions upon the mind; and to every person conversant with the subject, gives an immediate comprehension of what it represents.*

Hunter also praised 'the ingenious artists who made the drawings and engravings'. However, he does not mention Rymsdyk by name, while he does pay tribute to Robert Strange, who only produced three of the 34 illustrations.

Very little is known about Jan van Rymsdyk. There are no available diaries, letters, belongings or portraits of him. It is known that he was born in Holland and grew up there. He first appears in London in 1750, and no work of his can be traced before that date, although he was by then an accomplished artist and familiar with anatomical specimens. In the early 1750s he worked simultaneously with both Smellie and Hunter. In 1758 to 1759 he was a resident of Bristol, at that time a thriving centre of trade and commerce, where he advertised himself as a portrait painter:

> *JV Rymsdyk, portrait painter, at his rooms at the Registrar Office in All-Saints Lane, Bristol. Paints portraits at four guineas each: half lengths and full lengths in proportion. N.B. He instructs gentlemen and ladies in the art of drawing in its several branches, on reasonable terms: being likewise known for his drawings of anatomy, herbs, fossils, etc to the most eminent of faculty in London. His paintings may be seen at any time of the day at his lodging.*

Rymsdyk had only marginal success as a portrait painter and was constantly impoverished, such that he was reduced to painting signs for commercial establishments. He resented Hunter, whom he felt should have done more to promote his ability as an artist. He had one son, Andreas, who later anglicised his name to Andrew, was born in 1753 and died before his father in 1786, at the age of 33. Rymsdyk and his son published a slim volume entitled *Museum britannicum*, which was mainly drawings of natural history subjects in the British Museum. In the footnotes to these drawings, he criticises a variety of people including 'idle thieving plagiary drones and critick stinging wasps'. In his later years Rymsdyk made several drawings for Thomas Denman. His name was written with various spellings, including Riemsdyk, Rijmskyk, Remsdyk, Reimsdyk and often with the addition of a final 'e'. However, in his *Museum britannicum* and on Hunter's plates, his surname is spelt Rymsdyk. He probably died in 1788 or 1789, but there is no record of his passing. Thus, we have very limited information on an artist who raised the standard of anatomical illustration to an

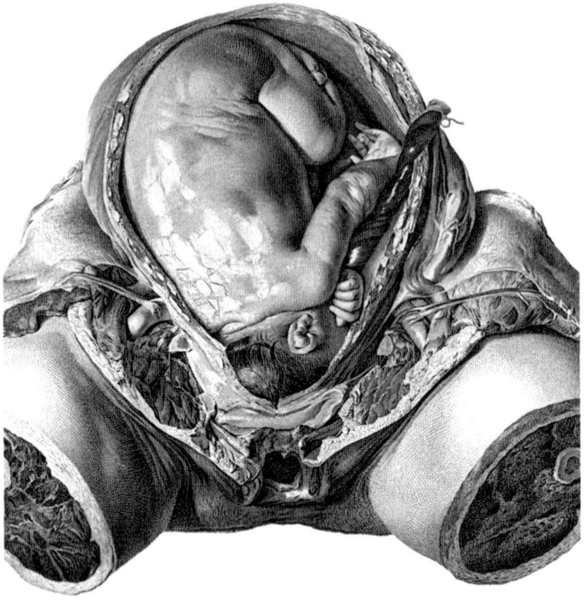

Anatomical plate VI from a drawing by Jan van Rymsdyk in William Hunter's *Anatomy of the Gravid Uterus*

art and whose work is still admired more than 200 years after his death. Indeed, no less a person than James Young Simpson described Plate VI of Hunter's atlas thus: 'as a mere work of art, perhaps the most beautiful anatomical plate that has ever been given to the world'.

Selected Publications

Smellie W. *A Sett of Anatomical Tables with Explanations and an Abridgement of the Practice of Midwifery*. London; 1754.

Hunter W. *The Anatomy of the Human Gravid Uterus*. Birmingham: John Baskerville; 1774. Also published in: *The Classics of Obstetrics and Gynecology Library*. Birmingham: Gryphon Editions; 1991 (facsimile).

Rymsdyk J and A van. *Museum britannicum*. London: J. Moore; 1778.

Bibliography References

239, 271, 405, 748, 749, 858, 1138, 1337, 1362, 1363, 1425, 1426, 1428, 1429, 1567, 1583.

S

Saling, Erich (b. 1925)

Fetal Scalp Blood Sampling

It is not uncommon during the search for a solution to one problem for those involved to find the answer to another. Such was the case with fetal scalp blood sampling in labour for the detection of fetal hypoxia and acidosis. In order to obtain rapid measurement of oxygen saturation to aid resuscitation of the asphyxiated newborn, Erich Saling and his biochemist colleague K Damaschke developed a technique for analysis of micro blood samples in the newborn. Saling then began to obtain fetal blood samples during labour in cases of rhesus isoimmunisation to guide the immediate treatment of the newborn. As he later wrote:

A decisive step forward came with the idea of withdrawing fetal blood samples from the presenting part of the fetus in cases of Rh-erythroblastosis, thus being able to perform, before delivery, the most important serologic and hematologic examinations, such as the Coombs test, hemoglobin concentration, and the blood groups.

The fast O_2 micro analysis, which had just been achieved, and the knowledge that blood samples could be taken so easily from the skin of the presenting part of the fetus provided us with the idea of also performing fetal blood gas analyses. This was the birth of fetal blood analysis (FBA). A short time later, equipment for measuring pH in micro blood samples came onto the market and we purchased one.

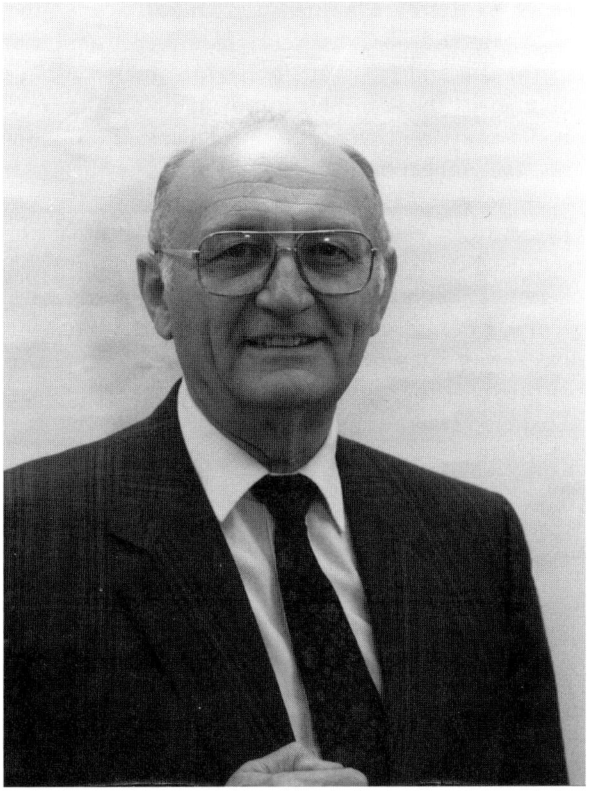

Erich Saling

The first FBA during labor with pH and O_2 saturation measurement and PCO_2 calculation were used clinically on June 21, 1960. Only one day later, an FBA was taken from the buttock of a fetus. In addition to the fetal blood analysis during labor, we performed, for the first time, an acidity measurement in the umbilical artery blood and umbilical vein blood of this infant. So on June 22, 1960 the complementary assessment of the newborn by also measuring the umbilical artery pH value, employed today by many obstetricians, was born.

Saling published the technique in 1962. In association with electronic fetal heart rate monitoring it has become an integral part of the surveillance of the high-risk fetus in labour.

Erich Saling was born in Stanislau, Galicia, the son of a forester. He studied medicine at the University of Jena and the Free University of Berlin, qualifying in 1952. He completed his specialty training in obstetrics and gynaecology at the Women's Hospital in Berlin-Neukölln. For more than 30 years he combined clinical obstetric practice with research in perinatal medicine. In addition to his pioneer work on fetal blood sampling, he has contributed original research on neonatal resuscitation, amnioscopy, fetal assessment, external version, prevention of prematurity and vacuum extractor design. He was appointed professor at the Free University of Berlin in 1968 and became director of the Institute of Perinatal Medicine in 1976. After his election as emeritus professor of perinatal medicine in 1991, he continued to work in the field of perinatal research. Saling has received widespread recognition for his work, including Fellowship ad eundem from the Royal College of Obstetricians and Gynaecologists in 1987. In 2005, at the 7th World Congress of Perinatal Medicine, a symposium on fetal assessment was held in honour of his eightieth birthday.

Selected Publications

Saling E, Damaschke K. Neue Mikroschnellmethode zur Messung des Blutsauerstoffs auf elektrochemischem Wege. *Klin Wochenschr* 1961; 39: 305–6.

Saling E. Neues Vorgehen zur Untersuchung des Kindes unter der Geburt: Einführung, Technik und Grundlagen. (New technique for examining the fetus during labour: introduction, technique and basics.) *Arch Gynäkol* 1962; 197: 108–22.

Saling E. Fetal blood analysis. In: Rooth G, Saugstad OD (eds) *The Roots of Perinatal Medicine*. New York, NY: Thieme-Stratton Inc; 1985, pp. 108–14.

Bibliography References

635, 819, 1536, 1731.

Sampson, John Albertson (1873–1946)

Endometriosis

In 1921 John Sampson gave the first of three presentations on endometriosis he was to make before the American Gynecological Society. In the first of these he graphically described the clinico-pathological findings of ovarian endometriosis:

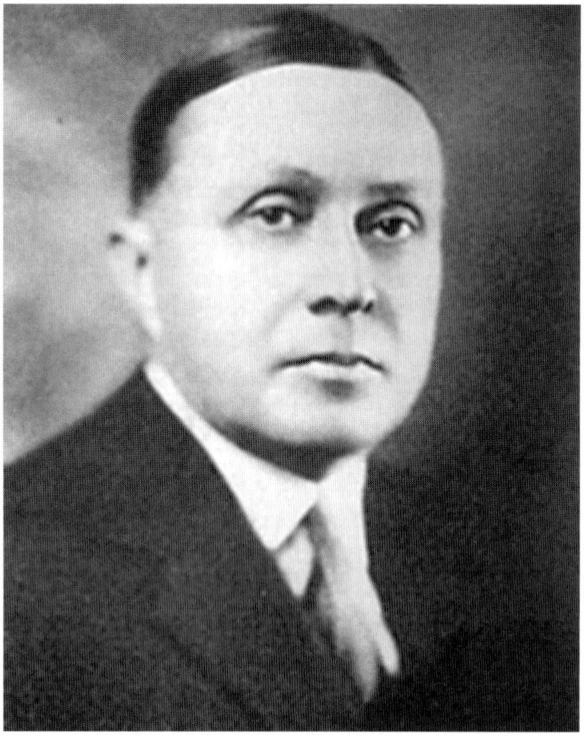

John Albertson Sampson

> *At operation the ovary containing such a cyst is found to be adherent and in freeing it the chocolate contents escape . . . Adhesions, due to the 'irritating' action of the material . . . may be found in any of the natural pockets and folds of the pelvis where such material would be apt to lodge and especially in the cul de sac . . . the adhesions in the cul de sac may be accompanied by such a marked reaction as to resemble malignancy . . . The histologic study of these hematomata shows that periodic hemorrhage occurs similar to that of menstruation. I have come to the conclusion that these ovarian hematomata are of endometrial type.*

Sampson continued to study endometriosis throughout the 1920s and developed the histogenic theory of retrograde menstruation as a causative factor. He had observed retrograde menstruation at laparotomy and felt that the blood contained viable endometrial cells capable of implantation and growth on the ovary and adjacent peritoneum. His opponents, including Emil Novak, favoured the theory of coelomic metaplasia propounded by Robert Meyer of Germany. In response to those who felt that the menstrual endometrial cells were dead and incapable of growth, Sampson said, 'If they are dead, then my theory is dead also and should be buried'. Sampson died before subsequent definitive studies supported his theory, showing that endometrial cells in menstrual blood were viable and capable of growth.

A small branch of the ovarian artery that runs with and usually inferior to the round ligament is called Sampson's artery. Although the name is attributed to him, there is no specific reference to it in his writings.

John Albertson Sampson was born at Troy, New York. He graduated MD from Johns Hopkins University in 1899 and completed his residency in obstetrics and gynaecology at the same institution. In 1905 he went to Albany, New York, where he was to spend the rest of his life. He became professor of gynaecology at the Albany Medical College. A bachelor, he was fond of animals and trees. It is said that he once changed a new car because his dog didn't like it.

Selected Publications

Sampson JA. Perforating hemorrhagic (chocolate) cysts of the ovary. *Am J Obstet Gynecol* 1921; 2: 525–33.

Sampson JA. Peritoneal endometriosis due to the menstrual dissemination of endometrial tissue into the peritoneal cavity. *Am J Obstet Gynecol* 1927; 14: 422–69.

Bibliography References

188, 289, 528, 801, 1003, 1246, 1480.

Sanger, Margaret Louise (1879–1966)

Birth Control

Margaret Sanger was born on 14 September 1879 in Corning, New York, the sixth of 11 children. Her mother was a strict Catholic who died from tuberculosis at the age of 48. Her father was an agnostic Irish immigrant stonemason with an independent streak who taught his daughter defiance of authority. She applied to a New York drama school but declined to attend when they wrote asking for her leg measurements. Instead she became a nurse. At the age of 19 she married William Sanger, an architect involved in the socialist movement. They had three children. In 1912 she began working as a nurse among the poor of the Lower East Side in New York. Here she came in contact with the reality of unlimited reproduction and crushing poverty. She found a desperate ignorance of contraceptive knowledge, except for the $5.00 back street abortion:

> *I heard over and over again of their desperate efforts at bringing themselves 'around' – drinking various herb-teas, taking drops of turpentine on sugar, steaming over a chamber of boiling coffee or of turpentine water, rolling down stairs, and finally inserting slippery-elm sticks, or knitting needles, or shoe hooks into the uterus.*

In her early years she was influenced by the radical feminist and anarchist Ellen Goodman (1869–1940). Sanger coined the term 'birth control' and her philosophy, 'Birth control is essentially an education for women' remains true on a global scale. She studied the available literature on contraception and visited France, where she was impressed that 'every married woman knew all there was to know about contraception as well as the art of love'.

In 1914 she started a magazine called *Woman Rebel*, in which she disseminated advice on birth control. This ran foul of the federal Comstock Law, named after Anthony Comstock (1844–1915), who was against most things and initiated the bill passed in 1873:

> *No article, or thing, designed or intended, for the prevention of conception, or notice of any kind in writing or print, giving information directly or indirectly, where or how, or of whom, or by what means either of the things before mentioned may be obtained or made, shall be carried in the mail.*

In August 1914 Sanger was indicted under this law but she fled to Europe on the eve of her trial. The charges were dropped when she returned to the United States one year later. In October 1916, along with her sister, she opened the first United States birth control clinic in Brooklyn. This was closed down and she was sentenced to 30 days in jail as a 'public nuisance'. The attendant publicity helped elevate her to celebrity status and confirmed the value of challenging authority with the concomitant media attention. When forbidden by the Catholic-dominated Boston civic authorities to speak on birth control, she stood on the stage with her mouth taped shut while a colleague read her prepared talk. She spoke out against the Catholic church's position on contraception, 'Church control or birth control . . . the dictatorship of celibates'.

Sanger helped organise the American Birth Control League, which developed into the Planned Parenthood Federation of America in 1942. She was also involved in the creation of the International Planned Parenthood Federation in 1952 and was appointed the first joint honorary president.

As are many who succeed against the odds, Sanger was self-absorbed, egotistical and relentless in pursuit of her goals. She was sometimes reluctant to acknowledge the contributions of others to 'her cause'. She once described herself as 'not a fit person for love, home, children, friends or anything which needs attention or consideration'. Her liberated attitude to sexuality led to many short-lived liaisons. In 1921, at her instigation, she divorced William Sanger. In the same she year married a senior millionaire, James

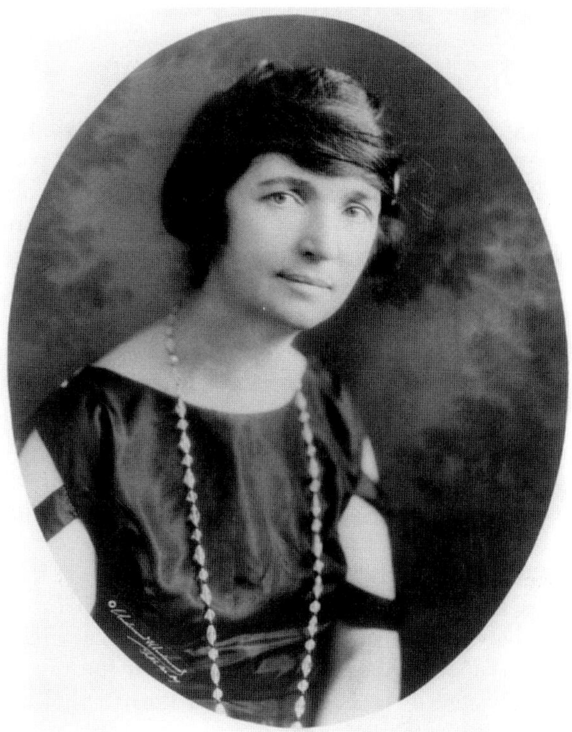

Margaret Louise Sanger

Noah Slee (1861–1943), president of the 3-in-One oil company, who substantially funded her work. Early in her first marriage she had two sons and one daughter, who died of pneumonia at the age of seven. The boys were sent to boarding school and later both became physicians.

She used her influence with the philanthropist Katharine McCormick to guide funding of the work of Gregory Pincus in the development of the oral contraceptive. She also collaborated with Robert Dickinson, working to disseminate information on sex education and contraception. In her later years, with the initial barriers overcome, she softened her radical approach and cultivated the social, political and medical establishments both at home and abroad. She established a Birth Control Clinical Research Bureau to promote sorely needed education on the topic among the medical profession. She had her first heart attack when she was 70 and had to reduce her travel and lecture schedule. She became addicted to demerol (pethidine), prescribed for chest pains. She retired to Tucson, Arizona and died there in her eighty-eighth year on 6 September 1966. There was no one in the first half of the twentieth century who matched her sustained and effective commitment to women's freedom over their own sexuality and reproduction.

Margaret Sanger advised women 'to look the whole world in the face with a go-to-hell look in the eyes'.

Selected Publications

Sanger M. *Family Limitation.* London and Glasgow: Bakunin Press; 1920.

Sanger M. *My Fight for Birth Control.* New York, NY: Brentano; 1931.

Bibliography References

31, 193, 197, 267, 288, 433, 516, 586, 596, 630, 667, 726, 792, 817, 866, 981, 1026, 1201, 1274, 1297, 1309, 1345, 1379, 1485, 1498, 1573, 1716.

Sänger, Max (1853–1903)

Classical Caesarean Section

In the early development of caesarean section, the uterine incision was made in every conceivable part and plane of the uterus, including the posterior wall. The uterine wound was not sutured and therefore haemorrhage was a common cause of death. In the latter part of the nineteenth century, the need for closure of the uterine wound gained acceptance. In 1882 Max Sänger brought together the advances on the site and closure of the uterine incision in his paper on caesarean section. This involved the vertical anterior wall incision and its careful layered closure by suture, the latter point being the most important in producing haemostasis. By undermining and carefully coapting the final musculo-peritoneal layer, he produced a watertight incision to reduce the risk of seepage of infected uterine contents into the peritoneal cavity. Sänger's operation, the classical caesarean section, allowed the safe conservation of the uterus and obviated the need for Edoardo Porro's subtotal caesarean hysterectomy:

> *Even though the technique is still considered to be lacking in certainty and completeness, nevertheless the classic caesarean section is the one and only universal method of operating which can be applied to all indications. The other methods which compete with it, including Porro's operation should be considered as appropriate for one indication at the most, for others they are not applicable.*

Sänger's paper and treatise were published with theoretical rather than practical insight. The first 'Sänger' classical caesarean section was performed on 25 May 1882 when Sänger assisted Christian Leopold – both mother and infant survived. He did not perform the operation himself until 1884. He did, however, forcefully and energetically promote his technique of uterine closure, which became widely accepted. Largely forgotten was the careful uterine closure of the transverse lower-segment incision proposed and performed by Ferdinand Kehrer a year earlier.

Max Sänger was born in Bayreuth. He took his medical studies in Würzburg and Leipzig, graduating

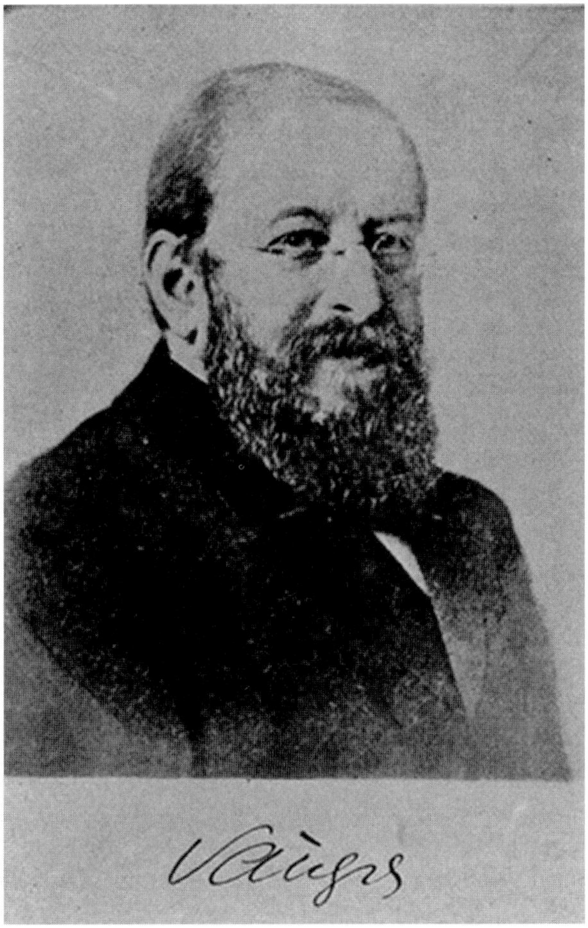

Max Sänger

in 1876. He did two years' postgraduate work in pathology before becoming assistant to Carl Credé in the Leipzig department of obstetrics and gynaecology. In addition to his work on caesarean section he was a noted vaginal surgeon. In 1899 he wasappointed professor and head of obstetrics and gynaecology in the German University of Prague. Soon after he moved his health failed, and he died of 'apoplexy' just before his fiftieth birthday. In his obituary it was said, 'he removed from the obstetric art probably the final reproach of the cruelty of ignorance'.

Selected Publications

Sänger M. Zur Rehabilitirung des classischen Kaiserschnittes. *Arch Gynäkol* 1882; 19: 370.

Sänger M. *Der Kaiserschnitt bei Uterusfibromen nebst vergleichender Methodik der Sectio Caesarea und der Porro-Operation*. Leipzig: W. Engelmann; 1882.

Bibliography References

99, 102, 548, 950, 987, 1205, 1261, 1290, 1333, 1346, 1347, 1480, 1595, 1631, 1734.

Santorini, Giovanni Domenico (1681–1737)

Vesical Venous Plexus

Those gynaecologists who perform urethrovesical tape suspensions will occasionally encounter significant haemorrhage in the paravesical space. When this happens, it will be of no solace to realise that one has encountered the venous plexus lateral and inferior to the bladder, first described by Giovanni Santorini in 1724. In women this plexus of veins communicates with the vaginal venous plexus and enters the internal iliac vein. Santorini also described the accessory pancreatic duct, among other anatomical eponyms.

Giovanni Santorini was born in Venice, the son of an apothecary. He studied medicine in Bologna, Padua and Pisa, graduating from the latter university in 1701. Among his contemporaries Santorini was

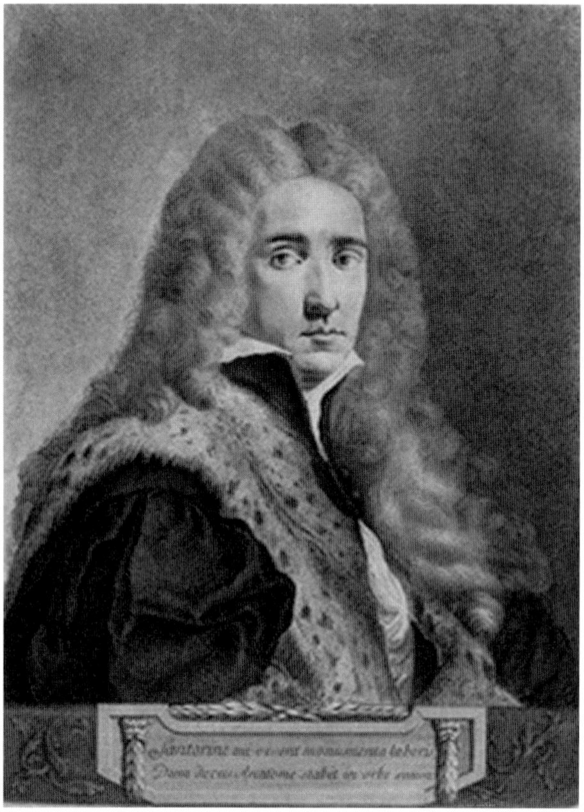

Giovanni Domenico Santorini

acknowledged as one of the greatest anatomists. He was professor of anatomy and medicine in Venice from 1703 to 1728. Santorini became chief physician at the Spedaletto Hospital in Venice, where he also taught obstetrics. He dedicated his major work, *Observationes anatomicae,* to Peter the Great of Russia.

Selected Publications

Santorini GD. *Observationes anatomicae.* Venice: GB Recurti; 1721

Bibliography References

397, 406, 563, 604, 1718.

Saxtorph, Matthias (1740–1800)

Saxtorph's Manoeuvre

Matthias Saxtorph was born in the village of Meirup, near Holstelro in Jutland, Denmark, on 1 June 1740. He received his MD in Copenhagen in 1762 and studied in Vienna, Strasburg and Paris from 1767–70. He concentrated on obstetrics and upon his return was appointed as *Stadtaccoucher* or 'town-obstetrician', as well as a member of the Royal Midwives Commission in Copenhagen. In 1785 he became obstetrician and lecturer, later professor, at the Friedrichs Hospital, Copenhagen.

Saxtorph made many useful observations on the mechanism of labour and the relationship of the fetal head to the pelvic curve. He was the first to advocate downward pressure on the shanks of obstetric forceps during traction to deliver the fetal head, reasoning that this brought the angle of traction into the plane of the pelvic curve. This manoeuvre is more commonly attributed to Charles Pajot, but Saxtorph advised it more than a century before Pajot's description. Saxtorph also designed a set of obstetric forceps with handles and articulation similar to that of William Smellie. Furthermore, the handles could be folded back over the blades, reducing the size such that the forceps could be carried in the pocket. These forceps were described posthumously in Saxtorph's works, which were edited by his son Johan Sylvester Saxtorph and published in 1804. Matthias Saxtorph died in Copenhagen on 29 June 1800.

Selected Publications

Saxtorph M. *Theoria de diverso partu*. Copenhagen: AH Godiche; 1772.

Saxtorph JS, Scheel P. *Matthias Saxtorph's Gesammelte Schriften*. Copenhagen: Brummer; 1804.

Bibliography References

99, 361, 399, 604, 648, 721, 763, 1261, 1291.

Scanzoni, Friedrich Wilhelm (1821–1891)

Scanzoni's Manoeuvre

The wider diameter presented by the occipito-posterior position is associated with prolonged labour and difficult forceps delivery. Attempts to assist delivery in the posterior position have usually involved manual or instrumental rotation to the more favourable, narrower occipito-anterior diameter. William Smellie was the first to use forceps to rotate the fetal head, and he was able to achieve this with relatively short, straight forceps, akin to the principles later put forward by Christian Kielland. With the advent of longer forceps with a pronounced pelvic curve, rotation became impossible without trauma to the mother, infant or both. In 1851 Friedrich Scanzoni devised a technique of performing the rotation in two stages, removing the forceps after rotation and reapplying them for traction and delivery. Scanzoni stated the problem thus:

> *If one considers the construction of the forceps, on the one hand, and the shape of the fetal head and the maternal pelvis, on the other, one sees at a glance that the instrument will function most effectively and least traumatically when it is applied to both temporal regions and is so situated in the pelvis that its pelvic curve corresponds exactly with the direction of the pelvic axis. This is possible, however, only when the anteroposterior diameter of the head lies parallel to the anteroposterior of the pelvis, in which case the blades, applied along both side walls of the pelvis, grasp the head at its two lateral surfaces ...*
>
> *If the forceps are applied to the sides of the head, however, when the anteroposterior diameter of the latter lies parallel to the transverse or an oblique diameter of the pelvis, then the tips of the instrument have to be turned more or less toward one of the pelvic side walls in order to bring the instrument into the relation to the pelvic axis necessary for extraction. Extraction may be very dangerous, often quite impossible, when attempted with improperly applied forceps.*

To overcome this conundrum, Scanzoni advocated the following. If, for example, the head was right occipito-posterior, the forceps were applied cephalically as though it were left occipito-anterior. The head was then rotated clockwise to right occipito-anterior, at which point the forceps were removed and reapplied correctly for traction and delivery in the occipito-anterior position. Scanzoni's manoeuvre was widely adopted in Europe and North America.

Friedrich Wilhelm Scanzoni was born in the village of Lichtenfels on the periphery of Prague. He graduated in medicine from the University of Prague in 1844. In 1850, after acting as an assistant to Franz Kiwisch he was appointed professor of obstetrics and gynaecology in Würzburg. Here his reputation as a teacher and private practitioner soared. He was called to St Petersburg to deliver the Empress of Russia. When he planned to resign his chair in 1863, the citizens of Würzburg petitioned the King of Bavaria, who responded with a personal request to Scanzoni to remain. The king also added the tangible reward of a baronetcy, so that Scanzoni could now use as his full

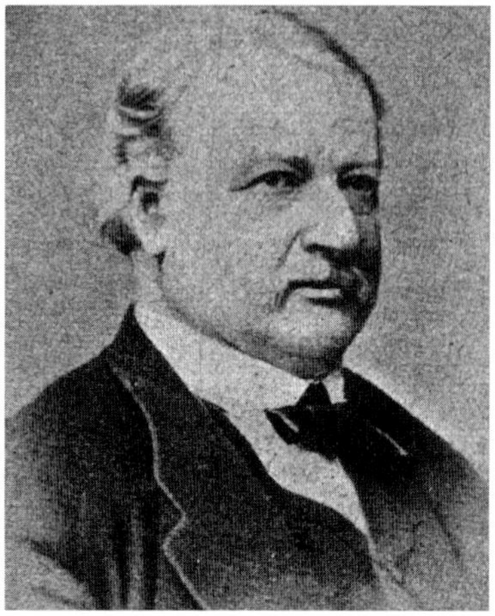

Friedrich Wilhelm Scanzoni

name, Friedrich Wilhelm von Lichtenfels Scanzoni. His main reputation was in the field of obstetrics, even though he was a bitter and vociferous opponent of Ignac Semmelweis' doctrine.

Scanzoni did not embrace the emerging field of surgical gynaecology, being of the school that applied leeches to the cervix for many gynaecological disorders.

At the age of 50 Scanzoni retired from medical practice and spent the last 20 years of his life at his estate in the Bavarian Alps.

Selected Publications

Scanzoni FW. Die Anwendung der Geburtszange als Mittel zur Verbesserung der Stellung des vorleigenden Kindeskopfes. *Verh Phys-Med Ges Würz* 1851; 2: 184–201

Scanzoni FW. *Lehrbuch der Geburtshülfe.* (Vol. 2.) Wien; 1853, pp. 838–40.

Bibliography References

361, 548, 648, 721, 1088, 1261, 1480.

Scarpa, Antonio (1752–1832)

Scarpa's Fascia

Antonio Scarpa was born in Motta di Livenza, Italy, the son of a boatman. He studied medicine under Giovanni Morgagni at Padua and graduated when he was 18. Two years later he was appointed professor of anatomy and theoretical surgery at the University of Modena. In 1783 he became professor of anatomy and surgery at the University of Pavia. He made many original anatomical and surgical discoveries, including work on hernia, club foot, ophthalmology and the nerve supply to the heart. Scarpa was an artist of the first order and illustrated his own texts.

Scarpa became quite wealthy and remained a bachelor. He reputedly fathered a number of sons from informal liaisons and supported their education. He had an articulate and sarcastic wit and could be quite ruthless and tyrannical. In his later years he was more feared then revered. He is remembered eponymously for Scarpa's (femoral) triangle and the deeper, membranous layer of the superficial fascia of the lower abdominal wall: 'Scarpa's fascia'.

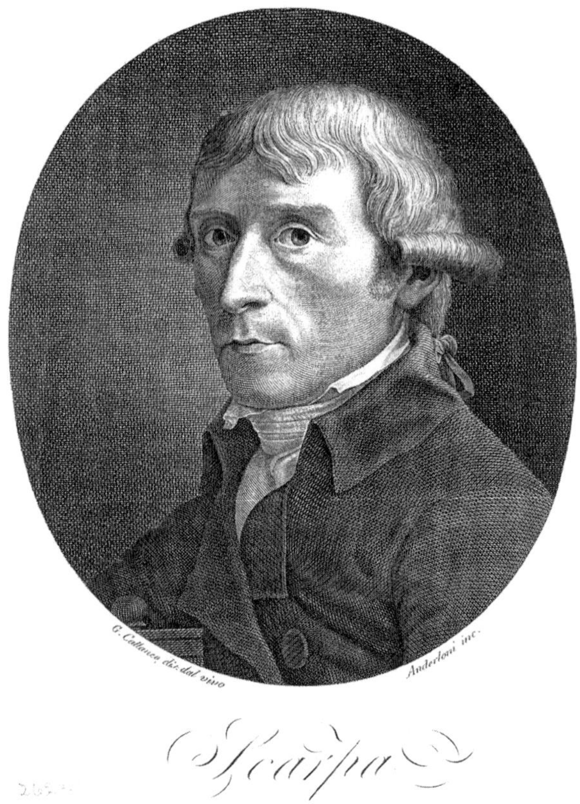

Antonio Scarpa

Selected Publications

Scarpa A. *Memoire anatomico-chirurgiche.* Milan; 1809.

Bibliography References

8, 271, 406, 579, 595, 648, 1074.

Schauta, Friedrich (1849–1919)

Radical Vaginal Hysterectomy

The earliest radical hysterectomies by the vaginal route were performed by Karl Pawlik and Karl Schuchardt. Friedrich Schauta carried out his modification of the technique for the first time on 1 June 1901. The advantage of the vaginal over the abdominal approach was a much lower operative mortality. The disadvantage, as Ernst Wertheim was to demonstrate, was the inability to perform a complete pelvic lymphadenectomy. Schauta's technique was later modified by Alfred Amreich (1885–1972) to enable more pelvic connective tissue to be removed. Thus, the procedure is often referred to as the Schauta–Amreich operation.

Friedrich Schauta took his MD at the University of Vienna in 1874. He was professor of obstetrics and gynaecology in Innsbruck from 1881–7 and at the German University in Prague from 1887–91. He returned to Vienna as the head of the first university department of obstetrics and gynaecology in 1891. By this time Schauta had an international reputation and did not accept any challenge to his authority. He and his assistant, Wertheim, increasingly disagreed. In 1897 Wertheim became head at the Elizabeth Hospital and later at the second university department, where he went on to develop the radical abdominal hysterectomy.

Schauta planned and oversaw the move of the first university department from the old Allgemeines Krankenhaus in 1908.

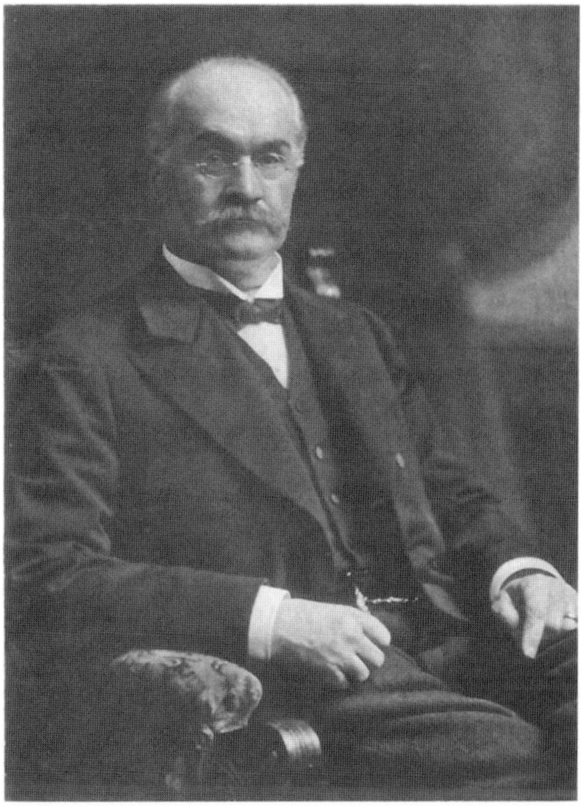

Friedrich Schauta

Selected Publications

Amreich A. Anatomie und Technik der erweiterten vaginalen Carcinomoperation. *Arch Gynäkol* 1924; 122: 497.

Schauta F. Die operation des gebärmutterkrebes mittels des Schuchardtschen paravaginalschnittes. *Mschr Geburtsh Gynäkol* 1902; 15: 133.

Schauta F. *Die erweiterte vaginale Totalextirpation des Uterus bei Kollumkarzinom.* Vienna: J. Sofar; 1908.

Bibliography References

97, 383, 501, 524, 541, 648, 896, 1071, 1107, 1291, 1292, 1412, 1641.

Schiller, Walter (1887–1960)

Schiller's Test

The diagnosis of cancer of the cervix depends on the histological interpretation of tissue taken from the appropriate biopsy site. In 1927–8, Walter Schiller carried out studies on the histogenesis of early cervical cancer which culminated in his test outlining the suspicious area by staining the cervix with iodine. He noted:

> *This glycogen, which is a physiologic component of normal portio epithelium is completely lacking in carcinomatous epithelium ... If the normal portio or vaginal epithelium is painted with iodine solution containing potassium iodide, such as Lugol's solution, the normal epithelium soon stains a deep dark brown after a few seconds. Pathologic epithelium, especially carcinomatous does not take up the stain, but instead remains light, or at most slightly yellowish.*

Schiller pointed out that failure to take up the stain was not pathognomic of cancerous epithelium but also the case with benign epithelial changes such as infection, hyperkeratosis or traumatic desquamation. However, he noted that dark brown staining always indicated well-glycogenated normal epithelium.

Walter Schiller was born in Vienna and received his MD from the University of Vienna in 1912. He worked in the medical laboratory of the Austrian Army during the First World War, following which he was appointed director of laboratories at the university clinic at the University of Vienna. It was here he defined the work leading to the Schiller test. Following a lecture tour of the United States in 1936 he was appointed Director of Laboratories at the Jewish Memorial Hospital in New York. He subsequently held similar positions at the Cook County Women's and Children's Hospitals in Chicago.

While speaking in favour of Hans Hinselmann's recently introduced colposcope he said:

> *In a crowded out-patient department it is hardly possible to examine a cervix for such minute detail and it is no doubt true that often cervices which appear to the naked eye as healthy, smooth and unsuspicious, really harbor small incipient carcinomata.*

Thus, in the days before cytology, Schiller's attempt to find a practical clinical screening test for cervical cancer was quite reasonable. It is still used today to help delineate areas for treatment of cervical intraepithelial neoplasia.

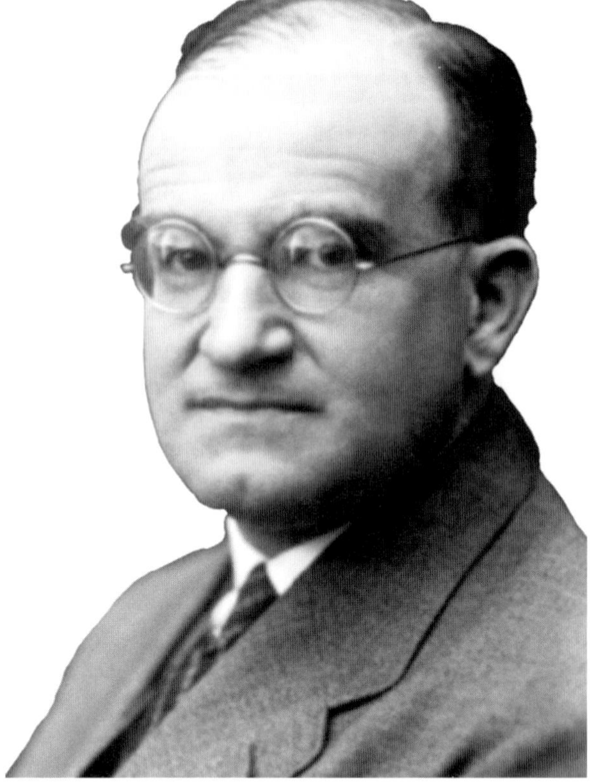

Walter Schiller

Walter Schiller died in his home in Chicago on 2 May 1960.

Selected Publications

Schiller W. Über Fruhstadien des Portiocarcinoms und ihre Diagnose. *Arch Gynäkol* 1928; 133: 211–83.

Schiller W. Zur histologischen Frühdiagnose des Portiokarzinoms. *Zentralbl Gynäkol* 1928; 52: 1562–7.

Schiller W. Early diagnosis of carcinoma of the cervix. *Surg Gynecol Obst* 1933; 56: 210–2.

Bibliography References

383, 664, 1354, 1389, 1480, 1676.

Schuchardt, Karl August (1856–1901)

Schuchardt's Incision

In the latter half of the nineteenth century, hysterectomy for cervical cancer was usually carried out by the vaginal route to avoid the huge mortality associated with abdominal hysterectomy. Many surgeons, including Conrad Langenbeck, Christian Leopold and Alfred Duhrssen, used perineal relaxing incisions to improve access to the uterus.

In 1893 Karl Schuchardt was operating on a woman with cervical cancer extending into the left parametrium. Confronted by inadequate access to achieve excision of the diseased parametrium and nodes, Schuchardt employed an extensive relaxing incision which he described as follows:

> *. . . a large, essentially sagittal incision is made, somewhat convex externally, beginning between the middle and posterior third of the labium majus on the side of the involved parametrium, extending posteriorly toward the sacrum, and stopping two fingersbreadths from the anus. The wound is deepened only in the fatty tissue of the ischiorectal fossa, leaving the funnel of the levator ani muscle, the rectum behind it, and the sacral ligaments intact. Internally the side wall of the vagina is opened into the ischiorectal fossa and the vagina divided in its lateral aspect by a long incision extending up to the cervix. There thus results a surprisingly free view of all the structures under consideration, and removal of the uterus as well as the cancerous nodes in the broad ligament on this side can be carried out with the greatest certainty and ease.*

He published this report within weeks of the operation, and thereafter it has been known as Schuchardt's incision.

Karl August Schuchardt was born in Göttingen, the son of a physician. He took his medical studies in Jena, Strasburg and Göttingen, graduating in 1878. He carried out eight years postgraduate training in pathology and surgery. He became professor and director of surgery in Stettin State Hospital. His death at 45 years of age was from sepsis following a surgical needle-stick injury.

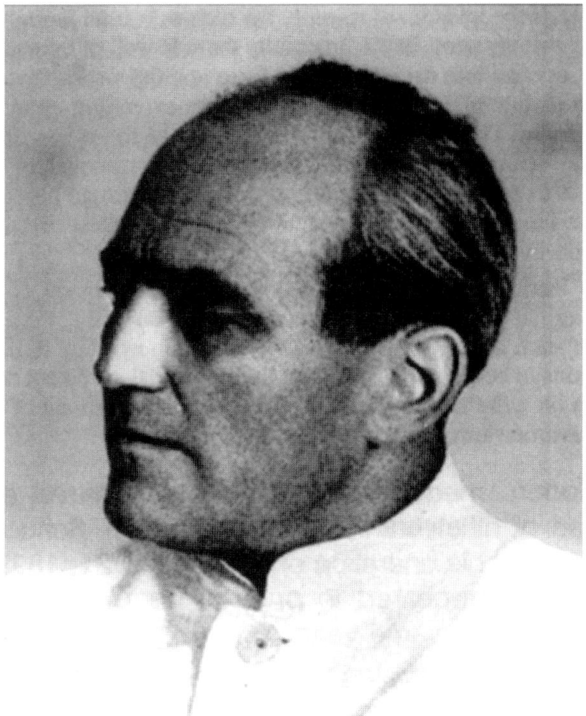

Karl August Schuchardt

Selected Publications

Schuchardt K. Eine neue Methode der Gerbärmutterexstirpation. *Zentralbl Chir* 1893; 20: 1121–6.

Bibliography References

553, 648, 1290, 1291, 1358, 1412, 1638.

Schultze, Bernhard Sigmund (1827–1919)

Placental Separation/Neonatal Resuscitation

In his superb obstetric atlas, published in 1865, Schultze illustrated his view of the normal mechanism of placental separation and expulsion. In the text accompanying the illustration, he wrote:

> *The labour contractions that expelled the fetus brought about such a diminution in size of the uterus, that the placenta was separated to a large extent from the uterine wall. The subsequent contractions and the considerable flow of blood that ensues from the torn vessels of the uterine wall, force the placenta completely off the uterine wall . . . and the inverted membranes forward, along with much clotted fluid blood, through the cervix . . .*

Schultze therefore felt that the shiny, fetal surface of the placenta normally presented at the introitus. This was later challenged by Matthews Duncan, who taught that, without interference, the more ragged maternal surface of the placenta presented. Since then generations of medical students have learned to distinguish between the two methods as 'shiny Schultze' and 'dirty Duncan'.

Schultze was also known for his contributions to neonatal resuscitation, work that he maintained over a 50-year period until his death. In 1871 he published his 179-page monograph, *Der Scheintod Neugeborener*, in which he described his method of artificial respiration for the asphyxiated newborn. He advocated his technique based on 12 years of experience, 'which I recommend warmly, because – if applied in time – it is rarely unsuccessful'. He described his method as follows:

> *The objective of this method is to simultaneously move the ribs and the diaphragm of the thorax in a passive way in order to alternately provide expansion and compression of the thoracic cavity . . . the child is taken with both hands at the shoulders such that both thumbs overlie the anterior surface of the thorax, the forefingers reach behind to the axillary fossae, and the other three fingers obliquely and lengthwise rest on the posterior surface of the thorax. In so doing, the head, which usually flops backwards, is comfortably supported by the palms. The obstetrician with legs astride and the upper part of the body bent forward, takes the floppy infant in the above way with the arms stretched downwards. Without delay the obstetrician swings the infant from this position upwards. When the arms of the obstetrician reach a position slightly above the horizontal, they slow and stop gently to avoid over-twisting the child; the body should sink down slowly, and due to the weight of the pelvis and abdomen is strongly compressed . . . This gradual flexion of the infant's pelvis above the abdomen results in a significant compression of the thoracic viscera, the diaphragm, and the entire chest wall. As a result of this passive expiratory movement, aspirated fluids often come out of the respiratory tract. The flexion of the child having been completed slowly but steadily, the obstetrician again moves his arms down between his legs. In so doing the infant's body is stretched with the acceleration and the thorax, without any pressure, due to its elasticity will now expand . . . The weight of the infant moving down, will also elevate the ribs, move the diaphragm down resulting in a passive but massive inspiration.*

Schultze's technique was described in many popular obstetric texts of the late nineteenth and early twentieth centuries. In these texts, sensible advice was given to dry the baby before applying the technique, thereby avoiding a slippy swinging neonate from becoming a flying neonate.

Bernhard Sigmund Schultze was born in Freiburg and followed his father and elder brother in the study of anatomy in Greifswald. He later studied obstetrics at the University of Berlin. In 1858 he assumed the chair of obstetrics in Jena, where he remained. His atlas and textbook of obstetrics were very popular, the latter going into 15 editions. Like many anatomists of his era, he was an accomplished artist and did the illustrations for his own papers and books.

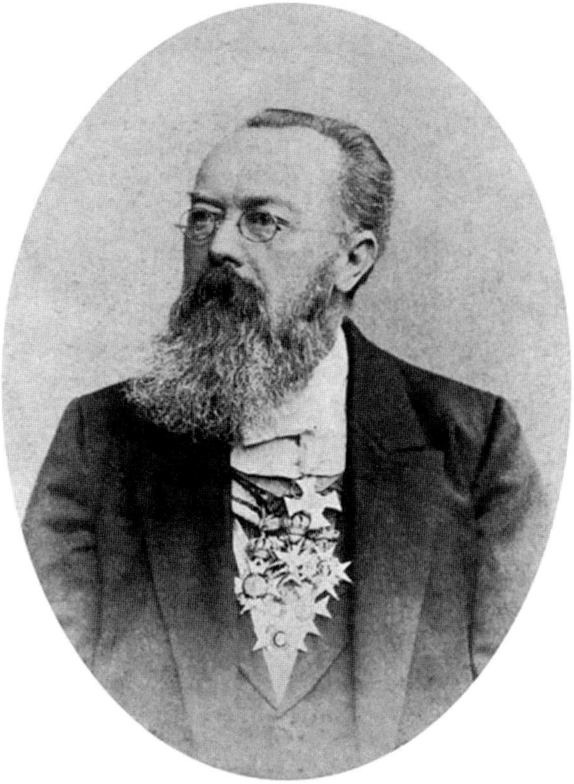

Bernhard Sigmund Schultze

Schultze retired from the chair at Jena in 1902 but continued to be active in research, particularly in the field of neonatal resuscitation. Although he was almost totally blind and deaf, he continued his work and published his last paper one day before his death at the age of 91. His obituary was written by Otto

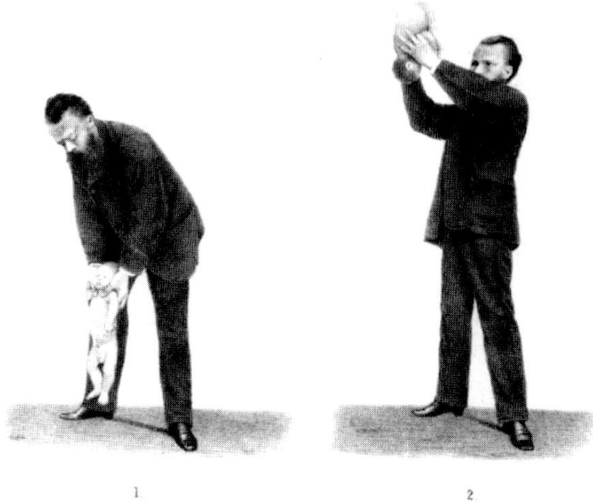

Illustration showing Schultze's method of neonatal resuscitation

Küstner, who said, 'He passed away not like an old, tired man who had done his work and was now relaxing, but death took him out in the middle of his productive activity'. Bernard Schultze died in Jena on 17 April 1919.

Selected Publications

Schultze BS. *Wandtafeln zur Schwangerschafts und Geburtskunde*. Leipzig: Gunther; 1865.

Schultze BS. *Der Scheintod Neugeborener*. Jena: Mauke's Verlag; 1781.

Bibliography References

74, 87, 548, 553, 648, 862, 1128, 1261, 1265, 1480.

Semm, Kurt Karl Stephan (1927–2003)

Operative Laparoscopy

Kurt Semm was born in Munich on 23 March 1927. After school, he worked briefly as a toolmaker before enrolling in medicine at Munich University, where he graduated MD in 1951. He did his postgraduate training in obstetrics and gynaecology at Munich and became associate professor in 1964. He was appointed professor and head of obstetrics and gynaecology at Kiel University in 1970.

In the early 1960s laparoscopic surgery was banned in German hospitals due to safety concerns with the crude equipment available at that time. The main limitations were with the insufflators used to produce the pneumoperitoneum, and thermal burns from monopolar electrocautery units with tubal ligation. Using his skills as a toolmaker, Semm produced the automatic CO_2 insufflator and an improved thermocoagulation unit. He formed his own medical instrument company, WISAP, to ensure that these innovations came to market. At this time the laparoscope was used mainly in the upper abdomen by internists and surgeons for diagnosis and liver biopsy; the pneumoperitoneum was created using air. In 1970, wishing to differentiate the procedure from this limited use, Semm introduced the word 'pelviscopy' to emphasise the pelvic and gynaecological dimension of the operation.

Semm went on to extend the boundaries of laparoscopic surgery in gynaecology in the 1970s and 1980s with adhesiolysis, ovarian cystectomy, oophorectomy, salpingotomy and salpingectomy for ectopic pregnancy, myomectomy and laparoscopic-assisted vaginal hysterectomy. He also carried out CO_2 hysteroscopy from the mid-1970s. During this innovative period Semm developed many new laparoscopic aids and instruments, including extra and intracorporeal knot tying, endoloop ligatures, acquapurator dissection and tissue morcellation.

In the early years, Semm's audacious laparoscopic endeavours were met with opposition and, in some cases, outright hostility. In the early 1970s at Kiel, his promotion of laparoscopic surgery prompted a request from colleagues that he undergo a brain scan. Unused to the laparoscope, they felt such extreme use must be a sign of brain damage. Semm tried to promote the use of operative laparoscopy by his general surgical colleagues, which stimulated a formal request that his medical licence be suspended. In September 1980, Semm carried out the first laparoscopic appendectomy, to the widespread opprobrium of his peers. His written report on this case was rejected by the *American Journal of Obstetrics and Gynecology* as 'unethical'.

In the mid-1980s, a major advance was the development of computer chip video cameras that could be attached to the scope. For the first time, others in the operating theatre could see the procedure, which led to a greater understanding and acceptance of laparoscopic surgery.

Semm published and taught relentlessly in Germany and abroad. He became the preeminent travelling teacher of laparoscopic surgery, particularly in the United States, where he was welcomed as a pioneer, in contrast to the more muted response in his homeland. Many regarded him as the father of laparoscopic surgery.

Kurt Semm retired from his position at Kiel in 1995. His first wife died in 1986 and he remarried in 1994. They moved to Tucson, Arizona in 1996. In his later years, Semm's dogged innovation was recognised by national and international endoscopic societies. He had the comfort of knowing that he had played a major role in the development and acceptance of minimally invasive surgery. Kurt Semm died from complications of Parkinson's disease on 16 July 2003.

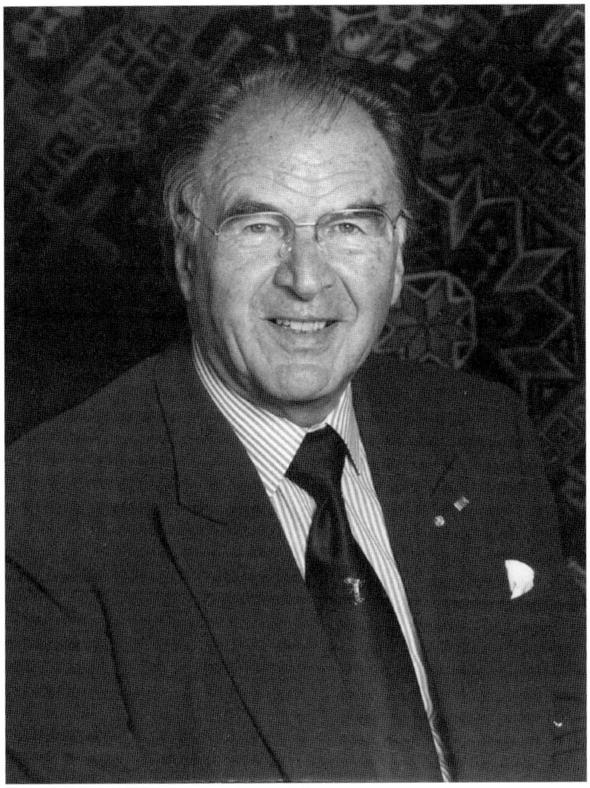

Kurt Karl Stephan Semm

Selected Publications

Semm K. *Pelviskopie und Hysteroskopie*. Stuttgart: Schattauer Verlag; 1976.

Semm K. *Atlas of Gynecologic Laparoscopy and Hysteroscopy*. Philadelphia, PA: Saunders;1977.

Semm K. Endoscopic appendectomy. *Endoscopy* 1983; 15: 59–64.

Bibliography References

146, 915, 1041, 1070, 1367, 1512, 1535.

Semmelweis, Ignac Philipp (1818–1865)

Puerperal Sepsis

It is not uncommon for the reputation of a person to be modified by later reappraisal of available information. Such is the case with Ignac Semmelweis, one of the best known and most romanticised characters in medical history. A reassessment dispels some of the myths surrounding his life and work but confirms the essence of his considerable achievement.

Ignac Philipp Semmelweis, the fifth of eight children and known to his family as Naci, was born in Buda, Hungary. His father was a grocer and the family was of German descent. He grew up speaking Swabian, a German dialect, and learned Hungarian in high school. As a result, he was not a polished speaker or writer in either Hungarian or German. To a degree this accounted for his lack of self-confidence in the more cultured medical circles of Vienna.

Semmelweis went to the University of Vienna in 1837 and studied law for one year. He transferred to medicine, graduated in 1844 and then did four months' extra training in obstetrics, for which he received his master's diploma in practical midwifery. While waiting for a job as an assistant in the department of obstetrics, he worked with three of the young rising stars of the medical faculty: Josef Skoda (1805–81), who taught general medicine and statistics, Ferdinand Hebra (1816–80), the dermatologist, and Carl Rokitansky (1804–78), the great pathologist. All these men influenced and supported Semmelweis during his training. He also admired and assisted the professor of forensic pathology, Jakob Kolletschka (1803–47), whose death was the catalyst for Semmelweis' doctrine.

In July 1846, Semmelweis was appointed assistant to the professor, Johann Klein (1788–1856), in the first obstetrical clinic at the Allgemeines Krankenhaus in Vienna. As such he was confronted with the appalling maternal mortality from 'childbed fever' that existed in the unit. As he later noted:

> *All was uncertain, all was doubtful, all was inexplicable, only the number of deaths was an indubitable fact.*

Semmelweis studied the records of the obstetrical unit back to the opening of the hospital in 1794. A number of relationships evolved from this scrutiny. In the early years of the hospital's existence the maternal death rate was less than 1 per cent. By the 1830s the importance of autopsy training for medical students and doctors was emphasised, and the death rate rose. In 1833 the unit was divided into two divisions, both staffed by medical students and midwives. From 1840, medical students and doctors worked only in the first division, while midwives staffed the second division. It was from this date that Semmelweis noted a discrepancy in the death rates between the two units, with a two- to four-, and in some months, a ten-fold increase in the first division's mortality.

In March 1847 Kolletschka died from sepsis following an accidental skin puncture inflicted by a student at autopsy. Semmelweis reviewed the postmortem findings on Kolletschka and concluded that the pathological picture was the same as that found in the victims of puerperal sepsis:

> *Day and night I was haunted by the image of Kolletschka's disease and was forced to recognise, ever more decisively, that the disease from which Kolletschka died was identical to that from which so many maternity patients died . . .*
>
> *I was forced to admit that if Kolletschka's disease was identical with the disease that killed so many maternity patients, then it must have originated from the same cause that brought it on in Kolletschka.*

It was Semmelweis' own extensive experience in pathology under the tutelage of Rokitansky and Kolletschka that had prepared him to grasp this association: 'I was accustomed before the morning visit of the professor, to examine for the benefit of my gynaecological studies almost every day all the female bodies in the dead house'. In establishing the link between infectious material carried on the hands of students and doctors from the autopsy room to patients in the maternity ward, Semmelweis had to confront his own role in this chain:

> *In consequence of my conviction I must affirm that only God knows the number of patients who went prematurely to their graves because of me. I have examined corpses to an extent equalled by few other obstetricians . . . No matter how painful and oppressive such a recognition may be, the remedy does not lie in suppression. If the misfortune is not to persist forever, then this truth must be made known to everyone concerned.*

Semmelweis noted that after ordinary soap and water washing, hands retained the cadaveric odour and reasoned that some infectious matter must remain. Thus, 'In the middle of May, 1847, without noting the exact day, I instituted chlorine washings'. All students and doctors entering the maternity ward had to wash their hands in a chloride of lime solution. Within one month, the mortality in the first division fell from 12.2% to 2.4%. In 1848, the first full year of chlorine prophylaxis, the death rate in the first division fell to 1.2%, comparable to the 1.3% rate in the second division. Semmelweis had proved his point comprehensively.

In the mythologised versions of history Semmelweis is often depicted as a lone voice railing against a blundering medical establishment. In fact, most of the young and increasingly influential faculty praised and supported Semmelweis, including Skoda, Hebra and Rokitansky. Hebra wrote two articles in the local medical society's journal emphasising the importance of the work. Skoda lectured at the Vienna Academy of Sciences, in support of Semmelweis' conclusions. Skoda also asked the faculty to establish a committee to review and report on the findings. Klein, who had instituted autopsy teaching for students, opposed the idea and influenced the senior faculty to reject the review. In addition, Klein refused to reappoint Semmelweis in March 1849. Semmelweis remained in Vienna as an unpaid midwifery instructor. It is at this point that Semmelweis failed to support his cause by writing up and publishing his data. Indeed, he first presented his work to the Medical Society of Vienna in May 1850, sponsored by Rokitansky. He acquitted himself well in this forum but did not present his lecture in written form for publication, as was the custom.

Slighted by the offer of a minor teaching post, Semmelweis abruptly left Vienna in October

1850 without telling his supporters. He returned home to Buda, and in 1851 took up a position as director of obstetrics at St Rochus Hospital in Pest, on the opposite side of the Danube river. Here he applied his methods and consistently kept the maternal mortality rate below 1 per cent. In 1855 he was appointed professor of theoretical and practical obstetrics at the University of Pest. It was to be ten years after his discovery that Semmelweis first published on the subject. His paper, *The Aetiology of Childbed Fevers,* was published in a Hungarian journal of limited circulation. The following year he began to write his full account, *Die Aetiologie, der Begriff und die Prophylaxis des Kindbettfiebers* (The Etiology, the Concept and the Prophylaxis of Childbed Fever), which bears the date 1861 but was actually published in August 1860.

Unfortunately, Semmelweis' writing style was long, repetitive and at times almost impenetrable. Frank Murphy who translated *Die Aetiologie* into English said, 'The style is wordy and repetitious; the argument flows back and forth without progressing to any logical point; the author is egotistic and bellicose'. While some accepted his reasoning, others did not. As one of his biographers, Sir William Sinclair, later put it, 'If he could have written like Oliver Wendell Holmes his *Aetiology* would have captured Europe in 12 months'.

Semmelweis attacked his detractors in this book, and after its publication he wrote a series of 'open letters' to those who dared question his conclusions. In these letters, phrases such as 'the puerperal sun which arose in Vienna in the year 1847 has not enlightened your mind', and 'I declare before God and the world that you are a murderer' did not serve to endear him to the academic community or support his work as that of a reasonable and logical man. His final publication, in 1862, was an *Open Letter to All Professors of Obstetrics,* in which he reiterated the points of his thesis with supporting data from various clinics: 'Such brilliant results prove to me that I am on the right road toward finally protecting the childbearing sex and its unborn fruits from an untimely and criminal death'.

By the early 1860s Semmelweis began to show signs of mental deterioration. Episodes of rage alternated with bouts of depression and periods of elation. His memory failed and he was liable to behave inappropriately. By 1865 he was intermittently psychotic. In July 1865 he was due to present his report at the faculty meeting. He rose and distractedly read out the text of the midwives' oath. His colleagues escorted him home, where his wife tried to care for him. On 31 July his wife and some friends took him by train to Vienna where, with the help of his old friend Hebra, he was committed to a private institution, The Lower Austrian Mental Home. He died two weeks later on 13 August 1865 and, after an autopsy, was buried in the local cemetery.

The cause of Semmelweis' death has been reevaluated. The romantic myth has always ascribed his death to sepsis following a needle-stick injury, the very condition he strove to prevent in pregnant women. However, a recent analysis suggests that Semmelweis suffered from premature organic brain disease, Alzheimer's dementia, and died as a result of injuries sustained when beaten or restrained by the attendants at the mental home. The autopsy showed that sepsis was indeed the cause of death but that the

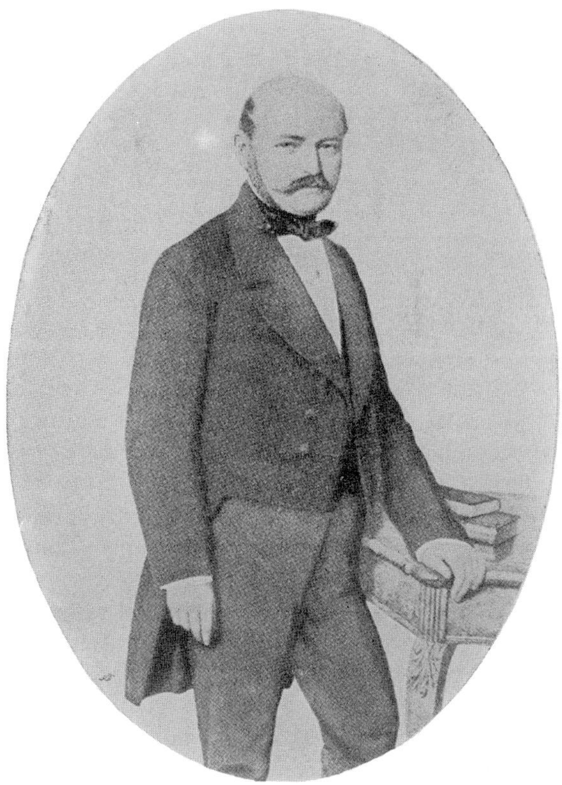

Ignac Philipp Semmelweis

portal of entry was the injuries he sustained in the mental home.

Semmelweis remains a tragic figure who, to some extent was the architect of his own failure and rejection, because of his inability to communicate the doctrine he so brilliantly deduced. In the concluding remarks of his treatise, he expressed confidence that his views would prevail and hoped he would live to see his methods universally accepted. It was not to be in his lifetime:

> *If I look back into the past with my present conviction, then I can banish the melancholy which overtakes me, looking at the same time into that happy future, in which within and without the lying-in hospitals over the entire world only cases of auto-infection will occur . . . But should it not be given to me, which God forbid, to behold this happy time with my own eyes, the conviction that this time will come without fail sooner or later after me, will still soothe the hour of my death.*

One hopes it did.

Selected Publications

Hebra F. Höchst wichtige Erfahrungen über die Aetiologie der in Gebäraustalten epidemischen Puerperalfieber. (Experience of the highest importance concerning the etiology of epidemic puerperal fever in lying-in hospitals). *Zeit Keiserlich-Koniglichen Gesellschaft Aerzte Wien* 1847–48; 4: 242–4.

Semmelweis IP. A Gyermekágyi lás Kóroktana (Etiology of Childbed Fevers). *Orvosi Hetilap* 1858; 2: 1, 17, 65, 81, 305, 337, 353.

Semmelweis IP. *Die Aetiologie, der Begriff und die Prophylaxis des Kindbettfiebers*. Pest-Vienna-Leipzig; CA Hartleben; 1861. Also published in: The Classics of Obstetrics and Gynecology Library Birmingham: Gryphon Editions; 1990 (facsimile).

Bibliography References

16, 29, 151, 219, 227, 244–246, 301, 360, 372, 421, 429, 508, 650, 681, 868, 869, 896, 939–941, 1020, 1109, 1119, 1122, 1188, 1426, 1598.

Sertoli, Enrico (1841–1910) Leydig, Franz von (1821–1908)

Sertoli–Leydig Cell Tumour

The sex cords and stroma of the ovary can have a female, granulosa-theca cell, or male, Sertoli–Leydig cell, differentiation. Sertoli–Leydig cell tumours (androblastoma, arrhenoblastoma) are very rare. They are usually of low-grade malignancy and one or other cell type may predominate. In androgen-secreting tumours, Leydig cells tend to prevail.

Enrico Sertoli was born at Sondrio, Italy. He graduated in medicine from the University of Pavia in 1865 and undertook postgraduate studies in physiology and biochemistry at Vienna and Tübingen. He returned to Milan in 1870 as professor of anatomy and physiology at the Royal School of Veterinary Medicine. He later established the Laboratory of Experimental Physiology. Here he carried out his study of spermatogenesis and the seminiferous tubules, the cells of which bear his name:

> *Special cells seen in a certain quantity and not previously described by anyone. These cells are irregularly cylindrical or conical with delicate borders and with nuclei that invariably contain a nucleolus. The cytoplasm is transparent, homogeneous, and always contains fine fat droplets. These cells are almost always furnished with very transparent fine processes in which fat droplets are found . . . In some of these cells one sees a bifurcation or other secondary processes. Other cells of this type send out more processes that branch and sometimes envelop other cells.*

Franz von Leydig was born at Rothenburg, Germany. His medical studies were taken at Munich and Würzburg. In 1857 he became professor of zoology at Tübingen and in 1875 professor of comparative anatomy in Bonn. It was in 1850, while still a lecturer at Würzburg, that he published his original description of the interstitial cells surrounding the seminiferous tubules:

> *Comparative studies of the testis led to the discovery of cells constantly surrounding the seminiferous tubules, vessels, and nerves. These special cells are sparse when they follow the course of blood vessels but increase in mass*

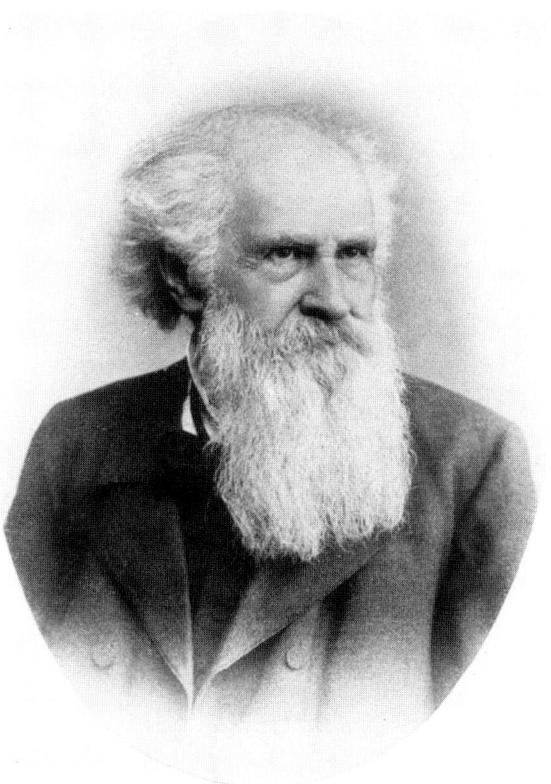

Franz von Leydig

when they surround seminferous tubules. They are lipoid in character, not altered by treatment with acetic acid or sodium bicarbonate. They can be either colorless or tinged slightly yellow; they have light vesicular nuclei, and their semifluid cytoplasm is surrounded by a sharply defined cell membrane.

Leydig retired to the town of his birth in 1887.

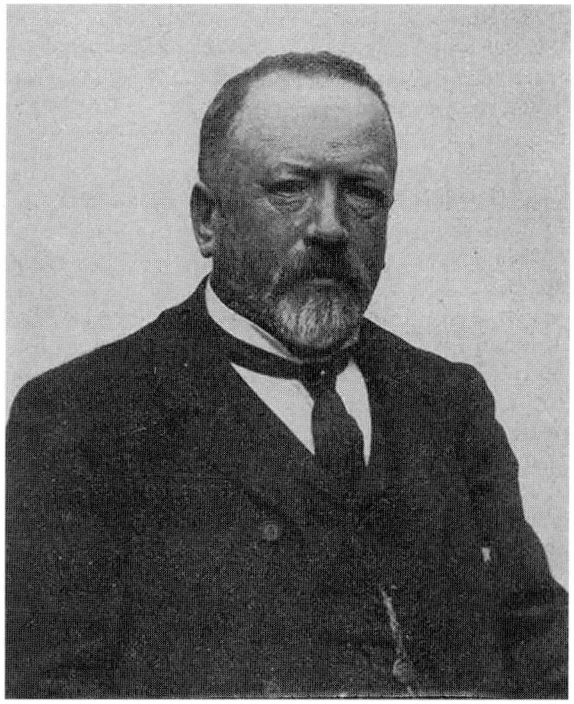

Enrico Sertoli

Selected Publications

Leydig F. Zur Anatomie der männlichen Geschlechtsorgane und Analdrüsen der Säugethiere. *Ztschr wiss Zool* 1850; 2: 1–57.

Sertoli E. Dell' esistenza di particolari cellule ramificate nei canalicoli seminiferi del testiculo umano. *Morgagni* 1865; 7: 31–40.

Bibliography References

623, 968, 1125, 1480, 1743.

Sharp, Jane (c. 1670)

Midwifery Text

In the seventeenth century, the main texts in English available to midwives were *The Byrth of Mankynde* and Nicholas Culpeper's *Directory for Midwives*. In 1671, Jane Sharp, 'practitioner in the art of midwifery above thirty years', published the first text in English written by a midwife. In the preface she put her case 'To the Midwives of England':

I have often sate down sad in the consideration of the many miseries women endure in the hands of unskilful midwives; many professing the art (without any skill in

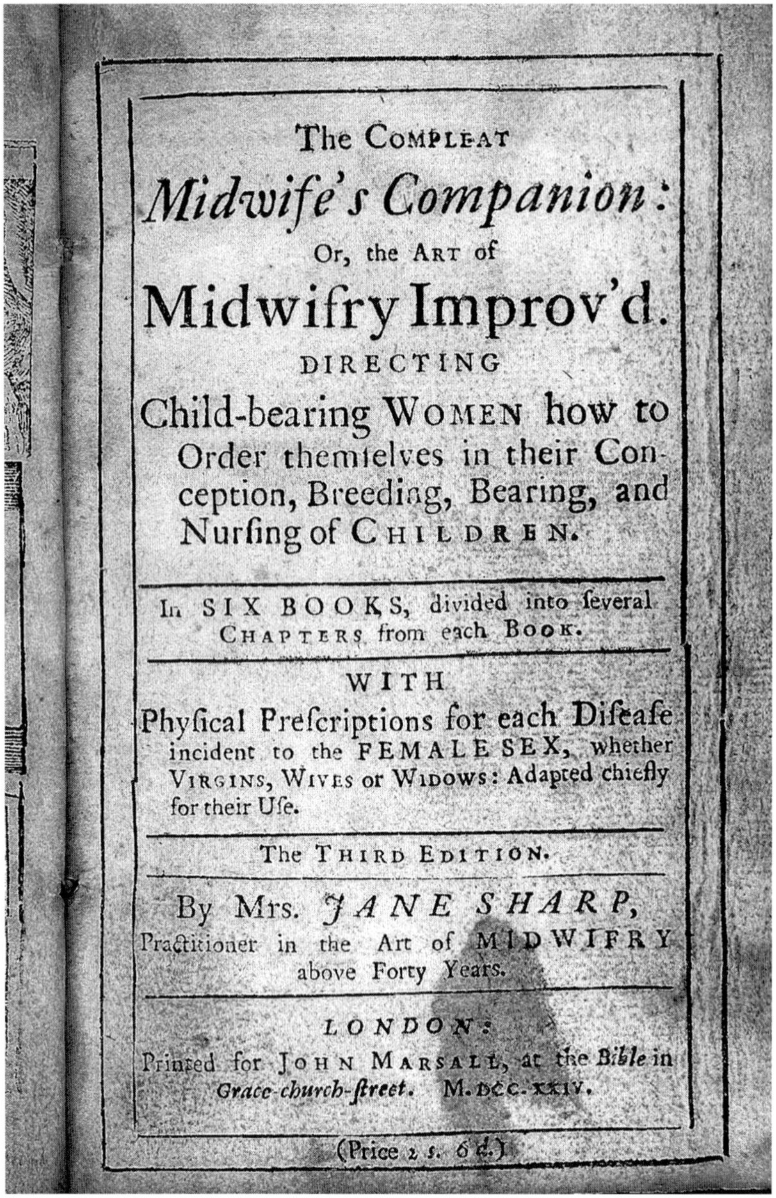

The COMPLEAT
Midwife's Companion:
Or, the ART of
Midwifry Improv'd.
DIRECTING
Child-bearing WOMEN how to
Order themſelves in their Conception, Breeding, Bearing, and Nurſing of CHILDREN.

In SIX BOOKS, divided into ſeveral CHAPTERS from each BOOK.

WITH
Phyſical Preſcriptions for each Diſeaſe incident to the FEMALE SEX, whether VIRGINS, WIVES or WIDOWS: Adapted chiefly for their Uſe.

The THIRD EDITION.

By Mrs. *JANE SHARP,*
Practitioner in the Art of MIDWIFRY above Forty Years.

LONDON:
Printed for JOHN MARSALL, at the *Bible* in *Grace-church-ſtreet.* M.DCC.XXIV.

(Price 2 *s.* 6 *d.*)

Title page of Jane Sharp's *The Compleat Midwife's Companion*, 3rd edition, 1724

anatomy, which is the principal part effectually necessary for a midwife) merely for lucres sake . . .

The art of midwifery is doubtless one of the most useful and necessary of all arts, for the being and well-being of mankind, and therefore it is extremely requisite that a midwife, be both fearing God, faithful, and exceeding well experience in that profession.

The book, like others of that era, was mainly a recycling of the works of the ancients, contemporary authors and, in particular, that of Culpeper. Jane Sharp was, like Culpeper, an astrologer and recommended her own table of the planets to calculate their influence on pregnancy and childbirth. In contrast to the texts written by physicians, who had little or no practical experience of labour and childbirth, Sharp was a practising midwife. Thus, although her book copied the errors of her contemporary physician authors, she wrote with humanity and gave clinical advice based on personal experience.

That said, she produced some surprising statements:

> *. . . it is not without reason maintained also, that a boy is sooner and easier brought forth than a girl . . . for women are lustier that are with child with boys, and therefore they will be better able to run through with it.*

While acknowledging that doctors had their place – 'I cannot deny the honour due to able physicians and surgeons' – she was opposed to the encroachment of men into the field of midwifery. She felt that the extra theoretical knowledge men gained from a university education, denied to women, was offset by the fact that 'yet farther knowledge may be gained by a long and diligent practice, and be communicated to others of our own sex'.

One passage in her text suggests that midwives carried out post-mortem caesarean section in an attempt to salvage and baptise infants:

> *But if the mother dye in child-bearing, and the child be alive, then you must keep the woman's mouth and privites open that the child may receive air to breath, or it will be presently stifled, then turn the woman on her left side, and there cut her open and take out the infant. This is also a Caesarian Birth.*

After Jane Sharp's death, John Marshall, a bookseller in London, published three further editions with the title *The Complete Midwife's Companion*: a second edition in 1720, of which there are no known copies, and third and fourth editions in 1724 and 1725 respectively.

Nothing is known of Jane Sharp. She was said to have been a respected and experienced midwife who practised in London, but even that is uncertain. It is possible that Jane Sharp was a pseudonym.

Selected Publications

Sharp J. *The Midwives Book or, the Whole Art of Midwifry Discovered.* London: Simon Miller; 1671. Annotated Edition, Hobby E (ed.). *Women's Writers in English.* New York, NY: Oxford University Press; 1999.

Sharp J. *The Compleat Midwife's Companion or, The Art of Midwifry Improved.* 3rd edn. London: John Marshall; 1724.

Bibliography References

46, 102, 169, 419, 515, 534, 548, 809, 982, 1386, 1682, 1710.

Sheehan, Harold Leeming (1900–1988)

Sheehan's Syndrome

Sheehan's syndrome is the occurrence of post-partum hypopituitarism associated with infarction of the anterior pituitary. The infarction is due to thrombosis of the vulnerable hypophyseal portal vessels secondary to hypotension, usually due to obstetric haemorrhage. In the full-blown case there is failure to produce all the trophic hormones, with subsequent impairment of thyroid, adrenal and ovarian function. The classical clinical picture is one of failure to lactate, rapid breast involution and amenorrhoea with later loss of axillary and pubic hair, genital and breast atrophy and signs and symptoms of hypothyroidism and adrenal insufficiency. However, the amount of pituitary infarcted can vary, and sufficient function may be maintained to allow resumption of ovulation and reproduction.

In 1914 Morris Simmonds, a German pathologist in Hamburg, described chronic hypopituitarism in a woman who died 11 years after surviving severe puerperal sepsis and in whom, at autopsy, the pituitary was severely atrophied. One year earlier LK Glinski, a Polish pathologist in Krakow, described extensive pituitary necrosis in two women who died some days after severe obstetric haemorrhage. However, it was Harold Sheehan who made a comprehensive study of post-partum necrosis and delineated the pathogenesis and consequences in more than ten publications between 1937 and 1968.

Harold Sheehan worked as pathologist to the Glasgow Royal Maternity Hospital in the 1930s and noted the association between necrosis of the anterior pituitary and post-partum haemorrhage in the not uncommon maternal deaths of that era:

The significance of necrosis of the anterior pituitary chiefly concerns its relationship to a series of disorders of pituitary function which culminate in Simmond's disease. As the lesion is an irreversible one its aetiology is of importance from the standpoint of possible prophylaxis.

In reviewing the contribution of obstetric deaths to anterior pituitary necrosis Sheehan performed autopsies on 76 consecutive maternal deaths at the Glasgow Royal Maternity Hospital. He found 12 cases of anterior pituitary necrosis with a distinct pattern:

The necrosis centres usually in the antero-inferior part of the anterior lobe in the mid-line and spreads out to involve most of the lobe. The parts which normally escape are the postero-superior angle beneath and in front of the stalk and a very thin layer on the surface . . . the situation of the necrosis suggests a peculiar distribution of blood supply to the anterior lobe during pregnancy.

Sheehan's careful studies showed that the cause of necrosis was thrombosis of the pituitary vessels, usually secondary to haemorrhagic shock:

It is significant that, in the few cases where haemorrhage is not recorded, collapse due to other causes occurred.

As Sheehan developed his interest in the relationship between obstetric haemorrhage and pituitary necrosis, it was the custom to summon him to the maternity unit when such cases occurred, so he could start the autopsy as soon as possible and avoid post-mortem autolysis. The story is told, apocryphal perhaps, of the patient with post-partum haemorrhage who remained near death for several hours. She eventually recovered and as she was leaving the hospital, knowing how close to death she had been, thanked the nursing sister and medical staff for saving her life. She also asked if they would convey her gratitude to the senior, grey-haired consultant whose hovering attendance she had noted during the critical hours of her care. She was referring to Sheehan, whose peripheral attendance was for a potential purpose other than her recovery.

It was also during his time in Glasgow that Sheehan described liver damage in pregnant women after chloroform anaesthesia, a condition known in France as *maladie de Sheehan.*

Harold Leeming Sheehan was born in Carlisle, England, the son of a general practitioner. He was a medical graduate of Manchester University in 1922 and followed this with six years' general practice in Carlisle before returning to Manchester as a lecturer in pathology. In 1934 he spent a year as a Rockefeller Fellow at the Johns Hopkins Hospital in Baltimore. He returned to an appointment as pathologist to the Royal Maternity Hospital in Glasgow. During the Second World War he served as a medical officer, directing the pathology services at the allied headquarters in Italy. In 1946 he was appointed professor of pathology at Liverpool University, which position he held until he retired in 1965. He spent the next 15 years analysing his collection of histological specimens and wrote two books, the last of which, *Post-partum Hypopituitarism,* was published when he was 82.

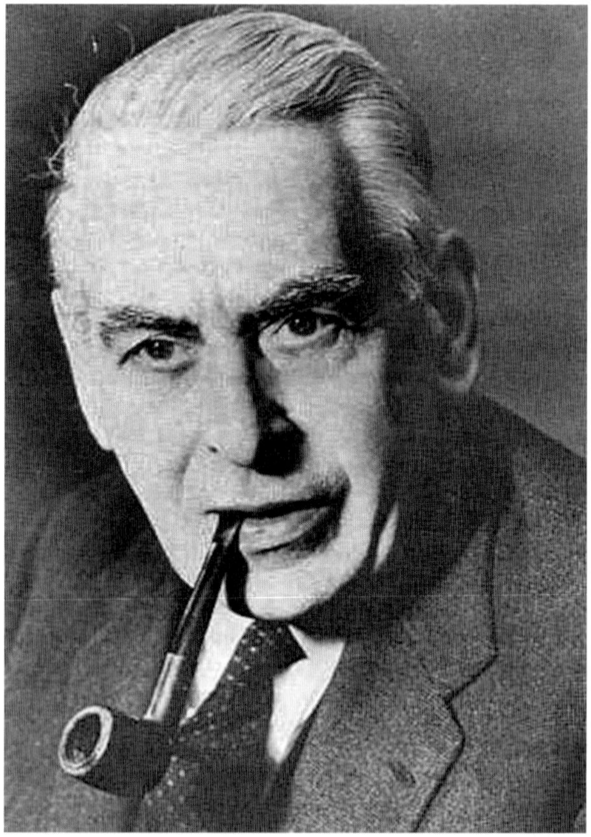

Harold Leeming Sheehan

Selected Publications

Glinski LK. Anatomische veranderungen der hypophyse. *Dtsch Med Wochenschr* 1913; 39: 473.

Sheehan HL. Post-partum necrosis of the anterior pituitary. *J Pathol Bacteriol* 1937; 45: 189–214.

Sheehan HL, Murdoch R. Post-partum necrosis of the anterior pituitary: Pathological and clinical aspects. *J Obstet Gynaecol Br Emp* 1938; 45: 456–72.

Sheehan HL. Simmonds disease due to postpartum necrosis of the anterior pituitary following postpartum haemorrhage. *Quart J Med* 1939; 32: 277–309.

Simmonds M. Über hypophysisschwund mit tödlichem Ausgang. *Dtsch Med Wochenschr* 1914; 40: 322–3.

Bibliography References

364, 661, 804, 855, 1396.

Shirodkar, Vithal Nagesh (1899–1971)

Shirodkar Cervical Suture

The problem of second trimester pregnancy loss was approached in a surgical manner by Shirodkar in 1955:

> *There are some unfortunate women who abort repeatedly between the fourth and seventh months; no amount of rest and treatment with hormones seem to help them in retaining the products of conception . . . My work so far has been confined to cases where one can, by repeated internal examinations, prove the existence of weakness of the internal os, which gradually yields to the rising intra-uterine pressure . . . All these cases can be saved by a simple operation, done during pregnancy, when one finds that the cervix is gradually yielding. I have operated upon them, even when they had entered the seventh month of pregnancy, with no ill effects and they have gone to full term.*

Shirodkar's technique involved removing a strip of fascia lata from the patient's thigh. Using anterior and posterior incisions in the cervix at the level of the internal os, an aneurysm needle was used to encircle the cervix with the fascial strip under the cervical mucosa. The fascia was then tightened and sutured to close the internal os and the cervical incisions were sutured over the fascia. Shirodkar advised delivery by caesarean section at term. He claimed success in 30 women so treated. Others modified his technique: one of the simplest being that devised by Ian McDonald.

Vithal Nagesh Shirodkar was born in Goa, in the village of Shiroda from which his family name was derived. He took his medical degree at Grant Medical College, Bombay, in 1923, and his specialist MD in obstetrics and gynaecology from the University of Bombay in 1927. He was consultant to several hospitals in Bombay and appointed professor of midwifery and

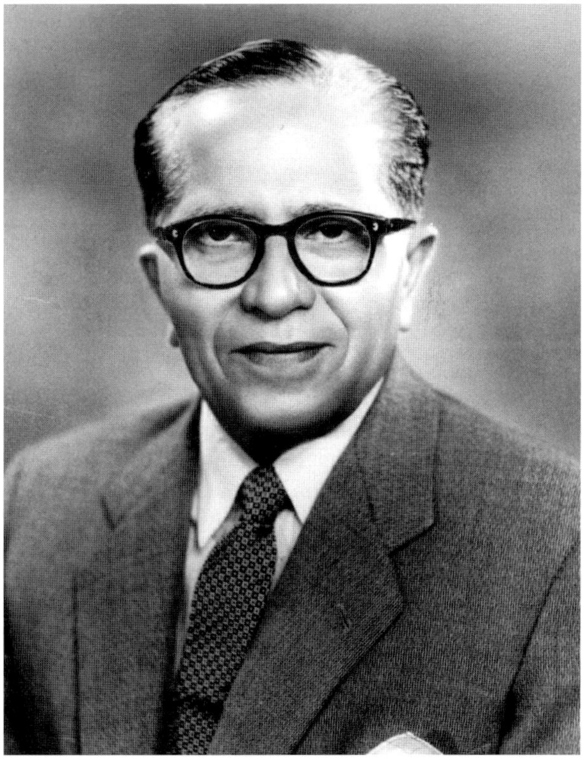

Vithal Nagesh Shirodkar

gynaecology at Grant Medical College in 1940. An innovative and celebrated surgeon who also devised two operations for genital prolapse, Shirodkar rarely operated without an audience of keen observers. He gained international recognition and lectured widely, being one of the first to show films of his operations. In 1963 he became president of the Federation of Obstetric and Gynaecological Societies of India and received the honorary fellowship of the Royal College of Obstetricians and Gynaecologists. In his day he was a good tennis and golf player. He also painted and exhibited his work at the Bombay Art Society. He died on 7 March 1971 from cardiac disease.

Selected Publications

Shirodkar VN. A new method of operative treatment for habitual abortions in the second trimester of pregnancy. *Antiseptic* 1955; 52: 299–300.

Shirodkar VN. Habital abortion in the second trimester. In: *Contributions to Obstetrics and Gynaecology.* Edinburgh and London: E & S Livingstone Ltd; 1960, pp. 1–15.

Bibliography References

1405, 1406, 1561.

Sigault, Jean René (b. 1740)

Symphysiotomy

In 1768, at a meeting of the Royal Academy of Surgery of France, Jean René Sigault proposed an operation to divide the symphysis pubis, thereby enlarging the pelvis and providing an alternative to caesarean section and destructive operations on the fetus. He claimed to have gained at least 2.5 cm in the pelvic diameters with this procedure in cadavers. The Academy was not impressed. He pursued the idea in his graduation thesis and later received support in principle from Pieter Camper. His opportunity came on 30 September 1777, when, with the assistance of one Alphonse le Roy, he performed symphysiotomy on a soldier's wife who had four previous stillborn infants and produced a live child. The patient was a rachitic dwarf 'three feet, eight inches high', said to have an obstetric conjugate of only 6.5 cm. Her postoperative course was stormy, with infection, vesicovaginal fistula and inability to walk for two months. However, following a committee review, the Faculty of Medicine of Paris enthusiastically endorsed the procedure. Sigault was widely praised, received a royal pension and a medal was struck to commemorate the event – not a bad haul for one short operation with severe complications. The patient, Madame Souchot, received admiration from the Faculty for 'her spirit and fortitude, the members being very sorry it was not in their power to allow her and her child a pension'.

Symphysiotomy was adopted in Europe but never received much support elsewhere and, as the attendant mortality and morbidity were high, it fell into disuse. It was revived in the late nineteenth century

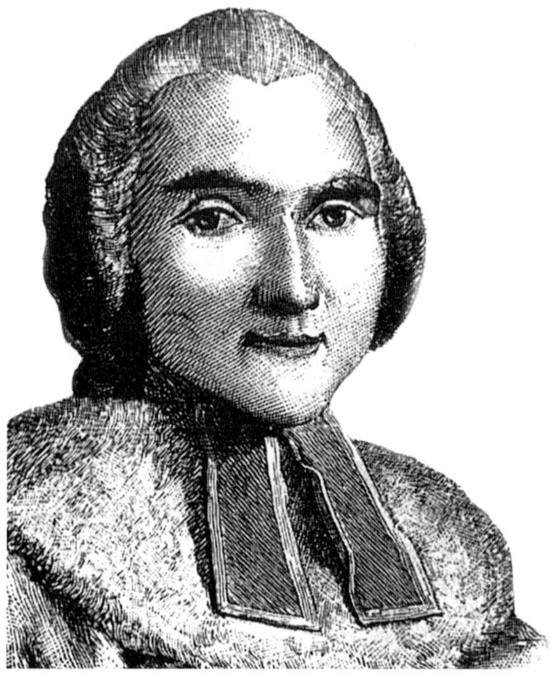

Jean René Sigault

and has had selected but diminishing application since then.

Jean René Sigault was born in Dijon in 1740. He received his mastership in surgery from the Collège de Saint-Côme at Paris in 1770. He entered the École de Médecine in 1772 and graduated in 1776. It was in this graduation thesis that he proposed symphysiotomy. He established a successful obstetric practice in Paris. The date of his death is unknown

Selected Publications

Sigault JR. Mémoire. In: *Aux assemblées du 3 et du 6 Décembre 1777*. Paris: Faculty of Medicine; 1777.

Sigault JR. *Discours sur les Avantages de la Section de la Symphyse dans les Accouchements*. Paris; Quillau; 1779.

Bibliography References

102, 298, 452, 548, 608, 609, 648, 692, 1261, 1408, 1728.

Simpson, James Young (1811–1870)

Chloroform in Obstetrics/Simpson's Forceps

At 2.45 p.m. on Friday 13 May 1870, a funeral procession one mile long and with 2,000 people set off from 52 Queen Street, Edinburgh. All activity ceased in the city and 30,000 citizens lined the route past the early blooms in the Edinburgh Botanical Gardens to Warriston Cemetery. There was no formal service at the graveside, only the words spoken by the minister: 'Such men are rare. We cannot hope to see his like again'. The object of this unprecedented city-wide show of respect was Sir James Young Simpson, late professor of midwifery at the University of Edinburgh.

Simpson first used ether anaesthesia during labour in January 1847. Because of the difficulties in administering it for a prolonged time he sought a simpler alternative. After much self-experimentation he discovered the anaesthetic properties of chloroform at his home during after-dinner tests with his assistants, Drs Matthews Duncan and George Keith, on 4 November 1847. Four days later he administered it during labour to a doctor's wife with such good effect that she christened the resultant daughter 'Anaesthesia':

> *The lady to whom it was first exhibited during parturition had previously been delivered in the country by perforation of the head of the infant, after a labour of three days duration. In this, her second confinement, pains supervened a fortnight before the full time. Three hours and a half after they commenced, and ere the first stage of the labour was completed, I placed her under the influence of the chloroform, by moistening, with half a teaspoon of the liquid, a pocket handkerchief, rolled up into a funnel shape, and with the broad or open end of the funnel placed over her mouth and nostrils. In consequence of the evaporation of the fluid, it was once more renewed in about ten or twelve minutes. The child was expelled in about twenty-five minutes after the inhalation was begun.*

He read this account to the Medico-Chirurgical Society of Edinburgh on 10 November 1847. Simpson emphasised the ease and safety of the technique, requiring only a small bottle of chloroform and a pocket handkerchief. Within a few days, he also gave chloroform anaesthesia for surgical procedures on children. Like Walter Channing in the United States, Simpson faced much criticism both within and without the medical profession. With his wide knowledge of literature and the scriptures, Simpson was well able to deal with his detractors. Religious objections were raised and the Bible quoted, Genesis 3:16: 'in sorrow thou shalt bring forth children'. Simpson quoted back, Genesis 2:21: 'And the lord God caused a deep sleep to fall upon Adam, and he slept: and he took one of his ribs, and closed up the flesh instead thereof'. He quoted the words of Galen: 'pain is useless to the pained'. In his own words he summed up his philosophy:

> *All pain is per se, and especially when in excess, destructive and even ultimately fatal in its action and effects . . . the great pain accompanying human parturition is no exception to this general pathological law.*

The debate continued for years until Queen Victoria had chloroform administered by Dr John Snow during her labour in April 1853. Later the Queen's physician, Sir James Clark, who attended the delivery, wrote to Simpson telling him:

> *The Queen had chloroform exhibited to her during her late confinement . . . Her Majesty was greatly pleased with the effect, and she certainly never has had a better recovery.*

Realising the importance of this influential event, he added:

> *I know this information will please you, and I have little doubt it will lead to a more general use of chloroform in midwifery practice in this quarter than has hitherto prevailed.*

After this widely publicised regal event, chloroform *à la reine*, the technique became widely accepted. Sir James Clark (1789–1876) was a graduate of Edinburgh who in his early career practised in Rome. Here he looked after the poet John Keats during his last illness.

James Young Simpson was the seventh son and eighth child born to a family in Bathgate, Scotland. He was not christened 'Young' but acquired and retained that appellation. His father was a baker and former whisky distiller and his mother was descended from French Huguenots. His mother was 40 when he was born, and she died nine years later. Although he came from working stock, this was a society that cherished education. Young James' propensity for learning was encouraged, and he went up to Edinburgh University when he was only 14. Initially enrolled in arts, he changed to medicine and finished the course when he was 18, though he could not take his MD until he was 20. For a time, he worked as an assistant to the professor of pathology and then turned his attention to obstetrics. He was appointed to the Leith Lying-in Hospital and began to lecture and write extensively. When only 29 years old he applied for the vacant chair of midwifery at Edinburgh. In a contest with Evory Kennedy, he was elected by one vote. He wrote home, 'I was elected professor today by a majority of one. Hurrah!' His lectures and writings were well received and he built a large private practice. As one biographer put it, 'his name was writ in chloroform, but he was first and last an obstetrician'. His energy and inventive output were enormous. Within a year of introducing chloroform anaesthesia he presented his 'air tractor', the forerunner of the modern vacuum extractor produced a century later, and his obstetric forceps that bear his name and continue in use. He also emphasised the use of bimanual pelvic examination and reintroduced the uterine sound to gynaecology. He was one of the best known and respected medical men of his era and was showered with many international honours. He was knighted in 1866.

In February of 1870 he became ill with angina and shortness of breath. By April he realised he would not recover, amended his will, and declared that he would die: 'Well, I have done some work. I wish I had been busier'. His family gathered, and he died peacefully at home on 6 May 1870. His wife refused the offer of burial in Westminster Abbey, and he was laid to rest in Warriston Cemetery in Edinburgh. Eight male Simpson relatives lowered the coffin into the grave. There is a marble bust of him in St Andrew's Chapel of Westminster Abbey with the inscription, 'To whose genius and benevolence the world owes the blessings derived from the use of chloroform for the relief of suffering'. In 1997 a memorial plaque to Simpson was placed in St Giles Cathedral, Edinburgh to mark the 150th anniversary of the introduction of chloroform to obstetrics. His home at 52 Queen Street, Edinburgh remains, and the dining room table below which he,

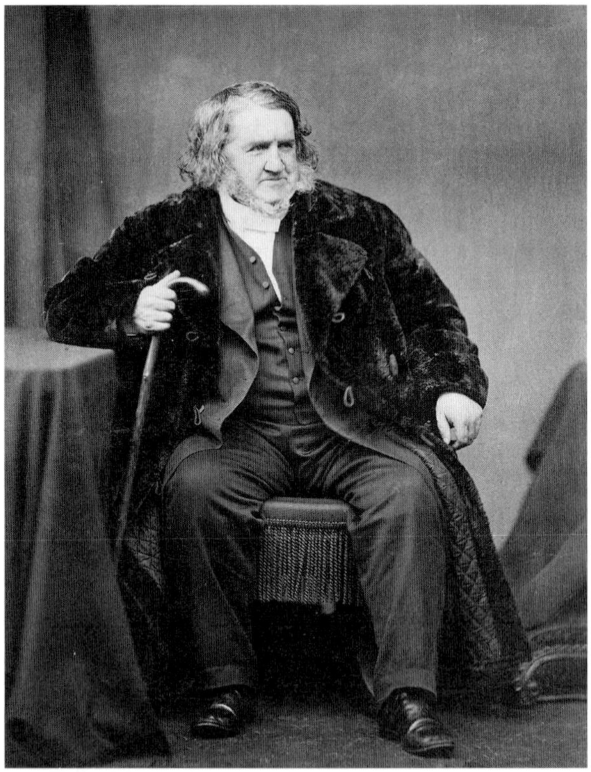

James Young Simpson

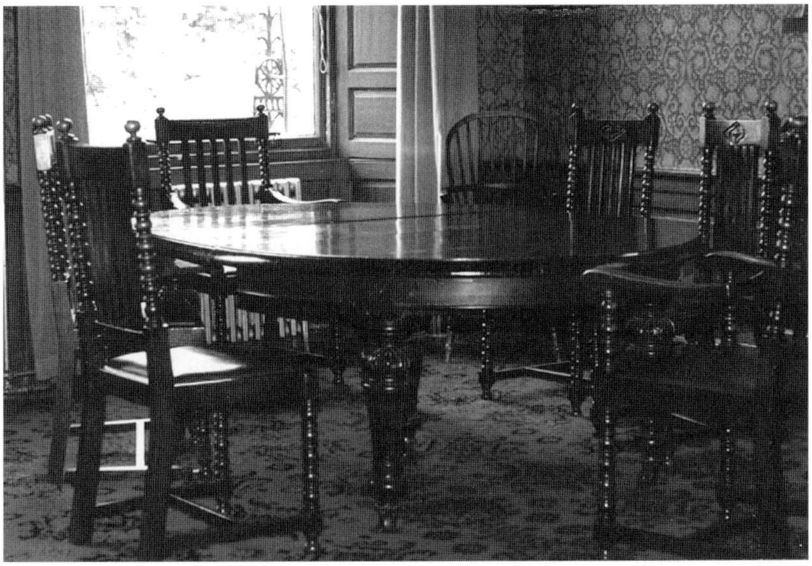

The dining table in the front room of 52 Queen Street, Edinburgh

Keith and Duncan gracefully slid after self-induced anaesthesia with chloroform, is still in the front room.

Selected Publications

Simpson JY. Notes on the equipment of sulphuric ether in the practice of midwifery. *Monthly J Med Sci.* 1847; 75: 638–40.

Simpson JY. *Answer to the Religious Objections Advanced Against the Employment of Anaesthetic Agents in Midwifery and Surgery.* Edinburgh: Sutherland and Knox; 1847, p. 23.

Simpson JY. Discovery of a new anaesthetic agent, more effective than sulphuric ether. *London Med Gazette* 1847; 40: 934–7, and *Lancet* 1847; 2: 549–51.

Simpson JY. On the mode of application of the long forceps. *Monthly J Med Sci* 1848; 26: 193–6.

Bibliography References

35, 56, 81, 92, 130, 252, 253, 259, 260, 287, 299, 319, 325, 327, 361, 363, 400, 435, 446, 453, 490, 521, 533, 558, 589, 641, 650, 696, 743, 807, 822, 956, 1017, 1048, 1062, 1065, 1263, 1338, 1403, 1421–1424, 1479, 1666.

Sims, James Marion (1813–1883)

Vesicovaginal Fistula/Sims' Speculum/Sims' Position

Although there were isolated successes in the surgical closure of vesicovaginal fistula by Gosset in England and John Mettauer and George Hayward in the United States, it was James Marion Sims of Alabama whose persistence achieved a reproducible surgical technique for cure. On 18 November 1857 Sims gave the anniversary discourse before the New York Academy of Medicine, entitled 'Silver Sutures in Surgery':

> *In 1845 I conceived the idea of curing vesicovaginal fistula, and entered upon the broad field of experiment with all the ardour and enthusiasm of a devotee. After nearly four years of fruitless labour, silver wire was fortunately substituted for silk as a suture, and lo! a new era dawns upon surgery. This was done on the 21st June, 1849; since which time I have used no other suture in any department of surgery.*

His route to this 'new era' necessitated almost pathological zeal and tenacity in the face of repeated failure over four years. It all started in 1845 in Montgomery, Alabama, where Sims had been in practice for ten years and had developed a reputation as an able doctor and surgeon. In attempting manual correction of uterine retroversion, Sims placed a patient in the knee-chest position. As he pressed down with his fingers the vagina ballooned open with air and he was able to see the entire length of the anterior vaginal wall. He had just recently seen two young slaves with vesicovaginal fistula and thought:

> *... why can I not take the incurable case of vesicovaginal fistula, which seems now to be so incomprehensible, and put the girl in this position and see exactly what are the relations of the surrounding tissues?*

Sims bought a malleable pewter spoon and fashioned it into a retractor for the posterior vaginal wall. This was the forerunner of Sims' speculum:

> *Introducing the bent handle of the spoon ... the fistula was as plain as the nose on a man's face. The edges were clear and well-defined ... the opening could be measured as accurately as if it had been cut out of a piece of plain paper.*

By this time, another young slave had been sent to see Sims, and others would follow. All had vesicovaginal fistulae secondary to obstetric trauma. This stalwart trio – Lucy, Betsey and Anarcha – would spend the next four years in a small hospital Sims built behind his home. He modified existing instruments or designed his own, including a malleable self-retaining tin catheter. Thus prepared and fired with enthusiasm he operated on Lucy on 10 January 1846 and 'expected at once a magical cure'. He failed, as he was to do on 40 occasions over the next three and a half years. Sims was obsessed with his 'mission of divine origin' and, in dramatic mode later wrote, 'My repeated failures brought about a degree of anguish that I cannot now depict even if it were desirable'. However, he added, 'never for one moment did I despair of eventual success'. One imagines that his patients must have despaired at times, although Sims stated they 'implored me to repeat operations so tedious, and at the same time so painful, that none but a woman could have borne them'. Personal tragedy also struck Sims at this time, when his three-year-old son died of gastroenteritis in October 1848.

There are those who have condemned Sims for 'experimentation' on these unfortunate women. His approach must be placed in the context of the almost indescribable, unremitting and incurable misery inflicted by a vesicovaginal fistula. Sims called it 'one of the most loathsome maladies that can possibly befall poor human nature'. Johan Friedrich Dieffenbach (1792–1847) of Königsberg, who laboured for years unsuccessfully to find a surgical cure summed up the wretched plight of these women:

> *A sadder situation can hardly exist than that of a woman afflicted with a vesicovaginal fistula. A source of disgust, even to herself, the woman beloved by her husband becomes, in this condition, the object of bodily revulsion to him; and filled with repugnance, everyone else likewise turns his back, repulsed by the intolerable, foul odour ... A vesicovaginal fistula is the greatest misfortune that can happen to a women, and the more so, because she is condemned to live with it, without the hope to die from it, to submit to all the sequelae of its tortures till she succumbs either to another disease or to old age.*

One problem Sims had to overcome was securing the knots of his sutures high in the vagina. Harking back to his fishing days as a youth, he perforated lead shot and compressed it on the suture, holding the knots in place. These sutures were placed to hold two thin lead cross-bars on either side of the fistulous opening which, when pulled together clamped shut the edges of the fistula. The final step was to have a local jeweller, Mr Swan, make a fine silver thread, Thus, on 21 June 1849, the long-suffering Anarcha underwent the first successful closure of a vesicovaginal fistula at the hand of Sims. In short order, the remaining slaves were cured and returned to their owners. As young, otherwise healthy women, who might have faced decades of incontinent misery, their courage and fortitude over four years had finally paid off.

Sims published an account of his surgical technique in 1852. His move to silver suture material might have occurred earlier had he been aware of Montague Gosset's successful case report in the *Lancet* 15 years before using silver-gilt wire. Gosset described the qualities of the silver-gilt suture as follows: 'It excites but little irritation and does not appear to induce ulceration with the same rapidity as silk or any other material of which I am acquainted'.

James Marion Sims was born on a farm near Hanging Rock, Lancaster County, South Carolina. He was apprenticed to a local doctor, whose daughter he would later marry, and then attended the medical college of Charleston for one year. He transferred to Jefferson Medical College in Philadelphia and graduated in 1835. He established his first practice in Mount Meigs, Alabama and in 1840 moved to Montgomery. During his years in Montgomery, Sims was ill with chronic dysentery. He found that the climate and water of New York improved his health, and he moved there in 1853. On 4 May 1855 he opened the first hospital devoted only to gynaecology and the surgical management of vesicovaginal fistula. The Women's Hospital of New York on 83 Madison Avenue had a ten-bed unit and treated about 250 fistula patients per year with a 75 per cent cure rate. He spent most of 1861 visiting Dublin, London, Edinburgh and Paris, demonstrating his surgical technique. He returned to New York in 1862, but because of the Civil War and his confederate loyalties, he went back to Europe, where he remained for the next five years. During the Franco-Prussian War of 1870 he returned to Europe as surgeon-in-chief of the Anglo-American Ambulance Corps. For his role in treating the wounded of both sides, he received the Legion of Honour from the French and the Iron Cross from the Germans.

Sims made many contributions to surgery in general as well as gynaecology. He studied infertility in detail, in particular the survival of spermatozoa in the cervical and vaginal secretions – the forerunner of the Sims–Hühner postcoital test. He would later recognise that the exhausting and undignified knee-chest position was unnecessary for most speculum examinations and procedures. Thus, the 'Sims position' evolved as follows:

The patient is to lie on the left side. The thighs are to be flexed at about right angles with the pelvis, the right being drawn up a little more than the left. The left arm is thrown behind across the back, and the chest rotated forwards, bringing the sternum very nearly in contact with the table . . . Indeed, the position must simulate that on the knees as much as possible, and for this reason the patient is rolled over on the front, making it a left lateral semiprone position.

Sims resigned from the Women's Hospital in 1874 after a dispute with the board of the hospital. They imposed a limit of 15 spectators at operations and refused to admit patients with cancer. Sims disagreed on both points. In 1876 he was elected president of the American Medical Association and in 1880 served as president of the American Gynecological Society. He died of a coronary thrombosis on 13 November 1883.

In the continuing debate about the motives and ethics of Sims' relentless pursuit of a surgical cure for vesicovaginal fistula, perhaps the testimony of one women cured by his surgery is the most symbolically relevant. Speaking in support of fund raising for the Women's Hospital in New York in 1857 she said:

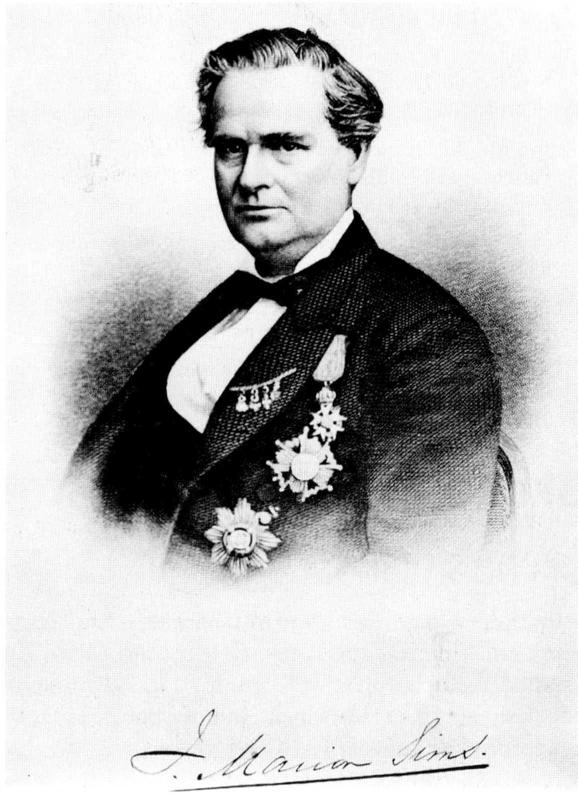

James Marion Sims

After sixteen years of the greatest anguish and suffering . . . a stranger. . . told me of the Women's Hospital in New York, and of the wonderful cures effected there. I am once more restored to my sex, my husband, my child and my home.

Professional recognition was renewed almost a century later by Chassar Moir, a subsequent master of the surgery of vesicovaginal fistulae:

To James Marion Sims, more than any man, is due the honour for this transformation. And, if a moment can be spared for sentimental reverie, look again, I beg, at his curious speculum and, gazing through the confused reflections from its bright curves, catch a glimpse of an old hut in Alabama and seven negro women who suffered, and endured, and had a rich reward.

A bronze statue of Marion Sims used to stand in Central Park, New York. Because of opposition to his surgical work involving slaves it has been moved to Greenwood Cemetery in Brooklyn, where Sims is buried.

Selected Publications

Dieffenbach J F. Über die Heilung der Blasen-Scheiden-Fisteln und Zerreissungen der Blase und Scheide. *Med Zeitung* 1836; 5: 117.

Gosset M. Calculus in the bladder-incontinence of urine-vesicovaginal fistula. Advantages of the gilt-wire suture. *Lancet* 1834; 1: 345–6.

Moir JC. J Marion Sims and the vesico-vaginal fistula: then and now. *BMJ* 1940; 2: 773–5

Sims JY. On the treatment of vesicovaginal fistula. *Am J Med Sci* 1852; 23: 59–82.

Sims JY. *Silver Sutures in Surgery. The Anniversary Discourse before the New York Academy of Medicine.* New York, NY: Samuel S and William Wood; 1858.

Sims J Y. *Clinical Notes on Uterine Surgery.* London: Robert Hardwicke; 1866. Also published in: The Classics of Obstetrics and Gynecology Library. Birmingham: Gryphon Editions; 1990 (facsimile).

Bibliography References

153, 184, 242, 356, 525, 631, 648, 657, 694, 725, 794, 811, 820, 931, 984, 1018, 1058, 1089, 1167, 1173, 1278, 1334, 1338, 1425, 1451, 1588, 1643, 1660, 1683, 1739, 1740.

Skene, Alexander Johnston Chalmers (1837–1900)

Skene's Glands

Alexander Skene was born in Aberdeenshire, Scotland, and emigrated to America at the age of 19. He studied medicine first at Toronto, 1860–1, then at the University of Michigan and finally graduated MD from the Long Island College Hospital, Brooklyn in 1863. He became professor of gynaecology and later dean at Long Island College Hospital. From 1899 he ran Skene's Hospital for self-supporting women.

The female urethra is surrounded by glands, considered the homologue of the male prostate. Some of these paraurethral glands enter the urethra directly and some via the paraurethral ducts, described by Skene in 1880. He wrote:

> *When I first described these glands I presumed they were mucous follicles that were accidently of unusual size in the subject examined, but having investigated more than one hundred of these, in many different subjects, and finding them constantly present, and so uniform in size and location, I became satisfied that they were worthy of a separate place in descriptive anatomy.*

In fact the paraurethral ducts were first described in 1672 by Regnier de Graaf in *De mulierum organis generationi inservientibus*, but had long disappeared from the anatomical texts of Skene's time. As an obstetrician, Skene was one of the early proponents of extraperitoneal caesarean section.

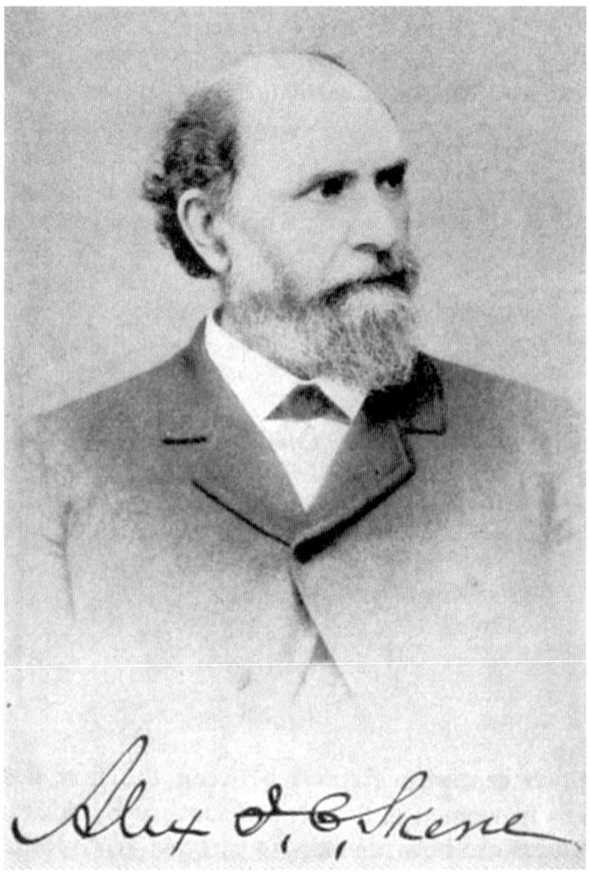

Alexander Johnston Chalmers Skene

Alexander Skene was a founding member of the American Gynecological Society and served as its tenth president in 1886. He received an honorary

LLD from Aberdeen University in 1897. He had an athletic physique and described himself as 'last in class, first in field sports'. A productive man, he did his writing before breakfast. Skene also served as mayor of Brooklyn before it became a borough of New York City. His statue stands in Prospect Park in Brooklyn.

Selected Publications

Skene AJC. The anatomy and pathology of two important glands of the female urethra. *Am J Obstet Dis Women Child* 1880; 13: 265–70.

Bibliography References

102, 406, 648, 968, 1428, 1429, 1472, 1480.

Smead, Louis (c.1940)
Jones, Thomas (c.1940)

Smead–Jones Suture

In the early days of abdominal surgery, wound dehiscence was common and associated with significant mortality. Better suture materials and wound closure techniques have reduced this complication. One of the methods with the lowest risk of wound dehiscence is the mass closure technique devised by Louis Smead. This was first reported from the Cleveland Clinic in 1941 by Thomas Jones and his colleagues, Newell and Brubaker. They used alloy steel wire and recorded no wound disruptions in 116 cases, at a time when figures of 3–5 per cent dehiscence were common. They clearly attributed the suture technique to Louis Smead:

> *This stitch was devised by Dr Louis Smead of Toledo, Ohio, during his residency in surgery under Dr John Finney, Sr of Baltimore. We have been advised by personal communication that a description of its use has not been published by him.*

The technique involves a figure-of-eight suture passing through anterior fascia, rectus muscle, posterior fascia and peritoneum on both sides. One end is then passed through the anterior fascia on both sides again. When tied, all layers act as one retention level and the anterior fascia as a second level. This suture technique is still used by many in patients at increased risk for wound dehiscence and has come to be known as the Smead–Jones suture. It is simple and effective and, although since modified, the principle remains intact.

Selected Publications

Jones TE, Newell ET, Brubaker RE. The use of alloy steel wire in the closure of abdominal wounds. *Surg Gynecol Obstet* 1941; 72: 1056–9.

Smellie, William (1697–1763)

Mauriceau–Smellie–Veit Manoeuvre/Obstetric Forceps

It is appropriate that much has been written on this diligent, honest and modest man, who achieved so much without privilege or hospital appointment. By working among the poor, he gained enormous clinical experience and, with critical appraisal of his own work, learned so much which he bequeathed to students through his classes and books. He has deservedly been accorded the title, 'the Master of British Midwifery'. Robert Johnstone, former professor of midwifery at the University of Edinburgh, and a biographer of Smellie, described his work as a bridge from 'blundering medievil [sic] midwifery to the beginnings of the science and art of obstetrics'.

William Smellie, an only child, was born in Lesmahagow near Lanark, Scotland, at that time a town of about 2,000 people. He was educated at Lanark Grammar School and then served a medical apprenticeship, probably with a Dr Gordon of Glasgow. He settled into general practice in Lanark in 1720, at the age of 23. From the outset he had an affinity for obstetrics and kept a record of all his cases, which later formed part of his treatise. He was admitted to membership as a surgeon in the Faculty of Physicians and Surgeons of Glasgow in 1733 and was awarded the MD by the University of Glasgow in 1745.

In 1739 he left Lanark for London, in the hope of learning more about obstetrics, and subsequently spent some months in Paris studying the methods of Grégoire. He was disappointed by the level of knowledge in both cities, returned to London and established his obstetric practice in the district of Pall Mall, 'around the slums and rookeries near St Pauls Cathedral'. His modest and logical approach to learning is captured in this comment:

> *When I first began to practice, I determined to follow the method of these gentlemen; but having by those means lost several children, and sometimes the mother, I began to alter my opinion, and consult my own reason.*

His own reason led him to do more to raise the knowledge and level of obstetric practice over the next 20 years than any other individual. Acknowledging and following the initial observations of Fielding Ould on the mechanism of entry of the fetal head into the pelvic brim during labour, Smellie established the method of descent and rotation. This was outlined by Pieter Camper in notes he took while attending Smellie's lectures in London:

> *He gives an entirely new theory of the fetus descending head first into the pelvis as the most usual condition, the head of the fetus undoubtedly descending obliquely so that one ear faces the pubes, the other the os sacrum; he concludes this to be the more natural because of the greater width of the pelvis, noting everywhere the diameter crossways of the head of the fetus is an inch shorter than the diameter lengthways. Then, when the head is in position in the pelvis, it gradually turns with the occiput towards the pubes until its diameter lengthways corresponds to the larger diameter in the lower part of the pelvis.*

Smellie emphasised a more scientific approach to evaluating the mechanism of labour, part of which was the pelvic measurements. He described the most important component of clinical pelvimetry, the diagonal conjugate, and its relevance:

> *... with the tip of my finger I could hardly reach the jutting forward of the last vertebra of the loins and upper part of the sacrum; from which circumstance I understood the pelvis at that part was not above half or three-quarters of an inch narrower than those that are well formed.*

Within two years of starting practice in London, Smellie began his courses of lectures and instruction for both midwives and physicians. Over a ten-year period, he gave 280 courses, involving 900 students in the management of over 1,000 labours. He also devised and built models and manikins of the pelvis and fetus to aid instruction:

> *I considered that there was a possibility of forming machines, which should so exactly imitate real women and children, as to exhibit to the learner, all the difficulties that happen in midwifery, and such I actually contrived, and made by dint of uncommon labour and application.*

Smellie became a master in the use of forceps, although he consistently cautioned how rarely they were necessary: 'only ten out of one thousand labours required instrumental delivery'. He started using Dusée's forceps but, like others, found them quite impractical. He also studied the models of Edmund Chapman and William Giffard and eventually devised his own short straight forceps and a longer version with a pelvic curve. He perfected the English lock, which is still in use. The basic rules he laid down for the application of forceps remain relevant.

Smellie was the first to use forceps for the after-coming head of the breech, as illustrated in his *Anatomical Tables*, published in 1754. He advocated his long forceps with the pelvic curve for this purpose: 'I have found them very serviceable in helping along the head in preternatural cases after the body and arms of the foetus were brought down'.

Like all obstetricians Smellie was faced with the conundrum of the obstructed occipito-posterior position. When applied in relation to the pelvis, the forceps would slip off and traumatise the head. Faced with such a case, Smellie introduced the blades of the forceps 'along the ears' and improvised:

> *I luckily thought of trying to raise the head with the forceps, and turn the forehead to the left side of the brim of the pelvis, where it was widest, an expedient which I immediately executed with greater ease than I expected. I then brought down the vertex to the right ischium, turned it below the pubes, and the forehead into the hollow of the sacrum, and safely delivered the head by pulling it up from the perineum over the pubes. This*

method succeeding so well, gave me great joy, and was the first hint, in consequence of which I deviated from the common method of pulling forcibly along, and fixing the forceps at random on the head. My eyes were now opened to a new field of improvement in the method of using the forceps at random in this position.

It was Smellie's careful study of the diameters of the pelvis and fetal head, as well as the mechanism of labour, that led him to this discovery. In this, the first description of forceps rotation, he would anticipate the work of Christian Kielland by almost two centuries.

Smellie's name is most often remembered in conjunction with the manual method of delivering the aftercoming head of the breech: the Mauriceau–Smellie–Veit manoeuvre. This had been described by Giffard in 1726. Smellie's own technique was very similar:

I introduced a finger into the mouth and by pulling quickly brought the forehead into the concave part of the sacrum; being afraid of overstraining the under-jaw, I quitted that hold and placed a finger on each side of the nose . . . Then I laid the body of the child on that arm and by slipping the fingers of the other hand over the shoulders and on each side of the neck, I got the head safely extracted.

Because of his increasing reputation as a teacher, Smellie was attacked by jealous colleagues and especially by prominent midwives, who saw their influence and role diminishing. Chief among the latter was Elizabeth Nihell, who was particularly against the use of forceps and aimed many vitriolic attacks against Smellie, who did not respond in kind.

Smellie published a three-volume work, *A Treatise of the Theory and Practice of Midwifery*, with the editorial assistance of the physician-writer and fellow Scot, Tobias Smollett (1722–1771). In 1759 Smellie retired back to Lanark. There he completed the third volume of his treatise. Smellie's works were among the first to be published in America, and his international reputation grew as the logic and safety of his teachings came to be appreciated. One of the premier historians of obstetrics, Heinrich Fasbender (1843–1914) of Berlin, said of Smellie, 'He was one of the most important obstetricians of all times and of all countries'.

Smellie was a fair painter and wood carver. Indeed, the picture illustrated in this book is a self-portrait. He was also fond of music, and played the violoncello, organ and flute. He was married but had no children. In March 1763 he died of 'asthma and lethargy'. He left his books to his old school, along with a sum of money for their storage and upkeep. These are now kept in the Lindsay Institute at the Public Library in Lanark. In 1938, Joseph DeLee of Chicago visited the library. He was much impressed and left funds with instructions for the purchase of two chairs. These mahogany chairs are still in place beside the bookcase holding Smellie's collection.

Smellie was buried near the wall of the old St Kentigern Kirk in Lanark. The grave was restored by the obstetrical and gynaecological societies of Glasgow and Edinburgh in 1931. At the base of the grave is a climbing rose with a plaque recording that this was planted by the Scottish Board of the Royal College of Midwives on the occasion of their centenary

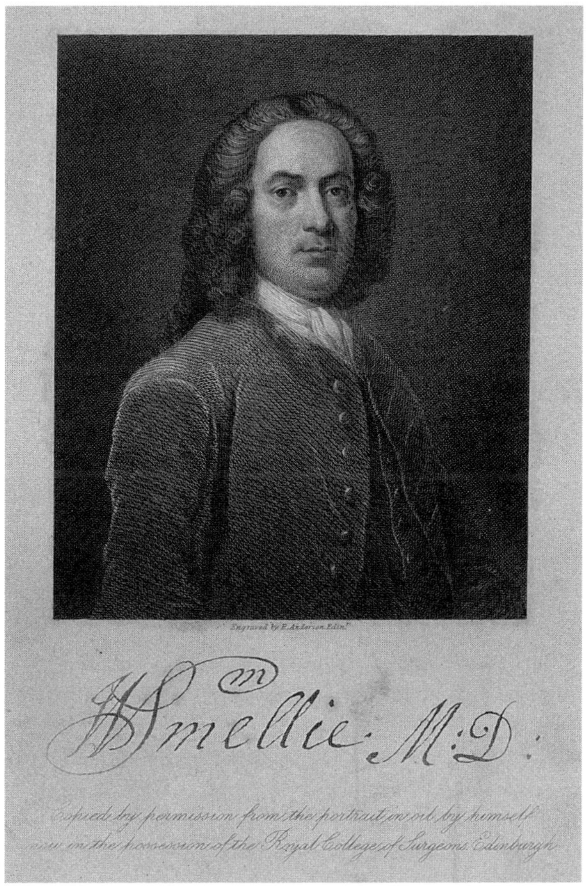

William Smellie

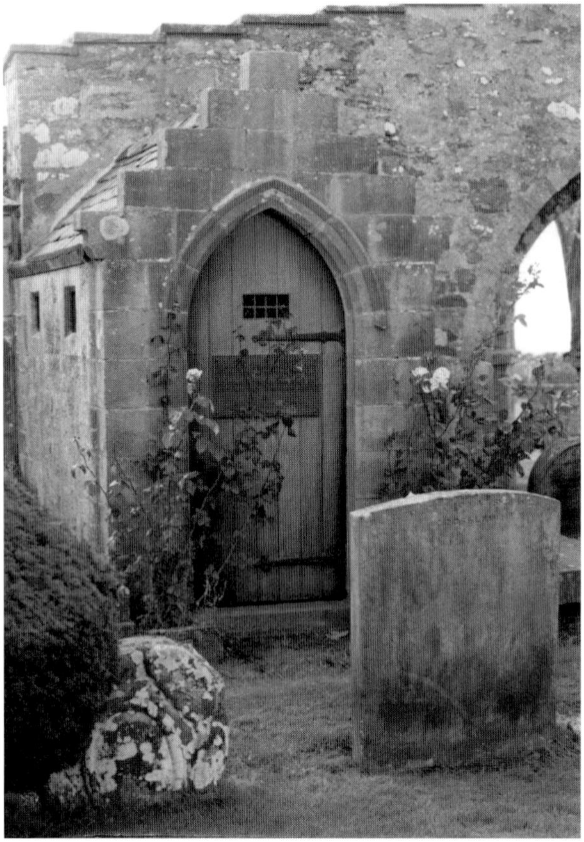

William Smellie's tomb by the wall of the old kirk of St Kentigern at Lanark

in 1981. Belated but touching recognition that William Smellie did so much to elevate the obstetric art for all and without favour taught both midwife and obstetrician.

Selected Publications

Smellie W. *A Treatise on the Theory and Practice of Midwifery* London: D. Wilson; 1752. Also published in: The Classics of Obstetrics and Gynecology Library. Birmingham: Gryphon Editions; 1990 (facsimile).

Smellie W. *A Sett of Anatomical Tables with Explanations and an Abridgement of the Practice of Midwifery.* London; 1754.

Smellie W. *A Collection of Cases and Observations in Midwifery.* (Vol. 2.) London: D. Wilson; 1754. Also published in: The Classics of Obstetrics and Gynecology Library. Birmingham: Gryphon Editions; 1990 (facsimile).

Smellie W. *A Collection of Preternatural Cases and Observations in Midwifery.* (Vol. 3.) London: D. Wilson & T. Durham; 1764. Also published in: The Classics of Obstetrics and Gynecology Library. Birmingham: Gryphon Editions; 1990 (facsimile).

Bibliography References

43, 44, 63, 99, 102, 108, 200, 223, 234, 235, 298, 361, 418, 425–428, 435, 449, 622, 721, 822, 847, 1034, 1261, 1299, 1543, 1575, 1639, 1710.

Smith, Albert Holmes (1835–1885)

Smith–Hodge Pessary

Albert Smith was a prominent obstetrician in Philadelphia during the latter half of the nineteenth century. Shortly after Hugh Hodge designed his pessary, Smith modified it by narrowing the anterior, subpubic end and widening the posterior limb. This became the commonly used Smith–Hodge pessary.

Albert Holmes Smith was born in Philadelphia, a descendant of Quaker ancestors from Yorkshire, England, who were among the earliest settlers of Pennsylvania. He entered the University of Pennsylvania at the age of 14, took his BA in 1853 and graduated MD in 1856.

He was a conservative obstetrician who spoke against the use of ergot in labour and the indiscriminate use of forceps, saying no obstetrician 'should drag a child from the mother except in rare instances'. The

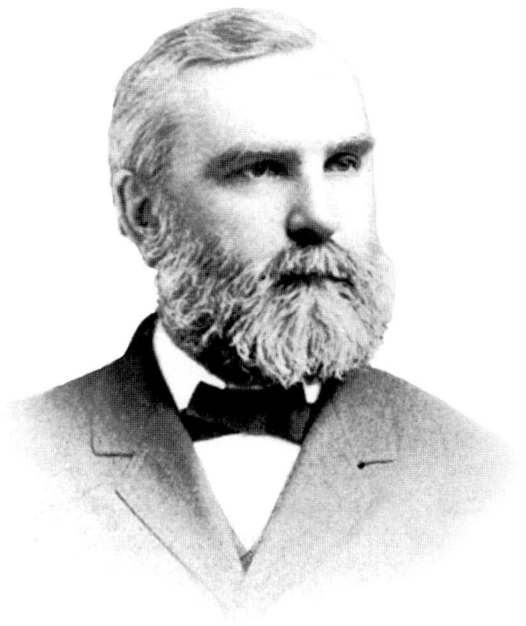

Albert Holmes Smith

Obstetrical Society of Philadelphia was founded at a meeting in his home in June 1868. He was president of the American Gynecological Society in 1884 and an early supporter of women doctors.

He died at his home on 14 December 1885.

Bibliography References

98, 376, 801, 810.

Smithells, Richard Worthington (1924–2002)

Neural Tube Defect Prophylaxis

Richard Smithells was born in Bushey, England, on 12 July 1924. He was educated at Rugby School and St Thomas' Hospital. After graduating in medicine, he did two years' national service in Germany. This was followed by training in paediatrics in Leeds and London. In 1959 he was appointed consultant paediatrician to Alder Hey Children's Hospital in Liverpool. It was here he began his life-long research interest in the prevention and management of congenital malformations.

In 1965 he reported his collaborative work with Elizabeth Hibbard of the department of obstetrics and gynaecology at Liverpool University. They found a five-fold increase in folic acid deficiency in women who had delivered an infant with a neural tube anomaly. They postulated:

> *The familial occurrence of serious nervous system malformations might be mediated, in some instances, through a genetically determined defect of folate metabolism.*

In 1968 Dick Smithells was appointed professor and head of paediatrics at Leeds University. As the evidence linking periconceptual nutritional deficiency and neural tube defects grew, Smithells planned the definitive double-blind controlled trial to assess the merit of vitamin supplementation. This was, however, rejected by three different research ethics committees. He therefore went ahead with two observational intervention studies by giving mothers, who had a previous infant with a neural tube malformation, a periconceptional multivitamin preparation. In the supplemented women the risk of neural tubal defect was reduced seven-fold.

In 1991, the Medical Research Council reported their randomised controlled trial (RCT) more than 10 years after Smithells was denied his own RCT by

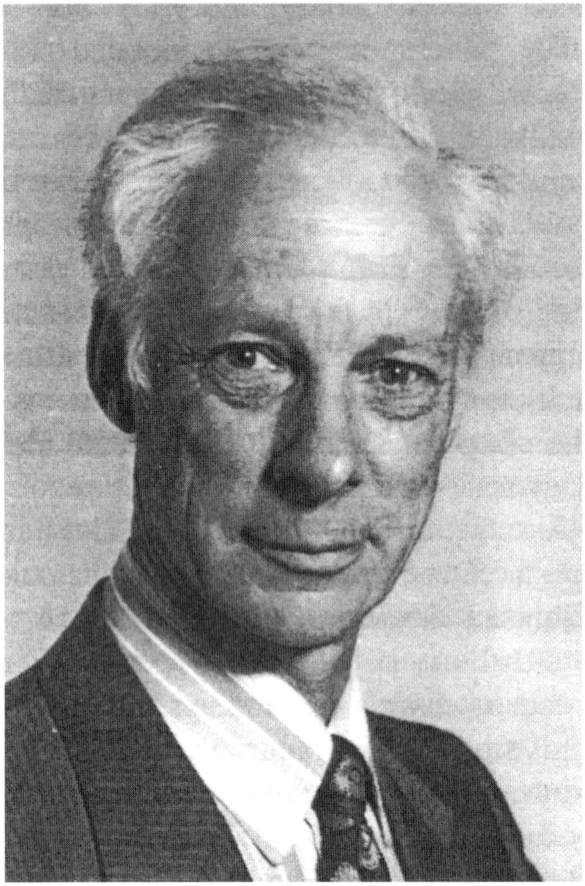

Richard Worthington Smithells

the ethics committees. They found a 72 per cent reduction in neural tube defects by giving mothers a daily supplement of 4 mg folic acid. They concluded:

> *Folic acid supplementation starting before pregnancy can now be firmly recommended for all women who have had an affected pregnancy, and public health measures should be taken to ensure that the diet of all women who bear children contains an adequate amount of folic acid.*

Within days of this report, departments of health in the United Kingdom, United States and many other countries recommended that all women planning pregnancy or becoming pregnant should take folic acid supplementation.

Smithells' work was not limited to his achievement as the prime mover in folic acid prevention of neural tube defects. He was either first or early in establishing congenital anomaly registries, genetic counselling services and rubella vaccination programmes. He was clinically involved in providing comprehensive services to thalidomide children. He worked to secure compensation for them and served as a trustee of the Thalidomide Trust.

In retirement he became an enthusiastic church bell ringer. Dick Smithells died of prostate cancer on 13 June 2002.

Selected Publications

Hibbard ED, Smithells RW. Folic acid metabolism and human embryopathy. *Lancet* 1965; 1: 1254.

Smithells RW, Sheppard S, Schorah CJ. Vitamin deficiencies and neural tube defects. *Arch Dis Child* 1976; 51: 944–9.

Smithells RW. Sheppard S, Schorah CJ. Possible prevention of neural tube defects by periconceptional vitamin supplementation. *Lancet* 1980; 1: 339–40.

MRC Vitamin Study Research Group. Prevention of neural tube defects: results of the MRC Vitamin Study. *Lancet* 1991; 338: 131–7.

Bibliography References

529, 720, 1130, 1442.

Smythe, Henry James Drew (1891–1983)

Drew Smythe Catheter

In the early part of the twentieth century, induction of labour was usually carried out by surgical methods: low amniotomy or insertion of bougies, stomach tubes or hydrostatic bags through the cervix. In reviewing these methods, Drew Smythe concluded that sepsis was the greatest associated risk. He therefore devised his own instrument to rupture the hindwaters, leaving no foreign body in the cervix:

> *For this purpose I have had made a double curved silver catheter similar to a prostatic catheter, with a blunt-ended stylet, which can be protruded at the distal end of the instrument.*

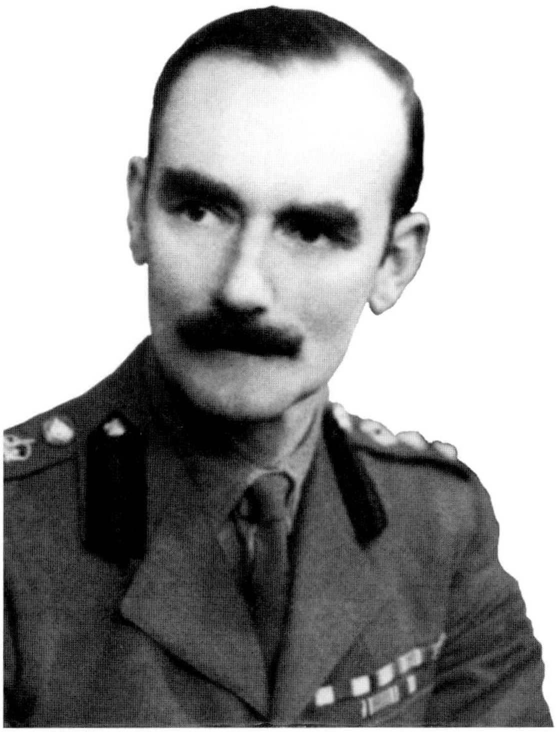

Henry James Drew Smythe

He described his technique at the Bath and Bristol branch meeting of the British Medical Association in March 1931:

> *The catheter, with the point of the stylet withdrawn, is passed up the cervical canal until it meets the child's head: the proximal end is then raised and the point of the catheter is passed behind the head, between the uterine wall and the membranes. When the point of the catheter has passed above the child's head the stylet is pushed home and the proximal end depressed; by so doing the distal end ruptures the membranes . . . liquor amnii commences to flow through the catheter . . . when sufficient has been collected the catheter is withdrawn.*

By retaining the integrity of the forewaters and leaving no foreign body through the cervix, Drew Smythe hoped to reduce the risk of sepsis. The Drew Smythe catheter was used extensively in obstetric practice until the 1960s and occasionally since in selected cases.

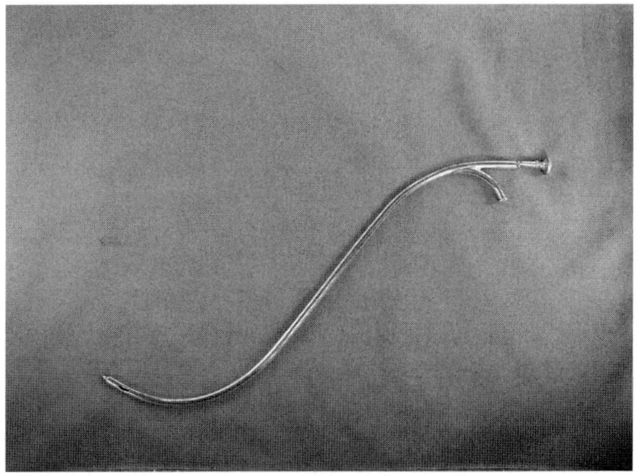

Drew Smythe catheter

Henry James Drew Smythe was born in Bristol and graduated in medicine from the University of Bristol in 1913. He served in the Royal Army Medical Corps in the First World War and received the Military Cross for valour. He became assistant and, later, consultant obstetrician to the Bristol General Hospital. Smythe was professor of obstetrics and gynaecology at the University of Bristol from 1935–50, a part-time appointment in those days.

Selected Publications

Smythe HJD. Indications for the induction of premature labour. *BMJ* 1931; 1: 1018–20.

Smythe HJD, Thompson DJ. Induction of labour by rupture or high puncture of the membranes. *J Obstet Gynaecol Br Emp* 1937; 44: 480–93.

Bibliography References

273, 1574.

Snow, John (1813–1858)

Chloroform *à la reine*/Neonatal Resuscitation

In the history of medicine, John Snow is best known for his investigation of the 1854 cholera epidemic in London and his meticulous epidemiological analysis of the outbreak that pinpointed the Broad Street water pump as the source of infection. In anaesthesia he is known as one of the first to apply scientific principles to what was in his day a mainly empirical craft. Snow's reputation was such that he was asked by the Queen's physician, Sir James Clark (1788–1876), to attend during Queen Victoria's delivery of Prince Leopold on 7 April 1853. Snow recorded the event in part as follows:

> *Thursday 7 April, administered chloroform to the Queen in her confinement ... At 20 minutes past 12 ... in the Queen's apartment I commenced to give a little chloroform with each pain by pouring 15 minims (0.9 ml) by measure on a folded handkerchief. The first stage of labour was nearly over when the chloroform was commenced. Her Majesty expressed great relief from the application, the pain being very trifling during the uterine contractions, while between the periods of contraction there was complete ease. The effect of the chloroform was not anytime carried to the extent of quite removing consciousness ... The chloroform was inhaled for 53 minutes. The placenta was expelled in a very few minutes and the Queen appeared very cheerful and well, expressing herself much gratified with the effect of the chloroform.*

Queen Victoria endorsed the whole procedure with enthusiasm: 'Blessed chloroform, soothing, quieting and delightful beyond measure'. This widely publicised event was known as *chloroform à la reine*. Six months later, on 20 October 1853, Snow administered chloroform to Mrs Thomas, the daughter of the Archbishop of Canterbury, during her confinement at Lambeth Palace. These two events had the symbolic effect of giving both Royal and the Church's blessing and removed many of the remaining medical, religious and lay objections to pain relief in labour. Snow was also called to administer chloroform during Queen Victoria's next confinement in 1857. The labour progressed so quickly that the Queen's husband, Prince Albert, started the administration of chloroform before John Snow arrived and took over. Presumably no one challenged Prince Albert's privileges in this matter and it must stand as an early example of 'family-centred maternity care'. Reputedly, when Snow was summoned to the palace for this event he left a note on his clinic door, which said, 'Out to attend the Queen'. Upon his return he found that someone had appended the words 'God save the Queen!'

Snow emphasised the importance of resuscitation of the newborn, stating, 'The number of children that die of asphyxia at the time of birth is very considerable ... one-twentieth of the children brought forth are still-born and of these a large proportion are asphyxiated from various causes, often at the very moment of birth'. He stressed the need for clearing the airway before initiating artificial respiration. He exhorted doctors to have equipment at hand to produce oxygen and also

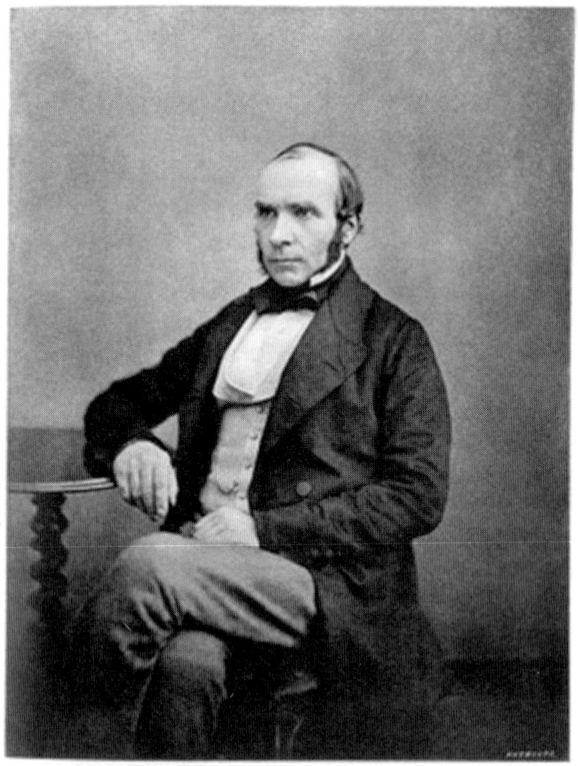

John Snow

modified a ventilation device used in adults so that it could be applied to the newborn. This consisted of two syringes operated simultaneously, one of which withdrew air from the lungs and the other returned a similar volume of fresh air. This device proved to be impractical but his general advice on assessment of the newborn and the underlying principles of artificial respiration were of value and ahead of their time.

John Snow was born into a working-class family on 15 March 1813 in the city of York. He served his medical apprenticeship with a doctor in Newcastle and then walked to London where he enrolled in the School of Medicine at Westminster Hospital. Following the principle that you can never have too many credentials for medical practice, he systematically acquired all of the medical qualifications available by examination, including those of the Royal College of Surgeons, Royal College of Physicians, London University and the Society of Apothecaries. Snow was a creative and hard-working medical scientist who helped establish the beginnings of anaesthesia as a specialty. He was an abstemious man, ate sparingly and died on 16 June 1858 at 45 years of age. Luckily, he wrote extensively, leaving a legacy of written material which continued to provide a valuable basis for the emerging specialties of anaesthesia and epidemiology. He is buried in the Brompton Cemetery in London; the original monument was destroyed during the 'blitz' of April 1940, and a replica was erected by the Association of Anaesthetists of Great Britain and Ireland in 1951.

Selected Publications

Snow J. On asphyxia and the resuscitation of still-born children. *Lond Med Gaz* 1841; 29: 222–7.

Snow J. *On Chloroform and Other Anaesthetics: Their Action and Administration.* London: John Churchill; 1858.

Bibliography References

34, 74, 128, 130, 230, 252–254, 446, 509, 540, 589, 594, 832, 850, 1120, 1283, 1295, 1399–1401, 1444–1447, 1540, 1579, 1582.

Soranus (c. 78–138)

Internal Version

The oldest published work on obstetrics and gynaecology is attributed to Soranus, who was born in Ephesus, Asia Minor towards the end of the first century AD. His medical training was at Alexandria, and he worked in Rome during the reigns of Trajan (AD 98–117) and Hadrian (AD 117–138). Many writings were attributed to him, and his main work, *Gynaecology,* brought together the knowledge of obstetrics, gynaecology and paediatrics of that era. It survived though many translations until a fifteenth century Greek manuscript was rediscovered in the nineteenth century at the Bibliothèque Royale in Paris, from which emanate the modern translations.

The obstetrical component of his work was written specifically for the instruction of midwives. He outlined the requirements for the ideal midwife:

> *Literate, with her wits about her, possessed of a good memory, loving work, respectable, sound of limb, robust and according to some people, endowed with long slim fingers and short nails at her fingertips.*

Among his writings were detailed instructions for the performance of internal version in cases of abnormal fetal lie:

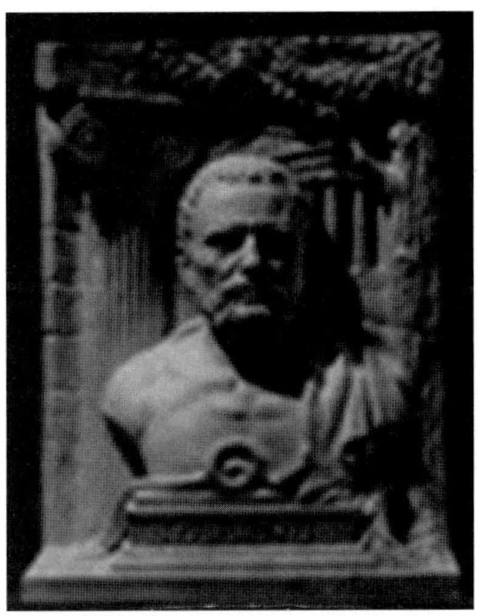

Soranus

> *... one should introduce the anointed left hand, the nails being pared so that they may not scratch, and the fingers extended, joined together at their tips to give them a tapering shape so that they may be introduced without causing laceration ... If the fetus is presenting by the knees, one must push it up and when thus the legs have been straightened, one should extract it by the feet ... If the fetus is spontaneously lying on its side one must put in the hand by the side and gently turn it ... One should do everything gently and without bruising, and should continually anoint the parts with oil, so that the parturient remains free from sympathetic trouble and the infant healthy: for we see many alive who have thus been born with difficulty.*

Soranus also included an extensive section on care of the newborn, including an initial appraisal at birth to 'consider whether it is worth rearing or not'. To a degree his advice on neonatal assessment was a forerunner of the Apgar score:

> *And the infant which is suited by nature for rearing will be distinguished by the fact that its mother has spent the period of pregnancy in good health, for conditions which require medical care, especially those of the body, also harm the fetus and enfeeble the foundations of its life. Second, by the fact that it has been born at the due time, best at the end of nine months, and if it so happens, later; but also after only seven months. Furthermore by the fact that when put on the earth it immediately cries with proper vigor; for one that lives for some length of time without crying, or cries but weakly, is suspected of behaving so on account of some unfavourable condition. Also by the fact that it is perfect in all its parts, embers and senses; that its ducts, namely of the ears, nose, pharynx, urethra, anus are free from obstruction; that the natural functions of every member are neither sluggish nor weak; that the joints bend and stretch; that it has due size and shape and is properly sensitive in every respect. This we may recognize from pressing the fingers against the surface of the body, for it is natural to suffer pain from everything that pricks or squeezes. And by conditions contrary to those mentioned, the infant not worth rearing is recognized.*

Soranus taught largely sensible midwifery and child care. Little new was added for the next 1,400 years, or if it was the writings were lost.

Selected Publications

Soranus' Gynaecology. Translated by Owsei Temkin. Baltimore, MD: Johns Hopkins University Press; 1956. Softshell Books edition; 1991.

Bibliography References

15, 88, 97, 125, 273, 439, 468, 494, 524, 593, 629, 632, 759, 762, 1021, 1045, 1131, 1264, 1289, 1411, 1502, 1588, 1595, 1619.

Spalding, Alfred Baker (1874–1942)

Spalding's Sign

Shortly after intrauterine death, liquefaction and shrinking of brain tissue lead to overlapping of the fetal skull bones, which Alfred Spalding demonstrated on X-ray. Spalding's sign is evident three to seven days after fetal death. In fact, this sign was first described by DA Horner in a lecture read before the Chicago Gynecological Society in December 1921:

> *It seems that very shortly after intra-uterine death, the brain tissue shrinks, which produces a typical overlapping of the foetal skull bones. This overlapping ... seems to be pathognomic of the condition of intra-uterine death and gives a picture quite different from the overlapping produced by molding ...*

Spalding described the same sign in April 1922, to the Society of the Alumni of the Sloane Hospital for Women. Both authors, unaware of the other's observations, published their papers in the same journal in 1922, but Spalding's was published one month (June) before Horner's. Thus, Spalding received the eponymous fame. From the original description in 1922, until the widespread use of ultrasound, this became one of the most commonly used signs to confirm fetal death.

Spalding also devised an operation for prolapse, in which the uterine corpus and cervix were amputated and the remaining isthmus was interposed between the bladder and anterior vaginal wall.

Alfred Baker Spalding was born in Kansas. He graduated from Columbia University's College of Physicians and Surgeons in 1900. He became professor and chairman of obstetrics at Stanford University in 1912. Beset by depression, he retired from practice in 1934.

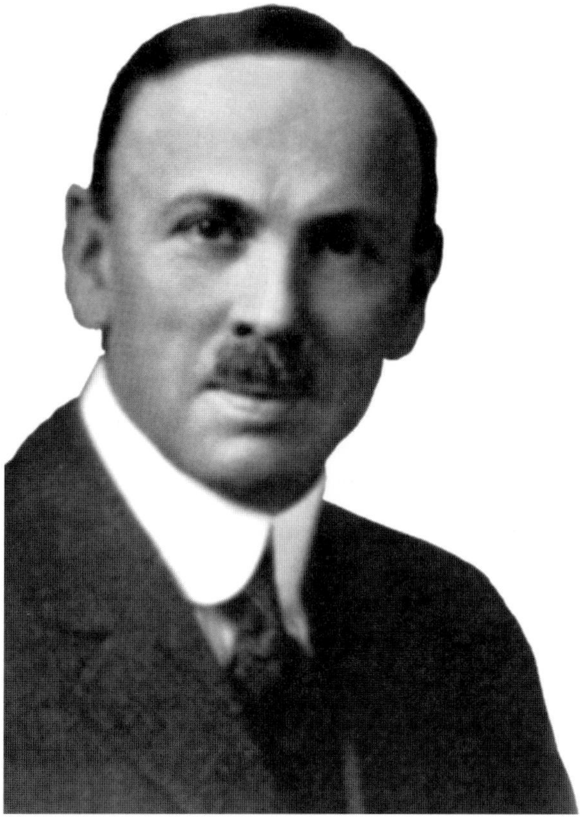

Alfred Baker Spalding

Selected Publications

Spalding AB. A pathognomic sign of intra-uterine death. *Surg Gynecol Obstet* 1922; 34: 754–7.

Bibliography References

523, 536, 801, 1464, 1480, 1485.

Spiegelberg, Otto von (1830–1881)

Spiegelberg's Criteria for Ovarian Pregnancy

In 1878, Professor Otto von Spiegelberg of Breslau published four criteria that must be fulfilled to establish the rare diagnosis of ovarian pregnancy: (1) the tube on the affected side must be intact, (2) the pregnancy sac must occupy the position of the ovary, (3) the ovary and sac must be connected to the uterus by the ovarian ligament, and (4) ovarian tissue must be present in the wall of the sac. In his paper Spiegelberg described the outcome of an extremely rare situation: a term ovarian pregnancy. He carried out the laparotomy in a small cellar apartment by kerosene lamp held by a midwife with the assistance of a resident who administered chloroform. The woman died, as expected, within a few hours. The infant, a girl, thrived initially on artificial feeding, but 'at three months old died, like most of the motherless babies of the poor because of atrophic disease'.

Otto von Spiegelberg was born in Hanover and was an 1851 medical graduate of the University of Göttingen. After postgraduate work in Berlin, Vienna and Prague, he settled in Göttingen as lecturer in obstetrics. In 1855 he visited medical centres in England, Scotland and Ireland. He was appointed professor of obstetrics and gynaecology at Freiburg in 1861, at Königsberg in 1864 and at Breslau in 1875. The University of Breslau honoured him in 1879 with the splendid title, *Rector magnificus*.

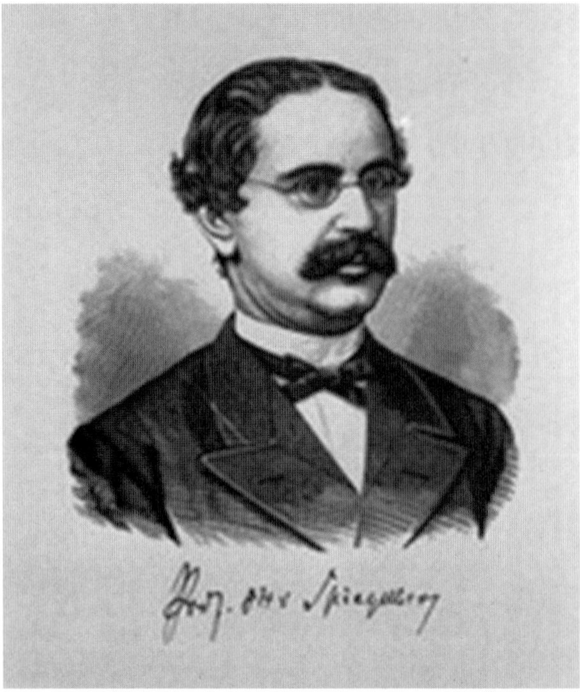

Otto von Spiegelberg

In his later career he concentrated on operative gynaecology and was one of the first to show the safety of replacing the ligated pedicle in the peritoneal cavity after ovariotomy. Spiegelberg was the first, in 1866, to describe the combination of ovarian fibroma, ascites and pleural effusion – later known as Meigs' syndrome. He died from chronic renal disease at the age of 51.

Selected Publications

Spiegelberg O. Zur Casuistik der Ovarialschwangerschaft. *Arch Gynäkol* 1878; 13: 73–9.

Bibliography References

548, 648, 1261, 1291, 1499.

Spinelli, Pier Giuseppe (1862–1929)

Spinelli's Operation

For the rare case of chronic uterine inversion, Spinelli adopted an anterior vaginal approach, incising the constricting cervical ring and anterior uterine wall. The uterus was then turned outside-in and the uterine wall and cervix sutured.

Pier Giuseppe Spinelli was born in Chieti, Italy, received his medical training in Naples and qualified in 1888. He sparked a transient revival of interest in symphysiotomy in 1892 when he presented the Naples experience of 24 cases without maternal loss. He practised obstetrics and gynaecology in Naples.

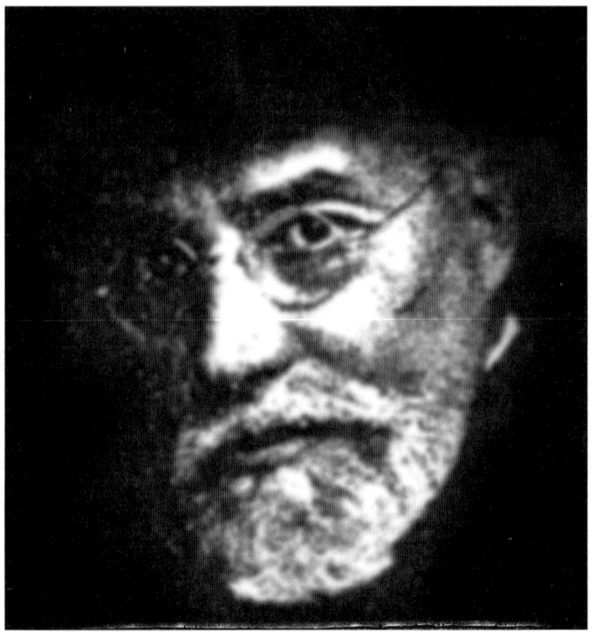

Pier Giuseppe Spinelli

Selected Publications

Spinelli PG. Les résultats de la symphyséotomie. *Ann Gynéc Obstet* 1892; 37: 2–15.

Spinelli PG. Cura chirurgica conservative dell' inversione cronica dell' utero col processo kehrer. *Arch Ital Ginecol* 1899; 2: 7.

Bibliography References

648, 1342, 1480, 1501.

Stearns, John (1770–1848)

Ergot

Epidemics of the disease 'ergotism' occurred at least 1,000 years ago. Indeed, even earlier (c. 600 BC), in Assyrian cuneiform tablets, there is reference to the 'noxious pustule in the ear of grain'. The name ergot is derived from the French *argot*, meaning the 'spur of a cockerel', which the fungus *Claviceps purpurea* resembles as it grows on the ear of the grain. Epidemics, related to wet seasons and damp crops favouring the growth of the fungus, occurred in areas of France and southern Germany, where the cereal rye was grown extensively. The vascular spasm associated with the chronic ingestion of contaminated rye bread caused abdominal pain, hallucinations and a typical, tingling and burning pain (fire) of the skin. At its worst, gangrene and autoamputation of digits and limbs would occur. A brotherhood of monks in France, the order of St Anthony, looked after the sufferers in hostels and the condition is often known as 'St Anthony's fire'. The link between bread made from rye contaminated with the fungus and ergotism was established by the medical faculty of Marburg University after studying an epidemic in 1595.

The recorded medicinal use of ergot goes back at least 400 years to a report from Germany in 1582 on ergot spurs, noting that:

> *they are held to be a special medicine for women in labour and for the purpose of awakening the pains three of the spurs are swallowed.*

Chassar Moir was later to show that three spurs contained about 0.5 mg ergometrine, the recommended dose in clinical practice. There are a number of references to the use of ergot for the augmentation of labour by midwives and physicians in France and Germany in the seventeenth and eighteenth centuries.

The modern use of ergot originated with John Stearns, a physician practising in Waterford, Saratoga County, New York. Stearns said he was 'informed of the powerful effects produced by this article in the hands of some ignorant Scotch women, in the county of Washington'. He had used ergot for several years when, in response to a request from a fellow physician in 1807, he sent a letter explaining the attributes of his *pulvis parturiens*, as he called it, and enclosed a sample of ergot:

> *It expedites lingering parturition, and saves to the accoucher a considerable portion of time, without producing any bad effects on the patient ... The pains induced by it are peculiarly forcing ... In most cases you will be surprised with the suddenness of its operation ... Since I have adopted the use of this powder I have seldom found a case that detained me more than three hours ...*
>
> *It is a vegetable, and appears to be a spurious growth of rye ... Rye which grows in low, wet ground, yields it in greatest abundance.*

With Stearns' agreement, this letter was published the next year in the *New York Medical Repository*. This was followed by many requests for samples from other physicians. Aware of the potential dangers of ergot, Stearns wrote:

> *My information was such as to impress upon my mind the necessity of extreme caution in my first experiments. The continued influence of this impression upon my subsequent practice, has been a source of much consoling reflection. It has tended to prevent those fatal errors which have so often occurred.*

Unfortunately, ergot was not used with the same 'consoling reflection' by other practitioners, and the sustained and excessive uterine action induced by ergot caused many stillbirths, ruptured uteri and maternal deaths. Opposition to its use in labour accumulated and was aptly summed up in 1822 by David Hosack (1769–1835) of the New York College of Physicians and Surgeons when he said the name *pulvis ad partum* should be changed to *pulvis ad mortem*.

Oliver Prescott Jr (1762–1827) of Massachusetts also advised extreme caution with its use before birth but emphasised its role in the prevention and treatment of post-partum haemorrhage:

> *The tendency of its operation is, I conceive, to constringe the uterine fibers, and lessen the caliber of its blood vessels; for when it is given to parturient patients, there has been no instance, within my knowledge, of undue hemorrhage after delivery.*

In his 1822 article, Stearns still advocated the use of ergot in 'lingering labours' but with extreme caution and circumspection. He also advised its use for inevitable abortion, retained placenta and in the prevention and treatment of post-partum haemorrhage. As the disasters associated with its use before delivery

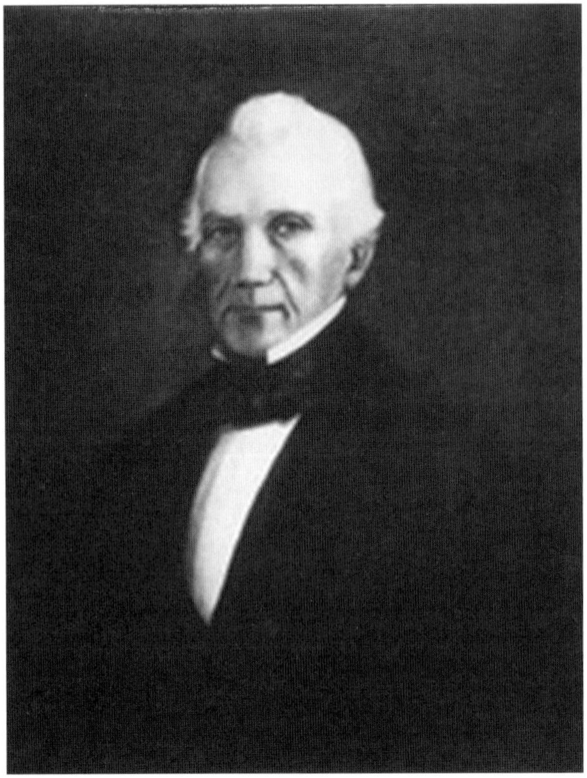

John Stearns

became evident, the prescription of ergot was restricted to abortion and post-partum cases. More than a century later, Harold Dudley and Chassar Moir in Britain and Edward Davis in the United States would isolate the rapid-acting fraction of ergot, known as ergometrine in Britain and ergonovine in the United States.

John Stearns was born on 16 May 1770 in Wilbraham, Massachusetts, and took his undergraduate degree at Yale College in 1789. He did his medical apprenticeship with a leading physician, Dr Erastus Sergeant of Stockbridge, Massachusetts, and later attended lectures at the University of Pennsylvania. In 1793 Stearns entered practice in Saratoga County, New York. He moved to Albany in 1810 and finally, nine years later, settled in New York City. He was well educated, prominent in his community, and in

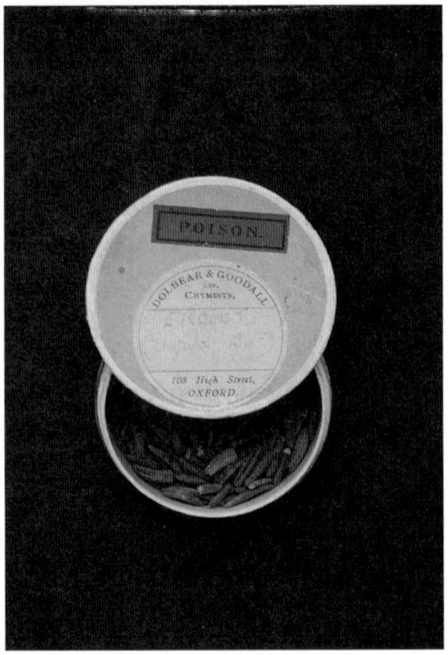

Spurs of ergot

1809 was elected to serve a four-year term as a state senator. He became president of the New York State Medical Society in 1817. When the New York Academy of Medicine was established in 1846, Stearns was elected the first president. He died on 18 March 1848 in New York at the age of 79 from septicaemia originating in a wound received while performing an autopsy.

Selected Publications

Lonicer A, *Kreuterbuch*. Frankfurt; 1582.

Prescott O. *A Dissertation on the Natural History and Medicinal Effects of Secale Cornutum or Ergot*. Andover: Flagg and Gould; 1813 and *Med Phys J* 1814; 32: 90.

Stearns J. Account of the pulvis parturiens, a remedy for quickening child-birth. *NY Med Repository* 1808; 11: 308–9.

Stearns J. Observations on the secale cornutum, or ergot, with directions for its use in parturition. *Med Rec* 1822; 5: 90.

Bibliography References

64, 82, 94, 560, 648, 680, 733, 810, 955, 1061, 1064, 1066, 1586, 1591, 1594, 1629, 1644, 1670.

Stein, Irving Freiler (1887–1976) Leventhal, Michael Leo (1901–1971)

Stein–Leventhal Syndrome

In November 1934, Irving Stein and Michael Leventhal presented their experience with seven patients treated by ovarian wedge resection for amenorrhoea associated with bilateral polycystic ovaries to the Central Association of Obstetricians and Gynecologists in New Orleans:

> *In the series of patients which we observed with bilateral polycystic ovaries and amenorrhea, the ovaries were found to be from two to four times the normal size and while they often maintained their original shape, they were sometimes distinctly globular. In one case, they were flat and soft, the so-called 'oyster ovaries'. The ovarian cortex was found to be hypertrophied in all of the cases and the tunica thickened, tough, and fibrotic.*
>
> *The cysts were follicle cysts, near the surface, and almost entirely confined to the cortex, and they contained clear fluid. There were 20 to 100 cysts in each ovary, varying in size from 1 mm to about 1.2 cm, but rarely larger. The color of the ovary was oyster gray with bluish areas where the cysts were superficial and appeared on the surface as sago-like bodies. On section, the variation in size of the cysts and the clear fluid contents were revealed. Corpora lutea were sometimes absent and when found, they were very small and deeply placed ...*
>
> *In some patients, there was observed a distinct tendency toward masculinizing changes.*

After treatment with a number of 'endocrine preparations' they tried a surgical approach, based on the previous finding that menstruation occurred in amenorrhoeic women after ovarian biopsy:

> *In the patients referred to in this series, we have resected from one-half to three-fourths of each ovary by wedge-resection, thereby removing the cortex containing the cysts, and have sutured the hilus with the finest catgut.*

They found that 'the only consistent pathologic finding is the presence of follicle cysts lined by these cells'. In discussing the possible etiology of the condition, they dismissed a congenital basis because the amenorrhoea was secondary. They postulated a mechanical factor:

> *It is our belief that a mechanical crowding of the cortex by cysts interferes with the progress of the normal graafian follicles to the surface of the ovary. This mechanical factor may account for the symptoms of amenorrhea and sterility.*

They followed the patients from one to four years: all had regular menstruation restored after wedge resection and two became pregnant.

Irving Freiler Stein was born in Chicago. He graduated in medicine from the Rush Medical College in Chicago in 1912. He spent his professional career at the Michael Reese Hospital where he became the senior staff gynaecologist. Stein was president of the American Society for the Study of Fertility and the International Fertility Association. He died on 18 October 1976.

Michael Leo Leventhal was born in Chicago and graduated from the Rush Medical College in 1924. He served as a medical officer with the United States Army during the Second World War. He also spent his whole career at the Michael Reese Hospital.

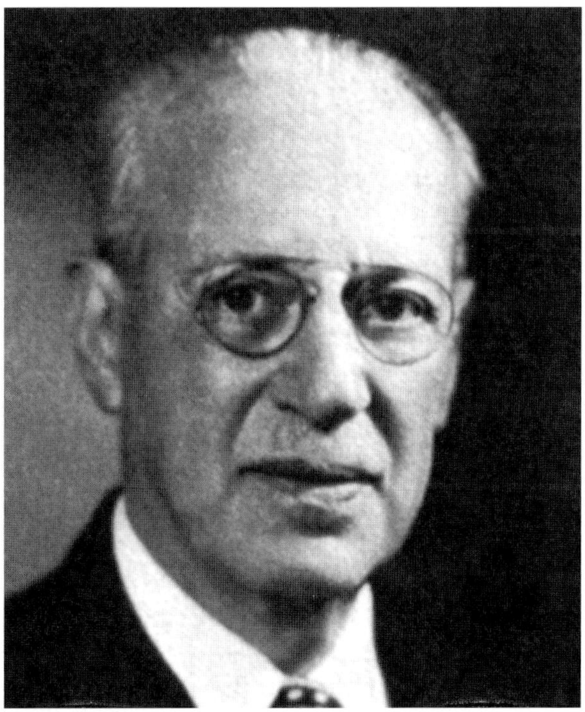

Irving Freiler Stein

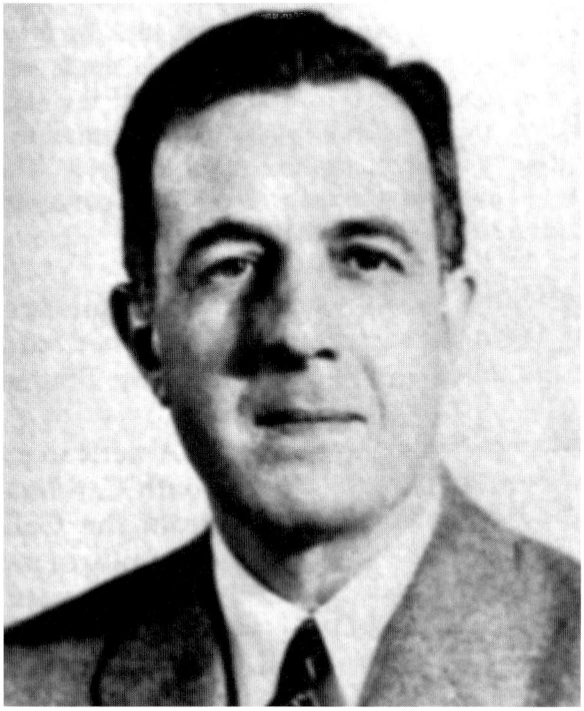

Michael Leo Leventhal

Selected Publications

Stein IF, Leventhal ML. Amenorrhea associated with bilateral polycystic ovaries. *Am J Obstet Gynecol* 1935; 29: 181–91.

Bibliography References

793, 1480, 1542.

Steinbüchel, Richard von (1865–1952)

Twilight Sleep

Richard von Steinbüchel followed the example of surgeons who had used a combination of morphine and scopolamine to achieve anaesthesia. He gave lower doses in labour, aiming to provide pain relief with 'seminarcosis' as opposed to full surgical anaesthesia. He used morphine 10 mg and scopolamine 0.4 mg, given by subcutaneous injection and repeated every two hours as necessary. With this regimen Steinbüchel found he could provide analgesia and perform operative vaginal delivery with little or no additional ether or chloroform anaesthesia. He reported a typical case history:

> *. . . although no further anaesthetic was given, the forceps operation and suture could be carried out without any notable complaint from the patient.*

He observed confusion and excitement in a number of patients, but only rarely was this excessive, although he described one who 'behaved like a raving lunatic'. He also pointed out that the advantage of using this technique was not having to remain with the patient during labour, compared to the need for inhalation analgesia with ether or chloroform. Steinbüchel briefly reported his method in 1902 and followed this with a more detailed publication in 1903, including the case histories of 20 patients.

Following Steinbüchel's lead, several clinics in Europe took up the method. Karl Gauss (1875–1957) in Freiburg studied the technique most comprehensively, and it was he who introduced the term 'twilight sleep' (*Dämmerschlaf*). He found that smaller doses sufficed and produced less neonatal depression:

> *. . . the end result of a skilfully given dosage is a kind of artificial twilight state, of which the chief characteristic is a complete amnesia extending over the whole labour.*

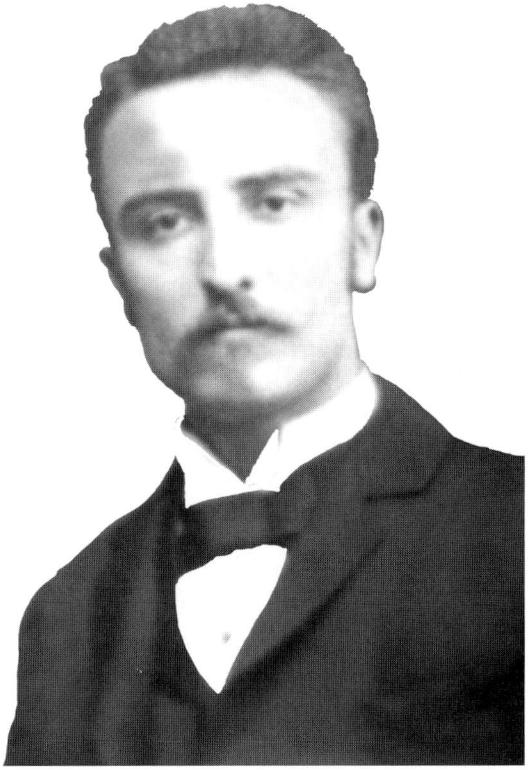

Richard von Steinbüchel

Gauss also described the marked mobility of the uterus in early pregnancy, which is sometimes known as 'Gauss' sign'.

Richard von Steinbüchel was born in Trieste. He studied medicine at Innsbruck University and received his MD in 1889. He was appointed assistant to the university women's clinic at the University of Graz in 1893 and became *privat dozent* in 1894. In 1896 he established his own practice of obstetrics and gynaecology in Graz, while continuing to lecture at the university. He served in the Austro-Hungarian army during the First World War.

Selected Publications

Gauss KJ. Geburten in künstlichen Dämmerschlaf. *Arch Gynäkol* 1906; 78: 579–631.

Steinbüchel R. Vorläufige mittheilung über die Anwendung von Skopolamin-Morphium injecktionen in der Geburtshilfe. *Zentralbl Gynäkol* 1902; 26: 1304–6.

Steinbüchel R. Die Skololamin-Morphium Halbnarkose in der Geburtschilfe. *Beitr Geburtsh Gynäkol* 1903; 1: 294–326.

Bibliography References

548, 648, 712, 848.

Steiner, Paul (1902–1978)

Amniotic Fluid Embolism

The first published report of amniotic fluid embolism was in 1926 by Dr JR Meyer from the pathology department at the University of Sao Paulo, Brazil. He described the case of a 21-year-old multiparous woman with a macerated fetal death who collapsed and died following acute respiratory distress, convulsions and haemorrhage. The pathology report showed squamous cells and caseous material in the maternal pulmonary vasculature. This single case report was published in the *Brazil-Medico* in Portuguese and seemed to go unnoticed in the rest of the medical world.

In 1941 Paul Steiner in the department of pathology at the University of Chicago published a report of eight women who died during or shortly after delivery, in which he noted the presence of epithelial squamous and amniotic fluid debris in the pulmonary blood vessels. Steiner was assisted in this work by Clarence Lushbaugh, a medical student. They carried out experiments on dogs and rabbits which showed that unfiltered amniotic fluid injected intravenously caused death, whereas the injection of filtered amniotic fluid was not lethal. The findings in the lungs of

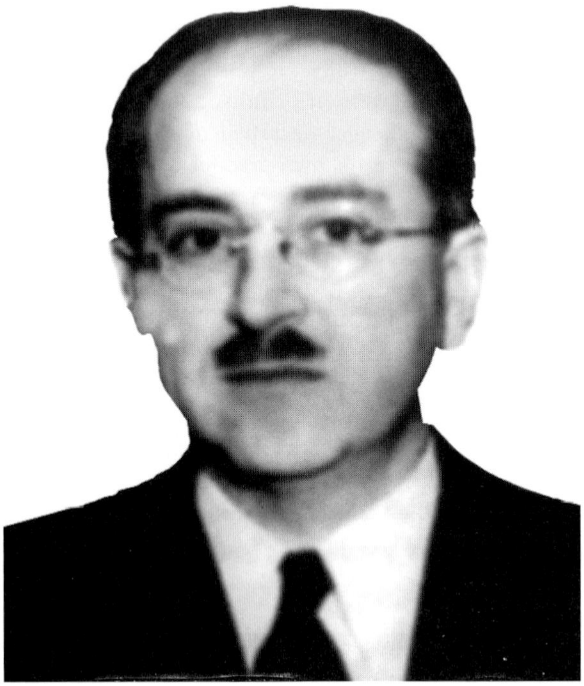

Paul Steiner

the animals who died, were similar to those of the eight women:

> *Pulmonary embolism by the particulate matter contained in amniotic fluid which gained entrance to the maternal circulation has been demonstrated by us at autopsy in 8 cases in which it seemed to be the cause of death . . . Having gained entrance to the maternal venous system, the emboli would be carried to the first filtered bed, in these instances the lungs, and would lodge in vessels corresponding to their size. Sudden showers of foreign particulate matter lodging in the lungs may produce severe systematic reactions resembling shock or anaphylactoid reactions.*

It is interesting that Steiner and Lushbaugh described the reaction as 'anaphylactoid', and this fits with the modern theory of pathophysiology of this enigmatic condition. It is now known that amniotic fluid and fetal squames often enter the maternal circulation without ill effect, but in certain susceptible women an anaphylactic type of response occurs, leading to the fully blown picture of amniotic fluid embolism. Steiner and Lushbaugh did not describe the coagulation defect, and it was only in the 1950s that it was realised that disseminated intravascular coagulation was an inevitable accompaniment of amniotic fluid embolism in women who survived beyond the first one to two hours.

Paul Steiner was born on 9 October 1902 in Columbus Grove, Ohio. He took his MD in 1932 at Northwestern University, Chicago. After his internship he joined the department of pathology at the University of Chicago and was promoted to professor in 1948. In 1959 he moved to the same position at the University of Pennsylvania and remained there until retirement in 1971. He was interested in the American Civil War and wrote two books on physician-generals and medical aspects of that conflict. He died on 24 October 1978 at the Mennonite Memorial Nursing Home in Bluffton, Ohio.

Selected Publications

Meyer JR. Embolia pulmonar amnio-caseosa. *Brazil-Medico* 1926; 2: 301–3.

Steiner PE, Lushbaugh CC. Maternal pulmonary embolism by amniotic fluid as a cause of obstetric shock and unexpected death in obstetrics. *JAMA* 1941; 117: 1245–54 and 1340–5.

Bibliography References

1480, 1485.

Steptoe, Patrick Christopher (1913–1988) Edwards, Robert Geoffrey (1925–2013)

In Vitro Fertilisation

Among the letters to the editor of the *Lancet* on 12 August 1978 was a report of the world's first infant conceived outside the mother's body. The birth of Louise Joy Brown by caesarean section, just before midnight on 25 July 1978, represented the culmination of ten years collaborative research between Patrick Steptoe and Robert Edwards. As Steptoe later recalled when he first handed Mrs Lesley Brown her baby:

> *She cradled the infant, then managed to whisper: 'Thank you for my baby. Thank you'. Louise Joy had arrived, a whole new person to make this family complete at last. I doubt if I shall ever share such a moment in my life again.*

The world of human reproductive medicine and infertility would never be the same.

Patrick Steptoe was a consultant obstetrician and gynaecologist in the district hospital of Oldham, Lancashire in the industrial north of England. The start of his journey to the first successful in vitro fertilisation (IVF) was his introduction to the laparoscope by Raoul Palmer of France in 1958. Steptoe also acknowledged the co-operation of another European pioneer of laparoscopy, Hans Fragenheim (1920–2001) in Wuppertal, Germany. Steptoe was quick to realise the laparoscope's potential and was the first to introduce it to Britain. He wrote the first text in English on the subject, *Laparoscopy in Gynaecology*, in 1967.

Steptoe presented his work on gynaecological laparoscopy at a meeting in the Royal Society of Medicine, London in February 1968. After the meeting he was approached by Bob Edwards, a geneticist and embryologist working in the University Physiology Laboratory at Cambridge. Edwards had published widely on IVF in animals and was anxious to pursue the possibility in humans. He saw the laparoscope as the way to recover oocytes from infertile women. Thus began the 20 years of collaboration between the two men, 250 kilometres apart, that led to the world's first 'test-tube' baby and ended only with Steptoe's death in 1988.

Their road to success was not easy. Edwards had to establish a laboratory in Oldham and frequently drive the 250 kilometres across country. Criticism about the ethics of their work was common. Research funding was sparse, and they never received support from the Medical Research Council. By 1970 they moved the small laboratory to the nearby Kershaw's Hospital in Royston, where they were given an operating theatre and two beds. Early progress was swift, and the first embryo transfer took place in 1971. However, the next four years brought repeated failure to achieve implantation. The first pregnancy was reported in April 1976 but had implanted in the wrong site, as their terse summary in the *Lancet* article outlined:

> *A human embryo in transition between a morula and blastocyst after culture in vitro was reintroduced into the mother's uterus via the cervix. The resulting pregnancy was closely monitored and was found to be located in the oviduct. The ectopic embryo was removed at 13 weeks of gestation.*

The second successful implantation aborted spontaneously. The follicle that produced Louise Brown was aspirated by Steptoe on 10 November 1977. The original oocyte aspirator was homemade in the Cambridge laboratory for $2.00. It was submitted for publication but apparently refused on ethical grounds. Ironically, just after Louise Brown was born, Steptoe reached retirement age for the National Health Service. Again, funding to continue their work was not forthcoming, so in 1980 Steptoe and Edwards founded the privately funded Bourn Hall Clinic, near Cambridge. It was here that Lesley and John Brown of Bristol sought help in conceiving again. Success led to the birth of their second IVF daughter, Natalie, four years after her sister Louise.

Both Edwards and Steptoe acknowledged the considerable contribution of Edward's assistant, Jean Purdy. A former nurse, Purdy joined them in 1969 and worked devotedly with the project until her death 15 years later.

Patrick Christopher Steptoe, the fifth of eight children, was born in Witney, Oxfordshire, where his father was the registrar of births, deaths and marriages. He was delivered by a Dr Patey, and Steptoe's mother, wishing to name her son after the doctor, chose Patrick as the closest acceptable variant. Patrick Steptoe was a talented musician, and by his early teens balanced two extremes of musical expression: playing the accompanying piano music for silent films in his local cinema and giving organ recitals at St Mary's church. Indeed, at the age of 18 he was appointed musical director and organist to the Christ Church Musical Society in Oxford. Thus, he did not begin his medical studies at King's College and St George's Hospital, London until he was 20, qualifying in 1939.

As a member of the Royal Naval Volunteer Reserve, he served as surgeon lieutenant-commander from 1939 to 1946. In 1941, his ship was torpedoed in the Mediterranean, and after some time in the water he was picked up by the Italians and held prisoner of war for two years. Part of his appreciation of Italian wine stems from this period. Apparently his captors approved of his love and knowledge of wine and provided him with samples. He went on to become a wine expert and later achieved the status of Chevalier du Tastevin de Bourgogne.

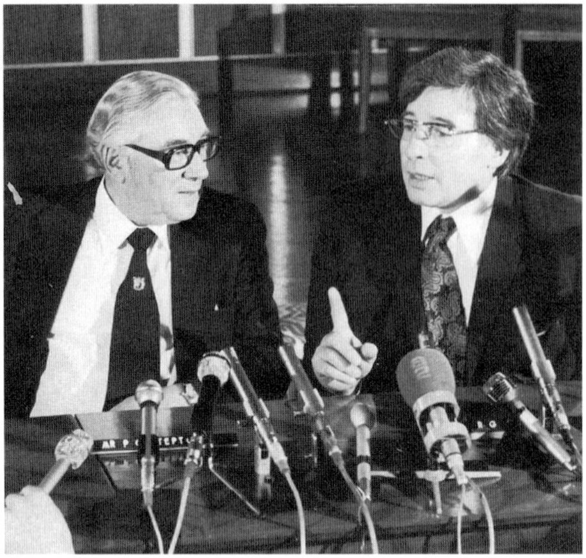

Patrick Christopher Steptoe (on the left) and Robert Geoffrey Edwards

Steptoe took his training in obstetrics and gynaecology in the London hospitals. Consultant posts in London were rare and he took up his position in Oldham in 1951 and established a first-class clinical and postgraduate training unit.

After he retired from the National Health Service, he spent the last eight years of his life training others at Bourn Hall and saw 1,000 successful IVF babies conceived in that programme. He died in Canterbury on March 21 1988 from prostate cancer. At his funeral, which was held in Bourn Hall Chapel, one of his own musical compositions, 'Requiem for a Dying Embryo', was played. He was buried in the Parish Church of Bourn.

Bob Edwards was born on 27 September 1925 in the small town of Batley in Yorkshire, England. After school in Manchester he studied agriculture at the University College of North Wales. This was interrupted by four years' army service in the Near East. After demobilisation he returned to university but transferred to zoology to pursue his interest in the biology of reproduction. Upon completion of his BSc, he gained a postgraduate scholarship to the Institute of Animal Genetics in Edinburgh and received his PhD during his six years there. Another grant enabled him to spend a year as a Population Council fellow studying immunology at the California Institute of Technology in Pasadena, California. He continued his research on the immunology of reproduction

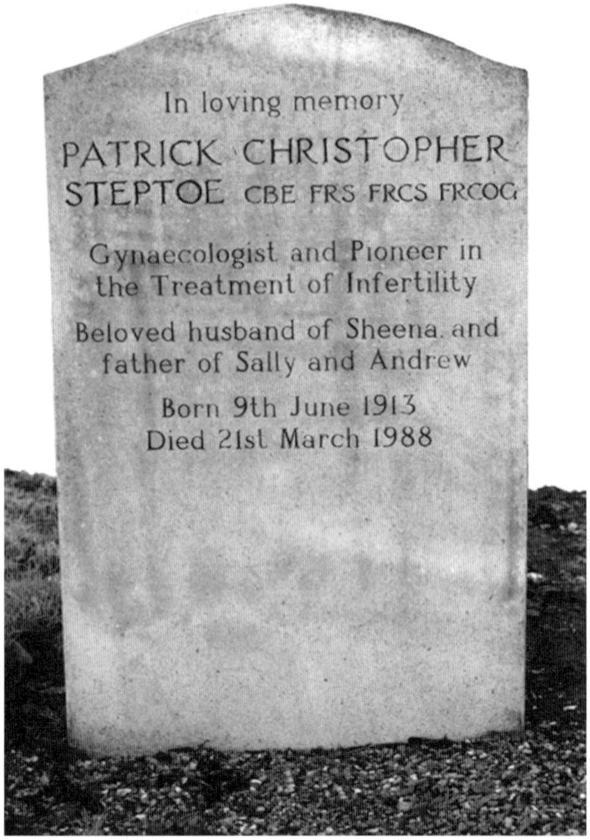
In loving memory
PATRICK CHRISTOPHER
STEPTOE CBE FRS FRCS FRCOG
Gynaecologist and Pioneer in
the Treatment of Infertility
Beloved husband of Sheena and
father of Sally and Andrew
Born 9th June 1913
Died 21st March 1988

Patrick Steptoe's grave, at the parish church of Bourn, near Cambridge

during the next five years, 1957–62, at the National Institute of Medical Research in London. In 1963 he moved to the Physiological Laboratory at Cambridge and conducted further research on induction of ovulation and IVF in animals. It was his need to move the application of his research to humans that led Edwards to seek out Steptoe as his clinical collaborator. The first few years of their collaboration involved dogged persistence in the face of repeated setbacks. As Edwards was to write later:

> *There was only one way to proceed, and that meant I had to travel to Oldham. Patrick displayed his force of character all over again in introducing human IVF into clinical practice with me. It was not an easy ride, indeed it was full of problems and opposition from all quarters. It would result in the elimination of most forms of human infertility within 25 years, the opening of genetic analyses on human embryos, fundamental studies on virtually every aspect of human conception, and in a vast change in social outlook on human fertilization and embryonic*

Letters to the Editor

BIRTH AFTER THE REIMPLANTATION OF A HUMAN EMBRYO

SIR,—We wish to report that one of our patients, a 30-year-old nulliparous married woman, was safely delivered by cæsarean section on July 25, 1978, of a normal healthy infant girl weighing 2700 g. The patient had been referred to one of us (P.C.S.) in 1976 with a history of 9 years' infertility, tubal occlusions, and unsuccessful salpingostomies done in 1970 with excision of the ampullæ of both oviducts followed by persistent tubal blockages. Laparoscopy in February, 1977, revealed grossly distorted tubal remnants with occlusion and peritubal and ovarian adhesions. Laparotomy in August, 1977, was done with excision of the remains of both tubes, adhesolysis, and suspension of the ovaries in good position for oocyte recovery.

Pregnancy was established after laparoscopic recovery of an oocyte on Nov. 10, 1977, in-vitro fertilisation and normal cleavage in culture media, and the reimplantation of the 8-cell embryo into the uterus 2½ days later. Amniocentesis at 16 weeks' pregnancy revealed normal α-fetoprotein levels, with no chromosome abnormalities in a 46 XX fetus. On the day of delivery the mother was 38 weeks and 5 days by dates from her last menstrual period, and she had pre-eclamptic toxæmia. Blood-pressure was fluctuating around 140/95, œdema involved both legs up to knee level together with the abdomen, back, hands, and face; the blood-uric-acid was 390 μmol/l, and albumin 0·5 g/l of urine. Ultrasonic scanning and radiographic appearances showed that the fetus had grown slowly for several weeks from week 30. Blood-œstriols and human placental lactogen levels also dropped below the normal levels during this period. However, the fetus grew considerably during the last 10 days before delivery while placental function improved greatly. On the day of delivery the biparietal diameter had reached 9·6 cm, and 5 ml of amniotic fluid was removed safely under sonic control. The lecithin: sphingomyelin ratio was 3·9:1, indicative of maturity and a low risk of the respiratory-distress syndrome.

We hope to publish further medical and scientific details in your columns at a later date.

Department of Obstetrics and Gynæcology,
General Hospital,
Oldham OL1 2JH — P. C. STEPTOE

University Physiology Laboratory,
Cambridge CB2 3EG — R. G. EDWARDS

Steptoe's and Edwards' report of the first successful case of in vitro fertilisation

growth. This knowledge was essential for so many purposes – for new methods and to understand current methods of contraception, to alleviate some forms of infertility, and even in time for the introduction of new genetic technologies into human conception such as the diagnosis of inherited defects in preimplantation embryos and, one day no doubt for the introduction of genetic modifications in embryos carrying a genetic affliction. And above all, there was the enormous responsibility of conceiving children in vitro, and of bringing early human life into the care of medical science.

In the midst of these endeavours, Edwards became politically active and was elected a Labour Councillor to the Cambridge City Council. He even held hopes of becoming a parliamentary candidate for the Labour Party. Luckily for the world of assisted reproduction, he narrowly missed achieving this goal.

When the Bourn Hall Clinic opened in October 1980, Bob Edwards was appointed scientific director. He was named professor of human reproduction at Cambridge University in 1985 and retired in 1989. He was made editor-in-chief of the journal *Human Reproduction* in 1986. Edward's sustained research and achievements have been widely recognised with multiple honours, including fellowship of the Royal Society, the CBE in 1988 and, belatedly, the Nobel Prize in 2010 and a knighthood in 2011. Bob Edwards died on 10 April 2013.

The breakthrough by Steptoe and Edwards only came after 10 years of tenacious endeavour with limited resources and in the face of opposition from much of the medical establishment. It represented a classic achievement of collaboration between basic science and clinical medicine. Their work has allowed couples to have children who were formerly denied this privilege – more than 5 million in the 35 years following the first IVF success. Unfortunately, as the technique became more of a commercial enterprise in some units, less disciplined teams began to return multiple embryos, leading to high-order multiple pregnancies with the inevitable legacy of prematurity and long-term morbidity in many of the offspring. Ironically, more thoughtful and ethical practitioners are returning to Steptoe and Edward's original practice of returning only one embryo in the majority of cases.

Selected Publications

Steptoe PC, Edwards RG. Reimplantation of a human embryo with subsequent tubal pregnancy. *Lancet* 1976; 1: 880.

Steptoe PC, Edwards RG. Birth after the reimplantation of a human embryo. *Lancet* 1978; 2: 366.

Bibliography References

15, 40, 106, 188, 286, 510–514, 670, 959, 1201, 1206, 1315, 1384, 1514, 1515, 1548, 1717.

Stoeckel, Walter (1871–1961)

Epidural Analgesia

The first report of regional analgesia in labour was by Oskar Kreis (1872–1958), an obstetrician from Basel, in 1900. He reported the successful use of spinal (subarachnoid) instillation of 10 mg cocaine at the lumbar 3–4 level in six women in labour.

Walter Stoeckel, an obstetrician in the Women's Hospital of Marburg, Germany was the first to use extradural injection of local anaesthetic via the caudal route for pain relief in labour. Stoeckel acknowledged that he chose the epidural route based on the 1901 publication of this technique by two French physicians: the radiologist, Jean-Anthanase Sicard (1872–1929), and the urologist Fernand Cathelin (1873–1945) who, within three weeks of each other, described the injection of cocaine into the epidural space vis the sacral hiatus for backpain and surgery respectively:

> *As I felt certain that the pain of labour was due to the uterine contractions, I decided to make use of Cathelin's epidural injections during parturition. By this means it might be possible to achieve the ideal of painless childbirth by a temporary interruption of the nerve pathways carrying labour pain, thus avoiding the need for a general anaesthetic.*

Stoeckel used novocaine and was very impressed with the results:

> *. . . the result exceeded my expectations, the labour pains vanished while the progress of labour remained unimpaired. The birth of the child followed so painlessly that the mother did not even notice it. Inspired by this success, I decided to abandon the morphine-scopolamine combination then in use at my clinic and to test sacral anaesthesia.*

The work of Stoeckel and other European pioneers was largely ignored elsewhere. Indeed, Stoeckel

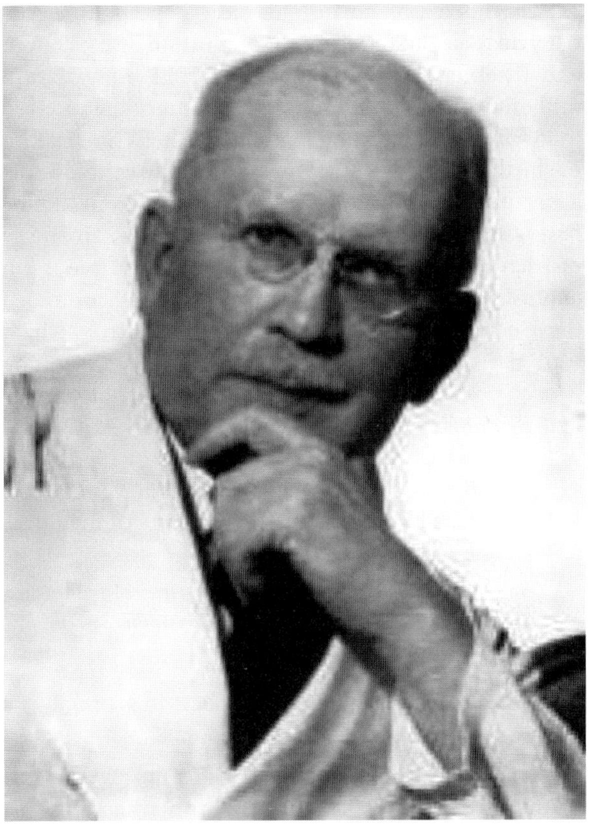

Walter Stoeckel

himself did not pursue the development of his technique. The widespread use of epidural analgesia in labour awaited its rediscovery and application in Canada and the United States.

Walter Stoeckel was the son of a farmer and grew up in Insterburg, East Prussia. His initial intention was to study veterinary medicine, but his father persuaded him to take up the human variety instead. He qualified in 1895 after studies at Königsberg, Munich and Leipzig. Following military service, he took training in obstetrics and gynaecology at Bonn and Berlin. In 1908 he was appointed to the chair of gynaecology at Marburg, where he carried out his work on epidural analgesia. After three years he left Marburg for Kiel, and in 1925 he succeeded Bumm in the chair at the University of Berlin. Here he was called upon to deliver two of Joseph Goebbels' children. He was one of the dominant German gynaecologists of his time and trained many other department heads.

Selected Publications

Cathelin MF. Une nouvelle voie d'injection rachidienne. Méthodes des injections épidurales par le procédé du canal sacré – applications à l'homme. *CR Soc Biol Paris* 1901; 53: 452–3.

Kreis O. Über Medullarnarkose bei Gebärenden. *Zentralbl Gynäkol* 1900; 28: 724–7.

Sicard JA. Les injections medicamenteuses extra-durales par voie sacrococcygienne. *CR Soc Biol Paris* 1901; 53: 396–8.

Stoeckel W. Über sacrale anästhesie. *Zentralbl Gynäkol* 1909; 33: 1–15.

Bibliography References

59, 60, 300, 430–432, 584, 1071, 1288, 1292, 1320, 1336, 1615, 1730.

Stopes, Marie Carmichael (1880–1958)

Birth Control

Marie Stopes was born in Edinburgh. Her mother was a Shakespearean scholar and her father an architect who specialised in the design of breweries. She received her initial schooling at home, with an underlying theme of severe Presbyterian teaching, until the age of 12. In 1902 her aptitude for science gained her a BSc in botany and geology from University College London, where she was also president of the Women's Debating Society. She took her PhD in Munich and returned to Britain as junior lecturer in botany at Manchester University. In 1905 she became the youngest DSc at the University of London and was elected a fellow of University College London in 1910. The following year she married a Canadian botanist,

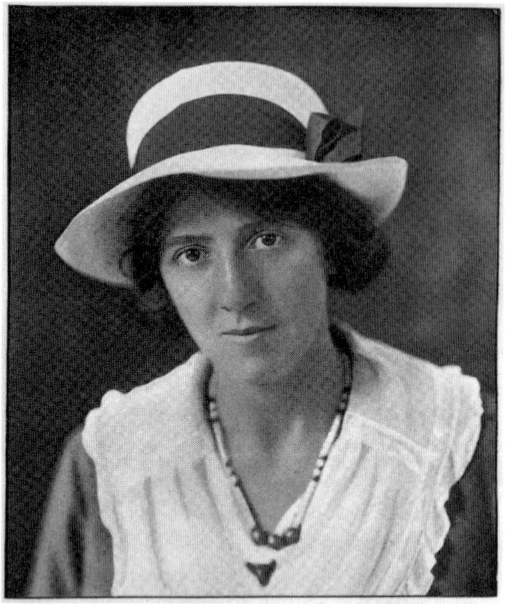

Marie Carmichael Stopes

accepting his proposal one week after they first met at a scientific conference. The marriage was unhappy and, according to her, unconsummated. In 1916, after extensive research in the library of the British Museum, she successfully argued her case in court and had the marriage annulled.

Based on her own unhappy experience and research, she wrote *Married Love: A New Contribution to the Solution of Sex Difficulties.* The book outlined, in plain English, the elements of human sexuality, albeit somewhat romanticised, and emphasised that sex should be as satisfying to women as to men. None of the major companies would publish it. It was eventually published by a small firm with the financial backing of Humphrey Roe of the Avro aeroplane company, who later became her second husband. She dedicated the book 'To young husbands and all those who are betrothed in love'. In the author's preface she wrote:

> *I have some things to say about sex, which, so far as I am aware, have not yet been said, things which seem to be of profound importance to men and women who hope to make their marriages beautiful.*

The book was an instant success, despite or partially because of the vehement opposition of the church and the medical establishment. It sold more than a million copies. In the thousands of letters she received following its publication, most requested information on birth control – a very small portion of the book. Thus, in 1921, she and her second husband opened the first scientific birth control clinic in the Holloway district of London. There they provided free birth control advice to married women. In 1922 she founded the Society for Constructive Birth Control, which was the forerunner of modern Family Planning Associations. In response to the requests for a comprehensive book on birth control, she published *Contraception: Its Theory, History and Practice* in 1923.

She wrote widely on science, travel and literature. In the preface of her first published book of mediocre poetry, she wrote:

> *Years ago I mapped out a life for myself . . . I planned to spend twenty years on scientific research, then twenty years on philosophy, and then twenty years in the direct service of humanity, meanwhile writing one poem in which to embody a lifetime's experience of the Universe, and when the poem was finished . . . to die!*

Her distrust of the medical profession was linked to the birth of her first stillborn son when she was 38 years old. Five years later she had a successful caesarean delivery of another son. She separated from her second husband in 1940 and later cut her son out of her will when he married against her advice. He had chosen to marry a short-sighted young woman who wore glasses. Stopes regarded this union to a 'goggle-eyed' girl as a 'eugenic crime'.

Marie Stopes stood firm against opposition from church and state, and once told George Bernard Shaw that she was speaking on behalf of God. Even her most ardent supporters acknowledged that she had an insensitive and arrogant side. That said, her writings and the attendant publicity served to educate and inform the general public about women's sexuality and contraceptive choices. To a degree, she forced the medical profession to face and acknowledge the impact of these factors on family life and health.

In late 1957 she ultimately accepted her obvious symptoms and belatedly and reluctantly consulted the medical profession: she had advanced inoperable breast cancer. She sought alternative treatment in Germany but was dead within the year.

Selected Publications

Stopes MC. *Married Love: A New Contribution to the Solution of Sex Difficulties*. London: AC Fifield; 1918.

Stopes MC. *Contraception: Its Theory, History and Practice*. London: John Ball, Sons & Danielsson Ltd; 1923. Also published in: The Classics of Obstetrics and Gynecology Library. New York, NY: Gryphon Editions; 1995 (facsimile).

Bibliography References

31, 101, 176, 263, 500, 516, 586, 656, 679, 726, 1004, 1026, 1077, 1297, 1309, 1327, 1716.

Storer, Horatio Robinson (1830–1922)

Caesarean Hysterectomy

Horatio Storer performed the first caesarean hysterectomy on 21 July 1869, some eight years before that of the celebrated Italian surgeon, Edoardo Porro. Unlike Porro, however, who planned the caesarean hysterectomy after careful thought and animal experimentation, Storer was forced into the situation when performing a caesarean section for obstructed labour due to a cervical fibroid He was compelled to perform hysterectomy because of unrelenting haemorrhage, the degree of which was described by one of his assistants as 'perfectly frightful'. Although he successfully accomplished a subtotal hysterectomy, the patient died three days later. Storer did not report the case himself but left this to his assistant, George Bixby, who presented it to the Gynaecological Society of Boston. It was subsequently published in the proceedings of that group. The patient in question was in labour with a fixed pelvis mass, 'either a fibro-cystic tumor of the uterus, or a multilocular ovarian cyst', which was obstructing vaginal delivery. Five doctors consulted and agreed that 'even with mechanical interference the escape of the foetus per *vias naturales* was utterly impossible'. Dr Storer therefore undertook laparotomy under chloroform anaesthesia and found the tumour was an impacted fibroid:

> *An exploratory incision was now undertaken in the tumor situated at the left. Each stroke of the knife revealed a regular series of concentric layers of fibrous tissue, not unlike that of the uterus. After cutting down to the distance of about two inches, the scalpel glided suddenly into a cavity, filled with a thick, brown, semi-fluid, putrilaginous substance, evidently resulting from degeneration of the fibroid. The hemorrhage being already very profuse, and the danger from shock and exhaustion imminent, with a few rapid strokes of the knife, Dr Storer extended his incision into the cavity of the uterus, and with all expedition removed a male child, weighing eight pounds; it being, as well as the placenta, in an advanced state of decomposition . . . It was apparent that the tumor in the uterine wall would necessarily prevent a perfect contraction of the organ, and thus render suppression of the hemorrhage impossible, contrary to what obtains in ordinary uncomplicated cases of Caesarean section. With his usual self-possession, Dr Storer decided to remove the whole mass as far as possible, which would include the uterus, as well as the fibro-cystic tumor of the left wall . . .*

The cervical stump was doubly ligated and 'seared by the hot iron'. The woman survived for three days but 'gradually sank and died':

> *The case now reported is probably the first one in which the removal of the puerperal uterus has ever been performed; and it is undoubtedly the most heroic of the bold procedures as yet resorted to by Dr Storer in extreme gynaecological emergencies. Nothing else could have been done; the patient begged for the chance of life, however small, and it was a matter of surprise to all concerned, in view of the terrific character of the operation, that she should have survived it at all, and still more so for so long a time.*

Horatio Storer was born to a prominent family in Boston. His father was professor of obstetrics and medical jurisprudence in Harvard University and president of the American Medical Association. While an undergraduate at Harvard University, Horatio Storer was president of the Harvard Natural History Society. He made two summer field trips: one to Russia and the other to Labrador and Nova Scotia. Following the latter trip, he published a monograph, *Observations on the fishes of Nova Scotia and Labrador, with description of a new species*. He graduated MD from Harvard in 1853 and later took his law degree, also at Harvard, so that he would be better

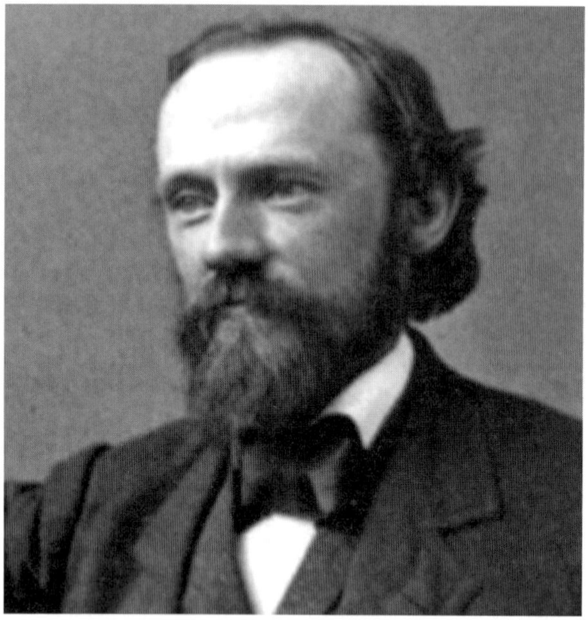

Horatio Robinson Storer

prepared to teach medical jurisprudence. After graduating in medicine, he went to Europe and spent two years studying at Paris, London and Edinburgh. For one year, he was an assistant in private practice to James Young Simpson. Upon his return to Boston he promoted the use of chloroform in labour, which brought him into conflict with the establishment in Boston, which favoured ether anaesthesia. Storer was one of the first physicians in the United States to limit his practice to gynaecology and was professor of obstetrics and medical jurisprudence at the Berkshire Medical School until its dissolution in 1869. He was among the early pioneers of hysterectomy and ovariotomy. Storer was among the first to use rubber gloves during surgery but was not wearing them in 1872 when he became seriously ill with septicaemia from an infected finger stick acquired at operation. In his retirement, he studied the history of medicine through numismatics and left a remarkable collection of more than 2,000 medical medals to the Boston Medical Library. Storer retired to Newport, Rhode Island and died there on 18 September 1922.

Selected Publications

Bixby GH. Extirpation of the puerperal uterus by abdominal section. *J Gynaecol Soc Boston* 1869: 1: 223–32.

Bibliography References

97, 102, 217, 345, 496, 690, 691, 693, 707, 987, 1333, 1586.

Stroganoff, Vasili Vasilievich (1857–1938)

Stroganoff's Method for the Treatment of Eclampsia

Eclampsia has always been one of the main causes of maternal death. At the end of the nineteenth century, the maternal mortality was about 25 per cent in most reports. Management varied from no intervention to *accouchement forcé*. In 1900, Vasili Stroganoff from Russia imposed a decisive voice on this debate. At an international medical congress in Paris, he reported his method of treating 92 eclamptics with the low maternal mortality of 5.4%. He observed, 'as the pathogenesis of eclampsia cannot as yet be considered definitely established, the treatment of it can only be empiric'. Stroganoff recognised that the prevention of further convulsions was the most important objective:

> *The oftener the attacks occur, the more disastrous their effects. After nine or ten attacks a woman, previously in the bloom of health, may be at the brink of the grave.*

Stroganoff first used his regimen in 1897 and modified it over the next 30 years. His method involved attention to detail in preventing convulsions and support of other body systems until labour supervened or could be safely induced. The patient was nursed in a quiet room and given morphia by subcutaneous injection under light chloroform narcosis. Chloral hydrate was given by mouth or rectally. Stroganoff felt that morphia sedated the sensory centre and chloral hydrate the convulsive centre of the brain. These drugs were repeated at 3- to 6-hour intervals. Digitalis was given if tachycardia occurred. The airway was kept clear and oxygen administered as required. In his early reports he advised cupping and bleeding for pulmonary oedema, but he later abandoned this.

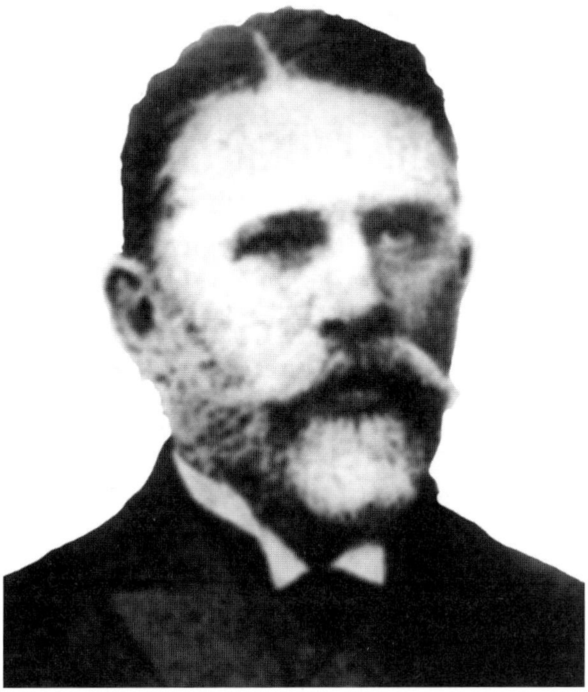

Vasili Vasilievich Stroganoff

Stroganoff recognised that 'delivery is another efficient means of interrupting fits' but spoke against caesarean section and *accouchement forcé* and only rarely used induction of labour. As other hospitals reproduced his success, Stroganoff's regimen was widely adopted and became the most common management of eclampsia in the first half of the twentieth century. The four- to five-fold reduction of maternal mortality from eclampsia represented an enormous advance.

Vasili Vasilievich Stroganoff was born in Vyazma, Russia. He graduated in medicine in 1880 and served as a medical officer for the district of Nezhinsk. In 1885 his interest in obstetrics took him to the research centre for obstetrics and gynaecology at the Povivalnyi Institut, where he was appointed professor 12 years later. He was the most influential obstetrical teacher of midwives and physicians in Russia. His book on the prophylactic treatment of eclampsia went into three Russian editions, the last of which was translated into English and French. He was recognised internationally by honorary membership in many medical societies around the world.

Selected Publications

Stroganoff VV. Lecheniyu eklampsii. *Vrach Delo* 1900; 21: 1137–40.

Stroganoff W. My improved method of the prophylactic treatment of eclampsia. *J Obstet Gynaecol Br Emp* 1923; 30: 1–31.

Stroganoff W. *The Improved Prophylactic Method in the Treatment of Eclampsia*. Edinburgh: E & S Livingstone; 1930.

Bibliography References

395, 542, 1083, 1480, 1482.

Sturmdorf, Arnold (1862–1934)

Sturmdorf Suture

In the early twentieth century, many pelvic symptoms were erroneously attributed to the lacerated or inflamed cervix. Cervical amputation (tracheloplasty) became a common operation. Prolonged suppuration and discharge from the healing cervical stump were frequent postoperative nuisances.

Marion Sims described using vaginal skin to cover the amputated cervix and promote rapid healing. The technique was perfected by Sturmdorf, and the suture he devised to cover the anterior and posterior portions of the cervix was widely adopted. This technique was extended to cover cervical amputation in operations for prolapse and some cases of cervical conisation:

> *Trimming the loose vaginal cuff to serve as an accurate lining to the interior of this muscular funnel, its retention in this position is secured in the following manner: Beginning with the anterior segment of the circular flap, a long strand of heavy silkworm gut is passed on its vaginal surface, transversely through the free border of its central*

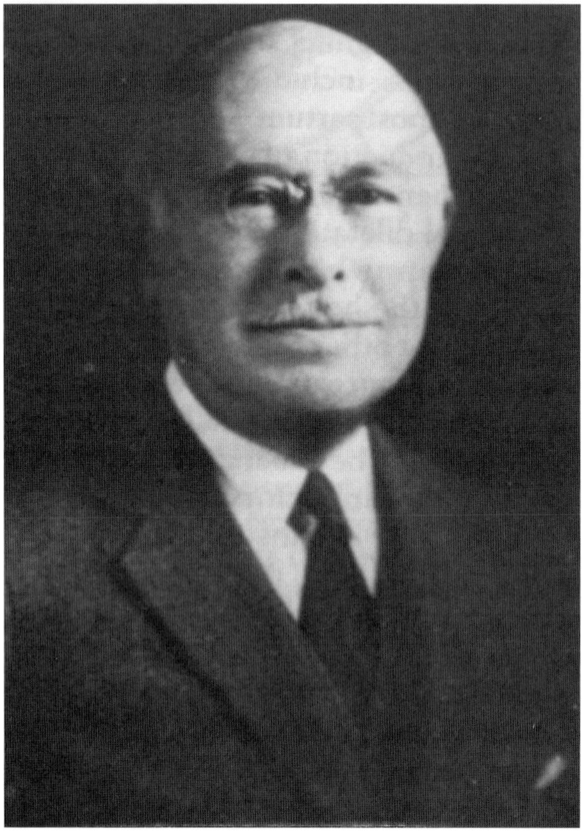

Arnold Sturmdorf

tip one-eighth of on an inch from the edge, like a mattress suture, the entrance and exit of the strand embracing a quarter inch of tissue.

The right free end of the suture is now carried into the cervical cavity to a point just above the internal os where, piercing all the tissues in a direction forward, upward, and to the right, emerges from the vaginal surface at the base of the flap.

The left free suture end after reaching the same point above the internal os, passes in the same manner forward, upward, and to the left, so that the two free ends, diverging in their transit, reappear on the surface of the anterior vaginal fornix, about one-fourth inch apart, where they are left loose for the time. The suture course for the posterior flap segment runs parallel to the above, but in a posterior direction, its free ends emerging on the surface of the posterior vaginal fornix. Now by tightening each individual set of suture ends, we draw the flap segments into the cervix, line its whole cavity with vaginal mucosa, the edge of which is thus approximated to the circumference of the internal os, where it is retained in apposition as long as desired.

Arnold Sturmdorf was born in Vienna and emigrated to New York as a youth. He received his MD in 1886 from the Columbia College of Physicians and Surgeons and practised both gynaecology and general surgery in New York. He was also an accomplished violinist. He died of myocardial infarction on 13 March 1934.

Selected Publications

Sturmdorf A. Tracheloplastic methods and results: A clinical study based upon the physiology of the mesometrium. *Surg Gynecol Obstet* 1916; 22: 93–104.

Bibliography References

536, 793, 1412, 1480, 1533.

T

Tait, Robert Lawson (1845–1899)

Ectopic Pregnancy

In the late nineteenth century, two out of three women with a ruptured tubal pregnancy died. Surgeons began to agree that the best potential for salvage was laparotomy and removal of the tube. However, by the time the diagnosis was certain, it was often too late to intervene. In 1881 Lawson Tait was consulted by a general practitioner, who suggested laparotomy. Tait procrastinated and the patient died. The autopsy confirmed the logic and feasibility of surgical treatment:

> *... I found that if I had tied the broad ligament and removed the ruptured tube I should have completely arrested the haemorrhage, and I now believe that had I done this the patient's life would have been saved.*

Two years later the chance presented itself, but the case was too far advanced and the patient was 'clearly dying'. Tait operated, but 'the patient never regained consciousness and died shortly after being removed from the operating table'. However, three months later, on 1 March 1883, Tait performed the first successful salpingectomy for a ruptured tubal pregnancy. By 1884 he reported the results of his first five cases:

> *I desire to place on record this, the first series, as I believe, of cases of extra-uterine pregnancy operated upon at the time of rupture ... I have been encouraged by my success in other abdominal diseases to try what surgery could do in these cases ... The results also confirm the soundness of interfering early in such cases, for four out of the five have been easily and completely cured of one of the most formidable conditions of pregnancy.*

Of the 40 patients Tait operated on following his first fatal case, only one died. Thus was established the life-saving operation that would become the mainstay of treatment for almost a century, until more conservative surgery and, in selected cases, medical treatment became available.

Robert Lawson Tait was born in Edinburgh and educated at Heriot's School. He attended the University of Edinburgh at the age of 15 and completed the medical course, but he took the medical licensing examination in 1866 rather than the university degree. One of his teachers was Sir James Young Simpson, whom he physically resembled and in whose house he lived for a time. As a student, 'he was fond of those diversions which appeal with such force to vigorous young manhood'.

In 1867 he was appointed house surgeon to the Wakefield Hospital in Yorkshire. There, in his twenty-fourth year, he carried out his first ovariotomy. The patient died, but the next four he performed all survived. He moved to Birmingham in 1870 and took his surgical fellowship in both the Edinburgh and English colleges. He was prominent in the movement to establish the Birmingham and Midland Hospital for Women in 1871.

Tait was one of the most audacious and talented surgeons of his era. He continually pushed back the boundaries of surgery, in particular abdominal surgery. He achieved many 'firsts', including oophorectomy for sepsis and bilateral oophorectomy for intractable menorrhagia in 1872, removal of hepatic hydatid cyst and appendicectomy for acute appendicitis in 1880, and salpingectomy for tubal pregnancy in 1883.

His advocacy of carefully considered laparotomy was known by some as Tait's Law:

> *In every case of disease in the abdomen or pelvis in which the health is destroyed or life threatened, and in which the condition is not evidently due to malignant disease, an exploration of the cavity should be made.*

When possible, he operated on patients in their own home rather than the hospital. In his early days he used Lister's technique of antisepsis. However, he soon abandoned this and used his own technique of obsessional cleansing of his hands and instruments. Without understanding the rationale completely, he used a strict aseptic technique. He always washed out the peritoneal cavity with water. Tait stopped using the clamp technique to exteriorise the ovarian pedicle and began ligating it and dropping it back into the peritoneal cavity. His results were excellent. In his second series of 50 ovariotomies, the mortality was only 6 per cent, well ahead of others at the time.

Tait was of short stature but large frame. He ate, drank and smoked excessively. He was articulate, opinionated, successful and often right – a combination guaranteed to make him enemies. He was an early admirer of Spencer Wells, but they later disagreed and became enemies. It was said that he showed 'a want of respect for age and authority remarkable even in Birmingham'. His interests and energy were enormous. As well as writing more than 200 medical papers and books, he produced leading articles for the *Birmingham Morning News* and served as president of the Birmingham Press Club. He was elected to Birmingham Town Council in 1876 and ran unsuccessfully for parliament in 1885. In the same year Tait founded and became president of the Medical Defence Union, the first litigation defence society for doctors. In 1884 he visited the United States, where he was held in high esteem. He was appointed professor of gynaecology at Queen's College, Birmingham. A founder member, he served as president of the British Gynaecological Society in 1886.

In the 1890s, the fortunes of Lawson Tait foundered. His health failed, owing to renal calculi and chronic pyelonephritis. He was sued for libel and also cited in a paternity case by one of his nurses. In 1897 he retired to Llandudno, with only occasional

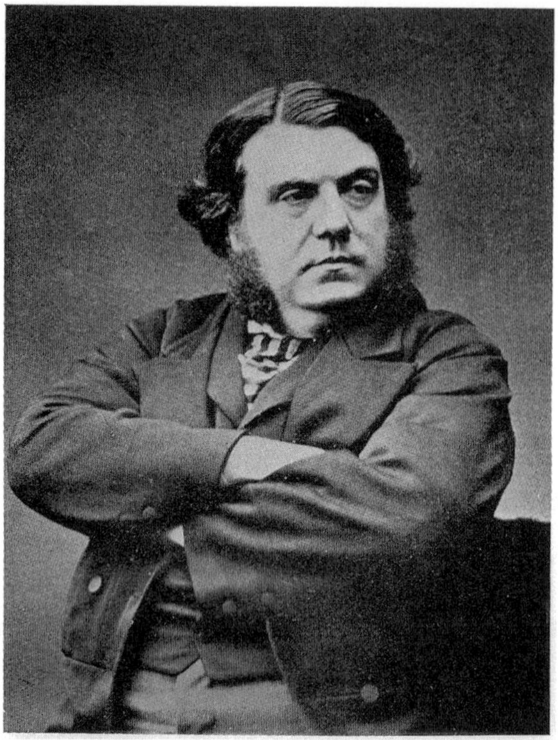

Robert Lawson Tait

consulting sessions in Birmingham. By early June 1899 he became anuric and knew he was dying. He smoked his final cigar, 'a very good Laranga – and the last I shall ever smoke', and died on 13 June 1899. Tait was cremated and his ashes laid in Warriston Cemetery, Edinburgh, close to the grave of Simpson. Hanging on the dining room wall of his house was the motto, 'Do the next thing'.

Selected Publications

Tait L. Five cases of extra-uterine pregnancy operated upon at the time of rupture. *BMJ* 1884; 1: 1250–2.

Tait L. *Lectures on Ectopic Pregnancy and Pelvic Haematocoele*. Birmingham: The 'Journal' Printing Works; 1888. Also published in: The Classics of Obstetrics and Gynecology Library. New York, NY: Gryphon Editions; 1992 (facsimile).

Bibliography References

88, 102, 177, 518, 519, 561, 753, 822, 948, 994, 1002, 1050, 1192, 1273, 1291, 1300, 1404, 1496, 1497, 1544–1546, 1552, 1645, 1734, 1746.

Tanner, James Mourilyan (1920–2010)

Tanner Stages

Jim Tanner was born on 1 August 1920 in Camberley, England, to a military family. As such he was enrolled at Marlborough College, the private school attended by his male ancestors over the previous 180 years. He started his medical studies at St Mary's Hospital Medical School in London at the beginning of the Second World War. As a student he was a nationally ranked hurdler. A Rockefeller Foundation scholarship enabled him to finish his training at the University of Pennsylvania, followed by an internship at Johns Hopkins Hospital, Baltimore.

Upon return to England, he took training posts in psychiatry, anatomy and physiology. He became interested in anthropology and auxology (the study of physical growth). The latter subject had added relevance with the need for food rationing during and following the Second World War. In 1949 he started the Harpenden Growth Study, a 25-year longitudinal study of successive generations of children whose growth was measured and assessed from childhood to adulthood.

The Tanner stages, also known as the Tanner scale, represent the physical measurements of childhood and adolescence, based on the external sex characteristics: size of breasts and genitals, testicular volume and development of pubic hair. The breast and pubic hair changes were each divided into five developmental stages. The overall study provided

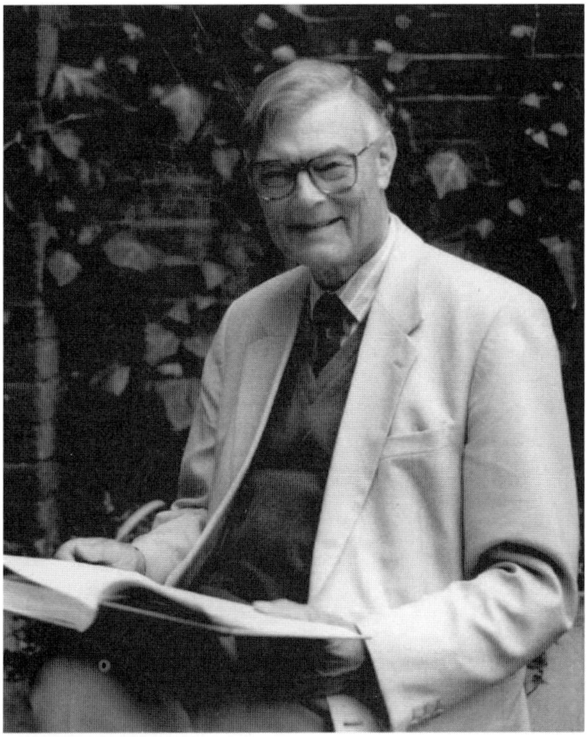

Photo: © Darrell Bock

James Mourilyan Tanner

growth charts against which the child's expected growth pattern could be assessed within its nutritional and social environment. As Tanner put it:

> *A child's growth rate reflects, better than any other simple index, his state of health and nutrition, and often indeed his psychological situation ... it is a powerful tool with which to monitor the health of a population or to pinpoint subgroups of a population whose share in economic or social benefits is less that it might be.*

In discussion of the pubertal changes in girls, Tanner noted the clinical relevance of the different stages:

> *It is important to recognize that the relation between the different events of puberty is a more significant index of normality than the chronological age at which they occur. For example, a 17-year-old girl who had not menstruated, but was growing rapidly and had breasts and pubic hair at Stage 3, could be regarded as an example of normal but late adolescence. Menarche would be expected in the near future. If, on the other hand, breasts and pubic hair had been mature for 2 or 3 years and growth had apparently ceased, the relation between events would be abnormal and a different explanation would have to be looked for. Yet other causes would have to be considered if there were no signs of puberty at all.*

Tanner's stage charts have been universally adopted as the best assessment of pubertal development.

The Harpenden Study was to be the core of Tanner's research career. He appointed a former regimental sergeant-major, Reginald Whitehouse (1911–87), as his research assistant. Their basement office leaked during rainstorms, and they often continued work under umbrellas.

In 1956 Tanner established the department of growth and development at the Institute of Child Health at London University, and in 1966 he was appointed as the first professor of child health and growth. Tanner's work was recognised by many international honours, including honorary degrees from universities in Madrid, Genoa and Budapest. He died on 11 August 2010 following a stroke.

Selected Publications

Tanner JM. *Growth at Adolescence*. Oxford: Blackwell Scientific Publications; 1955.

Marshall WA, Tanner JM. Variations in patterns of pubertal changes in girls. *Arch Dis Child* 1969; 44: 291–303.

Marshall WA, Tanner JM. Variations in patterns of pubertal changes in boys. *Arch Dis Child* 1970; 45: 13–23.

Bibliography References

565, 781, 1031, 1553, 1554, 1673.

Tarnier, Étienne Stéphane (1828–1897)

Tarnier's Axis-Traction Forceps/Neonatal Incubator

In the early nineteenth century, it was recognised that with high forceps delivery, traction in the axis of the upper pelvic curve was impossible. Thus, a lot of the traction was dissipated against the anterior pelvic wall, increasing the amount of force required for delivery. Manoeuvres such as that of Charles Pajot were used but could only partially compensate. Spurious attempts at developing axis-traction devices had been suggested by Hermann, Hubert and Pros of La Rochelle. However, it was Stéphane Tarnier who developed the first logical and effective axis-traction forceps. In his 1877 monograph on the subject Tarnier outlined his rationale:

> *All obstetricians know that in a proper application of the forceps, traction ought to be directed, as far as possible, in the axis of the pelvis; but all acknowledge that at the superior strait and above this strait it is impossible to pull far enough back, because the instrument is unavoidably maintained in the wrong direction by the resistance of the perineum. I will go farther and say that at the level of the inferior strait and of the vulval orifice, traction is always misdirected when one uses ordinary forceps, because of the very shape of the instrument . . .*

In his effort to produce the appropriate axis-traction forceps, Tarnier engaged two assistants: an artillery colonel and a craftsman. Some 30 different trial models were produced before Tarnier was satisfied. Two slim rods were attached by articulating joints to the blades beneath the fenestrae. These rods were combined in a separate handle below the forceps grip. Traction on the handle of the rods was therefore in the axis of the upper pelvis, resulting in much less force to achieve descent of the fetal head. These forceps were considered a great advance in reducing trauma to the fetus. Tarnier's forceps or other axis-traction modifications were used for the next century until the abandonment of high and difficult mid forceps.

Étienne Stéphane Tarnier was born on 29 April 1828 in the small town of Aiserey, near Dijon, France. His father was the local doctor. Tarnier did his medical studies in Paris, taking time out as a student to return to Dijon and help his father during a cholera epidemic. In 1856 he embarked upon further training in obstetrics at the Maternité in Paris, with a view to gaining enough experience to enter general practice in the country. Later he decided to specialise in obstetrics and made a study of puerperal sepsis. At one point he noted 31 deaths in 32 labours. He wrote his inaugural thesis on the subject in 1857 and, supported by his own studies, embraced the views of Ignac Semmelweis. After his training at the Maternité, Tarnier entered private practice in Paris. He was not successful and was on the verge of becoming a country doctor when his

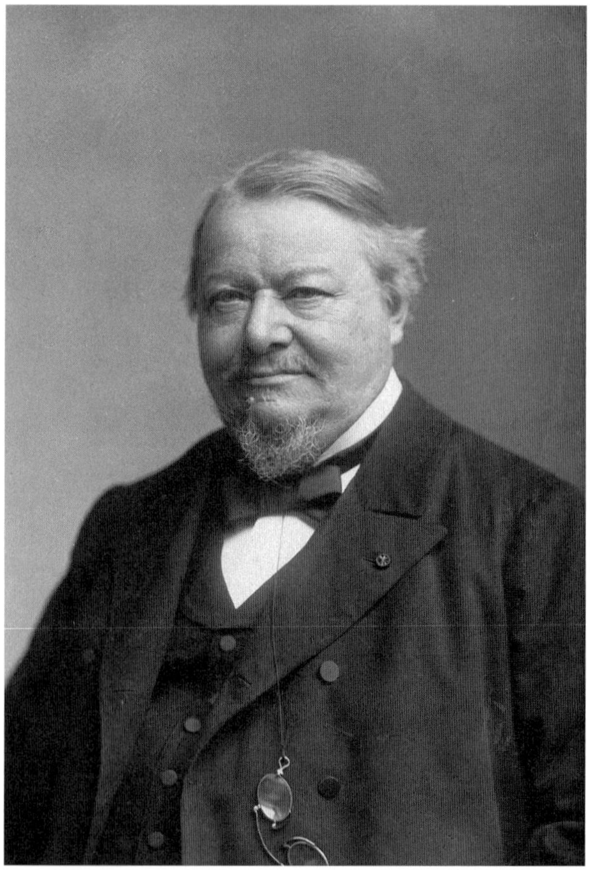

Étienne Stéphane Tarnier

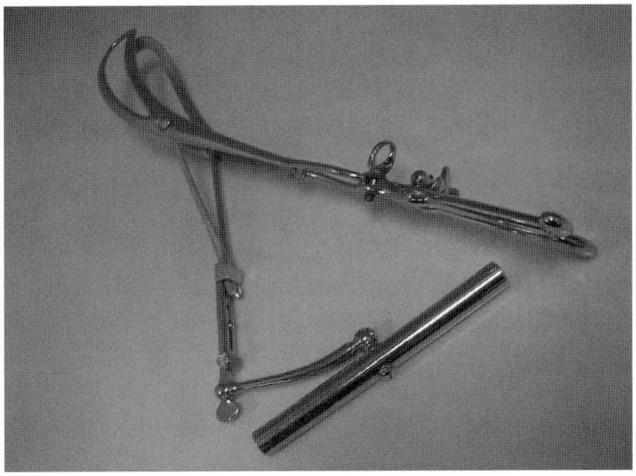

Tarnier's axis-traction forceps

work on puerperal sepsis gained attention and an appointment to the clinic at the Maternité. He became chief of the clinic in 1867 and in 1889 succeeded Pajot as the professor of obstetrics in the University of Paris. Pajot had strongly criticised Tarnier's axis-traction forceps and had received a tactful but clear rebuttal.

Tarnier's contribution to French obstetrics was considerable. In addition to his work on puerperal sepsis, he advanced the cause of the premature infant with heated incubators and gavage feeding. He was stimulated to produce the incubator when he saw a heated incubator used for hatching the eggs of exotic birds at the Paris Zoo in 1880. The following year he introduced a neonatal version to the Maternité.

Tarnier suffered a stroke on the day of his retirement and died soon after, on 23 November 1897. He was revered by his patients, colleagues and students. In 1905 a monument in his honour was unveiled on the side of the building where he worked at the corner of Rue d'Assas and the Avenue de l'Observatoire. The inscription reads: 'To the Master who devoted his life to the mothers and infants: from colleagues, his pupils, his friends, his admirers'.

Selected Publications

Tarnier ES. *Description de deux nouveaux forceps*. Paris: Martinet; 1877.

The new forceps of M. Tarnier. *BMJ* 1877; 1: 665–6.

Bibliography References

54, 67, 99, 183, 334, 451, 455, 478, 648, 721, 770, 1132, 1202, 1261, 1285, 1595, 1728.

Te Linde, Richard Wesley (1894–1985)

Operative Gynaecology Text

Richard Te Linde was born in Waupun, Wisconsin, to first-generation Americans of Dutch ancestry. His premedical studies were taken at Hope College in Holland, Michigan and at the University of Wisconsin. He received his medical degree from Johns Hopkins University in 1920 and carried out his residency in obstetrics and gynaecology at the same institution.

Te Linde was appointed professor and chairman of gynaecology, then a separate department from obstetrics, at Johns Hopkins in 1939 and retired in 1960. He continued in private practice in Baltimore until 1978 but gave up operating when he broke his hip in 1966. He helped pioneer fascial sling operations for stress incontinence in the United States and did much of the early work in delineating the diagnosis and appropriate treatment of cervical carcinoma in situ. In his early years, Te Linde carried out basic research with rhesus monkeys, which gave support to John Sampson's theory of histogenesis in endometriosis.

Feeling that there was no comprehensive text on gynaecological surgery, in 1946 he published *Operative Gynaecology*, which was destined to become a standard work. After retirement he enlisted his former resident, Richard Mattingly, as co-author for the fourth and fifth editions. It continues to be the standard American text under successive authors, who until recently were all his former residents.

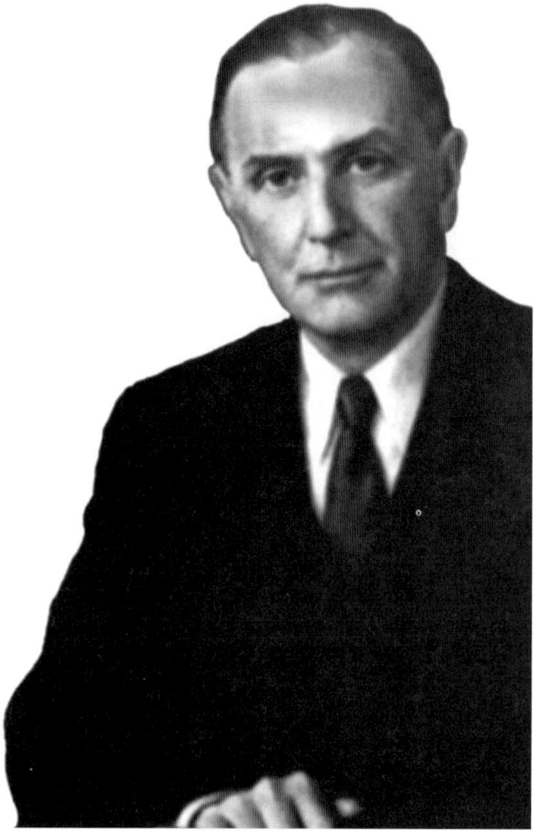

Richard Wesley Te Linde

Te Linde was a keen fisherman and spent many summers in Canada in pursuit of trout and Atlantic salmon. He was president of the American Gynecological Society in 1953. On 16 November 1989, at the age of 95, Richard Te Linde died at home in Baltimore.

Selected Publications

Te Linde RW. *Operative Gynecology*. 1st edn. Philadelphia, PA; Lippincott; 1946.

Bibliography References

135, 786, 1003, 1245, 1314, 1485, 1561, 1564, 1571, 1720.

Thoms, Herbert (1885–1972)

Thoms' X-Ray View of the Pelvic Brim

In the early days of X-ray pelvimetry, an accurate method of measuring the pelvic inlet was not available. The limiting factor was the inability to bring the incline of the pelvic brim parallel to the horizontal X-ray plate. Herbert Thoms devised a technique to overcome this problem:

> *... it is essential that the target shall be placed over the center of the superior strait and that all portions of the plane to this strait shall be equidistant from the sensitive plate. This is found possible with the patient in the semirecumbent position with the back of the patient arched ... Arching the back furthermore tends to throw the upper part of the trunk away from the vertical.*

Thoms found this technique produced accurate measurement of the pelvic brim in the non-pregnant patient and 'during the first six months of pregnancy'. He was a prolific contributor to the literature, with more than 50 articles on the pelvis. He tended to publish early, and some of his later papers were to correct previous errors after subsequent analytical reflection.

Herbert Thoms was born in Waterbury, Connecticut. He was of Scottish extraction on his father's side,

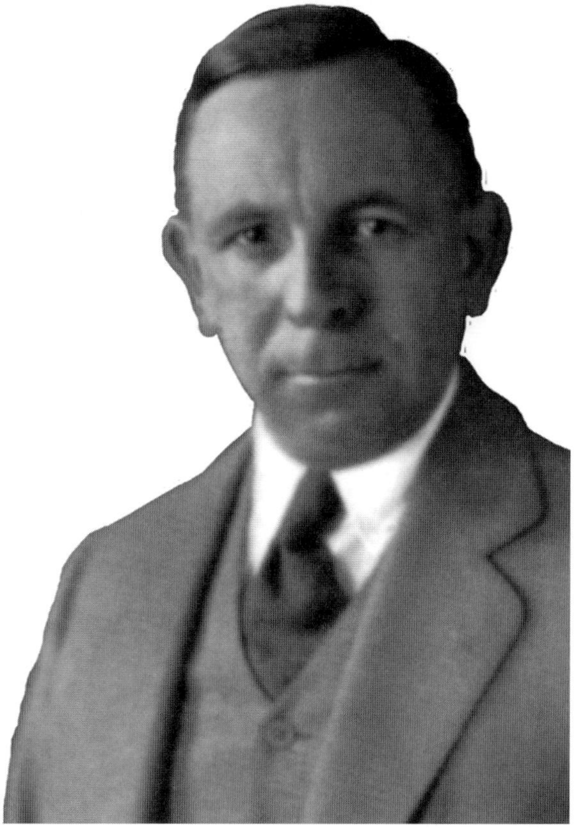

Herbert Thoms

and his mother was a descendant of Deacon Stephen Hart after whom Hartford, Connecticut was named. After school he worked in the laboratory of the American Brass Company for three years. In 1906 he entered Yale Medical College and graduated in 1910, having also been a member of the Yale choir during his student years. From 1911 to 1915 he trained in obstetrics and gynaecology at the Sloane Hospital for Women in New York and Johns Hopkins, Baltimore, interspersed with two years of general practice in New London, Connecticut. In 1915 he entered private practice in New Haven, with an appointment at Yale University. In 1927 he joined the Yale department of obstetrics and gynaecology as a full-time associate professor, becoming professor and head of the department in 1947. Thoms' productivity was legendary: he published several well-received books on medical history as well as taking courses in English literature, German, photography and etching – in all of which he became proficient.

Selected Publications

Thoms H. Outlining the superior strait of the pelvis by means of the X-ray. *Am J Obstet Gynecol* 1922; 4: 257–63.

Bibliography References

138, 497, 607, 801, 1485, 1561.

Torpin, Richard Ivan (1891–1976)

Torpin Packer/Vacuum Extractor

Richard Torpin was born in Oakdale, Nebraska, on 26 March 1891. He graduated MD from Rush Medical College, Chicago in 1917. After some general practice in rural Montana, he returned to Chicago as an assistant in obstetrics and gynaecology in 1928. He moved to Augusta, Georgia, in 1936 and one year later was appointed professor and head of the newly combined department of obstetrics and gynaecology. Torpin was a restless man with an inventive mind. From a workshop in his house, he produced prototypes of a number of obstetric devices including, an X-ray pelvimeter, neonatal insufflators, uterine packer and vacuum extractor. He was best known for his uterine packer, which he first reported in 1941 and which was still in use some 50 years later. He published his initial series of 11 successful cases using his uterine packer for severe post-partum haemorrhage unresponsive to pituitrin and ergot preparations. He had modified the uterine packer designed some 40 years earlier by another Rush Medical College graduate, Rudolph Holmes:

> *To facilitate the obstetric operation of uterine packing for postpartum haemorrhage so that within one or two*

minutes the pack may be introduced aseptically into the very apex and horns of the uterine cavity, the herein described instrument is offered. It is a large size modified Holmes packer with, as an integral part, a container for the requisite gauze pack. The length of the tube is about 6 inches and its diameter ¾ inches . . . The obstetrician introduces his right index and middle fingers into the finger holds and his thumb into the ring of the obturator piston. The introducing tube is then gently pushed through the vagina and cervix into the hollow of the left hand in the uterine cavity. The pack is then displaced by the obturator into the uterine cavity.

Two years earlier Torpin had published a preliminary report of a vacuum extractor. Apparently, the prototype was a 10 cm diameter toy rubber ball cut in half with the inner surface studded with projections from tyre patches, the latter based on the observation of James Young Simpson that the lining of the suckers of cuttlefish contained projections. He described the device as follows:

The device . . . is essentially a somewhat flexible concave hemisphere of a size to fit the fetal vertex rather snugly. In the center of the convex surface is a one-finger handle and adjacent toward one end is a hollow rubber tube leading from the vacuum pump and opening on to the concave surface. In addition, on the convex surface are two lugs for rotating . . . The concave surface is studded with rubber projections . . . the purpose of these is to keep the fetal scalp from blocking the small opening leading to the vacuum pump and thereby presenting as great an area as possible to the suction . . .

His paper reported ten cases of delay in the second stage of labour with successful use of his extractor. However, he later encountered many failures and ultimately abandoned its use.

Richard Torpin retired from the department in Augusta in 1958 and followed this with a two-year appointment as professor and head of obstetrics and gynaecology at Shiraz, Iran. He then retired back to Augusta and died there from a heart attack on 27 January 1976.

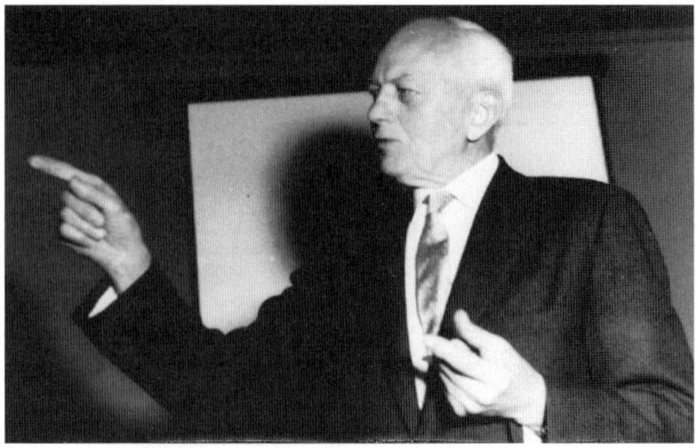

Richard Ivan Torpin

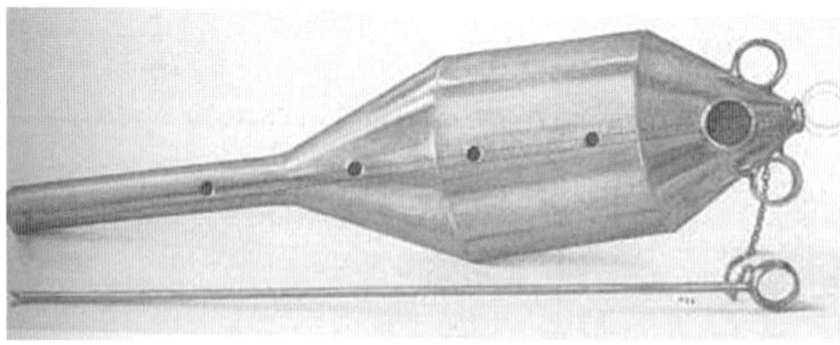

Torpin's uterine packer

Selected Publications

Torpin R. Preliminary report of obstetric device. *J Med Soc Georgia* 1939; 27: 96–8.

Torpin R. An automatic post-partum uterine packer. *Am J Obstet Gynecol* 1941; 41: 344–7.

Bibliography References

92, 122, 179, 971, 1453, 1621.

Trendelenburg, Friedrich (1844–1924)

Trendelenburg Position

The inclined position, with the head and chest lower than the pelvis, has been used since antiquity to reduce hernias and assist in the replacement of intestines with evisceration injuries. Trendelenburg was not the first to advocate this position for pelvic surgery but his academic stature brought it into general use and popularity. He first used the position to facilitate the abdominal transvesical approach in repair of vesicovaginal fistulae

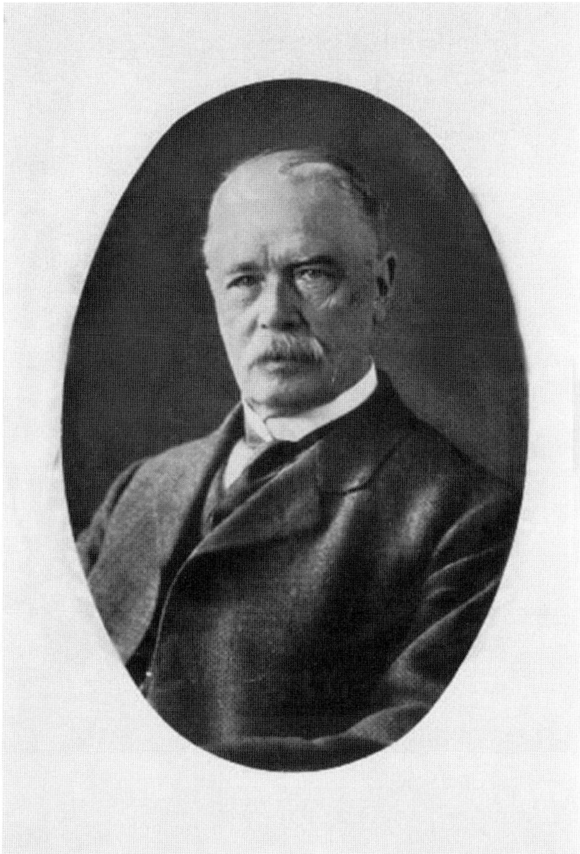

Friedrich Trendelenburg

that were not accessible by the vaginal route. He described the virtues of the position thus:

> *If the patient is placed on the operating table so that the pubic symphysis forms the highest point of the trunk and the long axis of the latter forms an angle of at least 45° with the horizontal, the abdominal organs fall into the concavity of the diaphragm.*

> *We work in the full light of the window, like the artist at his easel, without having to stoop . . . and without being burdened by protruding loops of bowel.*

Trendelenburg recognised the risks of this position on cardiac and respiratory function and advocated that the extreme angle only be used for five to ten minutes at a time. He designed an operating table with padded shoulder braces to accommodate the patient in this position. With modern anaesthesia and muscle relaxants, the full Trendelenburg position is not necessary, but minor degrees of this position remain helpful in pelvic surgery.

Friedrich Trendelenburg was born in Berlin and well educated in Latin and English. He studied medicine at the University of Berlin, graduating in 1866, but spent part of his student days in Edinburgh and Glasgow. When only 30 years of age, he was appointed director of the surgical ward in the Friedrichshain Hospital, Berlin. He later held successive appointments as professor of surgery at the Universities of Rostock, Bonn and Leipzig.

Trendelenburg was an energetic and productive surgical innovator. He has one of the largest lists of eponymous credits to his name. In addition to his position there are a sign, gait, test and four operations. He died from a malignant tumour of the lower jaw.

Selected Publications

Trendelenburg F. Über Blasenscheidenfisteloperationen und über Beckenhochlagerung bei Operationen in der Bauchhöhle. *Samml Klin Vortr* 1890; 355: 3372–92.

Bibliography References

140, 391, 553, 648, 1291, 1383, 1412, 1474, 1628.

Tucker, Ervin Alden (1862–1902) McLane, James Woods (1839–1912)

Tucker–McLane Forceps

James McLane was born in New York City and graduated in medicine from the College of Physicians and Surgeons in 1864. He became professor of obstetrics and diseases of women at his alma mater in 1878. McLane was instrumental in getting the Sloane Maternity Hospital built as a teaching hospital for the college and became the first president of the board of managers. He designed his solid bladed forceps in

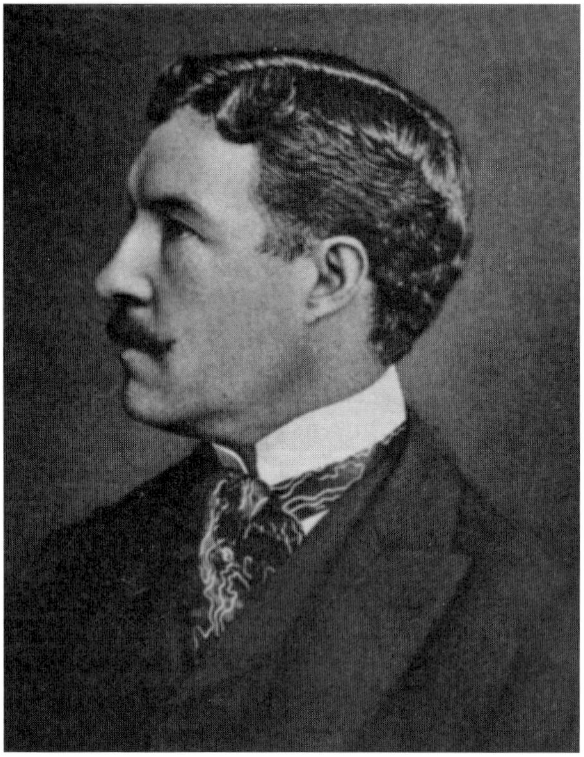

Ervin Alden Tucker

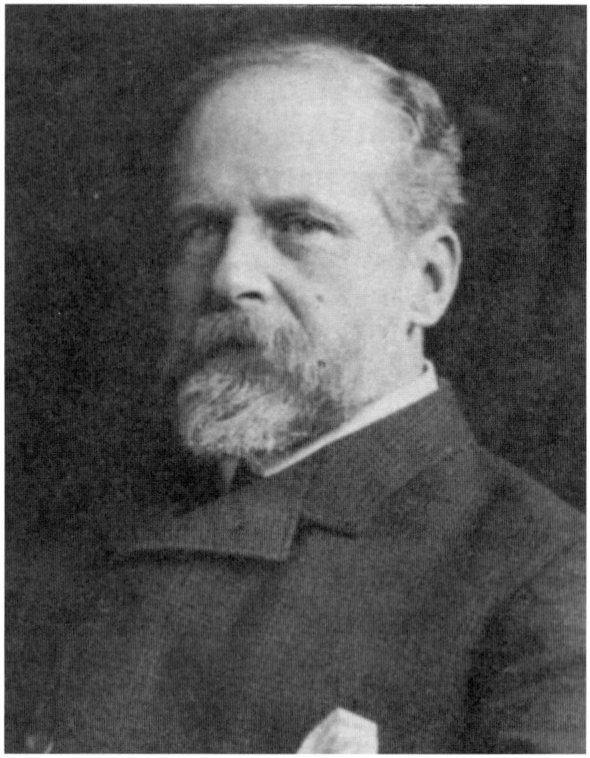

James Woods McLane

1868 but never published a description. They were manufactured by George Tiemann and Company and first appeared in their catalogue in 1880. McLane's first publication on the use of his forceps was in his 1891 report of the first 1,000 deliveries at the Sloane Maternity Hospital. There were 83 forceps deliveries, and his forceps were used in 81. When his original forceps were placed in the hospital museum he wrote:

> *This is the original 'McLane Forceps', designed by Dr McLane and made for him by Tiemann & Co. This instrument was used by him for 30 years, in private practice, and in this Hospital, and with it he delivered the first child by a forceps operation born in the Sloane Maternity Hospital, Dr Tucker – a Resident Physician thought the shank too short for high operations – and had it made slightly longer – as seen in the 'McLane–Tucker' instrument.*

McLane was elected president of the College of Physicians and Surgeons of New York in 1889. He died on 25 November 1912.

Ervin Tucker, of English descent, was born in Attleboro, Massachusetts. He graduated MD from the College of Physicians and Surgeons of New York in 1889. He took postgraduate studies at the Nursery and Child's Hospital of New York and also worked in Germany with Alfred Duhrssen. In December 1890 Tucker became a resident

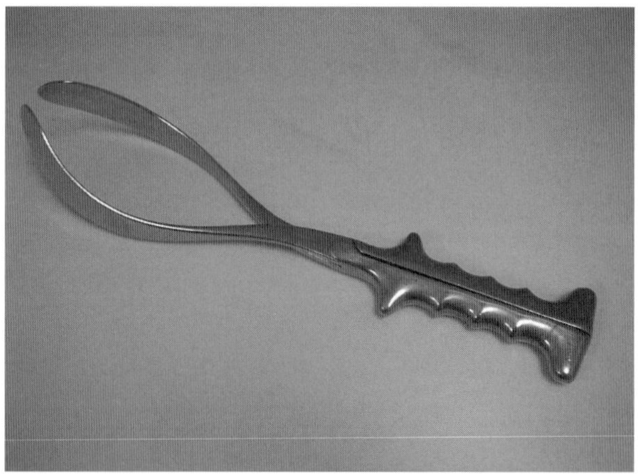

Tucker–McLane forceps

obstetrician at the Sloane Maternity Hospital and there modified McLane's forceps by lengthening the shank. In 1898 he helped found and was first president of the Society of the Alumni of the Sloane Maternity Hospital. He was the first doctor in New York to confine himself to obstetric practice. Tucker died at 40 years of age from pneumonia after an all-night obstetric case and exposure to a February storm.

Selected Publications

McLane JW. The Sloane Maternity Hospital. Report on the first series of one thousand successive confinements from January 1st, 1886 to October 1st, 1890. *Am J Obstet Gynecol* 1891; 24: 385–418.

Bibliography References

36, 361, 536, 554, 721, 801, 1025, 1480, 1484, 1485, 1634, 1658, 1669.

Tuohy, Edward Boyce (1908–1959)

Tuohy Needle

After the introduction of regional anaesthetic techniques in the early twentieth century, methods were devised to allow continuous infusion of local anaesthetics into the subarachanoid or epidural space. In 1939 William Lemmon of Philadelphia used a malleable needle, but it had the drawback of potential dislodgement and rare but serious breakage. For continuous spinal anaesthesia, Edward Tuohy introduced a ureteral catheter down a 15-gauge needle:

> *In an effort to obviate the difficulty of the malleable needle becoming displaced, a new method of performing continuous spinal anesthesia was devised utilizing a ureteral catheter . . . It was my feeling that a number 4 ureteral catheter would be less traumatic to tissues than a needle (malleable) when it is left in position for the duration of an operation, and if the catheter was satisfactorily introduced into the subarachnoid space it would not become dislodged as easily as a needle. The hazard of breakage of the catheter during any portion of the procedure did not appear to be as great as that with a needle, because of the flexibility and mobility of the catheter.*

With the normal exit bevel of a needle, the direction in which the catheter will advance, either cephalad or caudad, cannot be predicted. Tuohy therefore designed a needle with a lateral opening at the end to guide the catheter tip as it leaves the needle. Later the Tuohy needle was used by Manuel Curbelo, a Cuban anaesthetist, for continuous epidural block. It remains the standard needle guide for epidural catheter placement to provide analgesia in labour. The Tuohy needle was also used by William Liley and subsequent workers to place an epidural catheter in the fetal peritoneal cavity and allow transfusion in cases of severe isoimmunisation.

Edward Tuohy was born in Duluth, Minnesota, the son of a physician. He received his bachelor of science degree in 1929 from the University of Minnesota, and also played ice hockey for his university. He took his medical degree at the University of Pennsylvania in 1932. In 1933 he started as a fellow in

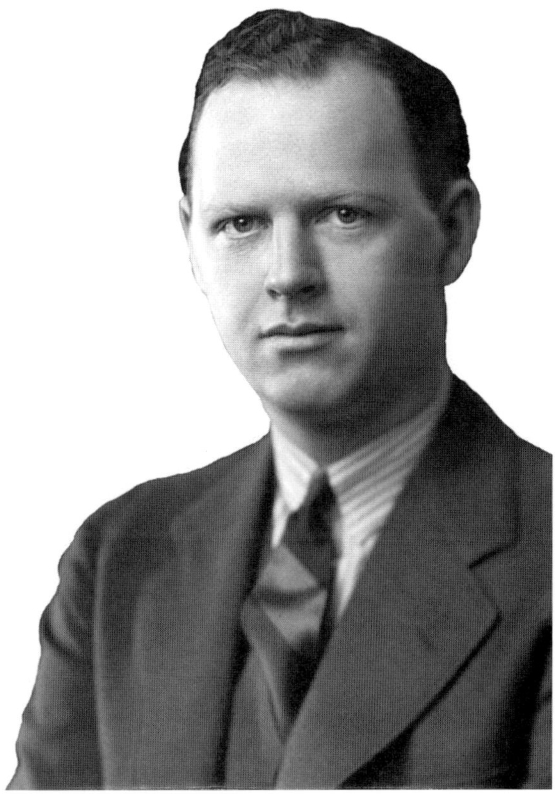

Edward Boyce Tuohy

medicine at the Mayo Clinic but transferred to anaesthesia and joined the staff as a consultant anaesthetist in 1935. From 1942–45 he served in the US Army Medical Corps in Washington DC and Battle Creek, Michigan, attaining the rank of major. He returned to the Mayo Clinic but left again in 1947 for Washington DC, where he became professor of anaesthesiology in the Georgetown University School of Medicine. His final move was to Los Angeles in 1951. Tuohy was elected president of the American Society of Anesthesiologists in 1947. He died of a cerebrovascular accident in his fiftieth year.

Selected Publications

Curbelo MM. Continuous peridural segmental anaesthesia by means of a ureteral catheter. *Curr Res Anesth Analg* 1949; 28: 12–23.

Tuohy EB. Continuous spinal anesthesia: its usefulness and technique involved. *Anesthesiology* 1944; 5: 142–8.

Tuohy EB. The use of continuous spinal anesthesia utilizing the ureteral catheter technic. *JAMA* 1945; 128: 262–4.

Bibliography References

60, 430, 431, 517, 584, 996, 1008, 1357, 1730.

Turner, Henry Hubert (1892–1970)

Turner's Syndrome

The association between small stature and defective ovarian development had been noted by the German physicians Funke and Rossle in the early part of the twentieth century. It was Henry Turner, in 1938, who described the full syndrome of small stature, sexual infantilism, webbed neck and cubitus valgus in seven young females seen over a five-year period:

> *This unusual phenomenon was observed exclusively in seven female patients, aged 15 to 23 years. Among the characteristic signs were retardation in growth and sexual underdevelopment. Webbing of the neck was slight to marked. Absence or fusion of the cervical vertebrae was not demonstrated, and the shortening of the neck was merely apparent, due to the webbing, and not real. The posterior hair margin extended well down on the neck. Deformity of the elbow, consisting of an increase in the carrying angle, or cubitus valgus, was constantly present.*

Later the associated chromosomal abnormality 45 XO was established. The term gonadal dysgenesis is also used.

Henry Hubert Turner was born in Harrisburg, Illinois. He graduated MD from the University of Louisville in 1921. Postgraduate study followed in the United States, London and Vienna. He became the doyen of clinical endocrinology in the United States. He diagnosed his own lung cancer as inoperable and worked on until his death on 4 August 1970.

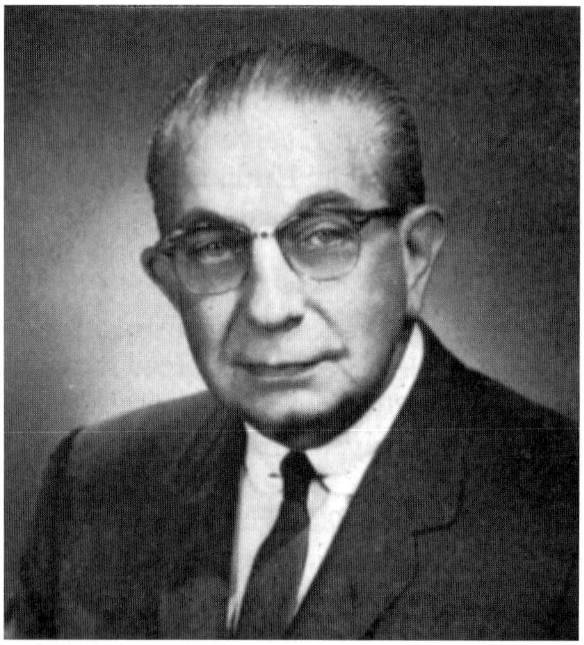

Henry Hubert Turner

Selected Publications

Turner HH. A syndrome of infantilism, congenital webbed neck, and cubitus valgus. *Endocrinology* 1938; 23: 566–74.

Bibliography References

406, 968, 1031, 1480, 1637.

U

Uchida, Hajime (1921–1996)

Uchida Tubal Ligation

In what must have been a career-long commitment to providing birth control services for women, Hajime Uchida was able to write, 'I have personally accomplished over 20,000 sterilisations during the past 28 years without a known failure and with minimal complications'. Uchida attributed the lack of failure to the fact that in his technique the proximal portion of the tube was buried beneath the serosa after ligation and the distal portion was ligated so that it was exterior to the serosa. In his 1975 article in the *American Journal of Obstetrics and Gynecology*, he described his technique as follows:

> *Uterine curettage should be carried out initially . . . the curet should be left in the uterus for manipulation of the fundus. An incision, 0.7 to 1 cm, is made in the skin between the umbilicus and symphysis . . . through this incision, which is held open with Uchida abdominal wall hooks, the entire length of the salpinx can be removed by use of a Uchida salpinx forceps. The curet which remains in the uterus and the salpinx forceps are handled with left and right hands respectively as a knife and fork . . . Epinephrine, saline solution (1:1000) is injected beneath the subserosa of the ampulla of the distal tube. This produces an ischemic fullness about the tube. The ballooned portion causes the muscular layer to separate from the serosa. When the edematous bleb is opened, the muscular tube will spring up in the shape of the letter 'U'. A 5 cm section of the tube toward the uterus is severed and ligated whereupon the ligated parts bury themselves beneath the serosa. The distal end is ligated together with the open fringe of the serosa.*

When the sterilisation was carried out post partum, or at the time of caesarean section, Uchida used the same technique but advised concomitant fimbriectomy. At a time when laparoscopic techniques of tubal ligation were becoming popular, Uchida claimed, 'This operation is simpler and safer than other methods of sterilisation, particularly laparoscopic sterilisation. No complicated apparatus is needed, and generally, it can be completed in about 5 minutes'.

Hajime Uchida was born on 26 July 1921 and graduated in medicine from Kyoto University in March 1945. He spent a short time training in the department of obstetrics and gynaecology at Kyoto University but then moved to his father's hospital, the Uchida Hospital in Ishikiwa. His father was a noted gynaecologist who ran his own private hospital of

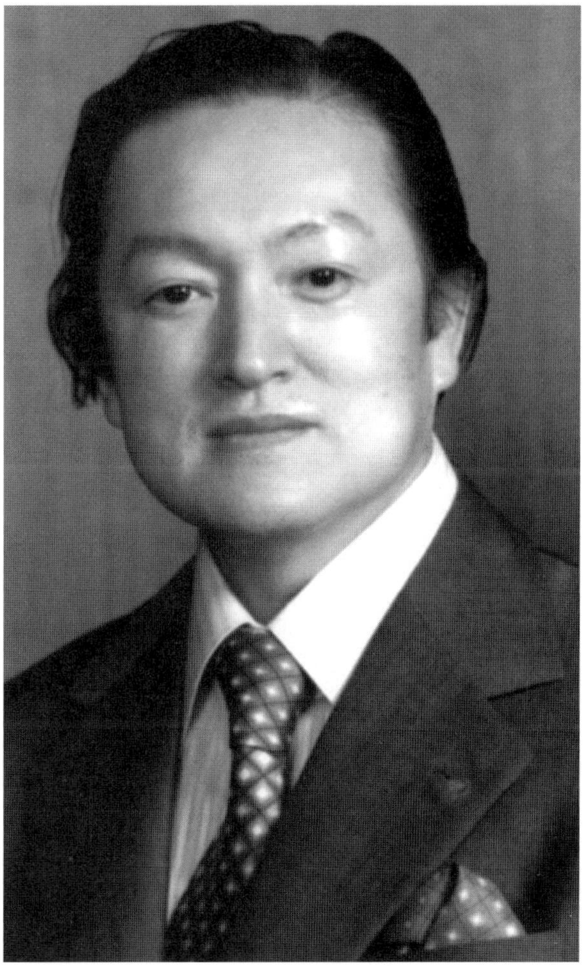

Hajime Uchida

obstetrics and gynaecology, which had more than 200 beds. Here Hajime Uchida learned his specialty and received his doctor of medical science in 1950. He spent his career working at the Uchida Hospital and ultimately succeeded his father as director of the hospital. He first presented his technique of abdominal tubal ligation in 1961 at the Third World Congress of Obstetrics and Gynaecology in Vienna, Austria. He served on a number of committees, including council of the Japan Society of Obstetrics and Gynaecology. He died on 22 September 1996 and was followed into the specialty by his son.

Selected Publications

Uchida H. *Uchida's abdominal sterilization technique.* Proceedings: Third World Congress of Obstetrics and Gynaecology, 1961, Vienna, Austria.

Uchida H. Uchida tubal sterilization. *Amer J Obstet Gynecol* 1975; 121: 153–8.

Bibliography References

168, 1235, 1410.

V

Vacca, Aldo (1941–2014)

Vacuum-Assisted Delivery

Aldo Vacca was born in the small town of Ingham, Northern Queensland, Australia, on 28 August 1941. Both his parents were born in Northern Italy. He graduated in medicine from the University of Queensland in 1965. Vacca worked in Papua New Guinea for eight years, initially as a general practitioner and later in obstetrics and gynaecology. It was here he worked with and was influenced by Geoffrey Bird, who trained him in the principles and practice of vacuum-assisted delivery. He completed his postgraduate training in Perth, Western Australia, and Portsmouth, England. It was in Portsmouth, from 1979 to 1981, that he conducted the definitive trial comparing vacuum with forceps assisted delivery, which helped popularise and establish the role of vacuum extraction.

Upon return to Australia, Vacca worked successively as director of obstetrics at the Mater Hospital, Brisbane, the Caboolture Hospital, Queensland, and consultant at the Royal Brisbane and Women's Hospital. He was appointed associate professor of obstetrics and gynaecology at the University of Queensland.

In 1990 he established Vacca Research to provide information on intrapartum care and interactive computer programmes for self-directed learning for obstetricians and midwives. He also wrote the definitive text, *Handbook of Vacuum Delivery*, which went to three editions between 1992 and 2009.

Vacca visited Tage Malmström on two occasions. By the mid-1990s he felt that the modern companies making vacuum extractors were missing the basic principles laid down by Malmström and Bird. They were, by producing a bell-shaped vacuum cup, reducing the ability of the accoucheur to place the cup over the flexion point of the fetal head, especially in the occipito-posterior position. One of his main teaching points was, 'It's always more posterior than you think', which he incorporated into a whimsical fifteen-verse poem to emphasise its importance. The first verse reads:

> *Vacuum extraction may drive some to distraction,*
> *While others may find comfort in a drink.*
> *Though life's replete with clichés, the answer is in the catch phrase:*
> *'It's always more posterior than you think'.*

Most of the companies manufacturing modern vacuum extractors did not heed his advice. The exception was Dean Wallace of Clinical Innovations in Utah; as a bioengineer, he understood the logic of Vacca's ideas. They first met in May 1998, and one year later the OmniCup vacuum extractor was produced, having been

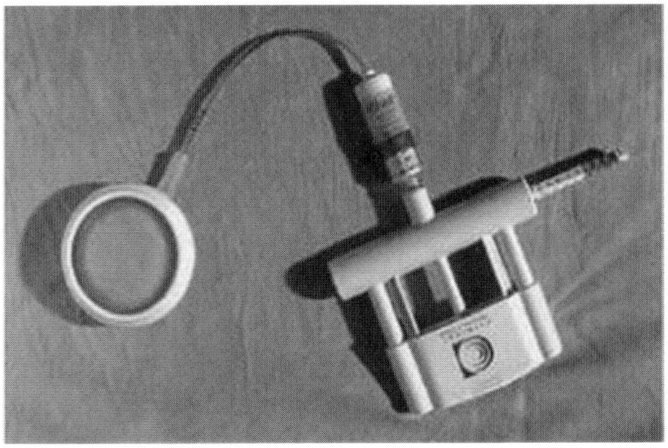

OmniCup vacuum extractor

tested and refined by Vacca in his clinical practice. The cup was combined with a handheld vacuum pump and produced by Clinical Innovations as a disposable unit. The name, OmniCup, was given by Vacca, as the cup could be used for any position of the fetal head. The name Kiwi was added by the marketing department of the company, ironically inappropriate for an Australian innovation. Vacca did not receive any proprietary gain and refused the offer to have the cup named after him. However, when, at his instigation the company produced a reusable device for low-resource regions, they named it the Vacca reusable OmniCup.

From 1999 Vacca split his time between teaching and clinical work. Assisted by his wife Janet, a registered nurse and midwife, he undertook an extensive schedule of seminars on vacuum-assisted delivery. Over a 15-year period he held teaching sessions in 33 countries involving thousands of doctors and midwives. Since 1999 some ten million OmniCups have been used to assist delivery.

Vacca's sustained commitment and contribution to obstetrics and safe vacuum-assisted delivery was recognised in 2007 with the award of the Medal of the Order of Australia, and by the Distinguished Service Medal from the Royal Australian and New Zealand College of Obstetricians and Gynaecologists (RANZCOG) in 2011. Aldo Vacca died on 16 March 2014, three months after his last teaching tour. In September 2015, at the Royal College of Obstetricians and Gynaecologists in London, a postgraduate symposium on operative vaginal delivery was held in his honour. The proceeds from this meeting were donated to the RANZCOG and helped support the Aldo Vacca Medal for original research at the college's annual scientific meeting, first awarded in 2016.

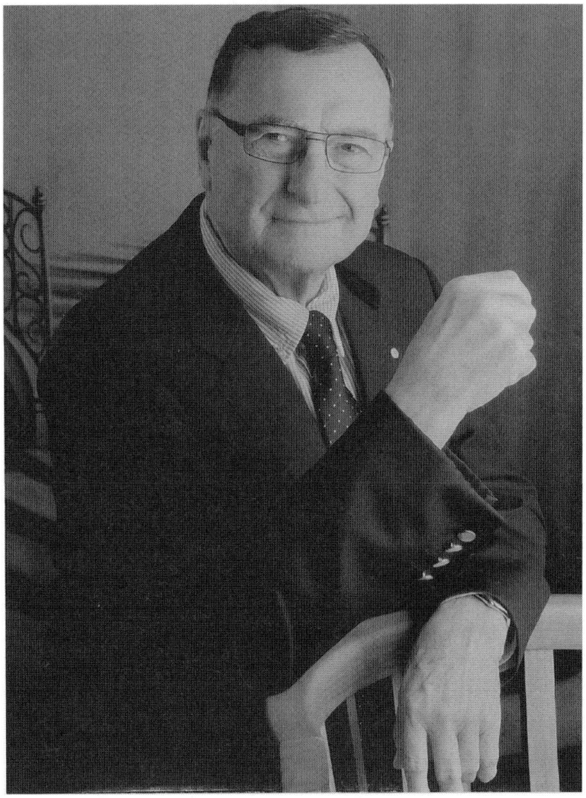

Aldo Vacca

Perhaps the most appropriate tribute to Aldo Vacca is embodied in this quote from Cicero (106–43 BC):

> *What nobler employment or more valuable to the state than that of the man who instructs the rising generation.*

Selected Publications

Vacca A, Grant A, Wyatt G, Chalmers I. Portsmouth operative delivery trial: a comparison of vacuum extraction and forceps delivery. *Br J Obstet Gynaecol* 1983; 90: 1007–1112.

Vacca A. It's always more posterior than you think. *Aust NZ J Obstet Gynaecol* 1999; 39: 136–7.

Vacca A, Operative vaginal delivery: clinical appraisal of a new vacuum extraction device. *Aust NZ J Obstet Gynaecol* 2001; 41: 156–60.

Vacca A, *Handbook of Vacuum Delivery in Obstetric Practice*. 3rd edn. Brisbane: Vacca Research; 2009.

Bibliography References

92, 99, 260, 532, 1133.

Veres, János (1903–1979)

Veres Needle

There can be few pieces of equipment with which the modern gynaecologist is more familiar then the Veres needle, used to introduce the pneumoperitoneum for laparoscopy. The needle was devised by János Veres, a chest physician, while he was chief of the department of internal medicine at the Regional Hospital, Kapuvar, Hungary. He used it to create a pneumothorax in cases of pulmonary tuberculosis in the 1930s.

The insufflation needle has a sharp outer canula and an inner blunt trocar with a spring mechanism. When the needle meets the resistance of the abdominal wall, the protruding blunt trocar retracts and the outer sharp canula penetrates. Once in the peritoneal space, the loss of resistance allows the spring-loaded blunt trocar to protrude once again, reducing the risk of trauma to intraperitoneal structures.

In his original publication Veres described the instrument as 'for the performance of chest and abdomen punctures and the treatment of pneumothorax'. He outlined the rationale thus:

> *An important moment for pleural and abdominal puncture is the instant when the needle perforates the pleura or peritoneum, because the easily injured lung or the intestines are exposed to injury by a pointed instrument. The sharp point is of great importance for the easy penetration of the pulmonary or abdominal wall, but only until the needle penetrates the cavity; once in the cavity the sharp point is unnecessary, even dangerous. The instrument to be described automatically prevents the injury of lung or intestine . . . The instrument is therefore suitable not only for exploratory punctures, but also for the emptying of exudates, empyemas, or for perfusions . . . For the treatment of pneumothorax I have used it for years (already almost 2000 cases).*

János Veres was born in Kismajtény, Hungary. In 1927 he received his medical degree from Debrecen University. His postgraduate training was in respiratory and internal medicine. From 1932–55 he was head of the departments of internal and respiratory medicine at the Regional Hospital in Kapuvar. In 1955 he moved to Budapest. He died from a myocardial infarction on 27 January 1979.

The spelling of his surname varied in his published papers between a single and double 's'. Apparently the single 's' spelling is correct. In 1997 the Hungarian Society of Gynaecological Endoscopists established the 'Veres Medal' in his honour, to be awarded for significant contributions to the advancement of laparoscopy. In addition, a memorial plaque was placed in the Kapuvar Hospital in 1999.

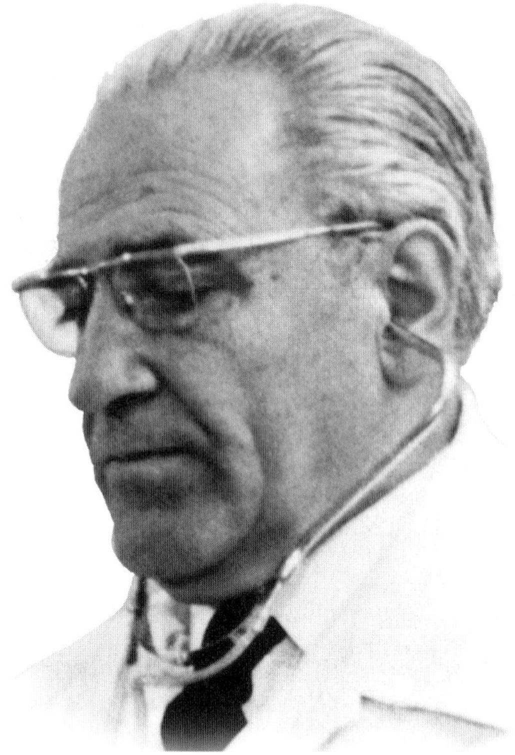

János Veres

Selected Publications

Veres J. Uj légmellkészit. *Orvosi Hetilap* 1936; 80: 536–7.

Veress J. Neues Instrument sur Ausfuhrung von Brust-oder Bauchpunktionen und Pneumothoraxbehandlung. *Dt Med Wochenschr* 1938; 64: 1480–1.

Bibliography References

580, 670, 1315, 1344, 1512, 1538, 1541.

Vigneaud, Vincent du (1901–1978)

Synthesis of Oxytocin

The identification and synthesis of oxytocin remains a landmark in the evolution of safe oxytocic drugs. In 1953, du Vigneaud and his colleagues, working in the biochemistry department of Cornell University Medical College, identified the structure of oxytocin and synthesised the hormone. Du Vigneaud was also the first to synthesise vasopressin.

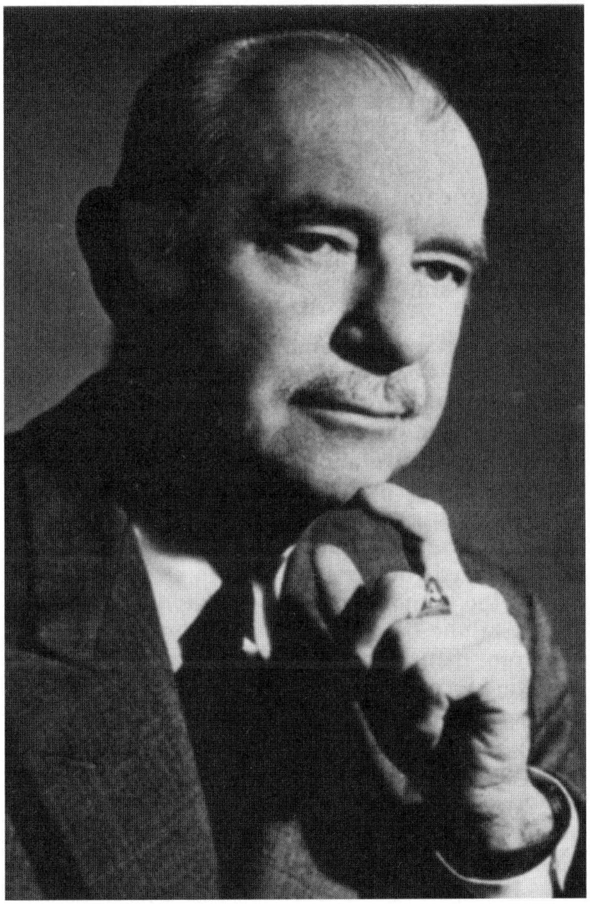

Vincent du Vigneaud

Vincent du Vigneaud was born in Chicago. His father was an inventor, and young Vincent grew up carrying out experiments with him in their basement laboratory. He received his chemistry degree from the University of Illinois in 1923 and his PhD from the University of Rochester in 1927. As a National Research Council fellow, he worked at Johns Hopkins University, in Dresden, Edinburgh and London from 1927–9. He became head of the department of biochemistry at George Washington University in 1932 and held the same position at Cornell University Medical College from 1938 to 1967. During the Second World War he worked on the synthesis of penicillin. Du Vigneaud received the Nobel Prize for chemistry in 1955 for the first synthesis of the posterior pituitary polypeptide hormones.

Selected Publications

Du Vigneaud V, Ressler C, Trippett. The sequence of amino acids in oxytocin, with a proposal for the structure of oxytocin. *J Biol Chem* 1953; 205: 949–57.

Du Vigneaud V, Ressler C, Swan JM, Roberts CW, Katsoyannis PG, Gordon S. The synthesis of an octapeptide with the hormonal activity of oxytocin. *J Am Chem Soc* 1953; 75: 4879–80.

Bibliography References

34, 82, 94, 576, 1452, 1485.

Voorhees, James Ditmars (1869–1929)

Voorhees' Bag

At the Sloane Maternity Hospital, New York, the de Ribes balloon for induction of labour was tried but found not to be durable or practical. In 1897 James Voorhees, resident obstetrician, modified the balloon and produced a rubber covered canvas bag, which he had manufactured locally for 25 cents each. In confronting the need to induce labour in the face of an unfavourable cervix Voorhees spoke against the more traumatic surgical incision or manual dilatation of the cervix:

> *The natural dilator of the cervix is a fluid wedge. If we can imitate it we respect all the physiological requirements, we help nature after her own dictates, and exactly to the measure of her needs. We use no violence, and such a measure ought to be very effective.*

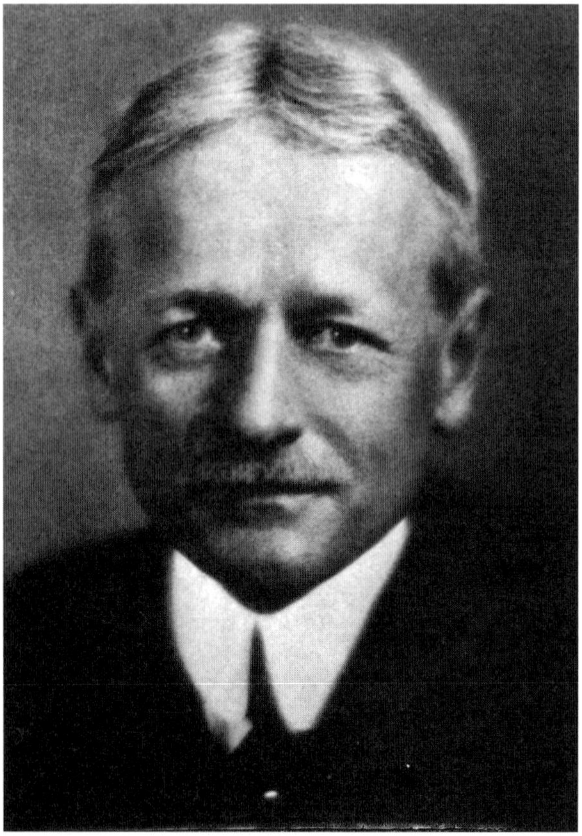

James Ditmars Voorhees

During a one-year study, Voorhees' bag was used in some 3 per cent of all deliveries at the hospital, mainly for induction of labour. It remained in clinical use until the 1930s.

James Ditmars Voorhees was born in Morristown, New Jersey, a descendant of the first Dutch settlers on Long Island. He was educated at Princeton University and gained his MD in 1893 from the College of Physicians and Surgeons of Columbia University. Postgraduate training followed at the Presbyterian and Foundling hospitals of New York, and he was appointed resident obstetrician at the Sloane Maternity Hospital in 1897. He later developed a very successful obstetric practice in New York.

In his private practice Voorhees was one of the first to advocate elective induction of labour:

> *Nothing pleases me more in my obstetrical work than to have a baby born a week or two ahead of time, especially in a primipara, because it means usually a quick, simple labor. Any baby weighing 6 to 7 pounds is plenty large enough, and getting into the world early, in my experience it does better than a larger child dragged out by a difficult forceps operation. Consequently it is not unusual for me to try to 'shake the apple off the tree' ahead of time . . . In multipara, who have had a previous difficult labor, or who have lost a baby in a previous confinement, without marked pelvic contraction, it is my custom to insert a bag one or two weeks before term with almost invariable good results.*

James Vorhees died following a stroke while on holiday in California.

Selected Publications

Voorhees JD. Dilatation of the cervix by means of a modified Champetier de Ribes balloon. *Med Rec* 1900; 58: 361–6.

Bibliography References

32, 88, 648, 983, 1462, 1480, 1484, 1485, 1559.

W

Walcher, Gustav Adolf (1856–1935)

Walcher's Position

Throughout the centuries, women have been advised to assume virtually all anatomically feasible positions to counteract abnormalities in labour. One which enjoyed popularity in the late nineteenth and early twentieth centuries was the hanging-legs position, advocated by Gustav Adolf Walcher in 1889. Walcher, as had others before him, felt that the sacrum had some antero-posterior mobility in pregnancy due to softening of the sacroiliac ligaments. He measured the diagonal conjugate of six women in late pregnancy in the lithotomy position and again with their hips extended by hanging their legs over the end of the examination couch-the Walcher position. He estimated an increase of 8–13 mm in the diagonal conjugate with the latter position:

> *While one is able to reach the promontory while the knees are drawn up, in cases of moderate pelvic contraction, he is no longer able to do so when the legs are extended.*

The Walcher position was therefore advocated in cases of pelvic contraction to assist entry of the presenting part through the pelvic brim and for assisted vaginal delivery. Like many discoveries, it was not new and had been described and illustrated in Scipio Mercurio's (1540–1615) obstetric text published in 1595, and even earlier by Abulcasis (936–1013) and Avicenna (979–1037).

Many endorsed the position, but others dissented, and subsequent radiographic studies did not confirm Walcher's observations. In the United States, Joseph DeLee, who initially advocated the Walcher position in earlier editions of his text, *The Principles and Practice of Obstetrics,* later rejected it, saying:

> *My results, curiously, have been better by the use of the exaggerated lithotomy position . . . the uterus and child are straightened out, the former thus being allowed to act with more directness, and the latter being brought into better position over the inlet.*

Ironically, these observations by De Lee outlined some of the advantages later found by William McRoberts with hyperflexion of the maternal hips for the management of shoulder dystocia.

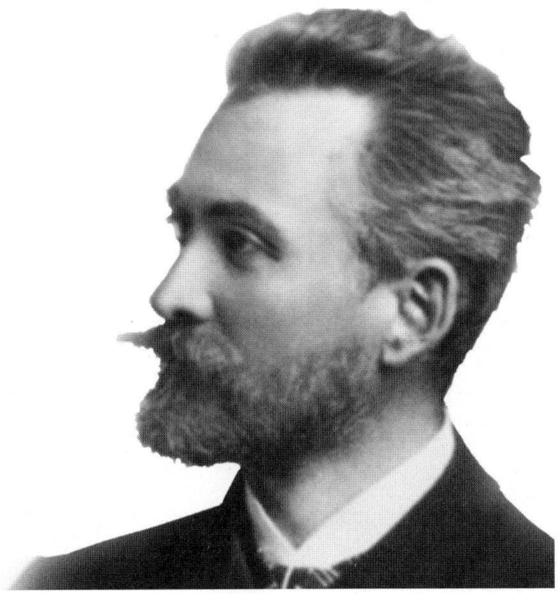

Gustav Adolf Walcher

Gustav Adolf Walcher was born in Ellwangen, Germany. He received his medical education in Leipzig, Berlin and Tübingen. Working as an assistant in the Tübingen Frauenklinik he completed his post-graduate studies in obstetrics and gynaecology. In 1887 he was appointed director of the Württenberg School of Midwifery in Stuttgart, where he remained until his retirement in 1918.

Selected Publications

Walcher G. Die conjugata eines eugen Beckens ist keine konstante Grösse, sondern lösst sich durch die Körperhaltung der Trägerin Verändern. *Zentralbl Gynäkol* 1889; 13: 892–3.

Bibliography References

648, 1005, 1480, 1631.

Waldeyer, Heinrich Wilhelm Gottfried (1836–1921)

Ovarian Fossa of Waldeyer/Germinal Epithelium of the Ovary

Wilhelm Waldeyer, also known as Waldeyer-Hartz, was born in Hehlen, Germany. He studied at Berlin and Göttingen, where he was a pupil of Jakob Henle. He became professor of anatomy at Strasburg in 1872 and worked there with other notables, Jakob von Recklinghausen (1883–1910) and Adolphe Kussmaul (1822–1902). In 1883 he was called to the chair of anatomy in Berlin.

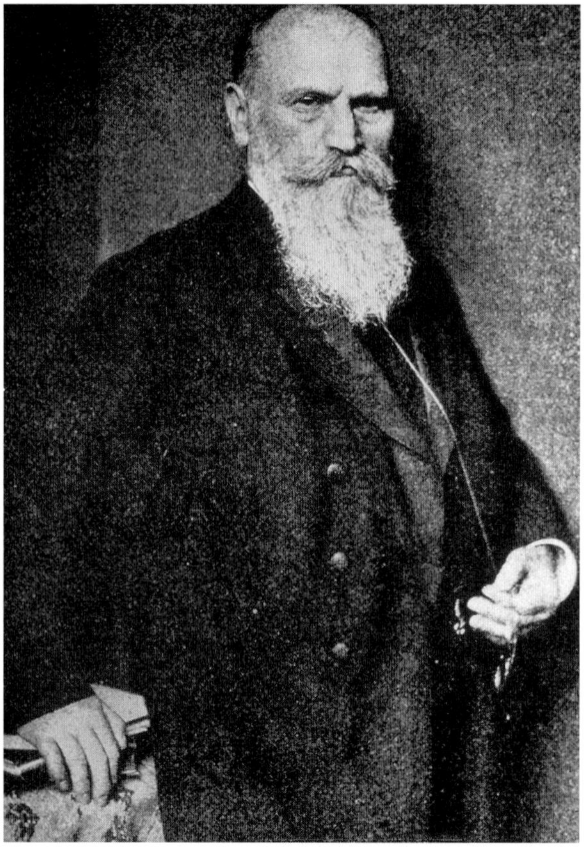

Heinrich Wilhelm Gottfried Waldeyer

The leading German anatomist of his era, he published a remarkable book on the ovary and ovum in 1870, in which he gave the first description of the germinal epithelium. He also described the slight depression on the pelvic sidewall between the divergent external and internal iliac vessels where the ovaries normally lie: the ovarian fossa of Waldeyer. Later, in 1884, he described the lingual, pharyngeal and palatine lymphatic drainage of the neck: Waldeyer's ring. He introduced the terms chromosome in 1888 and neurone in 1891.

Selected Publications

Waldeyer HWG. *Eierstock und Ei.* Leipzig: W. Engelmann; 1870.

Bibliography References

552, 604, 624, 648, 1480, 1703.

Walthard, Max (1867–1933)

Walthard's Cell Rests

Within the peritoneum covering the fallopian tube, the broad ligament and, less commonly, the ovary, may be seen small greyish nodules or cysts. They consist of cells resembling squamous epithelium, often with a cystic cavity lined by mesothelium. These were described in detail by Max Walthard and have become known as Walthard's cell rests, nests or islands. They may represent areas of focal metaplasia of the serosa and are felt by some to be the site of origin of Brenner tumours of the ovary.

Max Walthard was born in Bern, Switzerland. After medical qualification he served as an assistant to Theodor Kocher (1841–1917), and later studied in England, France and Germany. Upon return to Switzerland he combined private practice with basic studies in pathology and bacteriology. In 1920 he was appointed head of the Universitäts-Frauenklinik in Zurich, which post he held until his death on 29 September 1933.

Selected Publications

Walthard M. Zur Aetiologie der Ovarialadenome. *Ztschr Geburtshilfe Gynäkol* 1903; 49: 233–9.

Bibliography References

406, 1259, 1480.

Wassermann, August Paul von (1866–1925)

Wassermann Reaction

August von Wassermann was born in Bamberg, Bavaria, the son of a wealthy banker. He studied medicine at the Universities of Erlangen, Vienna and Munich and finally graduated from the University of Strasburg in 1888. He was a student of Robert Koch (1843–1910). In 1906, along with co-workers Albert Neisser and Carl Brück (1879–1944), he demonstrated antibodies to the syphilis antigen in the serum of syphilitic monkeys and later in humans:

> *The practical importance of these findings is obvious. We are in a position to determine in vitro whether a human or animal serum contains antibodies specific for substances of the syphilitic agent, and we should be able to quantify these antibodies.*

This evolved into the specific and sensitive complement fixation test or 'Wassermann reaction'. This was one year after Fritz Schaundin (1871–1906) and Erich Hoffmann (1868–1959) had isolated the causative organism, *Treponema pallidum*. Earlier, Wassermann had tried unsuccessfully to use the complement fixation test for the diagnosis of tuberculosis. He also proved that general paralysis of the insane was a late manifestation of syphilis.

In 1913 he was appointed director of the Kaiser Wilhelm Institute for Experimental Therapeutics in

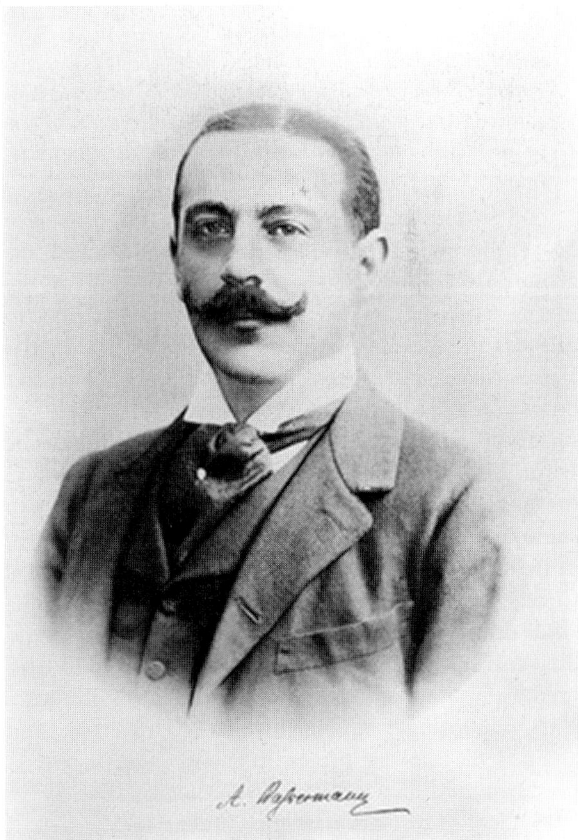

August Paul von Wassermann

Berlin but was never appointed professor at the university. He died in Berlin on 16 March 1925.

Selected Publications

Wassermann A, Neisser A, Brück C. Eine serodiagnostische Reaktion bei Syphilis. *Dt Med Wochenschr* 1906; 32: 745–6.

Bibliography References

618, 1146, 1254, 1525, 1667, 1672.

Watkins, Thomas James (1863–1925)

Watkins' Interposition Operation

The principle of using the uterus as a buttress for the bladder in cases of uterine prolapse and cystocoele was developed in the late nineteenth century by a number of European gynaecologists, including Ernst Wertheim. Following their lead, Thomas Watkins of Chicago devised his interposition operation, which he first reported to the Chicago Gynecological Society on 15 September 1899:

> *The bladder was separated from the uterus by blunt dissection and the peritoneal cavity opened in front of the uterus. The anterior wall of the uterus was grasped by bullet forceps and the organ anteverted. About two inches of the upper portion of the anterior vaginal wall was now sutured to the upper border of the broad ligaments lateral to the uterus, and to the fundus of the uterus with silkworm-gut sutures.*

With modifications, Watkins' operation proved to be simple and effective in the postmenopausal age group. Unfortunately, the acute anteversion of the uterus made access to the endometrial cavity very difficult in cases of postmenopausal bleeding. By the 1950s it had largely been replaced by the Manchester operation and vaginal hysterectomy with repair.

Thomas James Watkins was born on a farm outside Utica, New York. As a youth he worked long hours on the family farm but managed to get enough schooling to start the study of medicine at the University of Michigan in 1880. He transferred to the Bellevue Hospital Medical College, New York, in 1883 and received his MD in 1886. After three years further study in Utica, Brooklyn, and the Women's Hospital in New York, he moved to Chicago. He was appointed to the department of obstetrics and gynaecology of Northwestern University and attained the rank of professor in 1916. He served as president of the American Gynecological Society in 1915. He died of a coronary thrombosis.

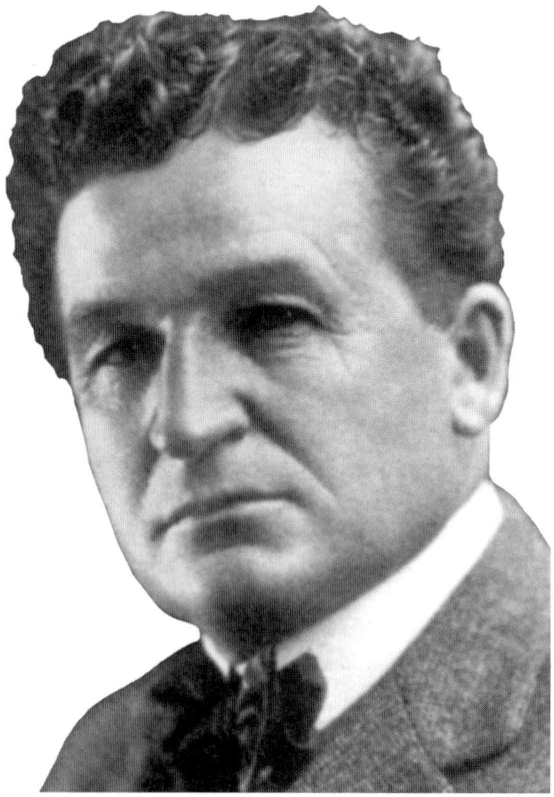

Thomas James Watkins

Selected Publications

Watkins TJ. The treatment of cystocele and uterine prolapse after the menopause. *Am J Obstet Gynecol Dis Women Child* 1899; 15: 420–3.

Bibliography References

342, 524, 801, 1480, 1485, 1561.

Wells, Thomas Spencer (1818–1897)

Ovariotomy/Spencer Wells' Forceps

In the early nineteenth century, both desirable and undesirable liquids were injected into ovarian cysts after tapping in an attempt to reduce the reaccumulation of fluid, usually to little or no avail. These included port wine, iodine and carbolic acid. Surgical removal of the cyst was reserved for extreme cases in debilitated patients. Thus, the high surgical mortality was to some extent a self-fulfilling prophesy.

It was into this surgical environment that Spencer Wells ventured in 1857. His first case died, but by 1880 he had performed 1,000 ovariotomies and had helped establish the role of the procedure. He was preceded by the pioneering efforts of Charles Clay in Britain and Washington Atlee in the United States, among others. In 1864 Wells published the first volume of his two-volume work on *Diseases of the Ovaries.* He displayed a conceited streak in dismissing the considerable efforts of Clay and Atlee, who had done many operations in the 15 years before Wells' first effort. Indeed, Wells' early mortality was high, and it was many years before his results improved. When he started in 1857, one French critic, Jacques Moreau, said ovariotomy 'should be placed among the prerogatives of the executioner'. As Wells himself put it, 'surgeons stood and trembled on the brink of ovarian waters'. However, Wells persisted and from the influence of his London base established himself as one of the most prolific ovariotomists of his era. He crossed swords in the literature with both Clay and Lawson Tait.

Wells devised a clamp to place across the ovarian pedicle and brought this out through the abdominal incision, which was carefully closed around it. The clamp usually came away within one to two weeks. He found this superior to leaving the ligatures on the pedicle out through the wound, which often led to a chronic infected sinus:

> *And it is a remarkable fact that in every case in which the pedicle was long enough to enable me to use the clamp the patient recovered.*

It was from this clamp that the smaller, more precise haemostatic artery forceps that bear his name were developed. Haemostatic forceps or pincers were used by many French surgeons, including Ambroise Paré in the sixteenth century. The French instrument maker Joseph Charrière (1803–76) devised the simple locking rachet on the shanks of the artery forceps in 1855. Before this date, the locking mechanisms were much more cumbersome. Wells described his own adoption of artery forceps as follows:

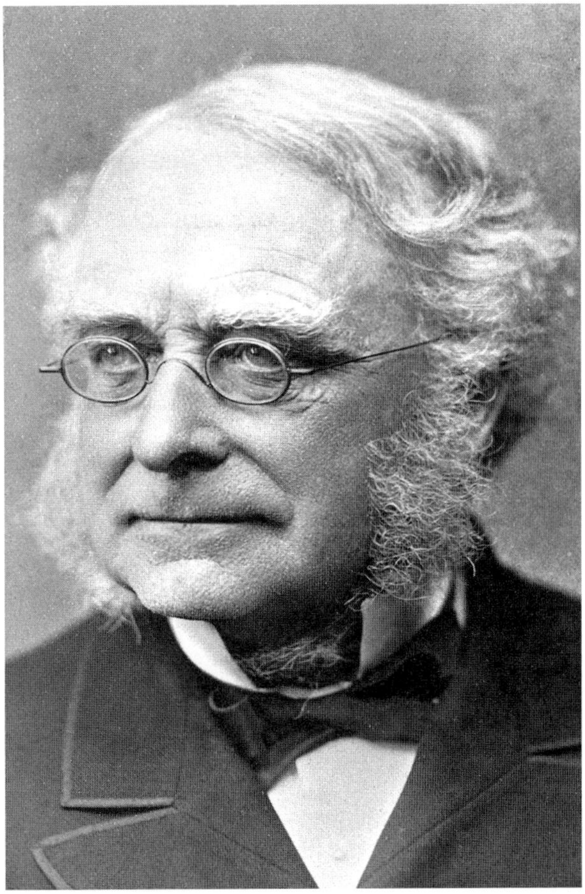

Thomas Spencer Wells

I can hardly recollect when I first began to use forceps instead of the fingers of an assistant for temporarily stopping bleeding during operations ... This must have been in 1854, because when I went to the Crimea in 1855 I took a number of 'bull-dogs' with me; and after my return in 1856, I never went to any serious operation without several.

Thomas Spencer Wells was born at St Albans, England, the eldest son of a builder. At the age of 17 he was apprenticed to a general practitioner in Barnsley. He later studied medicine at the Leeds General Infirmary, Trinity College Dublin and St Thomas' Hospital, London, qualifying in 1841. He then served six years as a surgeon in the Royal Navy, based at the Naval Hospital in Malta. Here he gained surgical and obstetrical experience, servicing both the naval and civilian populations. During the Crimean War, he served in the Dardanelles as a military surgeon. When he returned to London he practised as an ophthalmologist for a year and was then appointed to the Samaritan Hospital for Women and Children. It was there he began his career as an ovariotomist. In 1884 he was elected president of the Royal College of Surgeons and knighted by Queen Victoria. Sir Thomas Spencer Wells died of a stroke near Cannes on 31 January 1897.

Selected Publications

Wells TS. *Diseases of the Ovaries: Their Diagnosis and Treatment.* (2 vols). London: J. Churchill and Sons; 1865 and 1872.

Wells TS. Remarks on forcipressure and the use of pressure-forceps in surgery. *BMJ* 1879; 1: 9226–8.

Bibliography References

335, 428, 753, 822, 844, 1205, 1402, 1496, 1497, 1538, 1539, 1588, 1595.

Wertheim, Ernst (1864–1920)

Wertheim's Radical Hysterectomy

In the late 1800s a number of gynaecologists in Austria and Germany began to develop the abdominal approach to a more radical hysterectomy for cancer of the cervix. In the forefront of this movement was Ernst Wertheim, who diligently pursued perfection with this technique. Ultimately, he is said to have performed 1,300 such operations with complete follow-up.

The prevailing view that cancer of the cervix spread beyond the uterus only as a late manifestation of the disease had been discredited. As Wertheim noted in the introduction to his monograph, based on 500 cases:

... the realisation began to mature that one had to strive to remove as much as possible of the surrounding tissue together with the primary tumour in order to achieve better results as is the case with operative procedures for cancer of other organs.

His more radical approach was vindicated by the pathological findings in his series:

The correctness of our procedure was proved to us by histological examination of the extirpated organs. These showed the teaching to be false that cervical cancer transgresses the bounds of the uterus only late, for in a considerable number of apparently early cases the carcinoma had already sent its offshoots and advance guards to the parametrium and regional lymph nodes.

Confirming the superiority of the abdominal over the vaginal approach, Wertheim wrote:

Our knowledge of the behaviour of the regional lymphatics and parametrium, of the mode of spread of the carcinoma, and of what might be expected from a surgical operation, was put on a secure basis for the first time by the extended abdominal operation.

Ernst Wertheim was born in Graz, Austria and received his medical degree from that university. He then worked at the German University in Prague as assistant to Friedrich Schauta. In 1891, he accompanied Schauta when he left Prague to take up the chair in the first gynaecology clinic at the University of

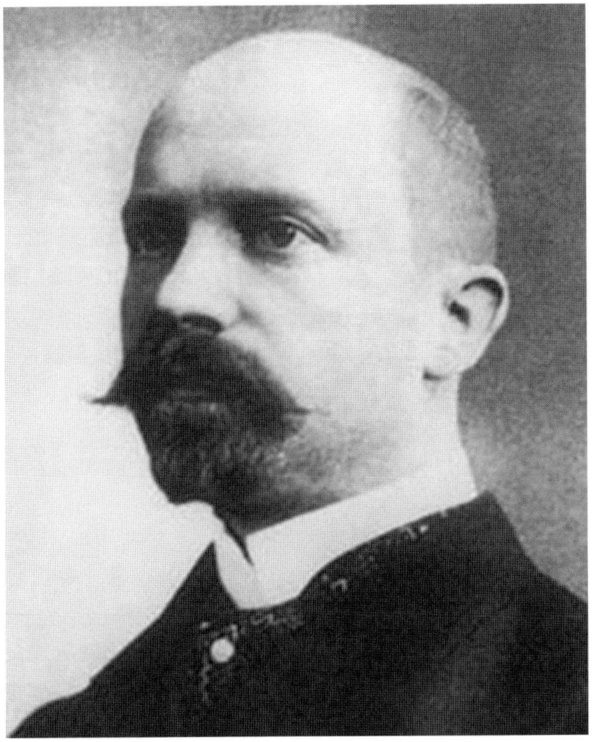

Ernst Wertheim

Vienna. However, increasingly they disagreed, and considerable antagonism developed between them. In 1897 Wertheim achieved his independence when he was appointed head at the Elizabeth Hospital and later at the second University Clinic in Vienna, where he become full professor.

Wertheim carried out the first full extended operation on 16 November 1898. He went on to become one of the most renowned gynaecological surgeons of his era. Although best known for his radical abdominal hysterectomy, he also made many contributions to vaginal surgery, especially for prolapse. Although rubber gloves were available for surgery from 1900, Wertheim refused to wear them, feeling they interfered with his sense of touch. He was a considerable sportsman, particularly in skiing and skating, and once crossed the alps in a balloon. Prone to bouts of depression, he had a defensive, abrupt manner. He died from influenza at 56 years of age. His grave is adjacent to that of Schauta in the Vienna City Cemetery.

Selected Publications

Wertheim E. Zur Frage der Radicaloperation beim Uteruskrebs. *Arch Gynäkol* 1900; 61: 627–8.

Wertheim E. *Die erweiterte abdominale Operation bei Carcinoma colli Uteri (auf Grund von 500 Fällen).* Berlin: Urban & Schwarzenberg; 1911.

Bibliography References

97, 383, 501, 541, 553, 648, 896, 1071, 1107, 1291, 1292, 1471, 1641, 1680, 1681.

Wharton, Thomas (1614–1673)

Wharton's Jelly

Thomas Wharton was born in Winston-on-Tees, County Durham, and studied at Cambridge, Bolton, London and Oxford, gaining his MD from the latter university in 1647. He was appointed physician to St Thomas' Hospital, London, in 1657. He is best known for his description of the duct of the submaxillary salivary gland, Wharton's duct, in his one published work. He also described the mucous connective tissue of the umbilical cord: Wharton's jelly. During the Great Plague of London in 1665, he was one of the few physicians to remain and treat patients in that city. Apparently, the Government promised an appointment as physician-in-ordinary to the King if he remained in London to look after the Guards. The promise was not fulfilled.

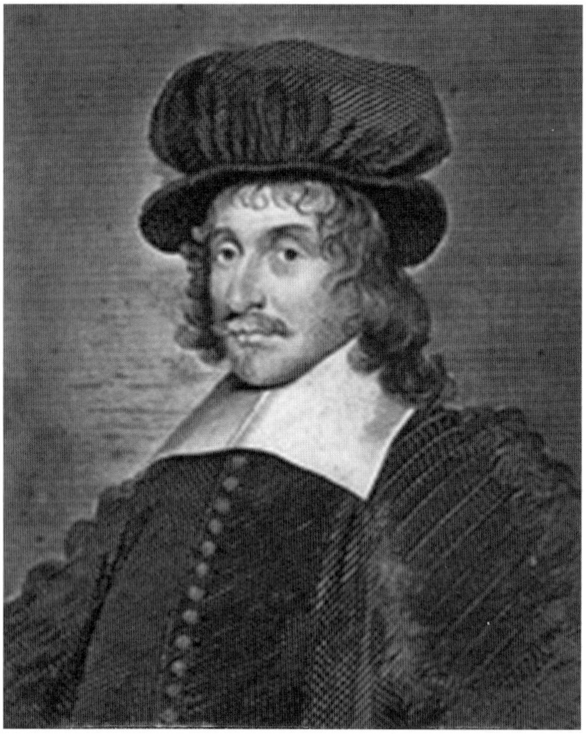

Thomas Wharton

Selected Publications

Wharton T. *Adenographia, sive glandularum totius corporis descriptio*. London: R. Marriot; 1656, pp. 243–4.

Bibliography References

406, 885, 1470, 1480, 1715.

White, Charles (1728–1813)

Puerperal Sepsis/Puerperal Deep-Vein Thrombosis

Charles White of Manchester was one of the first to make a concerted and organised effort to prevent the scourge of puerperal fever. He argued that it was an absorption fever and inadequate drainage of the lochia was a major factor. White used the term putrid fever rather than puerperal fever:

> *The danger does not arise from the smallness of the quantity of the discharge, but from its stagnation, whereby it becomes putrid and in this state is again absorbed into the circulation.*

To counteract this, he advocated a policy of strict cleanliness, fresh air, postural uterine drainage and early ambulation, in contrast to the horizontal 'confinement' to bed for several days as was then the fashion. He had a special bed constructed with an adjustable back-rest. He felt that by having the woman sit up in bed lochial drainage was promoted and its absorption prevented. A century later this principle was applied for postural surgical drainage by George Fowler (1848–1960) and became known as 'Fowler's position'.

In the second edition of his treatise, White also advocated uterine irrigation with a syringe of mild antiseptic solution in cases with 'putrid lochia'. When White's principles were followed, the incidence of puerperal fever was limited in his district, as he noted:

> *I have, however, the pleasure to observe that those fevers, in this neighbourhood at least, have of late years greatly decreased. This must chiefly be attributed to a system of*

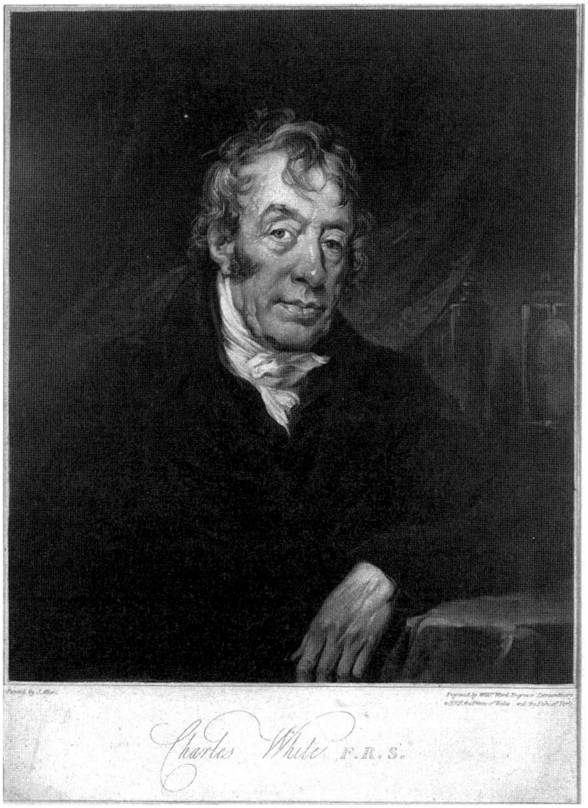

Charles White

management lately introduced, much to the honour of our present practitioners.

Charles White was born in Manchester, the son of a doctor and great-grandson of a knight who lost his estate in the great rebellion. He served an initial apprenticeship with his father and, at the age of 20, went to London and became a pupil of William Hunter and a friend of his brother, John. After four years in London, he returned to Manchester and founded a small hospital, which later developed into the Manchester Royal Infirmary. He was elected to Fellowship of the Royal Society and the Corporation of Surgeons in 1762. White's treatise had wide distribution with four English editions and separate publication in France, Germany and America.

White was also the first to fully describe post-partum deep-vein thrombosis and name it 'phlegmasia alba dolens puerperium'. It came to be called 'white leg' of pregnancy, the 'white' being descriptive and not eponymous. Appropriately, White's advice about early post-partum ambulation – 'the sooner she gets out of bed after her delivery the better' – revolutionary at the time, would have helped diminish the risk of thromboembolism.

In 1803 ophthalmia caused him to lose the sight of his left eye. He continued to work and operate until another attack in 1812 left him completely blind. He died on 20 February 1813, at the age of 84.

Selected Publications

White C. *A Treatise on the Management of Pregnant and Lying-in Women*. London: E & C Dilly; 1773.

White C. *An inquiry into the nature and cause of that swelling, in one or both of the lower extremities, which sometimes happens to lying-in women*. London: W. Eyres; 1784.

Bibliography References

10, 11, 211, 301, 336, 337, 377, 385, 681, 708, 808, 822, 927, 935, 940, 1180, 1207, 1261, 1595.

White, George Reves (1866–1926)

Paravaginal Repair

In 1909, George White of Savannah, Georgia, pointed out that many cases of cystocoele were due to lateral, paravaginal, fascial defects that may or may not be associated with a midline defect. In reviewing the frequent failure of the traditional midline anterior repair, he wrote:

The reason for failure seems to be that the normal support of the bladder has not been sought for and restored, but instead an irrational removal of part of the anterior vaginal wall has been resorted to, which could only result in disappointment and failure.

He studied the supports of the bladder in the cadaver, making the following observations:

The support of the bladder may readily be determined in the cadaver by making a suprapubic incision and attempting to push the bladder out through the vulva. It will be found to rest on the anterior vaginal wall to which it is slightly adherent. If the bladder be pushed aside and an attempt made to push the anterior vaginal wall back toward the perineum its support comes out very plainly. It is attached to the symphysis pubis and pubic bones in front, laterally to the white line of the pelvic fascia and ischiatic spine; and, above and behind, to the uterus . . . It is, therefore, evident that a cystocele is caused by the breaking loose of the vagina from the white line which can readily occur during labor and especially in an instrumental delivery.

White then described his technique for repairing the defects by reattaching the vagina to the white line of pelvic fascia. He concluded:

I have been surprised many times in working out this subject to follow the logic of many of the operations recommended for the cure of cystocele. Everything is recommended except repair of the anatomic supports of the bladder. The problem of keeping the bladder in place is solved in repairing the shelf on which it rests.

White then described his technique for repairing the defects by reattaching the vagina to the white line of pelvic fascia. His procedure did not gain acceptance, most gynaecologists preferring the simpler midline anterior repair. However, it has been rediscovered and is increasingly used, both by the vaginal and abdominal routes.

George Reves White was born on Long Island, New York in 1891. He graduated in medicine from the College of Physicians and Surgeons of Columbia in New York. His postgraduate studies were taken in New York and Europe, followed by surgical practice in New York. He served as a surgeon during the Spanish–American War. Following this he settled in Savannah and practised surgery from 1901 until his death in 1926. He was a tall, acromegalic man with long fingers, who reputedly operated often and at great speed. He died of tuberculosis.

Selected Publications

White GR. Cystocele: A radical cure by suturing lateral sulci of vagina to white line of pelvic fascia. *JAMA* 1909; 53: 1707–10.

White GR. An anatomical operation for the cure of cystocele. *Am J Obstet Dis Wom* 1912; 65: 286–90.

Bibliography References

13, 1086, 1255, 1724.

White, Priscilla (1900–1989)

White Classification of Diabetes in Pregnancy

Priscilla White joined the staff of the Joslin Clinic for the treatment of diabetes in Boston in 1924, just two years after the discovery of insulin. She was assigned to study diabetes in youth. As she wrote later:

Because of the size of the Joslin Clinic and the greater than average number of juvenile-onset diabetic patients surviving many years of diabetes, the abnormal course and outcome of pregnancy in diabetes became apparent. Although maternal survival was nearly assured, only half of these patients were delivered of live-born surviving infants. The classic occurrence was intrauterine fetal death, which peaked in week 36. This fetal loss was associated with symptoms of toxemia (gain in weight, rise of blood pressure, proteinuria) which subsided soon after the fetal death. When the timing of the delivery was changed to anticipate this occurrence, neonatal death replaced intrauterine death. The infant survival rate of 128 viable pregnancies between 1924 and 1938 was only 54 per cent.

She supervised the Joslin Pregnancy Clinic for 50 years and during that time managed more than 2,000 cases of overt diabetes in pregnancy. In order to facilitate comparison of different treatments, she developed her classification of diabetes in pregnancy in 1949. This was based on duration and age at onset of diabetes and the presence of vascular disease and renal complications. Her aim was to assist the accuracy of prognosis and management in individual cases. Gestational diabetes was not included, as this was rarely seen and treated at the Joslin Clinic. In her original publication she summed up her rationale as follows:

From the foregoing it is evident that our problem must concern the investigation of the causes and the means to

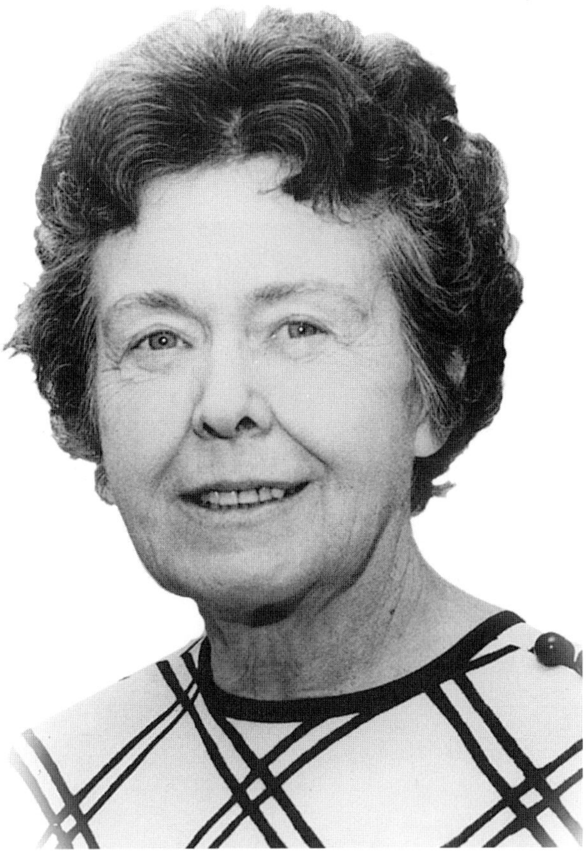

Priscilla White

prevent premature delivery of the infant of the diabetic mother prior to the period of its viability (which appears to be later than that of the normal woman) and, secondly, the termination of the pregnancy at the point of viability and before the dreaded late intrauterine accident can occur.

In addition to the chemical grading of patients, which has been previously reported upon, in 1948 clinical grading of the obstetric diabetic patient was made. This evaluation was based upon the pre-pregnancy state and the designation was alphabetical, A through F. Classes A through E referred to fetal risk and F to maternal risk. From the previous discussion it is evident that age at onset of diabetes, duration, severity and degree of maternal vascular disease all influence the fetal survival unfavourably. Renal disease carries with it maternal hazards in the diabetic population as well as the obstetric population at large.

Priscilla White was born in Boston on St Patrick's Day, 1900. She was educated at Radcliffe College and Tufts University Medical School, from which she graduated in 1923. She was assistant professor at Tufts and taught at Harvard Medical School. Her life's work was devoted to the management and research of juvenile diabetes. Her classification of diabetes in pregnancy has been applied worldwide and has facilitated more rational and precise management. During her career she saw perinatal survival in pregnant diabetics improve from 50 per cent to 97 per cent. Her work gained her international renown, and she was the first women to receive the Banting Medal, the highest scientific award of the American Diabetes Association. During her 50 years at the Joslin Clinic, she managed more than 2,200 diabetic pregnancies, often staying with the mother throughout labour. She never married and lived in an eighteenth-century home with her housekeeper and five dachshunds. She died following a coronary thrombosis at her home in Ashland, Massachusetts, on 16 December 1989.

Selected Publications

White P. *Diabetes in Childhood and Adolescence.* Philadelphia, PA: Lea and Febiger; 1932.

White P. Pregnancy complicating diabetes. *Am J Med* 1949; 7: 609–16.

White P. Classification of obstetric diabetes. *Am J Obstet Gynecol* 1978; 130: 228–30.

Bibliography References

591, 922, 1182, 1689.

Wigand, Justus Heinrich (1769–1817) Martin, August Eduard (1847–1934)

Wigand–Martin Manoeuvre

Many of the methods for delivering the aftercoming head of the breech advocate the use of suprapubic pressure by an assistant to ensure descent and flexion of the head. Justus Wigand proposed a technique for the physician working alone, which combined elements of the Mauriceau–Smellie–Veit manoeuvre with one hand and suprapubic pressure with the other. After delivery of the arms and shoulders, the infant is straddled upon one arm with the forefinger in the mouth flexing the head. The other hand provides downward suprapubic pressure on the head, further promoting flexion. As the head descends, the infant's body is raised up on the straddling arm and the occiput pivots beneath the symphysis. In a later generation, the technique was popularised by August Martin and is known as the Wigand–Martin manoeuvre.

Justus Heinrich Wigand was born in Revel, Estonia, the son of a minister. From 1788 he studied medicine at Jena and Erlangen, qualifying in 1793. He worked in Hamburg as a general practitioner and obstetrician for 20 years. He tried to move to St Petersburg but failed the Russian licensing examination. In 1814 he moved to Heidelberg, seeking a better climate because of his deteriorating health. Here he worked with Franz Naegele. Wigand was one of the first to use external version and the first to use vaginal packing for placenta praevia. He died on 10 February 1817 at the age of 47.

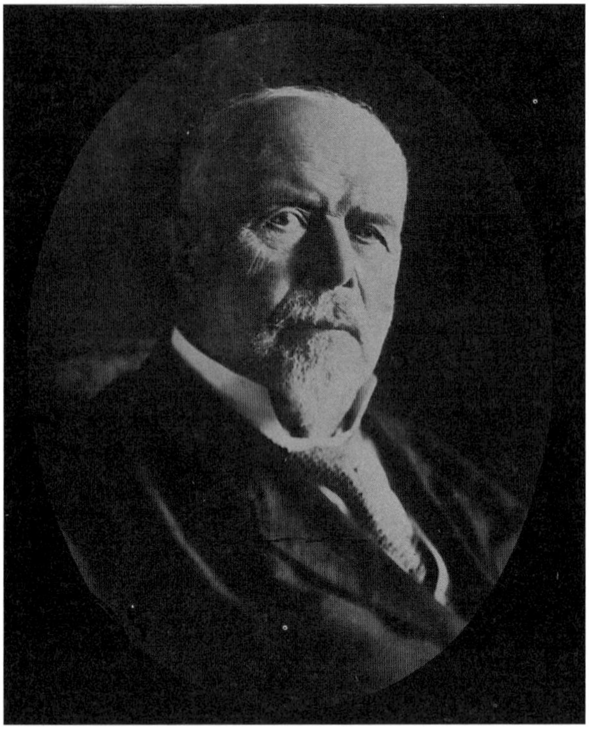

August Eduard Martin

August Eduard Martin was born in Berlin, the son of a prominent obstetrician. His father, Eduard Arnold Martin, delivered the grandson of Queen Victoria – later Kaiser Wilhelm II of Germany. The prince was in frank breech presentation and during breech extraction with extended arms suffered a permanent left brachial plexus paralysis.

The younger Martin took his medical degree at the University of Berlin, graduating in 1870. He became professor of gynaecology at the University of Greifswald, Prussia in 1899. He was a large imposing man, known to his students as 'August the strong'. One of the pioneers of abdominal myomectomy, Martin wrote a well-received text of gynaecology. In 1888 he was elected to honorary fellowship in the American Gynecological Society. He resigned his academic post in 1907 and returned to Berlin.

Selected Publications

Wigand JH. Über Wendung durch äussere Handgiffe. *Hamburg Med Mag* 1807; 1: 52.

Martin A. Über die Entwicklung des nachfolgende Kopfes bei räumlichem Missverhaltnis. *Zentralbl Gynäkol* 1886; 10: 758.

Bibliography References

88, 102, 548, 648, 713, 771, 983, 993, 1261, 1408, 1529.

Willett, John Abernethy (1872–1932)

Willett's Scalp Forceps

In the early part of the twentieth century, most cases of placenta praevia were delivered vaginally. The aim of management was to apply pressure on the lower uterine segment and placenta to control haemorrhage until vaginal delivery could be completed. This was usually achieved by podalic version and the bringing down of a leg, or the use of a de Ribes or similar bag. Both were effective as compressors of the placental site but could be traumatic and associated with increased blood loss during the requisite manipulation. Willett felt that in cases of vertex presentation it would be advisable to use the fetal head for tamponade, and he devised scalp forceps to apply traction to this end. In presenting his idea and early results to the Royal Society of Medicine in 1925, he said:

> *I had for some time thought that, could the requisite pressure be exerted by the forecoming head, the disadvantages of version and of de Ribes' bag might be obviated; and with the possible advantages of earlier treatment, less interference and so diminished risk of sepsis.*

Willett modified an existing pair of surgical scalp forceps and described them as follows:

> *It is of the t-shaped clip type, the holding bars being ½ in. long, narrow enough to pass where a finger will, and rigid enough to sustain the requisite weight where fixed in the foetal scalp. The holding teeth are rounded.*
>
> *The application of the forceps is easy and they can be applied to the scalp as soon as the os will admit a finger, thus ensuring early treatment . . . A weight varying from 1 lb to 2 lb, hanging over the end of the bed, is applied to the handles by a tape. Nothing further is done until the head is in the vagina, when the forceps are removed and the patient is allowed to deliver herself without further interference.*

This technique proved very effective in reducing blood loss and accelerating delivery. As the safety of caesarean section increased and fetal viability became a dominant consideration, Willett's scalp forceps were used only for the dead or pre-viable fetus.

John Abernethy Willett, one of five sons of a surgeon, was born in London. He studied medicine at Oxford and St Bartholomew's Hospital, qualifying in 1899. His postgraduate training in obstetrics and gynaecology was taken at St Bartholomew's and Queen Charlotte's hospitals in London. He held appointments at the City of London Maternity Hospital and the Samaritan Free Hospital. It was at the City of London Maternity Hospital that Willett did his work on placenta praevia and designed his scalp forceps.

Joe Willett, as he was known to his friends, was regarded as an able clinician and teacher who contributed substantially to the education of midwives. Having a personal income, he did not have to strive to develop a private practice. He was not possessed by upward angst, worked contentedly within his capabilities and did not seek or receive higher office.

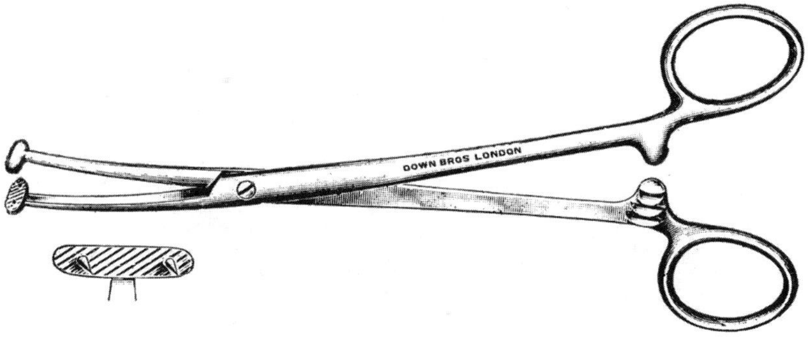

Willett's scalp forceps

Selected Publications

Willett JA. The treatment of placenta praevia by continuous weight traction: a report of seven cases. *Proc R Soc Med* 1925; 18: 90–4.

Bibliography References

88, 99, 102, 983, 985, 1261, 1696, 1697.

Williams, John Whitridge (1866–1931)

Williams' Obstetric Text

John Whitridge Williams was born in Baltimore, the son of a physician. He was educated at Baltimore City College and Johns Hopkins University, graduating MD in 1888. Following graduation, he studied gynaecological pathology in Berlin, Prague and Vienna for one year. He returned as assistant in the department of gynaecology at Johns Hopkins. In 1896 he was appointed associate professor of obstetrics. At this time Howard Kelly, who was primarily a gynaecological surgeon, was professor of obstetrics and gynaecology and confessed he had little interest in obstetrics. He asked Williams to take charge of obstetrics, and in 1899 Williams was appointed professor and obstetrician-in-chief at the hospital. Williams had been impressed by the combination of departments of obstetrics and gynaecology in the German Frauenkliniks and hoped to achieve the same model at Johns Hopkins. When Kelly retired, Williams asked the board to combine the two departments of obstetrics and gynaecology under his leadership. The board refused, one member bluntly telling Williams he was not a gynaecological surgeon. Gynaecology became a division of surgery with Thomas Cullen as head, while Williams remained head of the now separate department of obstetrics.

Williams acted as dean of the Johns Hopkins Medical School from 1911–23 and instituted clinical full-time university-based teachers. He continued to push for the amalgamation of obstetrics and gynaecology. In 1914 he stated:

> *I hope I may live to see the day when the term obstetrician will have disappeared and when all teachers, at least, will unite in fostering the broader gynecology, instead of being divided, as at present, into knife-loving gynecologists and equally narrow-minded obstetricians who are frequently little more than trained midwives.*

He remained thwarted in this ambition, and separate chairs of obstetrics and gynaecology existed at Johns Hopkins for 29 years after his death.

Williams was a man of strict routine. He arrived at the hospital at 9 a.m. and left at 6 p.m. In the evenings he worked in his study from 8.30 p.m. to 10 p.m. and had a glass of whiskey and water before retiring for the night. An inveterate pipe smoker, each week he used his pipes on a strict one-in-seven rotation. When he purchased a new pipe, he boiled it and carved the date on it.

Williams is remembered for his textbook of obstetrics, which he first published in 1903, four years after his appointment as obstetrician-in-chief. He started the preface with the following objectives:

> *In the following pages I have attempted to set forth, as briefly as seemed to be consistent with thoroughness, the scientific basis for and the practical application of the obstetrical art.*
>
> *Especial attention has been devoted to the normal and pathological anatomy of the generative tract in the hope that the book may prove serviceable as a laboratory guide for students. At the same time I have endeavoured to present the more practical aspects of obstetrics in such a manner as to be of direct service to the obstetrician at the bedside.*

The book was richly illustrated and included more than 1,100 references, many from the European literature, displaying his broad scholarship. From his pen six editions were published. It became the standard work on obstetrics in the United States and remains so under successive editors since his death. In 1997 the publishers released a facsimile limited-edition reprint of the first edition.

Williams is regarded as the father of academic obstetrics in the United States. He was a prodigious worker and a gentleman of the old school. His achievements were acknowledged at home and abroad

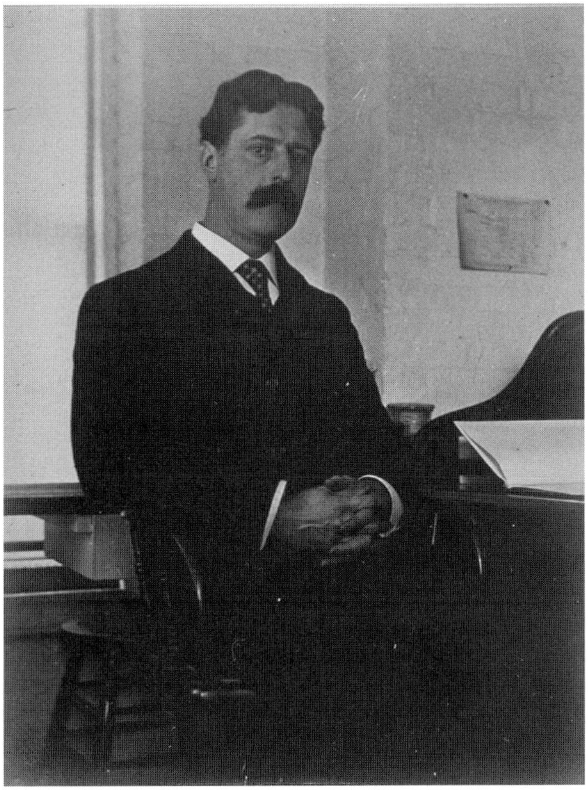

John Whitridge Williams

with honorary degrees, from Dublin, Maryland and Pittsburg, and honorary fellowship of the British (subsequently Royal) College of Obstetricians and Gynaecologists. Eleven of his former residents became departmental chairmen. He died on 21 October 1931 after an intestinal haemorrhage from an oesophageal ulcer.

Selected Publications

Williams JW. *Obstetrics: a Textbook for the Use of Students and Practitioners.* New York, NY: Appleton; 1903.

Bibliography References

88, 102, 131, 269, 358, 486, 498, 671, 813, 1407, 1434, 1485, 1487, 1564, 1700, 1701.

Willughby, Percivall (1596–1685)

Midwifery Text

The earliest textbook on midwifery in English was the *Byrth of Mankynde* in 1540, a translation by Richard Jonas from the Latin edition of Eucharius Rösslin. This popular text ran into 13 editions and advocated much physical interference by midwives. Percivall Willughby was one of the few physicians to confine his practice to obstetrics, and he therefore had considerable experience with midwives, being called in when labours were abnormal. He wrote his book, *The Country Midwife's Opusculum,* in an attempt to have midwives trust the natural process of labour and delivery, feeling that the safest conduct of labour was by 'the invisible midwife, Dame Nature'. His book was written in the seventeenth century and outlined 150 case reports. However, it was not printed in his time, and it was left to Henry Blenkinsop to publish it as *Observations in Midwifery* in 1863. He had this general advice for midwives:

> *I desire that all midwives may gain a good repute, and have a happy success in all their undertakings; and that their knowledge, charity, patience, with tender compassion, may manifest their worths among their women, and give their women just cause to love, honour and to esteem them. The midwife's duty in a natural birth is no more but to attend and wait on Nature and to receive the child, and (if need require) to help to fetch the afterbirth, and her best care will be Nature's servant. Let them always remember that gentle proceedings (with moderate warm-keeping and having their endeavours*

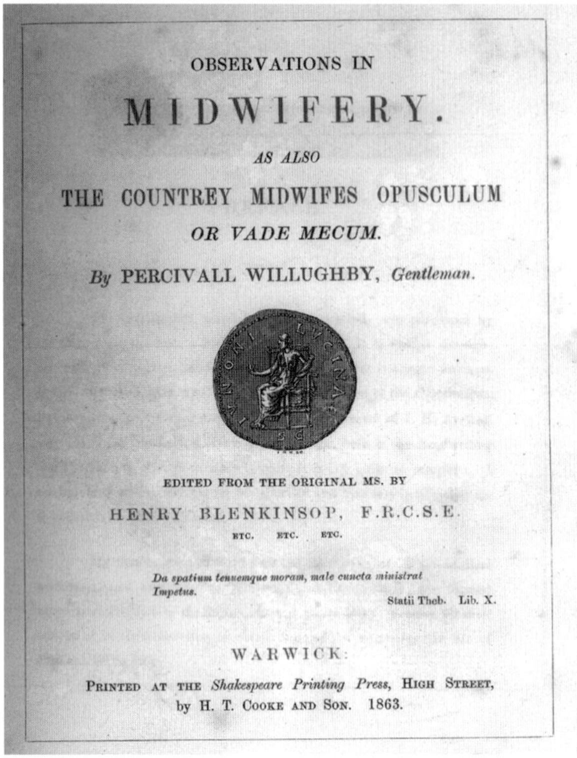

OBSERVATIONS IN

MIDWIFERY.

AS ALSO

THE COUNTREY MIDWIFES OPUSCULUM

OR VADE MECUM.

By PERCIVALL WILLUGHBY, *Gentleman.*

EDITED FROM THE ORIGINAL MS. BY

HENRY BLENKINSOP, F.R.C.S.E.

ETC. ETC. ETC.

Da spatium tenuemque moram, male cuncta ministrat Impetus.

Statii Theb. Lib. X.

WARWICK:

PRINTED AT THE *Shakespeare Printing Press*, HIGH STREET,
by H. T. COOKE AND SON. 1863.

Title page of Willughby's *Observations in Midwifery*

dulcified with sweet words) will best ease and relieve and soonest deliver their labouring women.

Willughby used ergot in non-progressive labour and described what may be one of the first cases of brachial plexus palsy following breech extraction: 'A week or more after delivery, the child was swelled in the right arm, and was weak in the wrist; and could not hold up the hand, but that it hung flagging down'.

Percivall Willughby was born in Wollaton Hall, Nottinghamshire in 1596. He received his formal education at Eton and Oxford, where he received his BA in 1620. He then became an apprentice to a barber-surgeon in London, moving to Derby in 1624 to work as a physician and man-midwife. From 1656 to 1660 he practised in London, 'among the meaner sort of women', and thereafter concentrated on obstetrics. One of his daughters became a midwife, and it is likely that he taught her. At this time the man-midwife was only brought into the lying-in chamber when major complications arose. Thus, when a man-midwife was summoned, the labouring woman usually knew that something was disastrously wrong. This reticence to accept man-midwives at labour and delivery is exemplified by a case when his midwife daughter was attending a woman with a breech presentation. She became uneasy and requested the assistance of her father. Willughby came to her aid and successfully delivered the infant with her but in a surreptitious manner: 'At my daughter's request, unknown to the lady I crept into the chamber upon my hands and knees and returned and it was not perceived by ye lady'.

Percivall Willughby returned to Derby in 1660 and continued a busy obstetric practice in that area. He died at the age of 89 in 1685.

Selected Publications

Willughby P. *Observations in Midwifery*, ed. H. Blenkinsop. Warwick: Shakespeare Printing Press; 1863.

Bibliography References

113, 115, 298, 347, 418, 469, 502, 503, 648, 1204, 1261, 1608, 1710.

Wolff, Caspar Friedrich (1733–1794)

Wolffian Body and Duct

Caspar Wolff was the first to describe the embryogenesis of the kidney in the chick embryo. In outlining the development of the mesonephros, Wolff wrote:

This cell substance on either side of the hind-gut gradually collects into mounds – on them small elevations are present, which become smaller and smaller in relation to the other parts but still result in an uneven, shaggy surface. Finally, small, sharply circumscribed, oval bodies arise, with a smooth surface, and supplied with filaments coursing from the kidneys back to the intestine.

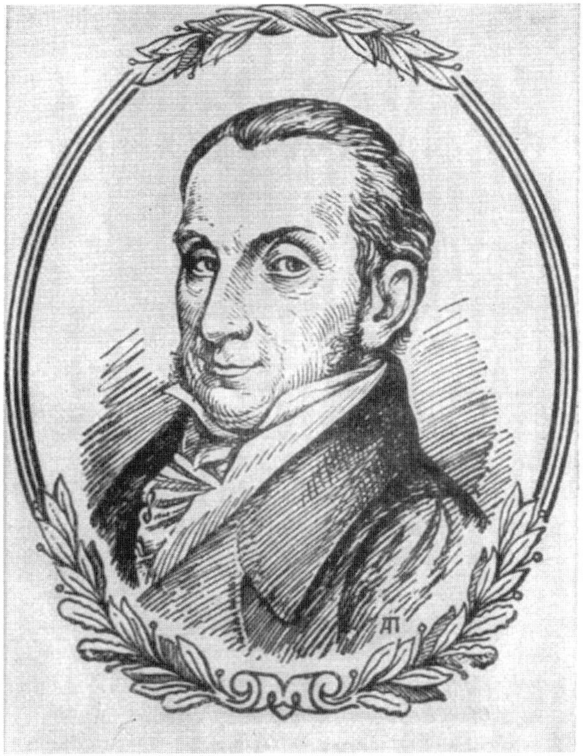

Caspar Friedrich Wolff

The cell substance that first appears along the surface of the spine on the third day and proceeds into the allantois on the fourth and fifth days, represents the first material that is destined to be transformed later into the kidneys.

Wolff reported his work at the age of 26 years in his doctoral thesis, *Theoria generationis.* The noted embryologist of the following century, Martin Rathke (1793–1860), designated the embryonic mesonephros the Wolffian body and its excretory duct the Wolffian duct.

The son of a tailor, Caspar Friedrich Wolff was born in Berlin. He began his medical studies there but transferred to Halle. His first academic appointment was teaching anatomy at Breslau. This he carried out with much success and returned to Berlin, hoping for academic advancement. There he met with hostility from many of his colleagues, based partly on academic jealousy and partly on religious opposition to his scientific studies that challenged the prevailing belief of preformation, which regarded the embryo as a completely formed miniature adult. Blocked in his academic ambitions in Berlin, Wolff left in 1769 for the Academy at St Petersburg, Russia, and remained there until his death from a brain haemorrhage on 6 March 1794.

Selected Publications

Wolff CF. *Theoria generationis.* Halle: Hendel; 1759, pp. 96–7.

Bibliography References

8, 39, 406, 592, 606, 615, 648, 676, 689, 1214, 1480, 1485, 1703.

Woods, Charles Edwin (1886–1946)

Woods' Screw Manoeuvre

In 1943 Woods published a paper outlining the application of a principle of physics to the clinical problem of shoulder dystocia. Using wooden models, he demonstrated that when the anterior fetal shoulder becomes impacted behind the symphysis pubis, direct propulsive or traction forces will not overcome the dystocia. He showed that the relationship between the fetal shoulders and the symphysis, sacral promontory and coccyx was like the threads of a screw. Thus, if the fetal shoulders were rotated through 180 degrees they could be 'corkscrewed' through the pelvis without trauma. He gave the rationale as follows:

After the head has been born the shoulders of the baby resemble a longitudinal section of a screw engaged in three threads, the 'pubic thread', the 'promontory thread' and the 'coccyx thread'. Any pulling on the baby's neck or axilla is mechanically incorrect because it violates a simple, well-known law of physics applicable to the screw.

Woods then outlined his screw manoeuvre:

A downward thrust is made with the left hand on the buttocks of the baby. At the same time two fingers of the right hand, on the anterior aspect of the posterior shoulder, make gentle clockwise pressure upward around the circumference of the arc, and past, twelve o'clock. The posterior shoulder is now delivered. With pressure applied downward from above with the left hand the two fingers

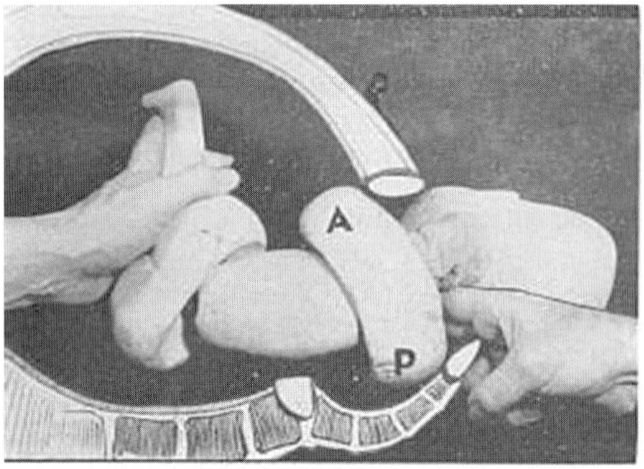

Fig. 5.

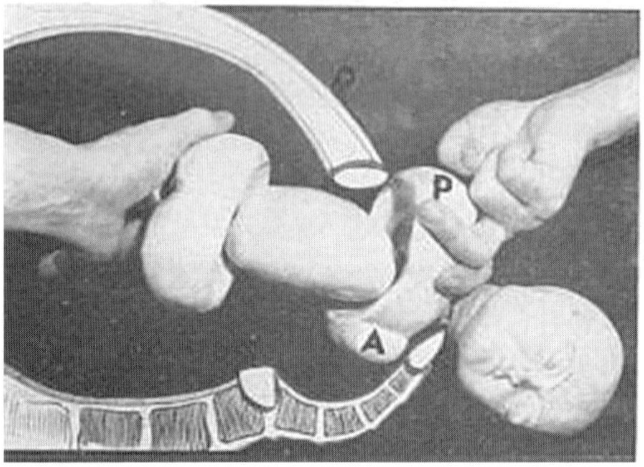

Illustration of wooden model in Woods' paper describing the screw manoeuvre

of the right hand make gentle counter-clockwise pressure upward around the circumference of the arc and past twelve o'clock, and the remaining shoulder is delivered.

A colleague later explained how Woods had come to believe this principle might apply to delivery of the shoulders in cases of shoulder dystocia. Apparently, Woods observed a furnaceman cleaning the wood-burning furnace at his home. To gain entry to the large furnace cavity through the circular porthole, the man first put his head, one arm and shoulder through the portal and then rotated his body 180 degrees to bring his other shoulder through. Observing this, Woods realised this principle could be applied to cases of shoulder dystocia, leading to his construction of wooden models to illustrate the point.

Woods' screw or corkscrew manoeuvre has been applied with success by many obstetricians over the last 60 years and remains one of the recommended methods for dealing with this stressful complication.

Charles Edwin Woods graduated from the Indiana University School of Medicine at Indianapolis in 1910. He served in France during the First World War. Living in Westbury, New York, he was on the staff of the Mercy Hospital, Rockville Centre and Meadowbrook Hospital, Hempstead. He died on 12 August 1946.

Selected Publications

Woods CE. A principle of physics as applicable to shoulder delivery. *Am J Obstet Gynecol* 1943; 45: 796–805.

Bibliography References

99, 113, 116.

Word, Samuel Buford (1907–1971)

Word Catheter

A cyst or abscess of Bartholin's gland duct is a common and annoying gynaecological problem. Definitive treatment is surgical marsupialisation, which often requires general or regional anaesthesia, particularly if infection is present. Simple incision and drainage under local anaesthesia may be unsuccessful in the long term, with recurrence due to the incision sealing over. Buford Word devised a technique that would allow incision and drainage under local anaesthesia and also the formation of a permanent epithelialised fistula to retain function of the gland and prevent recurrence:

A new permanent orifice to a duct of Bartholin's gland is easily created by making a stab wound in the cyst in the region of the original orifice, inserting the catheter, and inflating the bulb with water. The catheter is left in place

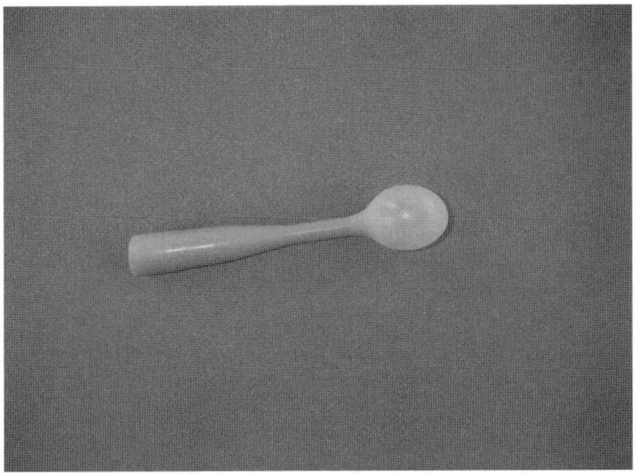

Word catheter

until epithelization of the new orifice is complete which usually takes 4–6 weeks. In essence, an epithelized fistula is created between the cyst and the vaginal vestibule. After the catheter is removed, the cyst shrinks and becomes a duct again and the resting gland resumes normal function.

Word first used a size 10F Foley catheter for this purpose in 1947. By 1963 he had a smaller version manufactured:

The catheter stem is 1-inch long, single-barreled and the size of 10F Foley catheter. A sealed stopper is attached to one end and a 5 cc capacity latex inflatable balloon is attached to the other stopper.

This has come to be known as the Word catheter. It is still widely used for the outpatient management of Bartholin's gland duct cyst and abscess, particularly in North America.

Samuel Buford Word was born in Aberdeen, Mississippi on 21 December 1907. He graduated MD from Louisiana State University in 1935 and carried out his internship at the Charity Hospital, New Orleans. He spent three years in private practice in Birmingham, Alabama and then served in the US Army Medical Corp in the Pacific during the Second World War. He retired from the army in 1946 with the rank of colonel. He spent his entire professional life as an obstetrician and gynaecologist in Birmingham, with an appointment as clinical associate professor in the department of obstetrics and gynaecology at the University of Alabama. Following his death on 4 January 1971, the Samuel Buford Word Annual Lectureship was established at the School of Medicine in the University of Alabama.

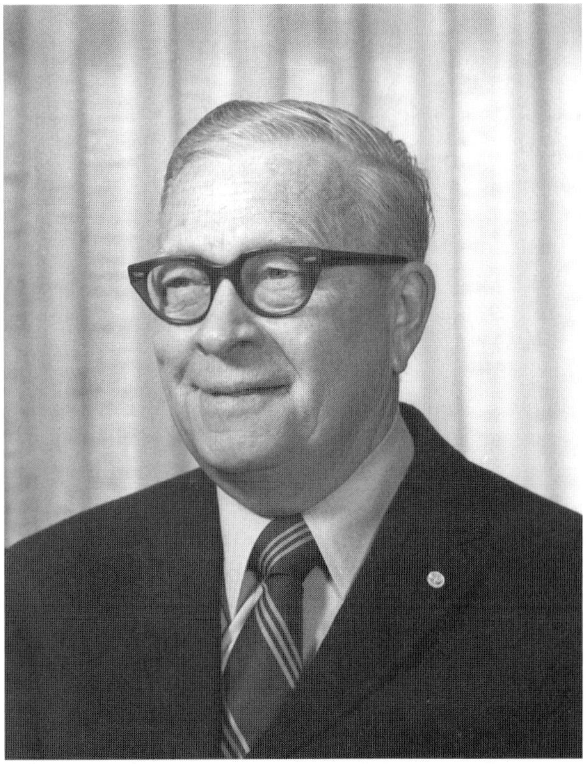

Samuel Buford Word

Selected Publications

Word B. New instrument for office treatment of cyst and abscess of Bartholin's gland. *JAMA* 1964; 190: 777–8.

Word B. A reappraisal of Bartholin's gland. *J Med Assoc State Ala* 1966; 35: 515–20.

Word B. Office treatment of cyst and abscess of Bartholin's gland duct. *South Med J* 1968; 61: 514–8.

Bibliography References

1725, 1726.

Wright, Marmaduke Burr (1803–1879)

Combined Cephalic Version

Marmaduke Wright was the first to advocate bimanual cephalic version in cases of shoulder presentation. The use of both internal and external hands to accomplish version is usually associated with Braxton Hicks. However, there were enough differences in their indications and techniques to acknowledge the contributions of both men. Wright first presented his work to the Ohio Medical Society on 6 June 1854, for which he was awarded the society's medal. His method was specifically for cases of shoulder presentation, as he outlined:

> *Suppose . . . the presentation to be the right shoulder, with the head in the left iliac fossa – the right hand to have been introduced into the vagina . . . We now apply our fingers upon the top of the shoulder, and our thumb in the opposite axilla, or on such part as will give us command of the chest, and enable us to apply a degree of lateral force. Our left hand is also applied to the abdomen of the patient, over the breech of the foetus. Lateral pressure is made upon the shoulders in such a way as to give the body of the foetus a curvilinear movement. At the same time, the left hand, applied as above, makes pressure so as to dislodge the breech, as it were, and move it towards the center of the uterine cavity. The body is thus made to assume its original bent position, the points of contact with the uterus are loosened, and perhaps diminished, and the force of adhesion is in a good degree overcome. Without any direct action upon the head it gradually approaches the superior strait, falls into the opening, and will, in all probability, adjust itself as a favourable vertex presentation.*

Marmaduke Burr Wright was born on 10 November 1803 in Pemberton, New Jersey, the eldest of eight children. He was apprenticed to Dr John McKelvey of Trenton, Ohio, and then studied at the University of Pennsylvania, receiving his MD in 1823. Wright initially practised medicine in Columbus, Ohio. In 1838 he was appointed professor of materia medica at the Medical College of Ohio in Cincinnati, transferring to the chair of obstetrics in 1840. He was removed from this position in 1850, following a quarrel between the faculty and university administration.

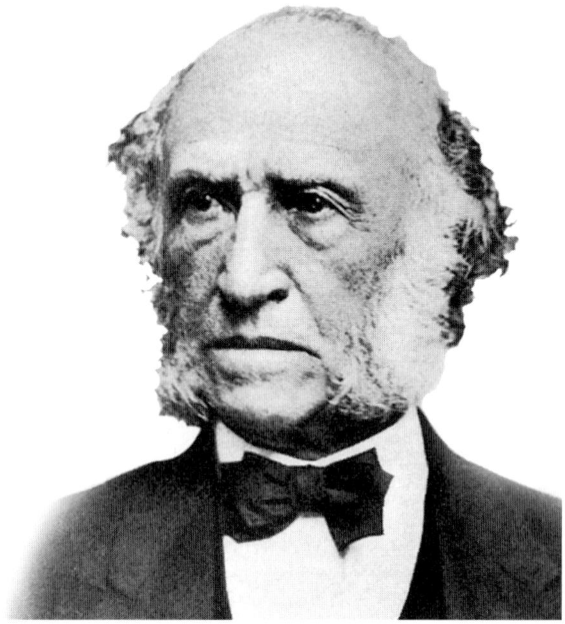

Marmaduke Burr Wright

Ten years later he was reappointed to the professorship and held the position until his retirement in 1868. A vigorous and opinionated man, Wright also served in the Ohio state legislature.

Wright's paper was first published in the transactions of the Ohio State Medical Society and issued separately later in the same year. He died on 15 August 1879 in Cincinnati.

Selected Publications

Wright MB. Difficult labours and their treatment. *Ohio State Med Soc Trans* 1854; 9: 59–88.

Wright MB. *Difficult Labours and Their Treatment.* Cincinnati, OH: Jackson White and Company; 1854.

Bibliography References

347, 648, 801, 810, 838, 1171, 1261, 1480, 1485, 1594, 1595.

Wrigley, Arthur Joseph (1902–1983)

Wrigley's Forceps

In 1935, Wrigley published his paper on 'The Forceps Operation', in which he went to some length to condemn the high application of forceps:

> *Today there should but rarely be the necessity to resort to any but the low forceps operation, which consists in the lifting of the fetal head past the perineum.*

He spoke against the long, curved, heavy forceps with axis-traction attachment that allowed application to the fetal head high in the pelvis. He echoed William Smellie's advice to use short forceps, which enforced safety by only being applicable to the fetal head low in the pelvis. Thus, Wrigley started to use James Young Simpson's short, straight forceps, but found that, without the pelvic curve, the application on the fetal head was incorrect and led to unsightly marks and bruising. He therefore took a pair of Smellie's straight forceps to the instrument makers, Allen and Hanburys, and bade them add a pelvic curve and shorten the handle. After a number of modifications, the final Wrigley forceps, weighing 285 g, was produced:

> *Its construction is such that it is impossible to exert a tremendous pull, and the risk to the child should in consequence be enormously decreased.*

Wrigley advocated use of the forceps to shorten the second stage of labour in cases of maternal distress with the head low on the pelvic floor. In such cases, his experience was that infant and perineal trauma was equivalent to that of spontaneous delivery. By the early 1970s the company had produced 1,500 pairs of Wrigley's forceps. He received no royalties.

Joe Wrigley, as he was known, was born in Lancashire. He entered St Thomas' Hospital Medical School in 1919 and qualified in 1925. He was awarded his MD with gold medal in 1928. After postgraduate training he was appointed to the department of obstetrics and gynaecology at St Thomas' in 1933 and rose to become head of the department in 1946. He was a major contributor to the first four *Reports on Confidential Enquiries into Maternal Deaths in England and Wales* produced between 1953 and 1965. In his spare time, he was a model train enthusiast and fisherman. In 1965, Joe Wrigley retired, unenamoured with the looming spectre of technology in obstetrics. In the same year he was

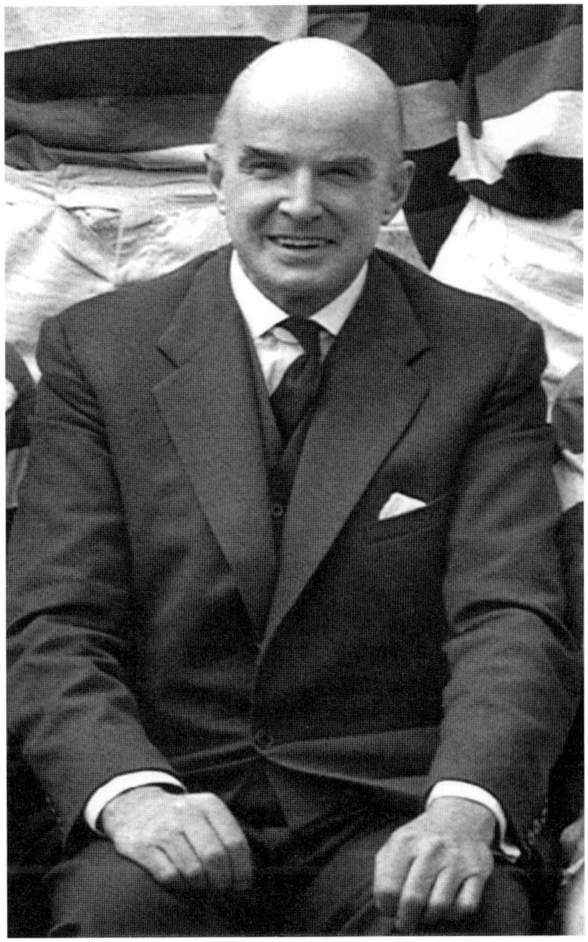

Arthur Joseph Wrigley

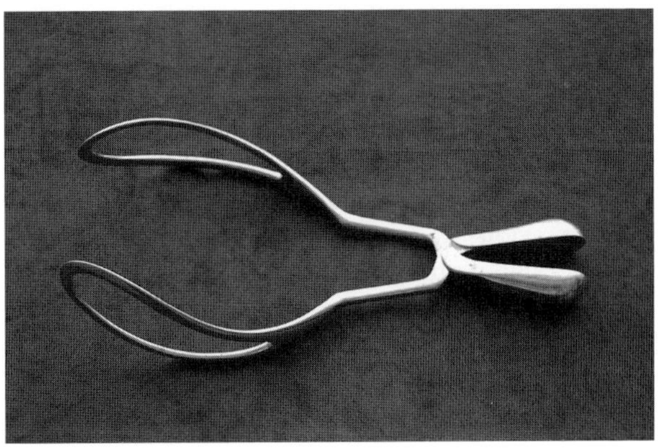

Wrigley's forceps

appointed CBE by the Queen. A northerner at heart and by birth, he retired back to Lancashire. He died on 18 December 1983.

His motto was that of a down-to-earth northern Englishman: 'Experience is the best of teachers – but his fees is very heavy'.

Selected Publications

Wrigley JA. The forceps operation. *Lancet* 1935; 2: 702–5.

Bibliography References

51, 263, 272, 361, 721, 822, 1186, 1285, 1566, 1729.

Youssef, Abdel Fattah (1924–2001)

Youssef's Syndrome

Vesicouterine fistulae associated with urinary incontinence may follow prolonged labour, operative vaginal delivery and gynaecological surgery. By the last half of the twentieth century, the majority of cases occurred after caesarean delivery.

In 1957, Abdel Youssef described a specific type of vesicouterine fistula following lower-segment caesarean section in which there was no urinary incontinence, apparent amenorrhoea with a patent cervical canal, and cyclical haematuria:

> *Very rarely, however, a different type of bladder fistula may complicate lower segment section which is, curiously enough, characterized by the complete absence of urinary incontinence. The patient, instead, presents herself some time after the operation complaining of amenorrhoea and of cyclic voiding of blood-stained urine at the expected time of her periods. Examination discloses that a vesicouterine fistula is present and that although no urinary leakage takes place and not a drop of menstrual blood passes through the natural passages, the cervical canal is perfectly patent.*

He introduced the term 'menouria' to describe this form of menstruation and the constellation of findings came to be known as 'Youssef's syndrome'. He noted that six similar case reports had been published previously.

To explain the paradoxical absence of urinary incontinence and the amenorrhoea, despite the fistula and patent cervical canal he postulated that:

> *The syndrome described in this paper, which may follow lower segment cesarean section in the rare event when a vesicouterine fistula above the anatomical internal os complicates the operation, can be satisfactorily explained only by assuming that a sphincter is present at the uterine isthmus which prevents the passage of urine or menstrual blood through the patent cervix . . . when a vesicocervical*

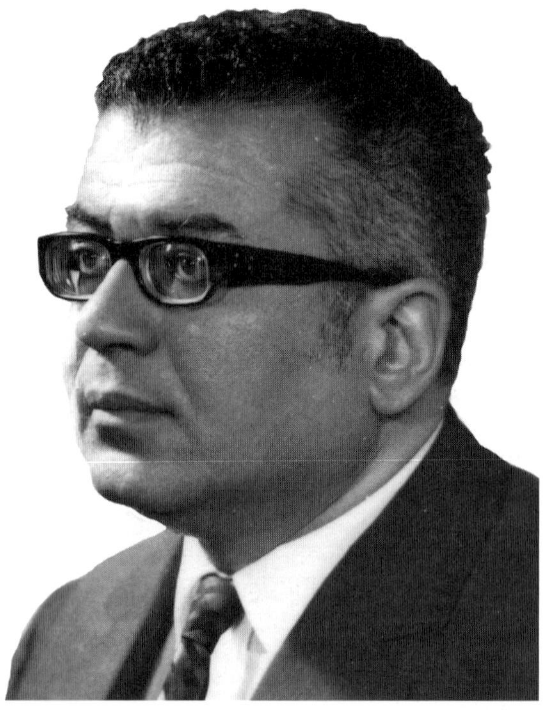

Abdel Fattah Youssef

fistula is present below the level of the isthmus, the usual picture of complete urinary incontinence occurs and the menstrual flow passes through the cervix and not through the fistula into the bladder.

In support of this theory, he filled the bladder with methylene blue but only got dye to leak through the cervix by applying strong suprapubic pressure. He felt that 'the resistance of the isthmic sphincter was overcome when the pressure to which it was subjected was markedly increased'.

Abdel Youssef was born on 21 June 1924 in Asyut, in Upper Egypt. He obtained his medical degree from Cairo University in 1946 and completed his postgraduate training in surgery, obstetrics and gynaecology by 1951. Youssef became the senior gynaecological surgeon at Kasr El-Aini Hospital, Cairo and, in 1967, was appointed professor and head of the department of obstetrics and gynaecology at Cairo University. He published widely, particularly in the field of urogynaecology. Abdel Youssef died in Cairo on 18 May 2001.

Selected Publications

Youssef AF. 'Menouria' following lower segment cesarean section. *Am J Obstet Gynecol* 1957; 73: 759–67.

Bibliography References

768, 968, 1551.

Z

Zavanelli, William Angelo (b. 1926)

Zavanelli Manoeuvre

At 2 a.m. on 18 January 1978, the obstetrician Bill Zavanelli, working in the small Valley Memorial Hospital, Livermore, California, was faced with a shoulder dystocia that he could not resolve by the usual means. The woman was a 30-year-old para 1 with a previous normal delivery of a 3.9 kg infant. On this occasion, her antenatal care, under Zavanelli's guidance, had been normal. She was admitted three days past term in spontaneous labour, progressed normally, and after 1½ hours in the second stage of labour, the head delivered spontaneously under pudendal block and with a right medio-lateral episiotomy. Restitution occurred, but the tight relationship of the vulval tissues to the fetal head signalled shoulder dystocia, which was unresponsive to the normal amount of downward traction and to suprapubic pressure. An attempt to reach the posterior arm failed, and from an interview with Dr Zavanelli it seems certain that this was a rare case of double shoulder dystocia with both shoulders arrested above the pelvic brim. In an attempt to gain further access, Zavanelli decided to rotate the fetal head to the anterior position, reversing the mechanism of delivery. As he did this, he applied pressure and flexion to the fetal head and found that, once rotated to the anterior position, the fetal head instantly recoiled into the vagina. The fetal heart had been monitored intermittently with an external handheld ultrasound device and had been normal during labour and was normal again following cephalic replacement into the vagina. He called in anaesthetic and obstetric colleagues from home, the patient was transferred from the second floor to the operating theatre on the first floor and, 67 minutes after reinsertion the fetal head, he performed a lower-segment caesarean section under general anaesthesia for a normal female infant weighing 5.5 kg with Apgar scores of 7 and 10. The recovery of mother and infant was uneventful.

At this time, Zavanelli was a clinical instructor in obstetrics and gynaecology at Stanford University, San Francisco. He mentioned the event to an obstetrical colleague at Stanford, Eugene Sandberg, who felt this case report should be published. However, Zavanelli was reluctant until development of the child was seen to be normal. The child continued to develop normally and, when she reached the age of seven

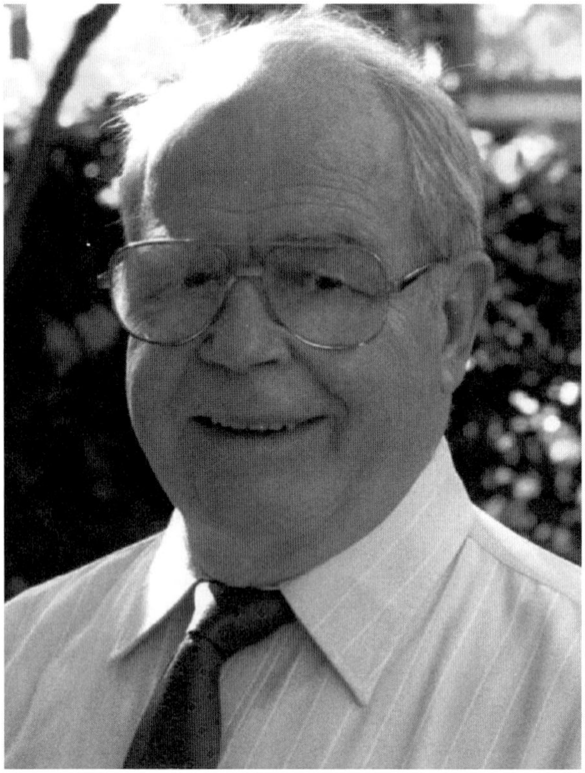

William Angelo Zavanelli

years, Sandberg published the case report. Zavanelli felt that the procedure should be called cephalic replacement, but Sandberg insisted on including the name 'Zavanelli manoeuvre' in the title, to honour the community obstetrician's innovative effort of desperation. Further informal follow-up by Zavanelli has shown that the child, now an adult, continues to be normal. The manoeuvre has subsequently been used on a number of occasions for those very rare cases of bilateral shoulder dystocia.

William Zavanelli, the youngest of three children, was born on 10 October 1926 in Martins Ferry, Ohio. His father was born in Canifilo, Italy, emigrated to the United States in his youth and later owned a bar and restaurant in Martins Ferry. His mother was of Welsh descent. After graduating from high school in 1944, he served in the United States Army in an administrative role in Hawaii during the Second World War. He received his bachelor's degree in bacteriology from the University of California at Los Angeles in 1951, following which he was recalled to service during the Korean War and stationed in Montana. He graduated as a doctor of osteopathy from the College of Osteopathic Physicians and Surgeons in Los Angeles in 1957 and was granted his MD from the California College of Medicine in 1962. From 1958–65 he worked as a general practitioner in Norwalk and Los Gatos, California. He then did a residency in obstetrics and gynaecology at St Mary's Hospital, San Francisco. From 1969 until the present, he has been in private obstetrical and gynaecological practice based at the Valley Memorial Hospital in Livermore, California, close to San Francisco.

Selected Publications

Sandberg EC. Zavanelli maneuver a potentially revolutionary method for the resolution of shoulder dystocia. *Am J Obstet Gynecol* 1985; 152: 479–84.

Sandberg EC. Zavanelli maneuver: twelve years of recorded experience. *Obstet Gynecol* 1999; 93: 312–7.

Bibliography References

99, 116.

Bibliography

1. Abell I. Professional attainments of Ephraim McDowell. *Bull Hist Med* 1950; 24: 161–7.
2. Abramovits A. Joseph Asherman, 60th anniversary celebration. *Harefuah* 1950; 38: 11.
3. Abramson DJ. Charles Bingham Penrose and the Penrose drain. *Surg Gynecol Obstet* 1976; 143: 285–6.
4. Abu-Hilal M, Newman JS. Sister Mary Joseph and her nodule: historical and clinical perspective. *Am J Med Sci* 2009; 337: 271–3.
5. Aburel, Eugen Bodgan (obituary). *Obstetrica si Ginecologia* (Bucharest) 1976; 24: 97–8.
6. Accardo PJ. Deformity and character: Dr Little's diagnosis of Richard III. *JAMA* 1980; 244: 2746–7.
7. Accardo P. William John Little and cerebral palsy in the nineteenth century. *J Hist Med Allied Sci* 1984; 44: 56–71.
8. Accardo P. *The Medical Almanac.* Clifton, NJ: Humana Press; 1992.
9. Adair FL. In memoriam: Joseph Bolivar De Lee (1869–1942) *Trans Am Gynec Soc* 1943; 67: 367–8.
10. Adami JG. The Manchester School: Charles White (1728–1813) and the arrest of puerperal fever. *J Obstet Gynaecol Br Emp* 1922; 29: 1–20.
11. Adami JG. *Charles White of Manchester (1728–1813) and the Arrest of Puerperal Fever.* London: Hodder and Stoughton Ltd; 1922.
12. Adams A. The family of Joseph Thomas Clover (1825–1882). In: Barr AM, Boulton TB, Wilkinson DJ (eds) *Essays on the History of Anaesthesia*: Royal Society of Medicine Press Ltd; 1996, pp. 141–5.
13. Adams EJ, Slack M. Anterior vaginal wall prolapse: an historical and anatomical perspective. In: Sturdee D, Olah K, Keane D (eds) *The Yearbook of Obstetrics and Gynaecology*. London: RCOG Press; 2001; 9: 61–70.
14. Adams HK. Joseph Thomas Clover: some aspects of his personal and professional life. In: Fink BR, Morris LE, Stephen CR (eds) *Proceedings of the History of Anaesthesia: Third International Symposium.* Park Ridge, IL: Wood Library-Museum of Anesthesiology; 1992, pp. 5–8.
15. Adler RE. *Medical Firsts: From Hippocrates to the Human Genome.* Hoboken, NJ: John Wiley & Sons; 2004.
16. Adriaunse AH, Pel M, Bleker OP. Semmelweis: the combat against puerperal fever. *Eur J Obstet Gynecol Reprod Biol* 2000; 90: 153–8.
17. Agarwal AK, Mukherjee R. Franz Kaspar Hesselbach (1759–1816). *Indian J Surg* 2008; 70: 96–8.
18. Alaily A. The history of the parturition chair. In: Studd J (ed.) *The Yearbook of Obstetrics and Gynaecology.* London; RCOG Press: 1996; 4: 23–32.
19. Allen E. In memoriam: Noble Sproat Heaney, 1880–1955. *Trans Am Gynec Soc* 1956; 79: 201–3.
20. Allen ED. Noble Sproat Heaney (obituary). *Proc Inst Med Chicago* 1956; 21: 43–5.
21. Allen PM, Setze TK. Howard Atwood Kelly (1858–1943): his life and his enduring legacy. *South Med J* 1991; 84: 361–8.
22. Allen WM. Recollections of my life with progesterone. *Gynecol Invest* 1974; 5: 142–82.
23. Allport WH. Louise Bourgeois: an old midwife's tale. *Am J Obstet Dis Women Child* 1912; 65: 820–51.
24. Ameline A. Antoine Basset (1882–1952). *Gynéc et Obstet* 1952; 51: 91–2.
25. Ancarani AGD. *L'Italia ostetrica.* 2nd edn. Siena: S. Bernadino; 1911.
26. Andrews BF. William Harvey in perinatal perspective. In: Smith GF, Vidyasagar D (eds) *Historical Review and Recent Advances in Neonatal and Perinatal Medicine* (vol. 2) New York, NY: Mead Johnson Ltd; 1981, pp. 165–78.
27. Andrews, Charles James (obituary). *Virginia Med Monthly*, September 1950.
28. Andrews HR. William Hunter and his work in midwifery. *BMJ* 1915; 1: 277–82.
29. Antall J. (ed.) *Pictures from the Past of the Healing Arts: Semmelweis Medical Historical Museum, Library and Archives.* Budapest: Semmelweis Museum; 1972.
30. Antoun M, Breen JL. Moschcowitz and the Moschcowitz procedure. *J Pelvic Surg* 1997; 3: 291–6.

31. Asbell B. *The Pill: A Biography of the Drug That Changed the World*. New York, NY: Random House; 1995.

32. Ashford JI. A history of *accouchement forcé*: 1550–1985. *Birth* 1986; 13: 241–9.

33. Ashwal S (ed.) *The Founders of Child Neurology*. San Francisco, CA: Norman Publishing; 1990.

34. Astrup P, Bie P, Engell HC. *Salt and Water in Culture and Medicine*. Copenhagen: Munksgaard; 1993.

35. Atkinson RS. *James Simpson and Chloroform*. London: Priory Press Ltd; 1973.

36. Atkinson WB. *The Physicians and Surgeons of the United States*. Philadelphia, PA: Charles Robson; 1878, pp. 343–4.

37. Attwood H. John William Ballantyne, perinatal pathology and antenatal care. In: *Proceedings of the XXIII International Congress of the History of Medicine*. London: Wellcome Institute of the History of Medicine; 1974, pp. 394–400.

38. Aubard Y, LeMeur Y, Grandjean MH, Baudet JH. Histoire de l'opération césarienne. *Rev Fr Gynécol Obstet* 1995; 90: 5–11.

39. Auli RP. Caspar Friedrich Wolff and his 'Theoria generationis', 1759. *J Hist Med Allied Sci* 1961; 16: 124–44.

40. Austin CR. Bob Edwards: a profile. *Hum Reprod* 1991; 6: 1–4.

41. Auvray M. Adolphe Pinard (1844–1934). *Bull Soc Obstét Gynéc Paris* 1934: 335–42.

42. Aveling JH. Immediate transfusion in England. *Obs J Gr Brit Irel* 1873; 5: 289–311.

43. Aveling JH. An account of the earliest English work on midwifery and the diseases of women. *Obstet J Gr Brit Irel* 1874; 2: 73–83.

44. Aveling JH. The curves of the midwifery forceps; their origins and uses. *Trans Obstet Soc Lond* 1879; 20: 130–51.

45. Aveling JH. *The Chamberlens and the Midwifery Forceps*. London: J & A Churchill; 1882.

46. Aveling JH. *English Midwives: Their History and Prospects. Reprint of the 1872 edition*. London: Hugh Elliott Ltd; 1967.

47. Aveling, James H (obituary). *Lancet* 1892; 2: 1477.

48. Aveling, James Hobson (obituary). *BMJ* 1892; 2: 1349–50.

49. Backman C. The Barton obstetric forceps. *Surg Gynecol Obstet* 1927; 45: 805–12.

50. Baer E von. *Autobiography of Dr Karl Ernest von Baer. Edited and translated from 1866 German edition by Jane M. Oppenheimer*. Canton, MA: Science History Publications; 1986.

51. Baird D. The evolution of modern obstetrics. *Lancet* 1960; 2: 557–64.

52. Baird, Dugald (obituary). *Aberdeen Press and Journal*. 11 November 1986.

53. Baird, Dugald (obituary). *Daily Telegraph*. 12 November 1986.

54. Baker JP. The incubator and the medical discovery of the premature infant. *J Perinatol* 2000; 20: 321–8.

55. Balchin J. *Quantum Leaps: 100 Scientists Who Changed the World*. London: Arcturus Publishing Ltd; 2007.

56. Ball C. James Young Simpson, 1811–1870. *Anaes Intens Care* 1996; 24: 639.

57. Ball C, Westhorpe R. Early blood transfusion equipment. *Anaes Intens Care* 2000; 28: 247.

58. Ball C, Westhorpe R. Local anaesthesia: early spinal anaesthesia. *Anaes Intens Care* 2003; 31: 493.

59. Ball C, Westhorpe R. Local anaesthesia: the early evolution of spinal needles. *Anaes Intens Care* 2003; 31: 611.

60. Ball C, Westhorpe R. Local anaesthesia: the continuing evolution of spinal needles. *Anaes Intens Care* 2004; 32: 3.

61. Ball OF. They made hospital history: Samuel Bard. *Modern Hospital* 1950; 75: 81–2.

62. Ballantyne, JW (obituary). *BMJ* 1923; 1: 213–6.

63. Bancroft-Livingstone G. Louise de la Vallière and the birth of the man-midwife. *J Obstet Gynaec Br Emp* 1956; 63: 261–4.

64. Barker BF. Report of committee on voluntary communication, on the comparative use of ergot and the forceps, in labor. *Trans Med Soc NY* 1858; 85: 113–30.

65. Barker DJP, Thornburg KL. The obstetric origins of health for a lifetime. *Clin Obstet Gynecol* 2013; 2: 4–11.

66. Barker, DJP (obituary). *BMJ* 2013; 347: f5703.

67. Barker F. Remarks on the obstetric forceps, with a description and demonstration of Tarnier's new instrument. *Am J Obstet* 1878; 11: 1–11.

68. Barkin J. Interstitial cystitis: the great imposter! Epidemiology, etiology, diagnosis and management. *J Sex Reprod Med* 2003; 3: 57–64.

69. Barnes, Robert (obituary). *J Obstet Gynaecol Br Emp* 1907; 11: 519–22.

70. Barr ML. Some notes on the discovery of the sex chromatin and its clinical application. *Am J Obstet Gynecol* 1972; 112: 293–5.

71. Barr, Murray Llewellyn (obituary). *Can Med Assoc J* 1995; 153: 992.

72. Barrow MV. A brief history of teratology to the early 20th century. *Teratology* 1971; 4: 119–30.

73. Bartlett J. Paul Portal: his true place in the literature of placenta praevia. *Clin Rev Chicago.* 1901; 14: 313–30.

74. Baskett PJF, Baskett TF (eds) *Resuscitation Greats.* Bristol: Clinical Press Ltd; 2007.

75. Baskett RJF. James Kenneth Wallace Ferguson: a life in Canadian medical research. *Ann R Coll Phys Surg Can* 1996; 29: 105–8.

76. Baskett TF. Ferguson's reflex: then and now. *J Soc Obstet Gynaecol Can* 1989; 11: 35–8.

77. Baskett TF. Thomas Cullen and the umbilical black eye. *J Soc Obstet Gynaecol Can* 1992; 14: 85–93.

78. Baskett TF. Roberts' sign of intrauterine fetal death. *J Soc Obstet Gynaecol Can* 1993; 15: 69–72.

79. Baskett TF. O'Sullivan's method of hydrostatic replacement of acute uterine inversion. *J Soc Obstet Gynaecol Can* 1994; 16: 1275–6.

80. Baskett TF. The first neonatal exchange transfusion for haemolytic disease of the newborn by Dr Alfred Hart of Toronto. *J Soc Obstet Gynaecol Can* 1995; 17: 153–5.

81. Baskett TF, Rishworth SK, Want PC. Historical perspective: cast of the head of the first infant delivered under ether anaesthesia by James Young Simpson. *ACOG Clin Rev* 1998; 3: 14–16.

82. Baskett TF. Some 20th century milestones in obstetrics and gynaecology. In: O'Brien PMS (ed.) *The Yearbook of Obstetrics and Gynaecology*. London: RCOG Press. 2000; 8: 1–9.

83. Baskett TF. Benjamin Pugh: the airpipe and neonatal resuscitation. *Resuscitation* 2000; 44: 153–5.

84. Baskett TF. Virginia Apgar and the newborn Apgar score. *Resuscitation* 2000; 47: 215–7.

85. Baskett TF. A flux of the reds: evolution of active management of the third stage of labour. *J R Soc Med* 2000; 93: 489–93.

86. Baskett TF, Nagele F. Naegele's rule: a reappraisal. *Br J Obstet Gynaecol* 2000; 107: 1433–5.

87. Baskett TF, Nagele F. Bernard Schultze and the swinging neonate. *Resuscitation* 2001; 51: 3–6.

88. Baskett TF. Of violent floodings in pregnancy: evolution of the management of placenta praevia. In: Sturdee D, Olah K, Keane D (eds) *The Yearbook of Obstetrics and Gynaecology*. London: RCOG Press 2001; 9: 1–14.

89. Baskett TF. James Blundell: the first transfusion of human blood. *Resuscitation* 2002; 52: 229–33.

90. Baskett TF. Edward Rigby (1747–1821) of Norwich and his *Essay on the Uterine Haemorrhage. J R Soc Med* 2002; 95: 618–22.

91. Baskett TF. *Pages of History in Canadian Obstetrics and Gynaecology*. Toronto: Rogers Media; 2003.

92. Baskett TF. The History of Vacuum Extraction. In: Vacca A. (ed.) *Handbook of Vacuum Delivery in Obstetric Practice*. Brisbane: Vacca Research; 2003, pp. 1–10.

93. Baskett TF. The development of prostaglandins. *Best Pract Res Clin Obstet Gynaecol* 2003; 17: 703–6.

94. Baskett TF. The development of oxytocic drugs in the management of postpartum haemorrhage. *Ulster Med J* 2004; 73: 2–6.

95. Baskett TF. Ambroise Paré and the arrest of haemorrhage. *Resuscitation* 2004; 62: 133–5.

96. Baskett TF. Edinburgh connections in a painful world. *JR Coll Surg Edinb Irel* 2005; 3: 99–107.

97. Baskett TF. Hysterectomy: evolution and trends. *Best Pract Res Clin Obstet Gynaecol* 2005; 19: 295–305.

98. Baskett TF. The history of pessaries for uterovaginal prolapse. In: Farrell SA (ed.) *Pessaries in Clinical Practice*. London: Springer-Verlag Ltd; 2006, pp. 1–9.

99. Baskett TF, Calder AA, Arulkumaran S. *Munro Kerr's Operative Obstetrics. 11th Centenary Edition.* Edinburgh: Elsevier; 2007.

100. Baskett TF. A tribute to Kieran O'Driscoll (1920–2007). *J Obstet Gynaecol Can* 2007; 29: 672–3.

101. Baskett TF. The Pill and the Pope. *West Engl Med J* 2016; 115: 1–14.

102. Baskett TF. *A History of Caesarean Birth: From Maternal Death to Maternal Choice*. Bristol: Clinical Press Ltd; 2017.

103. Bass FE. *Who's Who in Tennessee*. Hopkinsville, KY: Historical Record Association, 1961, p. 91.

104. Battey, Robert (obituary). *Chicago Med Rec* 1895; 9: 345.

105. Bauer AW. In memoriam: Kasper Blond. *Wein Klin Wochen* 1965; 1: 17.

106. Bavister BD. Early history of in vitro fertilization. *Reprod* 2002; 124: 181–96.

107. Bayon HP. William Harvey (1578–1657): his application of biological experiment, clinical observation, and comparative anatomy to the problems of generation. *J Hist Med Allied Sci* 1947; 11: 51–96.

108. Beaton JJ, Miller R, Boyle IT (eds) *Treasures of the College*. Glasgow: Royal College of Physicians and Surgeons of Glasgow; 1998.

109. Bechet PE. Hieronymus Fracastorius: a brief survey of his life and work on syphilis. *Arch Dermatol Syph* 1932; 26: 888–93.

110. Beecher HK. Oliver Wendell Holmes and anesthesia. *Anesthesiology* 1968; 29: 1068–70.

111. Beecher HK, Altschule MD. *Medicine at Harvard: The First Three Hundred Years.* Hanover, NH: University Press of New England; 1977.

112. Beer E. Memoir: Alexis Victor Moschcowitz. *J Mount Sinai Hosp* 1934; 1: 26–7.

113. Beer E, Folghera MG. Historical observations on shoulder dystocia. *Minerva Ginecol* 2001; 53: 219–22.

114. Beer E, Folghera MG. Early history of McRoberts' manoeuvre. *Minerva Ginecol* 2002; 54: 197–8.

115. Beer E. Shoulder dystocia and posture for birth: a history lesson. *Obstet Gynecol Surv* 2003; 58: 697–9.

116. Beer E, Mangiante G, Pecorari D. *Distocia delle spalle: storia ed attualità.* Roma: CIC Edizioni Internazionali; 2006.

117. Beer E. History of extraction of the posterior arm to resolve shoulder dystocia. *Obstet Gynecol Surv* 2006; 61: 149–51.

118. Beeson BB. Henri Hallopeau (biography). *Arch Derm Syphil* 1931; 23: 730–2.

119. Behbakht K, Mikuta JJ. Life and contributions of Otto Ernst Küstner (1848–1931). *J Pelvic Surg* 1998; 4: 108.

120. Belloni L. Giovanni Battista Morgagni. In: Gillispie CC (ed.) *Dictionary of Scientific Biography.* New York, NY: Charles Scribner's Sons;1974; 9: 510–2.

121. Benagiano G. History of adenomyosis. *Best Pract Res Clin Obstet Gynaecol* 2006; 20: 449–63.

122. Bernard GR, Allen L. Richard Torpin (1891–1976). *Anat Rec* 1976; 186: 256–7.

123. Bender GA. *Great Moments in Medicine.* Detroit, MI: Northwood Institute Press; 1966.

124. Bennett EP. The identity of erysipelas and certain forms of puerperal fever. *Am J Med Sci* 1850; 19: 376–83.

125. Benrubi GI. History of hysterectomy. *J Fla Med Assoc* 1988; 75: 533–8.

126. Benrubi GI. Labour induction: historic perspectives. *Clin Obstet Gynecol* 2000; 43: 429–32.

127. Berci G, Kont LA. A new optical system in endoscopy with special reference to cystoscopy. *Br J Urol* 1969; 41: 564–71.

128. Berci G, Forde KA. History of endoscopy: what lessons have we learned from the past? *Surg Endosc* 2000; 14: 5–15.

129. Bergman JA. The legacy of John Snow: an appreciation of his life and scientific contribution on the 100th anniversary of his death. *Anesthesiology* 1958; 19: 595–606.

130. Bergman NA. *The Genesis of Surgical Anesthesia.* Park Ridge, IL: Wood Library-Museum of Anesthesiology; 1998.

131. Berkeley C. In Memoriam: John Whitridge Williams. *J Obstet Gynaecol Br Emp* 1932; 39: 106–8.

132. Berkow SG. A visit with Dr Emil Novak. *Obstet Gynecol* 1956; 7: 107–13.

133. Berkow SG. 'Children unto God': notes on the life and work of Dr IC Rubin. *Obstet Gynecol* 1957; 9: 490–6.

134. Berkow SG. A visit with Dr Joe Vincent Meigs. *Obstet Gynecol* 1959; 13: 622–9.

135. Berkow SG. A visit with Dr Richard Wesley Te Linde. *Obstet Gynecol* 1959; 14: 257–66.

136. Berkow SG. A visit with Dr John Rock. *Obstet Gynecol* 1960; 15: 665–72.

137. Berkow SG. A visit with Dr George N. Papanicolaou. *Obstet Gynecol* 1960; 16: 243–52.

138. Berkow SG. The progress of a Connecticut Yankee: a visit with Dr Herbert Thoms. *Obstet Gynecol* 1962; 19: 137–44.

139. Berkowitz JS. *The College of Physicians of Philadelphia: Portrait Catalogue.* Philadelphia, PA: College of Physicians of Philadelphia; 1984.

140. Bernstein AM, Khoo HP, Bloom DA. Beyond Trendelenburg position: Friedrich Trendelenburg's life and surgical contributions. *Surgery* 1999; 126: 78–82.

141. Bernstein H, Novak D. Fetal nutrition and imprinting. In: Walker WA, Watkins JB, Duggan C. (eds) *Nutrition in Pediatrics.* 3rd edn. London: BC Decker Inc; 2003.

142. Bero L, Rennie D. The Cochrane Collaboration: preparing, maintaining and disseminating reviews of the effect of health care. *JAMA* 1995; 274: 1935–8.

143. Bevis, Douglas (obituary). *BMJ* 1994; 309: 1013–4.

144. Bevis, Douglas (obituary). *Daily Telegraph* 13 July 1994.

145. Bevis, Douglas (obituary). *The Times* 12 July 1994.

146. Bhattacharya K. Kurt Semm: a laparoscopic crusader. *J Min Access Surg* 2007; 3: 35–6.

147. Bickenbach W. Heinrich Martius (obituary). *Zentrabl Gynäk* 1965; 18: 594–5.

148. Bickers W. John Peter Mettauer of Virginia. *JAMA* 1963; 184: 870–1.

149. Billings JS. *The History and Literature of Surgery.* New York, NY: Argosy-Antiquarian Ltd; 1970.

150. Bing RJ. Doppler and his principle. In: *Past Truth and Present Poetry: Medical Discoveries and the People Behind Them*. Shrewsbury: tfm Publishing Ltd; 2006.

151. Birch CA. *Names We Remember*. Beckenham: Ravenswood Publications; 1979.

152. Bishop E. Ralph Hayward Pomeroy: an appreciation. *Brooklyn Hosp J* 1947; 5: 67–72.

153. Bissell DJ. Marion Sims: surgeon and humanitarian. *Am J Surg* 1929; 6: 561–5.

154. Bjornson O. Posterior position of the occiput in labour. *BMJ* 1933; 1: 311–13.

155. Black JW. Dr James Hobson Aveling. *Trans Obstet Soc London* 1893; 35: 67–71.

156. Blanton WB. *Medicine in Virginia in the Nineteenth Century*. Richmond, VA: Garrett & Massie Inc; 1933.

157. Blaschko HKF. Ulf von Euler. In: *Biographical Memoirs of Fellows of the Royal Society of London*, 1985; 31: 145–70.

158. Bloch H. Nicholas Culpeper MD (1616–1654), medical maverick in seventeenth-century England. *NY J Med* 1982; 82: 1865–7.

159. Blumenfeld-Kosinski R. *Not of Woman Born*. Ithaca, NY and London: Cornell University Press; 1990.

160. Blundell, James (obituary). *BMJ* 1878; 1: 351.

161. Blundell, James (obituary). *Lancet* 1878; 1: 255.

162. Bompeix ML. Mission de Mme du Coudray, sage-femme royale en 1770: école d'accouchement d'Auch. *Bull Soc Archeol du Gers* 1912; 13: 262–71.

163. Bonner TN. *Medicine in Chicago, 1850–1950*. New York, NY: American Book-Stratford Press Inc; 1957.

164. Bonney V. The late Professor Blair-Bell. *BMJ* 1936; 1: 342.

165. Bonney, Victor (obituary). *BMJ* 1953; 2: 99–100.

166. Bonney, Victor (obituary). *J Obstet Gynaecol Br Emp* 1953; 60: 566–9.

167. Bonney, Victor (obituary). *Lancet* 1953; 2: 93.

168. Børdahl PE. Tubal sterilization: a historical review. *J Reprod Med* 1985; 30: 18–24.

169. Bosanquet A. Jane Sharp. *The Practising Midwife*. 2009; 12: 33–5.

170. Boulton F. Sir Albert William Liley. *J Med Biog* 2005; 13: 71.

171. Boulton TB. Classical File: James Blundell MD, FRCP, and the introduction of the transfusion of human blood to man. *Surv Anesthesiol* 1986; 30: 100–3.

172. Bourne, Aleck W (obituary). *BMJ* 1975; 1: 99.

173. Bourne, Aleck W (obituary). *Lancet* 1975; 305: 115–7.

174. Bowen, John Templeton (obituary). *Arch Dermatol Syph* 1941; 43: 386–8.

175. Bowman JM. Maternal Rh blood group immunization: past, present, future. *J Soc Obstet Gynaecol Can* 1989; 11: 27–35.

176. Box M. *Birth Control and Libel: The Trial of Marie Stopes*. New York, NY: AS Barnes & Co; 1967.

177. Boyd ME. Lawson Tait and the surgical management of ectopic pregnancy. *J Soc Obstet Gynaecol Can* 1990; 12: 41–6.

178. Boyd ME. Ernest Ayre and the Ayre spatula. *J Soc Obstet Gynaecol Can* 1992; 14: 110–2.

179. Boyd W. Remarks on Richard Torpin. *Richmond Co Med Soc Bull* 27 June 1958.

180. Bracegirdle B. *A History of Microtechnique*. London: Heinemann; 1978.

181. Bracegirdle B. Famous microscopists: Antoni van Leeuwenhoek, 1632–1723. *Proc Roy Micr Soc* 1986; 21: 367–70.

182. Bradbury S. *The Evolution of the Microscope*. Oxford: Pergamon Press; 1967.

183. Braun GA. Über Tarnier's forceps. *Wien Med Wochenschr* 1880; 25: 681–5.

184. Breathnach CS. Biographical sketches No. 36: Sims. *Irish Med J* 1984; 77: 27.

185. Breathnach CS. Sir Thomas Browne (1605–1682). *J R Soc Med* 2005; 98: 33–6.

186. Breen JL, Chervenak D. A History of Ectopic Pregnancy. In: Langer A, Iffy L (eds) Littleton, MA: PSG Publishing Co Inc; 1986.

187. Breisky, August (obituary). *Am J Obstet Dis Women Child* 1889; 22: 717–8.

188. Brinsden PR, Rainsbury PA (eds) *A Textbook of In Vitro Fertilization and Assisted Reproduction*. Park Ridge, NJ: Parthenon Publishing Group; 1992, pp. 7–25.

189. Brock CH (ed.) *William Hunter (1718–1783): A Memoir by Samuel Foart Simmons and John Hunter*. Glasgow: University of Glasgow Press; 1983.

190. Brock CH. *Dr William Hunter (1718–1783)*. Glasgow's Past Academics Series. Glasgow: University of Glasgow Press; 1994.

191. Brock CH. The many facets of Dr William Hunter (1718–83). *Hist Sci* 1994; 32: 387–408.

192. Brock H. James Douglas of the pouch. *Med Hist* 1974; 18: 162–72.

193. Brodie JF. *Contraception and Abortion in 19th Century America*. Ithaca, NY: Cornell University Press; 1994.

194. Brody IA, Wilkins RH. Erb's palsy. *Arch Neurol* 1969; 21: 442–4.

195. Brody SA. The life and times of Sir Fielding Ould: man-midwife and master physician. *Bull Hist Med* 1978; 52: 228–50.

196. Brook RC. *The Life and Work of Astley Cooper*. Edinburgh: E & S Livingstone; 1952.

197. Brooke E. *Medicine Women: A Pictorial History of Women Healers*. Wheaton, IL: Theosophical Publishing House; 1997.

198. Brosens IA, Brosens JJ. Endometriosis. *Eur J Obstet Gynecol Reprod Biol* 2000; 90: 159–64.

199. Brown A. *Old Masterpieces in Surgery*. Omaha, NE: Omaha Printers; 1928.

200. Brown JR. A chronology of major events in obstetrics and gynaecology. *J Obstet Gynaecol Br Commonw* 1964; 71: 302–9.

201. Browne A (ed.) *Masters, Midwives and Ladies-in-waiting: The Rotunda Hospital 1745–1995*. Dublin: A & A Farmar; 1995.

202. Brun G. Léon Mansel and his solution. *Rev Hist Pharm (Paris)* 2009; 57: 193–200.

203. Brun GH. Antoine Lembert (1802–1851). *Bull Soc Pharm Bordeaux* 2009; 148: 129–34.

204. Brunn W. Die chirurgenfamilie Langenbeck. *Medizinische Welt* 1936; 1: 539–42.

205. Bruno E. Leonardo Gigli (1863–1908). *Arch Ital Ginecol* 1908; 1: 165–8.

206. Brunori A, Bruni P, Greco R, Giuffre R, Chiapetta F. Celebrating the centennial (1894–1994): Leonardo Gigli and his wire saw. *J Neurosurg* 1995; 82: 1086–90.

207. Buchanan JA. Lugol, his work and his solution. *Ann Med Hist* 1928; 10: 202–8.

208. Buchanan WW. William Hunter (1718–1783): the almost forgotten Hunter brother. *Ann R Coll Phys Surg Can* 1993; 26: 89–93.

209. Bulloch W. *History of Bacteriology*. London: Oxford University Press; 1938.

210. Burch D. *Digging up the Dead: Uncovering the Life and Times of an Extraordinary Surgeon*. London: Vintage Books; 2008.

211. Burgess AH. Development of provincial medical education illustrated in the life and work of Charles White of Manchester. *Lancet* 1941; 1: 235–41.

212. Burgess MA. Gregg and congenital rubella: lessons from history and clinical research. *Aust NZ J Ophthalmol* 1991; 19: 259–61.

213. Burgess MA. Gregg's rubella legacy 1941–1991. *Med J Aust* 1991; 155: 355–7.

214. Burnam CF. Howard Atwood Kelly. *Bull John Hopkins Hosp* 1943; 73: 1–22.

215. Burnham, Walter (obituary). *Boston Med Surg J* 1883; 107: 96.

216. Burrage WL. James Read Chadwick, MD. (1844–1905). *Trans Am Gynecol Soc* 1906; 31: 437–45.

217. Burrage WL. *A History of the Massachusetts Medical Society*. Boston, MA: Mass Medical Society; 1923.

218. Burrage WL. Walter Channing (1786–1876) In: *Dictionary of American Medical Biography*. New York, NY: D Appleton & Co; 1928, pp. 209–10.

219. Busby MJ, Rodin AE. Relative contributions of Holmes and Semmelweis to the understanding of puerperal fever. *Texas Rep Biol Med* 1976; 34: 221–37.

220. Butcher RG. Memoir of the life and writings of the late John Houston, MD. *Dublin Quarterly J Med Sci* 1846; 11: 294–302.

221. Butterfield J, Covey MJ. Practical epigram of the Apgar Score. *JAMA* 1962; 181: 353.

222. Butterfield LJ. Let's keep the Apgar Score in perspective. *ACOG Clin Rev* 1997; 2: 1.

223. Butterton JR. The education, naval service and early career of William Smellie. *Bull Hist Med* 1986; 60: 1–18.

224. Bynum WF. *Science and the Practice of Medicine in the Nineteenth Century*. Cambridge: Cambridge University Press; 1994.

225. Caffaratto TM. Ricardo di Edoardo Porro nel centenarion dell sua operazioni. *Minerva Ginecol* 1976; 28: 1033–40.

226. Calder I, Ovassapian A, Calder N. John Logie Baird: fibreoptic pioneer. *JR Soc Med* 2000; 93: 438–9.

227. Call EL. The evolution of modern maternity technic. *Am J Obstet Gynecol* 1908; 58: 392–404.

228. Call, Emma Louise (obituary). *N Engl J Med* 1937; 216: 999.

229. Calmes SH. Virginia Apgar: a woman physician's career in a developing specialty. *J Am Med Woman's Assoc* 1984; 39: 184–8.

230. Calverley RK. Classical file: John Snow: 'On asphyxia, and on resuscitation of still-born children'. *Surv Anesthesiol* 1992; 36: 397–400.

231. Cameron CA. On the anatomical knowledge and discoveries of Irish surgeons. *Dubl J Med Sci* 1885; 80: 453.

232. Cameron CA. *History of the Royal College of Surgeons in Ireland*. Dublin: Fannin and Co; 1916.

233. Cameron HC. Spasticity and the intellect: Dr Little versus the obstetricians. *Cerebral Palsy Bull* 1958; 1: 1–5.

234. Cameron SJ. William Smellie. *J Obstet Gynaecol Br Emp* 1929; 36: 521–36.

235. Cameron SJ. William Smellie. *Scottish Med J* 1957; 2: 439–44.

236. Campbell M. Victor Bonney's portable operating table. *Aust NZ J Obstet Gynaecol* 2003; 43: 190–1.

237. Campbell, K. An appreciation. *Aust Paediat J* 1974; 10: 48–52.

238. Campbell, Kate Isabel (obituary). *Med J Aust* 1987; 146: 161–2.

239. Camper, Pieter (Petrus). Itera in Angliam 1748–1785. *Opus Selecta Neerland de Arte Med* 1939; 15: 6.

240. Carlsson M, Lindskog G, Hammarskjöld F. The man behind the syndrome: Curtis Mendelson. *Läkartidningen*; 1998; 95: 400–1.

241. Carmichael DE. *The Pap Smear: Life of George N Papanicolaou*. Springfield: Charles C Thomas, IL; 1973.

242. Carmichael EB. J Marion Sims: inventor, physician, surgeon. *J Int Coll Surg* 1960; 33: 757–62.

243. Carr J, Carr I. The origin of cancer metastasis. *Can Bull Hist Med* 2005; 22: 353–8.

244. Carter KC. Ignaz Semmelweis, Carl Mayrhofer, and the rise of germ theory. *Med Hist* 1985; 29: 33–5.

245. Carter KC, Carter BR. *Childbed Fever: A Scientific Biography of Ignaz Semmelweis*. Westport, CT: Greenwood Press; 1994.

246. Carter KC, Abbott S, Siebach JL. Five documents relating to the final illness and death of Ignaz Semmelweis. *Bull Hist Med* 1995; 69: 255–70.

247. Carter PL. The life and legacy of William Bovie. *Am J Surg* 2013; 58: 109–10.

248. Cartwright FF. *A Social History of Medicine*. London: Longman; 1977.

249. Carwardine HH. The original obstetric instruments of the Chamberlens. *Trans Med-Chir Soc* 1818; 9: 181–4.

250. Castellani C. Spermatozoan biology from Leeuwenhoek to Spallanzani. *J Hist Biol* 1973; 6: 37–68.

251. Catchpole HR. Regnier de Graaf, 1641–1673. *Bull Hist Med* 1940; 8: 126–30.

252. Caton D. Obstetric anaesthesia: the first ten years. *Anesthesiology* 1970; 33: 102–9.

253. Caton D. *What a Blessing She Had Chloroform*. New Haven, CT: Yale University Press; 1999.

254. Caton D. John Snow's practice of obstetric anaesthesia. *Anesthesiology* 2000; 92: 247–52.

255. Cavanaugh R. Dr Girolamo Fracastoro (1478–1553) and the poetry of Syphilis. *J Med Biog* 2017; 25: 60–1.

256. Cefalo RC. Edward H. Bishop (1913–1995). *Trans Am Gynec Obstet Soc* 1996; 14: xxvii.

257. Chadwick, James (obituary). *Boston Med Surg J* 1905; 153: 376.

258. Chalmers I. Assembling comparison groups to assess the effects of health care. *J R Soc Med* 1997; 90: 379–86.

259. Chalmers JA. James Young Simpson and the 'suction-tractor'. *J Obstet Gynaecol Br Commonw* 1963; 70: 94–100.

260. Chalmers JA. *The Ventouse: The Obstetric Vacuum Extractor*. Chicago, IL: Year Book Medical Publishers; 1971.

261. Chamberlain G. *Victor Bonney: The Gynaecological Surgeon of the Twentieth Century*. London: Parthenon Publishing Group; 2000.

262. Chamberlain G. The master of myomectomy. *J R Soc Med* 2003; 96: 302–4.

263. Chamberlain G. *From Witchcraft to Wisdom: A History of Obstetrics and Gynaecology in the British Isles*. London: RCOG Press; 2007.

264. Chang MC. Gregory Goodwin Pincus. In: Gillispie CC (ed.) *Dictionary of Scientific Biography*. New York, NY: Charles Scribner's Sons; 1974, pp. 610–11.

265. Channing, Walter (obituary). *Bost Med Surg J* 1876; 95: 237–8.

266. Charlton C. Urological circles. In: Rolls R, Guy J, Guy JR (eds) *A Pox on the Provinces: Proceedings of the 12th Congress of the British Society for the History of Medicine*. Bath: Bath University Press; 1990, pp. 119–28.

267. Chesler E. *Woman of Valor: Margaret Sanger and the Birth Control Movement in America*. New York, NY: Simon & Schuster; 1992.

268. Chesley LC. A short history of eclampsia. *Obstet Gynecol* 1974; 43: 599–602.

269. Chesney AM. *The Johns Hopkins Hospital and the Johns Hospital University School of Medicine: A Chronicle. Vol. 1 Early Years 1867–1893*. Baltimore, MD: Johns Hopkins Press; 1943.

270. Chetwood GH, Wishard WN. Memorial to Edward Keyes. *Trans Am Assoc GU Surg* 1925; 18: 515–7.

271. Choulant L. *History and Bibliography of Anatomic Illustration. Leipzig: Rudolph Weigel*; 1852. English Translation by Mortimer Frank. Chicago, IL: University of Chicago Press; 1920.

272. Christie DA, Tansey EM (eds) *Origins of Neonatal Intensive Care in the UK. Wellcome Witnesses to Twentieth Century Medicine*. Vol. 9. London: Wellcome Trust; 2001.

273. Christie DA, Tansey EM (eds) *Maternal Care: Wellcome Witnesses to Twentieth Century Medicine.* Vol. 12. London: Wellcome Trust; 2001.

274. Christopherson WA. Surgical incisions and their anatomic basis. In: Buchsbaum HJ, Walton LA (eds) *Strategies in Gynecologic Surgery.* New York, NY: Springer-Verlag; 1986, pp. 29–44.

275. Churchill F. (ed.) *Essays on the Puerperal Fever and other Diseases Peculiar to Women.* London: Sydenham Society; 1849, pp. 445–500.

276. Cianfrani T. *A Short History of Obstetrics and Gynecology.* Springfield, IL: Charles C Thomas; 1960.

277. Cibils LA. Professor Roberto Caldeyro-Barcia (1921–1996) *Trans Am Gynec Obstet Soc* 1997; 15: xxvii.

278. Clapesattle H. *The Doctors Mayo.* Minneapolis, MN: University of Minnesota Press; 1941.

279. Clarke CA. The prevention of 'Rhesus' babies. *Scientific American* 1968; 219: 46–52.

280. Clarke CA. *Rhesus Haemolytic Disease: Selected Papers and Extracts.* Lancaster: MTP Medical and Technical Publishing; 1975.

281. Clarke CA. Prevention of Rh haemolytic disease by immunoglobulin anti-D. *Vox Sang* 1983; 44: 396–40.

282. Clarke CA. Preventing rhesus babies: the Liverpool research and follow-up. *Arch Dis Child* 1989; 64: 1734–40.

283. Clarke CA. Eighty-eight years of this and that: Part 1. *Proc R Coll Physicians Edinb* 1995; 25: 495–508.

284. Clarke, Cyril Astey (obituary). *BMJ* 2001; 322: 367.

285. Clarke EH. A century of American medicine: 1776–1876. *Am J Med Sci* 1876; 71: 127–64.

286. Clarke GN. ART and history, 1678–1978. *Hum Reprod* 2006; 21: 1645–50.

287. Claye AM. *The Evolution of Obstetric Analgesia.* London: Oxford University Press; 1937.

288. Cleland J. Contraception in historical and global perspective. *Best Pract Res Clin Obstet Gynaecol* 2009; 23: 165–76.

289. Clement PB. History of gynaecological pathology ix: Dr John Albertson Sampson. *Int J Gynecol Pathol* 2001; 20: 86–101.

290. Clover, Joseph Thomas (obituary). *BMJ* 1882; 2: 656.

291. Clover, Joseph Thomas (obituary). *Lancet* 1882; 2: 597.

292. Faulconer A, Keys TE. Clover, Joseph Thomas. In: *Foundations of Anesthesiology. Vol. I.* Springfield, IL: Charles E Thomas; 1965, pp. 607–11.

293. Coakley D. *The Irish School of Medicine: Outstanding Practitioners of the 19th Century.* Dublin: Town House; 1988.

294. Coakley D. *Irish Masters of Medicine.* Dublin: Town House; 1992.

295. Cochrane AL (with M Blythe). *One Man's Medicine.* London: BMJ (Memoir Club); 1989.

296. Cochrane AL. *Effectiveness and Efficiency: Random Reflections on Health Service (Memorial edition).* London: Nuffield Provincial Hospitals Trust; 1989.

297. Cockett WS, Cockett ATK. The Hopkins rod-lens system and the Storz cold light illumination system. *Urology* 1998; 51(Suppl): 1–2.

298. Cody LF. *Birthing the Nation: Sex, Science and the Conception of Eighteenth-Century Britons.* Oxford: Oxford University Press; 2005.

299. Cohen J. Doctor James Young Simpson, Rabbi Abraham De Sola, and Genesis Chapter 3, Verse 16. *Obstet Gynecol* 1996; 88: 895–8.

300. Cole F. *Milestones in Anesthesia: Readings in the Development of Surgical Anesthesia, 1665–1940.* Lincoln, NE: University of Nebraska Press; 1965.

301. Colebrook L. The story of puerperal fever: 1800 to 1950. *BMJ* 1956; 1: 247–52.

302. Collins J. Duchenne of Boulogne: a biography and an appreciation. *Med Rec* 1908;73:50–4.

303. Collins JA. Barr and the sex chromatin. *J Soc Obstet Gynaecol Can* 1991; 13: 52–6.

304. Colton FB. Steroids and 'the pill': early steroid research at Searle. *Steroids* 1992; 57: 624–30.

305. Comrie JD. *History of Scottish Medicine.* 2 vols. London: Bailliere, Tindall & Cox; 1932.

306. Cook B. *Contributions of the Hunter Brothers to Our Understanding of Reproduction: An Exhibition from the University Library's Collections.* Glasgow University Library, 1992.

307. Coombs RRA. History and evolution of the antiglobulin reaction and its application in clinical and experimental medicine. *Am J Clin Path* 1970; 53: 131–5.

308. Coombs, Robert Royston Amos (obituary). *Lancet* 2006; 367: 1234.

309. Cope Z. *A History of the Acute Abdomen.* London; Oxford University Press; 1965.

310. Copping-Corner B. Ibis and the artists: a sidelight upon Hunter's Atlas, *The Gravid Uterus. J Hist Med Allied Sci* 1951; 1: 1–21.

311. Cornella JL, Pereyra AJ. Historical vignette of Armand J Pereyra, MD, and the modified Pereyra procedure:

the needle suspension for stress incontinence in the female. *Int Urogynecol J* 1990; 1: 25–30.

312. Cornella JL, Ostergard DR. Needle suspension procedures for urinary stress incontinence: a review and historical perspective. *Obstet Gynecol Surv* 1990; 45: 805–16.
313. Corner GW. Howard Atwood Kelly (1858–1943) as a medical historian. *Bull Hist Med* 1943; 14: 191–200.
314. Corner GW, Danforth CH, Stone LS. Edgar Allen, 1892–1943. *Anat Rec* 1943; 86: 595–8.
315. Corner GW. The early history of estrogenic hormones. *J Endocrinol* 1965; 31: 3–17.
316. Corner GW. The early history of progesterone. *Gynecol Invest* 1974; 5: 106–12.
317. Corner GW. The discovery of the mammalian ovum. *Biol Reprod* 2013; 88: 4–11.
318. Cotte, Gaston (obituary). *BMJ* 1951; 2: 253.
319. Coues WP. Sir James Y Simpson (1811–1870): the prince of obstetricians. *N Engl J Med* 1928; 199: 221–4.
320. Coury C. *L'Hôtel-Dieu de Paris. Treize siècles de soins, d'enseignement et de recherche.* Paris; 1969.
321. Craig WS. *History of the Royal College of Physicians of Edinburgh.* Oxford: Blackwell Scientific Publications; 1976.
322. Crainz F. The editions and translations of Dr Matthew Baillie's Morbid Anatomy. *Med Hist* 1982; 26: 443–52.
323. Crainz F. *La Società Italiana di Ginecologica é Obstetrica nei primi cento anni dalla sua constituzione (1892–1992).* Roma: Peliti Associati; 1993.
324. Crainz F. *The life and works of Matthew Baillie (1761–1823).* Rome: Peliti Associati; 1995.
325. Creswell CH. *The Royal College of Surgeons of Edinburgh: Historical Notes from 1505 to 1905.* Edinburgh: Oliver & Boyd; 1926.
326. Crissey JT, Parish LC. *The Dermatology and Syphilology of the Nineteenth Century.* New York, NY: Praeger Publishers; 1981.
327. Croom H. Sir James Young Simpson's influence on the progress of obstetrics. *Edin Med J* 1911; 6: 523–33.
328. Cross J. *A Memoir of the Life of Edward Rigby, MD.* Norwich: Burks and Kinnebrook Printers; 1821.
329. Cullen TS. Dr Howard A Kelly. *Bull Johns Hopkins Hosp* 1919; 30: 287–93.
330. Cullen TS. The evolution of gynecology. *Ohio State Med J* 1924; 12: 484–95.
331. Cullen TS. In memoriam: John Albertson Sampson (1873–70) *Trans Am Gynecol Soc* 1947; 70: 273–4.
332. Cullen, Thomas Stephen (obituary). *JAMA* 1953; 151: 1218.
333. Cullingworth CJ. John Braxton Hicks. *Trans Obstet Soc London* 1898; 40: 65–78.
334. Cullingworth CJ. Biographical note on Étienne Tarnier. *Trans Obstet Soc London* 1898; 40: 79–89.
335. Cullingworth CJ. List of Sir Thomas Spencer Wells published writings, arranged chronologically. *Trans Obstet Soc London* 1898; 40: 91–5.
336. Cullingworth CJ. An address on Charles White, FRS. *Lancet* 1903; 2: 1071–6.
337. Cullingworth CJ. *Charles White FRS: A Great Provincial Surgeon and Obstetrician of the Eighteenth Century.* London: Henry J. Glaisher; 1904.
338. Cullingworth CJ. Oliver Wendell Holmes and the contagiousness of puerperal fever. *BMJ* 1905; 2: 1160–4.
339. Cumston CG. A brief résume of the life and work of Ambroise Paré. With biographical notes on men of his time. *Boston Med Surg J* 1901; 145: 395–400, 431–5, 464–8.
340. Cumston CG. Paul Portal, his life and treatise on obstetrics, with reflections on the science of the obstetrical art in France from the renaissance to the 18th century. *Am J Obstet Dis Women Child* 1905; 51: 778–804, 52: 110–25.
341. Curelaru I, Sandu L. Eugen Bogdan Aburel (1899–1975): the pioneer of regional analgesia for pain relief in childbirth. *Anaesthesia* 1982; 37: 663–9.
342. Curtis AH. Memoirs: Thomas J Watkins. *Surg Gynecol Obstet* 1925; 40: 712–3.
343. Curtis, Arthur Hale (obituary). *JAMA* 1955; 159: 1785.
344. Curtis Arthur Hale. In memoriam. *Trans Am Gynec Soc* 1956; 79: 119–200.
345. Cushing EW. The evolution in America of abdominal hysterectomy and total extirpation of the uterus. *Ann Gynaecol Paediatr* 1895; 8: 533–98.
346. Cutler EC. Ephraim McDowell, the surgeon. *N Engl J Med* 1930; 202: 276–8.
347. Cutter IS, Viets HR. *A Short History of Midwifery.* Philadelphia, PA: WB Saunders Co; 1964.
348. Cyr RM. Historical perspective: 'Once a caesarean . . . always a caesarean'. *ACOG Clin Rev* 2004; 9:12–14.
349. Cyr RM. Historical perspective: Irving W. Potter, MD, and his internal podalic version. *ACOG Clin Rev* 2006; 11: 12–14.
350. Cyr RM. Myth of the ideal caesarean section rate: commentary and historic perspective. *Am J Obstet Gynecol* 2006; 194: 932–6.
351. Cyr RM, Baskett TF. *Caesarean Birth: The Work of François Rousset in Renaissance France.* Cambridge: Cambridge University Press; 2010.

352. Daemmrich A. A tale of two experts: thalidomide and political engagement in the United States and West Germany. *Soc Hist Med* 2002; 15: 137–58.

353. D'Angelo GJ. Dilatation and curettage: a development covering 3,000 years. *Obstet Gynecol* 1953; 2: 322–5.

354. Dale HH. *Adventures in Physiology with Excursions into Autopharmacology*. London: Pergamon Press; 1953.

355. Dale, Henry Hallett (obituary). *Lancet* 1968; 2: 288–90.

356. Dally A. *Women Under the Knife*. London: Hutchinson Radius; 1991.

357. Dally A. Thalidomide: was the tragedy preventable? *Lancet* 1998; 351: 1197–9.

358. Danforth DD. Contemporary titans: JB DeLee and JW Williams. *Am J Obstet Gynecol* 1974; 120: 577–88.

359. Danforth WC. The influence of the French school in the sixteenth, seventeenth and eighteenth centuries upon the development of gynaecology and obstetrics. *Am J Obstet Gynecol* 1942; 44: 743–61.

360. Daniels IR. Historical perspectives on health. Semmelweis: a lesson to relearn? *J R Soc Med* 1998; 118: 367–70.

361. Das K. *Obstetric Forceps: Its History and Evolution*. Calcutta: The Art Press; 1929.

362. Davenport FH. In memoriam: Gilman Kimball. *Am J Obstet* 1892; 26: 560–6.

363. Davenport-Hines R. *The Pursuit of Oblivion: A Global History of Narcotics*. New York, NY: WW Norton & Co; 2002.

364. Davies C, Beazley JM. Harold Leeming Sheehan 1900–1988. *Trans Am Gynecol Soc* 1990; 9: 91.

365. Davis AW. *Dr Kelly of Hopkins*. Baltimore, MD: Johns Hopkins Press, 1959.

366. Davis CH. John Clarence Webster, 1863–1950. *Gynec Trans* 1950; 73: 263–5.

367. Davis G, Davidson R. 'A fifth freedom' or 'Hideous atheistic expediency'? The medical community and abortion law reform in Scotland, c.1960–1975. *Med Hist* 2006; 50: 29–48.

368. Davis HJ. *Intrauterine Devices for Contraception*. Baltimore, MD: Williams and Wilkins Co; 1971.

369. Dawes GS. Mont Liggins on birth, the fetal lung and the Weddell seal. In: Gluckman PD, Johnston BM, Nathanielsz PW (eds) *Advances in Fetal Physiology: Reviews in Honor of GC Liggins*. Ithaca, NY: Perinatology Press; 1989, pp. 1–12.

370. Dawes, Geoffrey Sharman (obituary). *BMJ* 1996; 2: 786

371. Dawes, Geoffrey Sharman (obituary). The *Times*. 20 May 1996.

372. Dawson PM. Semmelweis: an interpretation. *Ann Med Hist* 1924; 6: 258–79.

373. De Costa CM. A 'noble instrument': the obstetric forceps. *Med J Aust* 1999; 170: 78–80.

374. De Costa C. St Anthony's fire and living ligatures: a short history of ergometrine. *Lancet* 2002; 359: 1768–70.

375. De Costa CM. The King versus Aleck Bourne. *Med J Aust* 2009; 191: 230–1.

376. Deger RD, Menzin AW, Mikuta JJ. Vaginal pessary: past and present. *Postgrad Obstet Gynecol* 1993; 13: 1–7.

377. DeLacey M. Puerperal fever in eighteenth-century Britain. *Bull Hist Med* 1989; 63: 521–56.

378. Delauney P. François Poupart. *France médicale, Paris.* 1904; 51: 357–61.

379. DeLee, James Bolivar (obituary). *Lancet* 1942; 2: 114.

380. DeLee, James Bolivar (obituary). *JAMA* 1942; 118: 1314.

381. DeMoulin D. *A History of Surgery*. Dordrecht: Martinus Nijhoff Publishers; 1988.

382. Dennison WM. The Pierre Robin Syndrome. *Pediatr* 1965; 36: 336–41.

383. DePalo G. Cervical precancer and cancer, past, present and future. *Eur J Gynaecol Oncol* 2004; 25: 269–78.

384. Derry DE. Note of five pelves of women of the eleventh dynasty in Egypt. *J Obstet Gynaecol Br Emp* 1935; 42: 490–5.

385. Dewhurst J. Charles White of Manchester. *J Obstet Gynaecol* 1991; 11: 1–4.

386. Diamantis A, Magiorkinis E, Androutsos G. Alfred François Donné (1801–78): a pioneer of microscopy, microbiology and haematology. *J Med Biog* 2009; 17: 81–7.

387. Diamantis A, Magiorkinis E, Koutselini H. 50 years after the death of George Nicholas Papanicolaou (1883–1962): evaluation of his scientific work. *Acta Med Hist Adriat* 2014; 12: 181–8.

388. Diamond LK. The Rh problem through the retrospectoscope. *Am J Clin Path* 1974; 62: 311–24.

389. Diamond LK. Historic perspective on 'Exchange Transfusion'. *Vox Sang* 1983; 45: 333–5.

390. Dibble AW. John Christopher Burch (1900–1997). *Trans Am Assoc Obstet Gynecol* 1979; 89: 171.

391. Dick WF. Friedrich Trendelenburg (1844–1924). *Resuscitation* 2000; 45: 157–9.

392. Dickersin K, Manheimer E. The Cochrane Collaboration: evaluation of health care and services

using systematic review of the results of randomized controlled trials. *Clin Obstet Gynecol* 1998; 41: 315–31.

393. Dickinson RL, Bryant LS. *Control of Contraception.* Baltimore, MD: Williams and Wilkins Co; 1932.

394. Dickinson, Robert Latou (obituary). *New York Times.* 30 November 1950.

395. Dieckmann WJ. *The Toxaemias of Pregnancy.* 2nd edn. St Louis, MO: CV Mosby; 1952.

396. Dietal H. Hans Hinselmann (obituary). *München Med Wochenschr* 1959; 26: 1132–4.

397. Dietrich H. Giovanni Domenico Santorini (1681–1737) and Charles Pierre Denonvilliers (1808–1872): first description of urosurgically relevant structures in the pelvis. *Europ Urol* 1997; 32: 124–7.

398. Dildy GA, Scott JR, Saffer CS, Belfort MA. An effective pressure pack for severe pelvic hemorrhage. *Obstet Gynecol* 2006; 108: 1222–6.

399. Dill LV. *The Obstetric Forceps.* Springfield, IL: Charles Thomas; 1953.

400. Dingwall HM. *'A Famous and Flourishing Society': The History of the Royal College of Surgeons of Edinburgh 1505–2005.* Edinburgh: Edinburgh University Press Ltd; 2005.

401. Djerassi C. *The Politics of Contraception.* New York, NY: WW Norton and Company; 1979.

402. Djerassi C. The making of the pill. *Science* 1984; 5: 127–9.

403. Djerassi C. Steroid research at Syntex: 'the Pill' and cortisone. *Steroids* 1992; 57: 631–41.

404. Dobell C. *Antonj Van Leeuwenhoek and his 'Little Animals'.* London: John Ball, Sons and Danielsson Ltd; 1932.

405. Dobson J. John Hunter's artists. *Med Biol Illustration* 1959; 9: 138–49.

406. Dobson J. *Anatomical Eponyms.* 2nd edn. Edinburgh: E & S Livingstone; 1962.

407. Dods L. Norman Alister Gregg. *Med J Aust* 1966; 2: 1166–9.

408. Doe J. *A Bibliography of the Works of Ambroise Paré: Premier Chirurgien and Conseiller du Roy.* Chicago, IL: University of Chicago Press; 1937.

409. Doisy EA. An autobiography. *Ann Rev Biochem* 1976; 45: 1–9.

410. Dolan B (ed.) *Malthus, Medicine and Morality: 'Malthusianism' after 1798.* Atlanta, GA: Editions Rodopi BW; 2000.

411. Doll R. Hazards of the first nine months: an epidemiologist's nightmare. *J Irish Med Assoc* 1973; 66: 117–26.

412. Donald A. A short history of the operation of colporrhapy with remarks on the technique. *J Obstet Gynaecol Br Emp* 1921; 28: 256–9.

413. Donald, Archibald (obituary). *J Obstet Gynaecol Br Emp* 1937; 44: 527–38.

414. Donald, Archibald (obituary). *Lancet* 1937; 1: 1078–80.

415. Donald I. On launching a new diagnostic science. *Am J Obstet Gynecol* 1969; 103: 609–28.

416. Donald I. Apologia: how and why medical sonar developed. *Ann R Coll Surg Eng* 1974; 54: 132–40.

417. Donald I. Superfecundity: Simpson Oration: his problem and ours. *BMJ* 1977; 1: 555–60.

418. Donegan JB. *Women and Men Midwives.* London: Greenwood Press; 1978.

419. Donnison J. *Midwives and Medical Men.* London: Historical Publications; 1988.

420. Doolin W. The first hurdle: the arrest of haemorrhage. *J Irish Med Assoc* 1956; 38: 92–8.

421. Doolin W. The third hurdle: the conquest of sepsis. *J Irish Med Assoc* 1957; 40: 67–73.

422. Doran A. James Matthews Duncan. *Am J Obstet Dis Women Child* 1890; 23: 1090–8.

423. Doran A. A chronology of the founders of the forceps (1569–1799). *J Obstet Gynaecol Br Emp* 1910; 27: 154–72.

424. Doran A. Dusée: his forceps and his contemporaries. *J Obstet Gynaecol Br Emp* 1912; 22: 119–42.

425. Doran A. Dusée, DeWind and Smellie: an addendum. *J Obstet Gynaecol Br Emp.* 1912; 22: 203–7.

426. Doran A. Jointed obstetric forceps. *J Obstet Gynaecol Br Emp* 1913; 24: 197–210.

427. Doran A. A demonstration of some eighteenth-century obstetric forceps. *Proc R Soc Med* 1913; 6: 54–77

428. Doran AH. *Descriptive Catalogue of the Obstetrical Instruments in the Museum of the Royal College of Surgeons of England.* London; 1921.

429. Dormandy T. *Moments of Truth: Four Creators of Modern Medicine.* Chichester: John Wiley & Sons; 2003.

430. Doughty A. Epidural analgesia in labour: the past, the present and the future. *J R Soc Med* 1978; 71: 879–84.

431. Doughty A. Landmarks in the development of regional analgesia in obstetrics. In: Morgan BM (ed.) *Foundations of Obstetric Anaesthesia.* London: Farrand Press; 1987, pp. 1–17.

432. Doughty A. Walter Stoeckel (1871–1961): a pioneer of regional analgesia in obstetrics. *Anaesthesia* 1990; 45: 468–71.

433. Douglas ET. *Margaret Sanger: Pioneer of the Future.* Garrett Park, MD: Garrett Park Press; 1975.

434. Dow DA. *The Rotten Row: The History of the Glasgow Royal Maternity Hospital, 1834–1984.* Carnforth: Parthenon Press.

435. Dow DA. *The Influence of Scottish Medicine.* Park Ridge, NJ: Parthenon Publishing Group; 1988.

436. Dowd CN. Master surgeons of America: Edwin Bradford Craigin. *Surg Gynecol Obstet* 1925; 41: 845–7.

437. Down, John Langdon (obituary). *BMJ* 1896; 2: 1170–1.

438. Down, John Langdon (obituary). *Lancet* 1896; 2: 1104–5.

439. Drabkin IE. Soranus and his system of medicine. *Bull Hist Med* 1951; 25: 503–18.

440. Dreyfus C. *Some Milestones in the History of Hematology.* New York, NY: Grune and Stratton; 1957.

441. Drife J. The start of life: a history of obstetrics. *Postgrad Med J* 2002; 78: 311–5.

442. Drutz HP. The first century of urogynecology and reconstructive pelvic surgery: where do we go from here? *Int Urogynecol J* 1996; 7: 348–53.

443. Drutz HP, Morgan JE. Urogynecology and reconstructive pelvic surgery: Past, present and future. In: Drutz HP, Herschorn S, Diamant NE (eds) *Female Pelvic and Reconstructive Surgery.* London: Springer; 2002, pp. 1–10.

444. Ducachet HW. A biographical memoir of Samuel Bard MD, LLD. *Am Med Rec* 1821; 4: 609–33.

445. Dudley, Harold Ward (obituary). *BMJ* 1935; 2: 707–8.

446. Duffy J. Anglo-American reaction to obstetrical anaesthesia. *Bull Hist Med* 1964; 38: 32–44.

447. Duka WE, DeCherney AH. *From the Beginning: A History of the American Fertility Society, 1944–1994.* Birmingham, AL: American Fertility Society; 1994.

448. Dumont M, Morel P. *Histoire de L'Obstétrique et de La Gynécologie.* Lyon: Simep Editions; 1968.

449. Dumont M. Observations obstétricales curieuses de William Smellie. *J Med Lyon* 1975; 56: 1011–5.

450. Dumont M. Anecdotes sur François Mauriceau. *J Med Lyon* 1977; 58: 203–8.

451. Dumont M. Histoire et petite histoire du forceps. *J Gynecol Obstet Biol Reprod* 1984; 13: 743–57.

452. Dumont M. The long and difficult birth: from Severin Pineau to Jean René Sigault. *J Gynecol Obstet Biol Reprod* 1989; 18: 11–21.

453. Duncan JM. The controversy respecting the invention of the air-tractor. *Lond Med Gaz* 1849; 8: 609.

454. Duncan JM. On the life of William Hunter. *Edin Med J* 1876; 21: 1061–79.

455. Duncan JM. Discussion on Tarnier's forceps. *Trans Obstet Soc Lond* 1887; 19: 223–7.

456. Duncan, James Matthews (obituary). *Lancet* 1890; 2: 594–6.

457. Duncum BM. *The Development of Inhalation Anaesthesia.* London: Oxford University Press; 1947. Reprinted by Royal Society of Medicine Press Ltd; 1994.

458. Dunn LJ. Prevention of isoimmunization in pregnancy developed by Freda and Gorman. *Obstet Gynecol Surv* 1999; 54: S1–6.

459. Dunn PM. Dr James Blundell (1790–1878) and neonatal resuscitation. *Arch Dis Child* 1989; 64: 494–5.

460. Dunn PM. Dr William Harvey (1578–1657): physician, obstetrician and fetal physiologist. *Arch Dis Child* 1990; 65: 1098–100.

461. Dunn PM. Francois Mauriceau (1637–1709) and maternal posture for parturition. *Arch Dis Child* 1991; 66: 78–9.

462. Dunn PM. Dr Langdon Down (1828–1896) and 'mongolism'. *Arch Dis Child* 1991; 66: 827–8.

463. Dunn PM. Dr Thomas Denman of London (1733–1815): rupture of the membranes and management of the cord. *Arch Dis Child* 1992; 67: 882–4.

464. Dunn PM. Dr John Ballantyne (1861–1923): perinatologist extraordinary of Edinburgh. *Arch Dis Child* 1993; 68: 66–7.

465. Dunn PM. Dr Alfred Hart (1888–1954) of Toronto and exsanguination transfusion of the newborn. *Arch Dis Child* 1993; 69: 95–6.

466. Dunn PM. Sir Thomas Browne (1605–1682) and life before birth. *Arch Dis Child* 1994; 70: 75–6.

467. Dunn PM. Dr Grantly Dick-Read (1890–1959) of Norfolk and natural childbirth. *Arch Dis Child* 1994; 71: 145–6.

468. Dunn PM. Soranus of Ephesus (circa AD 98–138) and perinatal care in Roman times. *Arch Dis Child* 1995; 73: 51–2.

469. Dunn PM. Dr Percivall Willughby, MD (1596–1685): pioneer 'man'-midwife of Derby. *Arch Dis Child Fetal Neonatal Ed* 1997; 76: F212–3.

470. Dunn PM. Thomas Malthus (1766–1834): population growth and birth control. *Arch Dis Child Fetal Neonatal Ed* 1998; 78: F76–7.

471. Dunn PM. Dr Alexander Gordon (1752–99) and contagious puerperal fever. *Arch Dis Child Fetal Neonatal Ed* 1998; 78: F232–3.

472. Dunn PM. Dr William Hunter (1718–83) and the gravid uterus. *Arch Dis Child Fetal Neonatal Ed* 1999; 80: F76–7.

473. Dunn PM. The Chamberlen family (1560–1728) and obstetric forceps. *Arch Dis Child Fetal Neonatal Ed* 1999; 81: F232–5.

474. Dunn PM. Sir Joseph Barcroft of Cambridge (1872–1947) and prenatal research. *Arch Dis Child Fetal Neonatal Ed* 2000; 82: F75–6.

475. Dunn PM. Dr Edward Rigby of Norwich (1747–1821) and antepartum haemorrhage. *Arch Dis Child Fetal Neonatal Ed* 2000; 82: F169–70.

476. Dunn PM. Dr Carl Credé (1819–1892) and the prevention of ophthalmia neonatorum. *Arch Dis Child Fetal Neonatal Ed* 2000; 83: F158–9.

477. Dunn PM. Jacob Rueff (1500–1558) of Zurich and *The Expert Midwife*. *Arch Dis Child Fetal Neonatal Ed* 2001; 85: F222–4.

478. Dunn PM. Stéphane Tarnier (1828–1897), the architect of perinatology in France. *Arch Dis Child Fetal Neonatal Ed* 2002; 86: F137–9.

479. Dunn PM. John Chassar Moir (1900–1977) and the discovery of ergometrine. *Arch Dis Child Fetal Neonatal Ed* 2002; 86: F152–4.

480. Dunn PM. Louise Bourgeois (1563–1636): royal midwife of France. *Arch Dis Child Fetal Neonatal Ed* 2004; 89: F185-F187.

481. Dunn PM. Dr Priscilla White (1900–1989) of Boston and pregnancy diabetes. *Arch Dis Child Fetal Neonatal Ed* 2004; 89: F276–8.

482. Dunn PM. Jean-Louis Baudelocque (1746–1810) of Paris and *L'art des accouchemens*. *Arch Dis Child Fetal Neonatal Ed* 2004; 89: F370–2.

483. Dunn PM. Dr Christian Kielland of Oslo (1871–1941) and his straight forceps. *Arch Dis Child Fetal Neonatal Ed* 2004; 89: F456–7.

484. Dunn PM. Ignac Semmelweis (1818–1865) of Budapest and the prevention of puerperal fever. *Arch Dis Child Fetal Neonatal Ed* 2005; 90: F345–8.

485. Dunn PM. Paul Portal (1630–1703), man-midwife of Paris. *Arch Dis Child Fetal Neonatal Ed* 2006; 91: F385–7.

486. Dunn PM. John Whitridge Williams, MD (1866–1931) of Baltimore: pioneer of academic obstetrics. *Arch Dis Child Fetal Neonatal Ed* 2007; 92: F74–7.

487. Dunn PM. Oliver Wendell Holmes (1809–1894) and his essay on puerperal fever. *Arch Dis Child Fetal Neonatal Ed* 2007; 92: F325–7.

488. Dunn PM. Professor Munro Kerr (1868–1960) of Glasgow and caesarean delivery. *Arch Dis Child* 2008; 93: 167–9.

489. Dunn PM. Dr Leonard Colebrook (1883–1967) and the chemotherapeutic conquest of puerperal infection. *Arch Dis Child* 2008; 93: 246–8.

490. Duns J. *Memoir of Sir James Young Simpson*. Edinburgh: Edmonton and Douglas; 1873.

491. Durand MA. The safety of home birth: the Farm study. *Am J Public Health* 1992; 82: 450–2.

492. Durfee RB. Evolution of caesarean hysterectomy. *Clin Obstet Gynecol* 1969; 12: 575–89.

493. Dyer FN. Autobiographical letter from Horatio Robinson Storer, MD, to his son, Malcolm Storer, MD, discussing the 'History of Gynaecological Teaching'. *J Hist Med* 1999; 54: 439–58.

494. Dyer KA. Curiosities of contraception: a historical perspective. *JAMA* 1990; 264: 2818–9.

495. East MC, Steele PRM. Laparoscopic incisions at the lower umbilical verge. *BMJ* 1988; 296: 753.

496. Eastman NJ. The role of frontier America in the development of cesarean section. *Am J Obstet Gynecol* 1932; 24: 919–29.

497. Eastman NJ. Pelvic mensuration: a study in the perpetuation of error. *Obstet Gynecol Surv* 1948; 3: 301–29.

498. Eastman NJ. The contributions of John Whitridge Williams to obstetrics. *Am J Obstet Gynecol* 1964; 90: 561–4.

499. Easton L. Herman Johannes Pfannenstiel (1862–1909). *Br J Obstet Gynaecol* 1984; 91: 538–41.

500. Eaton P, Warnick M. *Marie Stopes: a checklist of her writings*. London: Croam Helm; 1977.

501. Eby MW, Longo LD. Furthering the profession: the early years of the American Gynecological Club and its first European tours. *Obstet Gynecol* 2002; 99: 308–15.

502. Eccles A. Obstetrics in the 17th and 18th centuries and its implications for maternal and infant mortality. *Bull Soc Hist Med* 1977; 20: 8–11.

503. Eccles A. *Obstetrics and Gynaecology in Tudor and Stuart England*. Kent, OH: Kent State University Press; 1982.

504. Edelman DA, Berger GS, Keith L. *Intrauterine Devices and Their Complications*. Boston, MA: GK Hall & Co; 1979, pp. 3–27.

505. Eden A. Johann Christian Doppler. *Ultrasound Med Biol* 1985; 11: 537–9.

506. Eden A. The beginnings of Doppler. In: Aaslid R (ed.) *Transcranial Doppler Sonography*. New York, NY: Springer-Verlag; 1986, pp. 1–9.

507. Eden A. *The Search for Christian Doppler*. Vienna: Springer-Verlag; 1992.

508. Edgar II. Ignatz Philipp Semmelweis: outline for a biography. *Ann Med Hist* 1939; 1: 74–96.

509. Edwards G. John Snow MD (1813–1858). *Anaesthesia* 1959; 14: 113–26.

510. Edwards R, Steptoe PC. *A Matter of Life: The Story of a Medical Breakthrough*. London: Hutchinson & Co; 1980.

511. Edwards RG. Tribute to Patrick Steptoe: beginnings of laparoscopy. *Hum Reprod* 1989; 4: 1–9.

512. Edwards RG. The early days of invitro fertilization. In: Alberda AT, Gan RA, Vemer HM (eds) *Pioneers in In Vitro Fertilization*. New York, NY: Parthenon Publishing Group; 1995, pp. 7–23.

513. Edwards RG. Biography of Patrick Steptoe. In: Edwards RG, Beard HK, Howles CM (eds) *Human Conception In Vitro, 1995*. Hum Reprod (Suppl) 1996, pp. 215–34.

514. Edwards RG. The current clinical and ethical situation of human conception in vitro. In: Jones S, Keyes M (eds) *Twelve Galton Lectures*. London: Galton Institute; 2008.

515. Ehrenreich B, English D. *Witches, Midwives and Nurses*. 2nd edn. New York, NY: Feminist Press; 2010.

516. Eig J. *The Birth of the Pill*. New York, NY: WW Norton & Co; 2014.

517. Eldor J. Huber needle and Tuohy catheter. *Reg Anesth* 1995; 20: 252–3.

518. Ellis H. *Famous Operations*. Media, PA: Harwell Publishing Co; 1984.

519. Ellis H. *Operations That Made History*. London: Greenwich Medical Media Ltd; 1996.

520. Ellis H. *A History of Surgery*. London: Greenwich Medical Media Ltd; 2001.

521. Ellis RH. The introduction of ether anaesthesia to Great Britain. *Anaesthesia* 1976; 31: 766–77.

522. Elverdam B, Wielandt H. The duration of a human pregnancy: medical fact or cultural tradition? *Int J Prenatal and Perinatal Psychology and Medicine* 1994; 6: 239–46.

523. Emge LA. Alfred Baker Spalding, 1874–1942. *Trans Am Gynecol Soc* 1945; 68: 287–90.

524. Emge LA, Durfee RB. Pelvic organ prolapse: four thousand years of treatment. *Clin Obstet Gynecol* 1966; 9: 997–1032.

525. Emmett TA. A memoir of Dr James Marion Sims. *NY Med J* 1884; 39: 1–5.

526. Engelmann G. History of vaginal extirpation of the uterus. *Am J Obstet Dis Women Child* 1895; 31: 295–7.

527. Epstein E, Maibach HI. Monsel's solution: history, chemistry and efficacy. *Arch Dermatol* 1964; 90: 226–8.

528. Eskes TKAB, Longo LD. *Classics in Obstetrics and Gynecology: Innovative Papers That Have Contributed to Current Clinical Practice*. New York, NY: Parthenon Publishing Group; 1994.

529. Eskes TKAB. From anemia to spina bifida: the story of folic acid. A tribute to Professor Richard Smithells. *Eur J Obstet Gynecol Reprod Biol* 2000; 90: 119–23.

530. Estes WL. *Dr William L. Estes, 1855–1940, The First Superintendent, Director and Chief Surgeon of St Luke's Hospital: An Autobiography*. Bethlehem, PA; 1967.

531. Euler US von. Pieces in the puzzle. *Ann Rev Pharmacol* 1971; 11: 1–12.

532. Eustace D. The origins and development of the ventouse. *The Diplomate*. 1999; 5: 260–5.

533. Eustace DLS. James Young Simpson: the controversy surrounding the presentation of his Air Tractor (1848–1849). *J R Soc Med* 1993; 86: 660–3.

534. Evenden D. *The Midwives of Seventeenth-Century London*. Cambridge: Cambridge University Press; 2000.

535. Everett HS. In Memoriam: Guy LeRoy Hunner. *Trans Am Gynec Soc* 1958; 81: 225–7.

536. Everett HS, Taylor ES. The history of the American Gynecological Society and the scientific contributions of its Fellows. *Trans Am Gynecol Soc* 1976; 99: 170–8.

537. Farlow JW. *The History of the Boston Medical Library*. Norwood, MA: Plympton Press; 1918.

538. Farmar T. Holles Street 1894–1994: The National Maternity Hospital. *A Centenary History*. Dublin: A & A Farmar; 1994.

539. Farmar T. *Patients, Potions and Physicians: A Social History of Medicine in Ireland 1654–2004*. Dublin: A & A Farmar; 2004.

540. Farr AD. Early opposition to obstetric anaesthesia. *Anaesthesia* 1980; 35: 896–907.

541. Fasbender H. *Geschichte der Geburtshülfe*. Jena: Gustav Fischer; 1906. (Reprinted Hildesheim: G. Olms; 1964).

542. Fehling H. *Entwicklung der Geburtshilfe und Gynäkologien im 19. Jahrhundert*. Berlin: Verlag von Julius Springer; 1925.

543. Feigenbaum A. Description of Behçet's syndrome in the Hippocratic third book of endemic diseases. *Br J Ophthal* 1956; 40: 355–7.

544. Figdor PP. *Philipp Bozzini: The Beginning of Modern Endoscopy. Vol. I*. Turrlingen: Verlag Endo-Press; 2002.

545. Figl M, Pelinka LE. Karl Landsteiner, the discoverer of blood groups. *Resuscitation* 2004; 63: 251–4.

546. Finch JS. *Sir Thomas Browne: A Doctor's Life of Science and Faith*. New York, NY: Collier Books; 1950.

547. Findley P. The forgotten man in obstetrics. *Trans Am Assoc Obstet Gynecol Abd Surg* 1937; 44: 259–70.

548. Findley P. *Priests of Lucina: The Story of Obstetrics*. Boston, MA: Little, Brown & Co; 1939.

549. Finkelstein M. Professor Bernhard Zondek: an interview. *J Reprod Fertil* 1966; 12: 3–19.

550. Finn R. Clarke CA (obituary). *University of Liverpool Recorder* 2001; 122: 18–19.

551. Finn, Ronald (obituary). *Lancet* 2004; 363; 2195.

552. Firken BG, Whitworth JA. *Dictionary of Medical Eponyms*. Park Ridge, NJ: Parthenon Publishing Group; 1987.

553. Fischer J. *Geschichte der Geburtshilfe in Wien*. Leipzig: Franz Deuticke; 1909.

554. Fish SA. The Tucker-McLane forceps: a history. *Am J Obstet Gynecol* 1953; 65: 1042–7.

555. Fish SA. The Barton obstetric forceps: a history. *Am J Obstet Gynecol* 1953; 66: 1290–6.

556. Fishbein M, DeLee ST. *Joseph Bolivar De Lee: Crusading Obstetrician*. New York, NY: E P Dutton and Co; 1949.

557. Fisher GJ. Historical and biographical notes: V. Gabriello Fallopio, 1532–1562. *Ann Anat Surg Soc* 1880; 2: 200–2.

558. Fisher W. Physicians and slavery in the antebellum Southern Medical Journal. *J Hist Med Allied Sci* 1968; 23: 36–49.

559. Fitch CD. In memoriam: Edward A. Doisy, PhD. *J Clin Endocrinol Metab* 1988; 66: 1094–5.

560. Fitzgerald WJ. Evolution of the use of ergot in obstetrics. *NY J Med* 1958; 4081–3.

561. Flack IH. *Lawson Tait, 1845–1899*. London: Wm Heinemann Medical Books Ltd; 1949.

562. Flam F, Larson B, Silverswärd C. Mannen bakom tumoreu: Friedrich Krukenberg. *Läkartidningen* 1993; 90: 2311–2.

563. Flati G, Andren-Sandberg A. Wirsung and Santorini: the men behind the ducts. *Pancreatology* 2002; 2: 4–11.

564. Fletcher WF. William Blair-Bell (obituary). *J Obstet Gynaecol Br Emp* 1936; 43: 303–6.

565. Floud R. James Tanner (obituary). *BMJ* 2010; 341: c5374.

566. Flynn VT, Spurrett BR. Sister Joseph's nodule. *Med J Aust* 1969; 1: 728–30.

567. Forbes JA. Rubella: Historical aspects. *Am J Dis Child* 1969; 118: 5–11.

568. Forbes TR. The regulation of English midwives in the sixteenth and seventeenth centuries. *Med Hist* 1964; 8: 235–44.

569. Ford BJ. Revelation and the single lens. *BMJ* 1982; 285: 1822–4.

570. Ford BJ. *The Leeuwenhoek Legacy*. Bristol: Biopress; 1991.

571. Ford JMT. Sir Thomas Browne (1605–1682). *J Med Biog* 2007; 15: 62.

572. Forster FMC. *Progress in Obstetrics and Gynaecology in Australia*. Sydney: John Sands; 1967.

573. Forster FMC. Robert Barnes and his obstetric forceps. *Aust NZ J Obstet Gynaecol* 1971; 11: 139–47.

574. Fothergill, William (obituary). *J Obstet Gynaecol Br Emp* 1927; 34: 102–6.

575. Fowler GR. *Diffuse Septic Peritonitis, With Special Reference to a New Method of Treatment, Namely, the Elevated Head and Trunk Posture, to Facilitate Drainage into the Pelvis, With a Report of Nine Consecutive Cases of Recovery*. In: *Medical Classics* 1940; 4, pp. 531–74.

576. Fox DM, Meldrum M, Rezak I (eds) *Nobel Laureates in Medicine or Physiology: A Biographical Dictionary*. New York, NY: Garland Publishing Inc; 1990.

577. Fox RH. *William Hunter, Anatomist, Physician, Obstetrician (1718–1783). With Notes of his Friends Cullen, Smellie, Fothergill and Baillie*. London: HK Lewis; 1901.

578. Fradin DB. *We Have Conquered Pain: The Discovery of Anesthesia*. New York, NY: Margaret K McElderry Books; 1996.

579. Franceschini P. Antonio Scarpa. In: Gillispie CC (ed.) *Dictionary of Scientific Biography*. New York, NY: Charles Scribner's Sons. 1975, pp. 136–9.

580. Frangenheim H. History of endoscopy: In: Gordon AG, Lewis BV (eds) *Gynecological Endoscopy*. London: JB Lippincott; 1988, pp. 2–3.

581. Frangos CC. Medical statues: George N Papanicolaou (1883–1962) MD. *J Med Biog* 2009; 17: 134.

582. Freinkel N. Of pregnancy and progeny. *Diabetes* 1980; 29: 1023–35.

583. Friedman EA. Evolution of graphic analysis of labor. *Am J Obstet Gynecol* 1978; 132: 824–7.

584. Frölich MA, Caton D. Pioneers in epidural needle design. *Anesth Analg* 2001; 93: 215–20.

585. Frost EAM. A history of nitrous oxide. In: Eger EL (ed.) *Nitrous Oxide*. New York, NY: Elsevier; 1985, pp. 1–22.

586. Fryer P. *The Birth Controllers*. New York, NY: Stein and Day; 1966.

587. Fukagawa M, Nemeth EF. Frontiers in parathyroid physiology. *Kidney International* 2006; 70: s1–2

588. Fuller JG. *The Day of St Anthony's Fire.* New York, NY: The Macmillan Company; 1968.

589. Fülöp-Miller R. *Triumph Over Pain.* New York, NY: Literary Guild of America; 1938.

590. Fulton JF, Wilson LG. *Selected Readings in the History of Physiology.* 2nd edn. Springfield, IL: Charles C Thomas; 1966.

591. Gabbe SG. A story of two miracles: the impact of the discovery of insulin on pregnancy in women with diabetes mellitus. *Obstet Gynecol* 1992; 79: 295–9.

592. Gaissinovitch AE. Caspar Friedrich Wolff. In: Gillispie CC (ed.) *Dictionary of Scientific Biography.* New York, NY: Charles Scribner's Sons. 1978, pp. 524–6.

593. Galanakis E. Apgar score and Soranus of Ephesus. *Lancet* 1988; 352: 2012–3.

594. Galbraith S. *Dr John Snow (1813–1858): His Early Years.* London: Royal Institute of Public Health; 2002.

595. Gambacorta G. *Antonio Scarpa: anatomico, chirugo, oculisto.* Milan: Asclepio; 2000.

596. Gamson J. Rubber wars: struggles over the condom in the United States. *J Hist Sex* 1990; 1: 262–82.

597. Garceau E. Vaginal hysterectomy as done in France. *Am J Obstet Dis Women Child* 1895; 31: 305–46.

598. Garcia CR. Gregory Goodwin Pincus (1903–1967). *Endocrinology* 1968; 82: 651–4.

599. Gardner DL. McDowell's saucer. *J R Coll Surg Edinb* 2001; 46: 277–8.

600. Gardner WV. Edgar Allen (obituary). *Science* 1943; 97: 368–9.

601. Garrett AP, Wenham RM, Sheats EE. Monsel's solution: a brief history. *J Lower Genital Tract Dis* 2002; 6: 225–7.

602. Garrison FG. Two pictures of Emil Noeggerath (1827–1895). *Ann Med Hist* 1928; 10: 210–11.

603. Garrison FH. Samuel Bard and the King's College School. *Bull NY Acad Med* 1925; 85–91.

604. Garrison FH. *An Introduction to the History of Medicine.* 4th edn. Philadelphia, PA: WB Saunders Company; 1929.

605. Gartner, H. Looking back. *Lancet* 1904; 2: 1527–8.

606. Gaskings E. *Investigations into Generation, 1651–1828.* Baltimore, MD: Johns Hopkins University Press; 1967.

607. Gebbie DAM. *Reproductive Anthropology: Descent Through Woman.* Chichester: John Wiley and Sons; 1981.

608. Gebbie D. Symphysiotomy. *Clin Obstet Gynaecol* 1982; 9: 663–83.

609. Gelbart N. Midwife to a nation: Mme du Coudray serves France. In: Marland H (ed.) *The Art of Midwifery: Early Modern Midwives in Europe.* London: Routledge; 1987, pp. 131–51.

610. Gelbart NR. *The King's Midwife: A History and Mystery of Madame du Coudray.* Los Angeles, CA: California Press; 1998.

611. George MS. Changing nineteenth century views on the origins of cerebral palsy. WJ Little and Sigmund Freud. *J Hist Neurosci* 1992; 1: 29–37.

612. Ghirardini G, Golinelli F. Bozzini and the birth of endoscopy. *Clin Exp Obstet Gynecol* 1992; 19: 70–2.

613. Giangrande de PL. The history of blood transfusion. *Br J Haematol* 2000; 110: 758–67.

614. Gigli, Leonardo. *Enciclopedia italiana* 1933; 17: 105.

615. Gilbert SF (ed.) *A Conceptual History of Modern Embryology.* New York, NY: Plenum Press; 1991.

616. Gilbert-Barness E. Profiles in Pediatrics: Edith Potter. *J Pediat* 1995; 126: 845–6.

617. Gill RS. About Emil Novak. *Obstet Gynecol Surv* 1954; 9: 1–13.

618. Gillert KE. August von Wasserman. In: Gillispie CC (ed.) *Dictionary of Scientific Biography.* New York, NY: Charles Scribner's Sons. 1978; 15: 521–4.

619. Gilliam, David Tod (obituary). *JAMA* 1923; 81: 1378.

620. Gillmer M. The oral contraceptive pill: a product of serendipity. *Diplomate. RCOG Press.* 1997; 4: 231–5.

621. Gilman SL. *Making the Body Beautiful: A Cultural History of Aesthetic Surgery.* Princeton, NJ: Princeton University Press; 1999.

622. Glaister J. *Dr William Smellie and His Contemporaries.* Glasgow: James Maclehose and Sons; 1894.

623. Glees P. Franz von Leydig. In: Gillispie CC (ed.) *Dictionary of Scientific Biography.* New York, NY: Charles Scriber's Sons. 1973; 8: 301–3.

624. Glees P. Heinrich Wilhelm Waldeyer. In: Gillispie CC (ed.) *Dictionary of Scientific Biography.* New York, NY: Charles Scribner's Sons. 1976; 14: 125–7.

625. Gleichert JE. Étienne Joseph Jacquemin, discoverer of 'Chadwick's Sign'. *J Hist Med Allied Sci* 1971; 26: 75–80.

626. Goellnicht DC. *The Poet-Physicians: Keats and Medical Science.* Pittsburgh, PA: University of Pittsburgh Press; 1984.

627. Golditch IM. Lawson Tait: the forgotten gynecologist. *Obstet Gynecol* 2002; 99: 152–6.

628. Goldstein A. The moral psychiatry of imperial Rome as practiced by Soranus of Ephesus. *Psychiatr Q* 1969; 43: 535–54.

629. Goldstein PJ. Birth asphyxia. In: Smith GF, Vidyasagar D (eds) *Historical Review and Recent Advances in*

Neonatal and Perinatal Medicine (Vol. 1). New York, NY: Mead Johnson Ltd; 1981, pp. 177–83.

630. Goldzieher JW. How the oral contraceptives came to be developed. *JAMA* 1974; 230: 421–5.
631. Gonzalez D. Sculpture of paradox: doctor as hero and villain. *New York Times.* 3 March 2014.
632. Gonzalez-Crussi F. *On Being Born and Other Difficulties.* Woodstock, NY: Overlook Press; 2004.
633. Goodell W. *A Sketch of the Life and Writings of Louyse Bourgeois.* Philadelphia, PA: Collins; 1876.
634. Goodell, William (obituary). *JAMA* 1894; 23: 697.
635. Goodlin RC. History of fetal monitoring. *Am J Obstet Gynecol* 1979; 133: 323–52.
636. Goodlin RC. On the protection of the maternal perineum during birth. *Obstet Gynecol* 1983; 62: 393–4.
637. Goodlin RC, Joseph B. DeLee and his textbook, *Principles and Practice of Obstetrics. ACOG Clin Rev* 1997; 2: 14–16.
638. Goodman H. Profile: Emil Noeggerath, first gynecologist to the Mount Sinai Hospital. *J Mt Sinai Hosp* 1957; 24: 26–30.
639. Goodwin JW. A personal reflection of Virginia Apgar. *J Obstet Gynaecol Can* 2002; 24: 248–9.
640. Goodwin WE. William Osler and Howard A. Kelly. *Bull Hist Med* 1946; 20: 611–52.
641. Gordon HL. *Sir James Young Simpson and Chloroform (1811–1870).* London: T. Fisher Unwin; 1897.
642. Gosden RG. Biosketch: George Washington Corner. *Biol Reprod* 2013; 88: 1–3.
643. Gould T, Uttley D. *A Short History of St George's Hospital and the Origin of its Ward Names.* London: Athlone Press; 1997.
644. Gow JG. Harold Hopkins, (obituary). *Br J Urol* 1995; 75: 263–4.
645. Graff, Erwin von. Tubal sterilization by the Madlener technique. *Am J Obstet Gynecol* 1939; 38: 295–300.
646. Graff L. Arthur H. Curtis, MD: Portrait of a professional perfectionist. *J Mich Med Soc* 1955; 54: 484–5.
647. Graham H. *The Story of Surgery.* New York, NY: Doubleday, Doran & Co; 1939.
648. Graham H. *Eternal Eve: The History of Gynaecology and Obstetrics.* New York, NY: Doubleday & Co; 1951.
649. Grandin EH. In memoriam: Ludwig Bandl. *Am J Obstet Dis Women Child* 1887; 20: 46–8.
650. Grant GJ, Grant AH, Lockwood CJ. Simpson, Semmelweis, and transformational change. *Obstet Gynecol* 2005; 106: 384–7.
651. Gray LA. *Ephraim McDowell: Father of Ovariotomy and Founder of Abdominal Surgery.* Philadelphia, PA and London: JB Lippincott Co; 1921.
652. Gray LA. Ephraim McDowell, 1809. *Obstet Gynecol* 1960; 16: 503–16.
653. Gray LA. *The Life and Times of Ephraim McDowell.* Louisville, KY: VG Reed and Sons; 1987.
654. Green GH. Historic perspective on Liley's 'fetal transfusion'. *Vox Sang.* 1985; 48: 184–7.
655. Green GH. William Liley and fetal transfusion: a perspective in fetal medicine. *Fetal Ther* 1986; 1: 18–2.
656. Green S. *The Curious History of Contraception.* London: Ebury Press; 1971.
657. Greenspan RE. *Medicine: Perspectives in History and Art.* Alexandria, VA: Ponteverde Press; 2006.
658. Gregg, Norman McAlister (obituary). *BMJ* 1966; 2: 364.
659. Gregg, Norman McAlister (obituary). *Lancet* 1966; 2: 347.
660. Gregg, Norman McAlister (obituary). *Med J Aust* 1966; 2: 1166–9.
661. Grimes HG, Brooks MH. Pregnancy in Sheehan's syndrome: report of a case and review. *Obstet Gynecol Surv* 1980; 35: 481–8.
662. Groskop V. Birth the way nature intended. *The Guardian Weekly.* 20 November 2009, pp. 28–9.
663. Gross SD. *Memorial Oration in Honor of Ephraim McDowell. Trans Kentucky State Med Soc.* Louisville, KY: John J. Morton & Co; 1879.
664. Gruhn JG, Roth LM. History of gynecological pathology: Dr Walter Schiller. *Int J Gynecol Path* 1998; 17: 380–6.
665. Grunze H, Spriggs AI. *History of Clinical Cytology.* 2nd edn. Baden: Verlag; 1983.
666. Guilly PJL. *Duchenne de Boulogne.* Paris: Baillière; 1936.
667. Gunn ADG. *Oral Contraception in Perspective.* Carnforth: Parthenon Publishing Group; 1987.
668. Gunn AL, Wood MC. The amplification and recording of foetal heart sounds. *Proc R Soc Med* 1953; 46: 85–90.
669. Gunn AL. James Young Simpson: the complete gynaecologist. *J Obstet Gynaecol Br Commonw* 1968; 75: 249–63.
670. Gunning JE. The history of laparoscopy. *J Reprod Med* 1974; 12: 222–6.
671. Guttmacher AF. Recollections of John Whitridge Williams. *Bull Hist Med* 1935; 3: 19–30.

672. Gwen FT. 'Posterior culdeplasty': revisited. *Am J Obstet Gynecol* 1985; 153: 135–9.

673. Haberling W. *German Medicine*.(Translated by Jules Freund) New York, NY; AMS Press; 1978.

674. Hacquin F, Joseph C. Anthèlme Récamier de la morine à la gynécologie (1774–1852). *Hist Sci Med* 1987; 21: 345–9.

675. Hadden DR. The development of diabetes and its relation to pregnancy: the long-term and short-term historical viewpoint. In: Sutherland HW, Stowers JM (eds) *Carbohydrate metabolism in pregnancy and the newborn. Proceedings of the 4th Aberdeen Colloquium*. 1989, pp. 1–8.

676. Hagelin O. *The Womans Booke: An Illustrated and Annotated Catalogue of Rare Books in the Library of the Swedish Society of Medicine*. Stockholm: Svenska Läkaresällskapet; 1990.

677. Hajdu SI. Cytology from antiquity to Papanicolaou. *Acta Cytologica* 1997; 21: 668–76.

678. Hall JJ, Hall DJ. The forgotten hysterectomy. *Obstet Gynecol* 2006; 107: 541–3.

679. Hall R. *Marie Stopes: A Biography*. London: André Deutsch; 1977.

680. Haller JS. Smut's dark poison: ergot in history and medicine. *Trans Studies Coll Phys (Philadelphia)* 1986; 3: 62–78.

681. Hallett C. The attempt to understand puerperal fever in the eighteenth and early nineteenth centuries: the influence of inflammation theory. *Med Hist* 2005; 49: 1–28.

682. Hamby WB. *Ambroise Paré: Surgeon of the Renaissance*. St Louis, MO: Warren H Green Inc; 1967.

683. Hamilton GR, Baskett TF. Mandrake to morphine: anodynes of antiquity. *Ann R Coll Phys Surg Can* 1999; 32: 403–6.

684. Hamilton GR, Baskett TF. In the arms of Morpheus: the development of morphine for postoperative pain relief. *Can J Anesth* 2000; 47: 367–74.

685. Hamilton HG. Postpartum labial or paravaginal hematomas. *Am J Obstet Gynecol* 1940; 39: 642–8.

686. Hamlin C. *The Hospital by the River*. Sydney: Macmillan; 2001.

687. Hamlin EC, Woldemichael A, Muleta M, Tafesse B, Aytenfesa H, Browning A. Obstetric fistula in the 21st century. In: Hillard T, Purdie D (eds) *The Yearbook of Obstetrics and Gynaecology*. London: RCOG Press. 2004, pp. 210–23.

688. Hanson MA. Tribute to Professor Geoffrey Dawes. *Ped Res* 1996; 40: 774–5.

689. Harder TJ, Witkowski JA, Wylie CC. (eds) *A History of Embryology*. New York, NY: Cambridge University Press; 1986.

690. Harris RP. The operation of gastro-elytrotomy (true caesarean section), viewed in the light of American experience and success. *Am J Med Sci* 1878; 75: 313–42.

691. Harris RP. Lessons from a study of the cesarean operation in the city and state of New York and their bearing upon the true position of gastro-elytrotomy. *Am J Obstet Dis Women Child* 1879; 12: 82–91.

692. Harris RP. The revival of symphysiotomy in Italy. *Am J Med Sci* 1883; 85: 17–32.

693. Harris RP. Results of the Porro caesarean operation in all countries. *BMJ* 1890; 1: 68–72.

694. Harris S. *Women's Surgeon: The Life Story of J. Marion Sims*. New York, NY: The MacMillan Co; 1950.

695. Harris S, Naina HV. Cullen's sign revisited. *Am J Med* 2008; 121: 682–3.

696. Hart DB. James Young Simpson. An appreciation of his work in anaesthesia and some of his outstanding papers. *Edin Med J* 1911; 6: 543–53.

697. Harvey AM. The 'Kensington colt' and the development of female urology. *Johns Hopkins Med J* 1974; 295–302.

698. Harvey J, Ogilvie M. Elizabeth Maplesden Ramsey. In: Ogilvie M, Harvey J, Rossiter M (eds) *Biographical Dictionary of Women in Science: Pioneering Lives from Ancient Times to the Mid-20th Century*. New York, NY: Routledge; 2000, pp. 1071–2.

699. Harvey TW. OW Holmes: his work in establishing the contagious nature of childbed fever. *Med Rec* 1911; 24: 102–9.

700. Haubrich WS. Krukenberg of the Krukenberg tumor. *Gastroenterology* 2005; 129: 1844.

701. Haultain, Francis (obituary). *J Obstet Gynaecol Br Emp* 1921; 28: 315–8.

702. Hawgood BJ. Professor Sir William Liley (1929–83): New Zealand perinatal physiologist. *J Med Biog* 2005; 13: 82–8.

703. Haymaker W, Schiller F. *The Founders of Neurology*. 2nd edn. Springfield, IL: Charles C Thomas; 1970.

704. Heagney B. *Rubella: Essays in Honour of the Centenary of the Birth of Sir Norman McAlister Gregg 1892–1966*. Sydney: Royal Australian College of Physicians; 1992.

705. Heaney NS. John Clarence Webster, 1863–1950. *Proc Inst Med Chicago* 1950; 18: 174.

706. Heaney, Noble Sproat: in memoriam. *Trans Am Gynec Soc* 1956; 79: 201–3.

707. Heaton CE. Obstetrics in Colonial America. *Am J Surg* 1939; 45: 606–10.

708. Heaton CE. Control of puerperal infection in the United States during the last century. *Am J Obstet Gynecol* 1943; 46: 479–86.

709. Heaton CE. The history of anesthesia and analgesia in obstetrics. *J Hist Med* 1946; 1: 567–72.

710. Heaton C. Fifty years of progress in obstetrics and gynecology. *NY State J Med* 1951; 51: 83–5.

711. Hecht, J. *City of Light: The Story of Fiber Optics.* New York, NY: Oxford University Press; 1999.

712. Hellman AM. *Amnesia and Analgesia in Parturition (Twilight sleep).* London: HK Lewis and Co. Ltd; 1915.

713. Hellman LM. Three deliveries that changed the history of the world. *Maryland Med J* 1972; 21: 41–8.

714. Helmkamp BF, Krebs HB. The Maylard incison in gynecologic surgery. *Am J Obstet Gynecol* 1990; 163: 1554–7.

715. Henle J. On miasmata and contagia. Translated by George Rosen. *Bull Hist Med* 1938; 6: 907–83.

716. Herman JR. *Urology: A View Through the Retrospectroscope.* New York, NY: Harper & Row Publishers; 1973.

717. Hertig A. Allen and Doisy's 'An Ovarian Hormone'. *JAMA* 1983; 250: 2684–8.

718. Hibbard BN. *The Obstetric Forceps: A Short History and Descriptive Catalogue of the Forceps in the Museum of the Royal College of Obstetricians and Gynaecologists.* 2nd edn. London: RCOG Press; 1992.

719. Hibbard B. Pioneers in Obstetrics and Gynaecology: Peter Chamberlen. *The Diplomate* 1994; 1: 309–11.

720. Hibbard B. William Blair-Bell: the enigmatic torch bearer. In: O'Brien PMS (ed.) *The Yearbook of Obstetrics and Gynaecology.* London: RCOG Press; 1997; pp. 12–19.

721. Hibbard B. *The Obstetrician's Armamentarium.* San Anselmo, CA: Norman Publishing; 2000.

722. Hicks, John Braxton (obituary). *BMJ* 1897; 11: 618–9.

723. Hicks, John Braxton (obituary). *Lancet* 1897; 2: 692.

724. Hillis, David Sweeney (obituary). *JAMA* 1942; 120: 1055.

725. Hilton P. Sims to SMIS: an historical perspective on vesico-vaginal fistulae. In: Studd J (ed.) *The Yearbook of the Royal College of Obstetricians and Gynaecologists.* London: RCOG Press; 1994, pp. 7–16.

726. Himes NE. *Medical History of Contraception.* New York, NY: Gamut Press Inc; 1963.

727. Hirsch A. *Biographisches lexicon der hervorragenden aertze aller zeiten und völker. Zweiter band.* Vienna and Leipzig: Urban and Schwarzenberg; 1885.

728. Hirst BC. Edmund Piper: 1891–1935. *Trans Am Gynecol Soc* 1936; 60: 331–4.

729. Hodge, Hugh (obituary). *Am J Med Sci* 1873; 63: 576–8.

730. Hoefnagel D, Lüders D. Ernst Moro (1874–1951). *Pediatrics* 1962; 29: 543–5.

731. Hoffman NY. Edith Potter, MD, PhD: pioneering infant pathology. *JAMA* 1982; 248: 1551–3.

732. Hoffman W. Who is Poupart? *Surg Gynecol Obstet* 1990; 170: 78–80.

733. Hofman A. Historical review of ergot alkaloids. *Pharmacology* 1978; 16(Suppl): 1–11.

734. Hohlweg W. In memoriam: Prof Selmar Aschheim. *Zentrabl Gynacol* 1965; 87: 1025–6.

735. Holland E. William Blair-Bell (obituary). *BMJ* 1936; 1: 287–9.

736. Holland E. The Princess Charlotte of Wales: a triple obstetric tragedy. *J Obstet Gynaecol Br Emp* 1951; 58: 905–19.

737. Holley HL. *A History of Medicine in Alabama.* Birmingham, AL: University of Alabama Press; 1982.

738. Holmes OW. *Medical Essays.* Vol. IX. Boston, MA: Haughton, Mifflin & Co; 1895.

739. Holmes, Rudolph Wieser (obituary). *JAMA* 1953; 152: 255.

740. Horine EF. The stage setting for Ephraim McDowell, 1771–1830. *Bull Hist Med* 1950; 24: 149–60.

741. Houtzager HL. Hendrik Van Deventer. *Eur J Obstet Gynecol Reprod Biol* 1986; 21: 263–70.

742. Houtzager HL. Reinier De Graaf and his contribution to reproductive biology. *Eur J Obstet Gynecol Reprod Biol* 2000; 90: 125–7.

743. Hovell BC, Wilson J. The history of anaesthesia in Edinburgh. *J R Soc Med Edin* 1969; 14: 107–16, 1165–79.

744. Howard SS. Antoine van Leeuwenhoek and the discovery of sperm. *Fert Steril* 1997; 67: 16–17.

745. Howard-Jones, N. On the diagnostic term 'Down's syndrome'. *Med Hist* 1979; 22: 102–4.

746. Huard P. André Levret 1705–1780. *Consours Méd* 1962; 84: 2035–41.

747. Hudson MM, Morton RS. Fracastoro and Syphilis: 500 years on. *Lancet* 1996; 348: 1495–6.

748. Huffman JW. Jan van Riemskdyk: medical illustrator extraordinary. *JAMA* 1969; 208: 121–4.

749. Huffman JW. The great eighteenth-century obstetric atlases and their illustrator. *Obstet Gynecol* 1970; 35: 971–6.

750. Hughes T. The medical education of Sir Thomas Browne, a seventeenth-century student at Montpellier, Padua and Leiden. *J Med Biog* 2001; 9: 70–6.

751. Hühner, Max (obituary). *JAMA* 1948; 136: 485.

752. Hunt T. *The Medical Society of London 1773–1973*. London: William Heinemann Medical Books Ltd.; 1972.

753. Hunting P. *The History of the Royal Society of Medicine*. London: Royal Society of Medicine Press; 2002.

754. Huntington, James Lincoln (obituary). *Boston Herald Traveler*. 10 May 1968.

755. Huntley FL. Sir Thomas Browne, MD, William Harvey, and the metaphor of the circle. *Bull Hist Med* 1951; 25: 326–42.

756. Hurt R. *The History of Cardiothoracic Surgery from Early Times*. New York, NY: Parthenon Publishing Group; 1996.

757. Huston P. Cochrane Collaboration helping unravel tangled web woven by international research. *Can Med Assoc J* 1996; 154: 1389–92.

758. Hutchin MD. History of blood transfusion. *Surgery* 1968; 64: 685–700.

759. Iceton S. The Soranus score. *Can Med Assoc J* 2001; 164: 674.

760. Illingworth C. *The Story of William Hunter*. Edinburgh: E & S Livingstone Ltd; 1967.

761. Illingworth C. William Hunter's manuscripts and letters: the Glasgow Collection. *Med Hist* 1971; 15: 181–6.

762. Ingerslev E. Rösslin's 'Rosengarten': its relation to the past (the Musico Manuscripts and Soranus), particularly with regard to podalic version. *J Obstet Gynaecol Br Emp* 1909; 15: 1–25, 73–92.

763. Ingerslev E. Mathias Saxtorph et ses contemporains. *Arch Mens Obstet Gynéc (Paris)*. 1914; 28: 192–232.

764. Irvin A. Professional attainments of Ephraim McDowell. *Bull Hist Med* 1950; 24: 161–7.

765. Irving FC. *Safe Deliverance*. Boston, MA: Houghton Mifflin Co; 1942.

766. Irving FC. Fifty years of medical progress. Medicine as a science: obstetrics. *N Eng J Med* 1951; 244: 91–100.

767. Israel SL. Andrew A Marchetti, 1901–1970 (obituary). *Trans Am Assoc Obstet Gynecol* 1970; 81: 153–5.

768. Issa MM, Schmid HP, Stamey TA. Youssef's syndrome: preservation of uterine function with subsequent successful pregnancy following surgical repair. *Urol Int* 1994; 52: 220–2.

769. Jackson JD. The first ovariotomy. *BMJ* 1874; 1: 466–7.

770. Jacobson AC. Evolution in axis-traction: an advance upon the method of utilizing the principle of axis-traction in vogue in obstetric practice unimproved since its introduction by Tarnier in 1877. *Am J Obstet Dis Women Child* 1906; 35: 326–45.

771. Jacoby MG. The birth of Kaiser Wilhelm II (1859–1941) and his birth injury. *J Med Biog* 2008; 16: 178–83.

772. James LS. Fond memories of Virginia Apgar. *Pediatrics* 1975; 55: 1–4.

773. James P. *Population Malthus, His Life and Times*. London: Routledge and Kegan Paul; 1976.

774. Janssens J, Kuijjer PJ. Petrus Camper (1722–1789): a physician of international repute and a universal scholar. In: Houtzager HL, Lammes FB (eds) *Obstetrics and Gynaecology in the Low Countries: A Historical Perspective*. Zeist: Medical Forum International; 1996.

775. Jarcho J. *The Pelvis in Obstetrics*. New York, NY: Paul B Hoeber Inc; 1933.

776. Jeanselme E. L'oeuvre scientifique d'Hallopeau. *Ann Dermat Syphil* 1918–19; 7: 232–5.

777. Jeffcoate N. Medicine versus nature. *J R Coll Surg Edin* 1976; 21: 263–77.

778. Jelliffe SE. Madame Dejerine-Klumpke. *J Nerv Ment Dis* 1928; 67: 644–7.

779. Jirka FJ. *American Doctors of Destiny*. Chicago, IL: Normandie House; 1940.

780. Johns Hopkins University School of Medicine. *Johns Hopkins University School of Medicine 1893–1943: A Brief Account of Its Founding and of Its Achievements During the First Fifty Years of Its Existence*. Baltimore, MD; 1943.

781. Johnston FE. James Mourilyan Tanner (1920–2010): a tribute. *Am J Hum Biol* 2011; 23: 1–3.

782. Johnston RD. The history of human infertility. *Fertil Steril* 1963; 14: 266.

783. Johnstone RW. James Young Simpson and chloroform. *Edin Med J* 1947; 54: 324–7.

784. Johnstone RW. William Harvey: 'The Father of British Midwifery'. *J Obstet Gynaecol Br Emp* 1948; 55: 293–302.

785. Johnstone RW. *William Smellie: The Master of British Midwifery*. Edinburgh: E & S Livingstone; 1952.

786. Jones HJ, Jones GS, Ticknor WE. *Richard Wesley Te Linde*. Baltimore, MD: William & Wilkins; 1986.

787. Jones HW, Mackmull G. The influence of James Blundell on the development of blood transfusion. *Ann Med Hist* 1928; 10: 242–8.

788. Jones HW. Chorionic gonadotrophin: a narrative of its identification and origin and the role of Georgeanna Seegar Jones. *Obstet Gynecol Surv* 2006; 62: 1–3.

789. Jonkman EJ. An historical note: Doppler research in the nineteenth century. *Ultrasound Med Biol* 1980; 6: 1–5.

790. Jotkowitz MW, Picton FCR. On the Bracht manoeuvre. *Aust NZ Obstet Gynaecol* 1970; 10: 151–4.

791. Judd GE. *History of the Los Angeles Obstetrical and Gynecological Society, 1914–1972*. Los Angeles, CA: LA Obstetrical and Gynecological Society; 1973.

792. Junod SW, Marks L. Women's trials: the approval of the first oral contraceptive pill in the United States and Great Britain. *J Hist Med Allied Sci* 2002; 57: 117–60.

793. Kagan SR. *Jewish Contributions of Medicine in America*. Boston, MA: Boston Medical Publishing Company; 1939.

794. Kaiser IH. Reappraisals of J. Marion Sims. *Am J Obstet Gynecol* 1978; 132: 878–84.

795. Kalisch PA, Scobey M, Kalisch BJ. Louyse Bourgeois and the emergence of modern midwifery. *J Nurse Midwifery* 1981; 26: 3–17.

796. Kass AM. The obstetrical case book of Walter Channing, 1811–1822. *Bull Hist Med* 1993; 67: 494–523.

797. Kass AM. Boston Lying-in Hospital: the early years. *ACOG Clin Rev* 1998; 3: 12–16.

798. Kass AM. 'My brother preaches, I practice': Walter Channing, MD. Antebellum obstetrician. *Mass Hist Rev* 1999; 1: 78–94.

799. Kass AM. *Midwifery and Medicine in Boston: Walter Channing, MD, 1786–1876*. New York, NY: Northeastern University Press; 2001.

800. Kaufman M, Galishoffs R, Savitt TL (eds) *Dictionary of Medical Biography*. 2 vols. London: Greenwood Press; 1984.

801. Keene FE (ed.) *Album of the Fellows of the American Gynecological Society, 1876–1930*. Philadelphia, PA: Wm Dornan; 1930.

802. Keep P. Nathan Keep: William Morton's Salieri? *Anaesthesia* 1995; 50: 233–8.

803. Kegel, Arnold Henry (obituary). *JAMA* 1972; 221: 314.

804. Keirns CC. Susan and the Simmonds-Sheehan syndrome: medicine, history and literature. In: Duffin J (ed.) *Clio in the Clinic: History in Medical Practice*. Oxford: Oxford University Press; 2005, pp. 116–27.

805. Keirse MJN. The history of tocolysis. *Br J Obstet Gynaecol* 2003; 110: 94–7.

806. Keith A. Duchenne of Boulogne as orthopedist. In: *Menders of the Maimed*. New York, NY: Robert E. Krieger Publishing Co; 1975, pp. 91–105.

807. Kellar RJ. Sir James Young Simpson: victor dolore. *J R Coll Surg Edin* 1966; 12: 1–6.

808. Kelleher ME, Swan KG, Kelleher DP. George Ryerson Fowler: Brooklyn's surgical pioneer. *Ann Surg* 2011; 253: 1230–2.

809. Keller E. Mrs Jane Sharp: midwifery and the critique of medical knowledge in seventeenth-century England. *Women's Writing* 1995; 2: 101–8.

810. Kelly HA. *A Cylopedia of American Medical Biography (2 volumes)*. Philadelphia, PA: WB Saunders Company; 1912.

811. Kelly HA. The history of vesicovaginal fistula. *Trans Am Gynecol Soc* 1912; 37: 3–29.

812. Kelly HA, Ward GE. *Electrosurgery*. Philadelphia, PA: WB Saunders Company; 1932.

813. Kelly HA. John Whitridge Williams (1866–1931). *Am J Surg* 1932; 15: 169–74.

814. Kelly HA. Reminiscences in the development of gynecology. *J Conn Med Soc* 1936; 1: 459–68.

815. Kelly J. The Addis Ababa Fistula Hospital for poor women with childbirth injuries. In: Studd J (ed.) *The Yearbook of the Royal College of Obstetricians and Gynaecologists*. London: RCOG Press; 1994, pp. 2–6.

816. Kelsey, Frances (obituary). *The Globe and Mail*. 7 August 2015.

817. Kennedy DM. *Birth Control in America: The Career of Margaret Sanger*. New Haven, CT and London: Yale University Press; 1970.

818. Kennedy, E (obituary). *BMJ* 1886; 1: 911.

819. Kennedy RG. Electronic fetal heart rate monitoring: retrospective reflections on a twentieth-century technology. *J R Soc Med* 1998; 91: 244–50.

820. Kenny SC, Word JL, Bryan CS. James Marion Sims and the rise of gynaecological surgery. *J Med Biog* 1999; 7: 217–23.

821. Keppie L. *William Hunter and the Hunterian Museum in Glasgow, 1807–2007*. Edinburgh: Edinburgh University Press; 2007.

822. Kerr JMM, Johnstone RW, Phillips MH(eds) *Historical Review of British Obstetrics and Gynaecology, 1800–1950*. Edinburgh and London: E & S Livingstone; 1954.

823. Kerr, John Munro (obituary). *BMJ* 1960: 2; 1166.

824. Kerr, JM. (obituary). *J Obstet Gynaecol Br Commonw* 1961; 68: 510–14.

825. Key JD, Shephard DAE, Walters W. Sister Mary Joseph's nodule and its relationship to diagnosis of

carcinoma of the umbilicus. *Minnesota Med* 1976; 59: 561–6.

826. Keynes G. The history of blood transfusion. *Br J Surg* 1943; 31: 38–50.
827. Keynes G (ed.) *The Apologie and Treatise of Ambroise Paré Containing the Voyages Made into Divers Places. With Many of His Writings upon Surgery*. Chicago, IL: University of Chicago Press; 1952.
828. Keynes G. Sir Thomas Browne. *BMJ* 1965; 2: 1505–10.
829. Keynes G. Tercentenary of blood transfusion. *BMJ* 1967; 4: 410–11.
830. Keynes G. *The Life of William Harvey*. London: Oxford Press; 1978.
831. Keynes M. Battle of eponymy. *BMJ* 1954; 1: 96.
832. Keys TE. *The History of Surgical Anesthesia*. New York, NY: Dover Publications; 1963.
833. Khattab AD. Dances with microscopes: Antoni van Leeuwenhoek (1632–1723). *Cyto Path* 1995; 6: 215–18.
834. Kight JR. John Peter Mettauer and the first successful closure of vesicovaginal fistula in the United States. *Am J Obstet Gynecol* 1967; 99: 885–92.
835. Kight JR. In rural Virginia, world-class medicine. John Peter Mettauer, 1787–1878. *Va Med* 1989; 116: 66–70.
836. Killiam H, Krämer G. *Meister der Chirurgie und die Chirurgenschulen im deutschen Raum*. Stuttgart: Georg Thieme Verlag; 1951.
837. Kinch RA. Dr JB Collip and the development of premarin. *J Obstet Gynaecol Can* 2008; 30: 244–5.
838. King AG. *The Cincinnati Obstetrical and Gynecological Society, 1876–1976*. Cincinnati, OH: 1976.
839. King JF. A short history of evidence-based obstetric care. *Best Prac Res Clin Obstet Gynaecol* 2005; 19: 3–14.
840. Kingsland S. Raymond Pearl: on the frontier in the 1920s. *Hum Biol* 1984; 56: 1–18.
841. Kirchhoff H, Polacsek R. *Gynäkologen deutscher Sprache: Biographie und Bibliographie*. Stuttgart: Georg Thieme Verlag; 1960.
842. Kirkland AS. Dr John Clarence Webster. *Can Med Assoc J* 1950; 62: 521.
843. Kirkup J. The history and evolution of surgical instruments. VII. Catheters, hollow needles and other tubular instruments. *Ann R Coll Surg Eng* 1998; 80: 81–9.
844. Kirkup J. Spencer Well's forceps. *J Med Biog* 2005; 13: 127.
845. Kirkup J. *The Evolution of Surgical Instruments*. Novato, CA: History of Science; 2006.
846. Kirkup J. Who made what? John Aitken's chain saw. *J Med Biog* 2009; 17: 80.
847. Klukoff PJ. Smollett's defence of Dr Smellie in *The Critical Review*. *Med Hist* 1970; 14: 31–41.
848. Knipe WHW. The Freiburg method of dämmerschlaf or twilight sleep. *Am J Obstet Gynecol* 1914; 70: 884–909.
849. Knörr K. Classic illustration: Kleihauer–Betke test. *Eur J Obstet Gynec Reprod Biol* 1985; 19: 333–5.
850. Koch T. John Snow, hero of cholera: RIP. *Can Med Assoc J* 2008; 178: 1736.
851. Kompanje EJO. A remarkable case in the history of obstetrical surgery: a laparotomy performed by the Dutch surgeon Abraham Cyprianus in 1694. *Eur J Obstet Gynecol Reprod Biol* 2005; 118: 119–23.
852. Kosmak GW. Ralph Hayward Pomeroy, MD, 1867–1925. *Trans Am Gynecol Soc* 1926; 51: 302–5.
853. Koss LG. George N Papanicolaou (1883–1962). *Acta Cytol* 1963; 7: 143–5.
854. Koss LG. On the history of cytology. *Acta Cytol* 1980; 24: 475–7.
855. Kovacs K. Sheehan syndrome. *Lancet* 2003; 361: 520–2.
856. Kresge N, Simori RD, Hill RL. The prostaglandins, Sune Bergström and Bengt Samuelsson. *J Biol Chem* 2006; 282: e9.
857. Krukenberg FE. What's in a name. The Krukenberg tumour. *Midwives Chronicle and Nursing Notes* 1966; 79: 101.
858. Krumbhaar EB. The early history of anatomy in the United States. *Ann Med Hist* 1922; 4: 271–86.
859. Kuh S. Wilhelm Erb, 1840–1921. *Arch Neur Psych* 1922; 7: 250–1.
860. Kurjak A. Ultrasound scanning: Prof Ian Donald (1910–1987). *Eur J Obstet Gynecol Reprod Biol* 2000; 90: 187–9.
861. Kurzrok R. The prospects for hormonal contraception. *J Contraception* 1937; 2: 27–9.
862. Küstner O. Bernhard Sigmund Schultze, Jena. *Zentralbl Gynäkol* 1919; 43: 393–8.
863. Kwasnik EM. William T Bovie: the surgical spark behind modern biophysics. *Current Surg* 2001; 58: 109–10.
864. Kyle RA, Shampo MA. Hulusi Behçet. *JAMA* 1982; 247: 1925.
865. Lacomme M. Alexandre Couvelaire (1873–1948). *Gynéc Obstét.* 1948; 47: 603–12.
866. Lader L. *The Margaret Sanger Story*. Westport, CT: Greenwood Press; 1955.
867. Lamont-Brown R. *Royal Poxes and Potions: The Lives of Court Physicians, Surgeons and Apothecaries*. Stroud: Sutton Publishing Ltd; 2001.

868. Lancester HO. Semmelweis: a rereading of *Die Aetiologie* Part I: Puerperal sepsis before 1845. *J Med Biog* 1994; 2: 12–21.

869. Lancester HO. Semmelweis: a rereading of *Die Aetiologie* Part II: Medical historians and Semmelweis. *J Med Biog* 1994; 2: 84–8.

870. Landsteiner, Karl (obituary). *Am J Clin Path* 1943; 13: 566–8.

871. Landsteiner, Karl (obituary). *JAMA* 1943; 122: 761.

872. Langhans, Theodor (obituary). *Lancet* 1916; 1: 161.

873. Langley LL (ed.) *Benchmark Papers in Human Physiology: Contraception.* Stroudsburg, PA: Dowden, Hutchinson and Ross; 1973.

874. Langstaff JB. *Dr Bard of Hyde Park.* New York, NY: EP Dutton & Co; 1942.

875. Larsell O. Anders Adolf Retzius (1796–1860). *Ann Med Hist NY* 1924; 6: 16–24.

876. Latzko, William Francis (obituary). *JAMA* 1945; 127: 942.

877. Laufe LE, Berkus MD. *Assisted Vaginal Delivery: Obstetric Forceps and Vacuum Extraction Techniques.* New York, NY: McGraw-Hill Inc; 1992.

878. Lavazzo C, Gkegkes ID, Gkegke XE, Karamanou M, Androutsos G. Konstantinos Logothetopoulos (1878–1961): the controversial life of an eminent gynaecologist. *Arch Gynecol Obstet* 2015; 292: 383–6.

879. Leavitt JW. *Brought to Bed: Childbearing in America, 1750–1950.* New York, NY: Oxford University Press; 1986.

880. Leavitt JW. Joseph B. DeLee and the practice of preventive obstetrics. *Am J Pub Health* 1988; 78: 1353–9.

881. Lee JA. Joseph Thomas Clover and the contributions of surgery to anaesthesia. *Ann R Coll Surg Eng* 1960; 26: 280–99.

882. Lee RJ. The Goulstonian Lectures on puerperal fever. *BMJ* 1875; 1: 304–6.

883. Lee, R. A biographical sketch. *Lancet* 1851; 1: 332–7.

884. Lee S (ed.) *Dictionary of National Biography.* London: Smith, Elders and Co.; 1893, pp. 1–4.

885. LeFanu W. Thomas Wharton. In: Gillispie CC (ed.) *Dictionary of Scientific Biography.* New York, NY: Charles Scribner's Sons. 1976; 14: 286–7.

886. Lehfeldt H. Ernst Gräfenberg and his ring. In: Van der Pas HFM, Dieben OM (eds) *State of the Art of the IUD.* Dordrecht: Kluwer Academic Publishers; 1989, pp. 1–7.

887. Lehman PA, Bolivar A, Quintero R. Russell E. Marker: Pioneer of the Mexican steroid industry. *J Chem Ed* 1973; 150: 195–9.

888. Lehman PA. Early history of steroid chemistry in Mexico: the story of three remarkable men. *Steroids* 1992; 57: 403–8.

889. Leiber B, Olbert T. *Die klinischen Eponyme.* Munich-Berlin-Vienna:Urban & Schwarzenberg; 1968.

890. Lenz W. A short history of thalidomide. *Teratology* 1988; 38: 203–15.

891. Leonard VN. The difficulty of producing sterility by operating on the fallopian tubes. *Am J Obstet Dis Women* 1913; 67: 443–50.

892. Leopold, Gerhard (obituary). *Boston Med Surg J* 1912; 165: 777–8.

893. Lepage F. Alexandre Couvelaire (1873–1948). *Paris Méd* 1948; 38: 181–2.

894. Lepage F. Eugen Aburel, 1899–1975. *J Gynéc Obstét Biol Reprod* 1976; 5: 473–4.

895. Lesky E. Die Wiener Experimente mit dem Lichtleiter Bozzinis (1806/1807). *Clio Medica* 1970; 5: 327.

896. Lesky E. *The Vienna Medical School of the 19th Century.* Baltimore, MD: Johns Hopkins University Press; 1976.

897. Levack ID. Aberdeen, archives and anaesthesia. In: Barr AM, Boulton TB, Wilkinson DJ (eds) *Essays on the History of Anaesthesia.* London: RSM Press Ltd; 1996, pp. 74–7.

898. Lever, JCW (obituary). *Lancet* 1859; 1: 75.

899. Levine P. The discovery of Rh hemolytic disease. *Vox Sang* 1984; 47: 187–90.

900. Levinson A. *Pioneers of Paediatrics.* New York, NY: Froben Press; 1943.

901. Levret, Andre. *BMJ* 1912; 1: 746–7.

902. Ley G. Utero-placental (accidental) haemorrhage. *J Obstet Gynaecol Br Emp* 1921; 28: 69–108.

903. Liggins G. Geoffrey Sharman Dawes (obituary). *Biographical Memoirs of Fellows of the Royal Society.* 1998; 44: 111–25.

904. Liley, Albert William (obituary). *Lancet* 1983; 1: 59.

905. Liley, Albert William (obituary). *NZ Med J* 1983; 96: 631–2.

906. Lindeboom GA. Pieter Camper. In: Gillispie CC (ed.) *Dictionary of Scientific Biography.* New York, NY: Charles Scribner's Sons; 1971, pp. 37–8.

907. Lindeboom GA. *Dutch Medical Biography: A Biographical Dictionary of Dutch Physicians and Surgeons, 1475–1795.* Amsterdam: Rodopi; 1984.

908. Lindemann HJ. Historical aspects of hysteroscopy. *Fertil Steril* 1973; 24: 230–42.

909. Lippes J. Intrauterine contraception: history and world impact. *J Intl Health* 1966; 2: 17–24.

910. Little DM. Classical file: CL Mendelson. *Surv Anesthesiol* 1966; 10: 598–9.

911. Little DM. Classical file: Virginia Apgar. *Surv Anesthesiol* 1975; 19: 399–401.

912. Little HM. Louise Bourgeois and some others. *Montreal Med J* 1910; 39: 172–87.

913. Little, William John (obituary). *Lancet* 1894; 2: 168–9.

914. Little, W. A biographical sketch. *Lancet* 1854; 1: 16–22.

915. Litynski GS. Kurt Semm and the fight against scepticism. *J Soc Laparoendo Surg* 1998; 2: 309–13.

916. Lockwood CJ. Homage to an obstetric legend: Edward H. *Hon. Contemp Ob Gyn* 2006; 51: 8–15.

917. Longo LD. Classic pages in obstetrics and gynecology. Anton J Nuck: Adenographia curiosa et uteri foeminei anatome nova. *Am J Obstet Gynecol* 1975; 123: 66.

918. Longo LD. Classic pages in obstetrics and gynecology. John Braxton Hicks: On the contractions of the uterus throughout pregnancy. *Am J Obstet Gynecol* 1975; 123: 442.

919. Longo LD. Classic pages in obstetrics and gynecology. Matthew Baillie: an account of a particular change of structure in the human ovarium. *Am J Obstet Gynecol* 1975; 123: 770.

920. Longo LD. Classic pages in obstetrics and gynecology. Franz Carl Naegele: Das schräg verengte Becken nebst einen Anhange über die wichtigsten Fehler das weiblichen Beckens überhaupt. *Am J Obstet Gynecol* 1976; 125: 561.

921. Longo LD. Classic pages in obstetrics and gynecology. Experimental studies on the prevention of Rh haemolytic disease. *Am J Obstet Gynecol* 1977; 127: 537.

922. Longo LD. Classic pages in obstetrics and gynecology. Priscilla White: *Pregnancy complicating diabetes. Am J Obstet Gynecol* 1978; 130: 227.

923. Longo LD. Classic pages in obstetrics and gynecology. Emanuel A Friedman: *The Graphic Analysis of Labor. Am J Obstet Gynecol* 1978; 132: 822–3.

924. Longo LD. The rise and fall of Battey's operation: a fashion in surgery. *Bull Hist Med* 1979; 53: 244–67.

925. Longo LD. Classic pages in obstetrics and gynaecology. Francois Mauriceau: Des maladies des femmes grosses, et accouchées. *Am J Obstet Gynecol* 1979;133:455–6.

926. Longo LD. John Whitridge Williams and academic obstetrics in America. *Trans and Studies Coll Physicians Philadelphia* 1981; 3: 221–54.

927. Longo LD. *Introduction to: A Treatise on the Management of Pregnant and Lying-in Women by Charles White.* Canton, MA; Science History Publications; 1987.

928. Longo LD, Ashwal S. William Osler, Sigmund Freud and the evolution of ideas concerning cerebral palsy. *J Hist Neurosci* 1993; 2: 255–82.

929. Longo LD. Classic pages in obstetrics and gynecology. Fielding Ould: *A Treatise of Midwifery in Three Parts. Am J Obstet Gynecol* 1995; 172: 1317–19.

930. Longo LD. Classic pages in obstetrics and gynecology. Three cases of extirpation of diseased ovaria. *Am J Obstet Gynecol* 1995; 172: 1632–3.

931. Longo LD. Classic pages in obstetrics and gynecology. James Marion Sims: *On the treatment of vesico-vaginal fistula. Am J Obstet Gynecol* 1995; 172: 1936–7.

932. Longo LD, Meschia G. Elizabeth M. Ramsey and the evolution of ideas of uteroplacental blood flow and placental gas exchange. *Eur J Obstet Gynecol Reprod Biol* 2000; 90: 129–33.

933. Longo LD, Ashwal S. William Osler and the cerebral palsies of children. In: Barondess JA, Roland CG (eds) *The Persisting Osler-III. Selected Transactions of the American Osler Society 1991–2000.* Malabor, FL: Krieger Publishing Company; 2002, pp. 125–140.

934. Longo LD. Howard A. Kelly's development as an academician: some insights from his letters to Robert P. Harris. *Trans and Studies Coll Physicians Philadelphia* 2002; 24: 93–136.

935. Loudon I. Deaths in childbed from the eighteenth century to 1935. *Med Hist* 1986; 30: 1–41.

936. Loudon I. Obstetric care, social class and maternal mortality. *BMJ* 1986; 293; 606–8.

937. Loudon I. Some historical aspects of toxaemia of pregnancy: a review. *Br J Obstet Gynaecol* 1991; 98: 853–8.

938. Loudon I. *Death in Childbirth.* Oxford: Clarendon Press; 1992.

939. Loudon I. *Childbed Fever: A Documentary History. Diseases, Epidemics and Medicine Series.* New York, NY and London: Garland Publishing; 1995.

940. Loudon I. *The Tragedy of Childbed Fever.* Oxford: Oxford University Press; 2000.

941. Loudon I. Ignaz Phillip Semmelweis' studies of death in childbirth. *J R Soc Med* 2013; 106: 461–3.

942. Løvset's manoeuvre for breech delivery. *BMJ* 1946; 2: 974.

943. Løvset, Jørgen (obituary). *Acta Obstet Gynecol Scand* 1982; 61: 193–4.

944. Lowbury EJL. Leonard Colebrook (1883–1967). *BMJ* 1983; 87: 727–8.

945. Lowis GW. Epidemiology of puerperal fever: the contributions of Alexander Gordon. *Med Hist* 1993; 37: 399–410.

946. Lowis GW, Minagar A. Alexander Gordon of Aberdeen and the discovery of the contagiousness of puerperal fever. *J Med Biog* 2002; 10: 150–4.

947. Lucas MC, Taylor RR. Joe Vincent Meigs and the evolution of Meigs' syndrome. *J Pelvic Surg* 2001; 7: 191–5.

948. Lurie S. The history of the diagnosis and treatment of ectopic pregnancy: a medical adventure. *Eur J Obstet Gynecol Reprod Biol* 1992; 43: 1–7.

949. Lurie S. Meig's syndrome: the history of the eponym. *Eur J Obstet Gynecol Reprod Biol* 2000; 92: 199–204.

950. Lurie S, Glezerman M. The history of cesarean technique. *Am J Obstet Gynecol* 2003; 189: 1803–6.

951. Lyman GH. History and statistics of ovariotomy, and the circumstances under which the operation may be regarded as safe and expedient. *Am J Med Sci* 1865; 49: 389–401.

952. Lyons JB (ed.) *Dublin Surgeon-Anatomists and other Essays by William Doolin: A Centenary Tribute.* Dublin: Royal College of Surgeons in Ireland; 1987.

953. Macafee, Charles Horner Greer (obituary). *Lancet* 1978; 1: 485.

954. MacCallum WG. Marcello Malpighi, 1628–1694. *Johns Hopkins Hosp Bull* 1905; 16: 275–84.

955. MacDonald RR. Classical illustrations: from St Anthony's fire to ergometrine (ergonovine). *Eur J Obstet Gynec Reprod Biol* 1982; 13: 325–7.

956. MacGregor TN. The rise and development of the Edinburgh School of obstetrics and gynaecology, and its contribution to British obstetrics. *J Obstet Gynaecol Br Emp* 1959; 66: 998–1006.

957. MacGregor WG, Bracken A. Improved analgesia for women in labour. *Midwives Chronicle and Nursing Notes.* 1966; 79: 179–81.

958. Macintosh RR. Historical note: the graves of John Snow and Joseph Thomas Clover. *Anaesthesia* 1969; 24: 269–70.

959. Macintyre I, MacLaren I (eds) *Surgeons' Lives.* Edinburgh: Royal College of Surgeons of Edinburgh; 2005.

960. Mackenrodt, Alvin (obituary). *Zentralbl Gynäkol* 1926; 50: 1041–50.

961. Mackinley CJ. Who is Houstoun? A biography of Robert Houstoun. *J Obstet Gynaecol Br Commonw* 1973; 80: 193–200.

962. Maclean AB. Paget's disease of the vulva. *J Obstet Gynaecol* 2000; 20: 7–9.

963. Maclean AB. Vulval cancer: the past 100 years and into the next century. *J Obstet Gynaecol* 2004; 24: 491–7.

964. Maclean JS. The life of Hans Hinselmann. *Obstet Gynecol Surv* 1979; 34: 788–9.

965. MacLeod D. Then and now: a tribute to Victor Bonney. *Proc R Soc Med* 1959; 52: 223–30.

966. MacPherson R. The curious stories of drugs with two lives: a new paradigm in drug development. *J R Soc Med* 2015; 108: 255–8.

967. Maehle AH. Pharmacological experimentation with opium in the eighteenth century. In: Porter R, Teich M (eds) *Drugs and Narcotics in History.* Cambridge: Cambridge University Press; 1995, p. 61.

968. Magalini SI, Magalini SC, de Francisci G. *Dictionary of Medical Syndromes.* 3rd edn. Philadelphia, PA: JB Lippincott Co., 1990.

969. Magner LN. *A History of the Life Sciences.* (3rd edn). New York, NY: Marcel Dekker Inc; 2002.

970. Mahfouz N. Urinary fistulae in women. *J Obstet Gynaecol Br Emp* 1957; 64: 24–34.

971. Maier RC. Control of postpartum hemorrhage with uterine packing. *Am J Obstet Gynecol* 1993; 169: 317–23.

972. Maisel AQ. *The Hormone Quest.* New York, NY: Random House; 1965.

973. Majno G. *The Healing Hand: Man and Wound in the Ancient World.* Cambridge, MA: Harvard University Press; 1975. (Paperback edition, 1991).

974. Major RH. Hieronymus Fracastorius (1483–1553): Syphilis or the French Disease. In: *Classic Descriptions of Disease.* 2nd edn. Baltimore, MD: Charles C Thomas; 1939, pp. 41–8.

975. Maltby JR. Mendelson's syndrome. In: Maltby JR (ed.) *Notable Names in Anaesthesia.* London: Royal Society of Medicine Press; 2002, pp. 138–40.

976. Maluf NSR. History of blood tranfusion. *J Hist Med* 1954; 9: 59–107.

977. Manuel DE. Robert Lee, the uterine nervous system and a wrangle at the Royal Society 1839–1849. *J R Soc Med* 2001; 94: 645–7.

978. Marchetti, A (obituary). *Washington Post.* 27 June 1970.

979. Marker RE. The early production of steroid hormones. *CHOC News.* Pennsylvania, PA: Center for History of Medicine, University of Pennsylvania. 1987; 2: 3–6.

980. Marland H. *Dangerous Motherhood: Insanity and Childbirth in Victorian Britain.* Basingstoke: Palgrave Macmillan; 2004.

981. Marks LV. *Sexual Chemistry: A History of the Contraceptive Pill.* New Haven, CT: Yale University Press; 2010.

982. Marland H (ed.) *The Art of Midwifery: Early Modern Midwives in Europe*. London: Routledge; 1993.

983. Marr JP. Historical background of the treatment of placenta praevia. *Bull Hist Med* 1941; 9: 258–93.

984. Marr JP. *Pioneer Surgeons of the Women's Hospital* Philadelphia, PA: FA Davis Company; 1957.

985. Marshall CH. Willett's forceps in placenta praevia. *J Obstet Gynaecol Br Emp* 1935; 42: 199–203.

986. Marshall CM. Neglected shoulder presentation: decapitation by the Blond-Heidler instrument. *J Obstet Gynaecol Br Emp* 1937; 44: 735–40.

987. Marshall CM. *Caesarean Section: Lower Segment Operation*. Bristol: John Wright & Sons Ltd; 1939.

988. Marshall, Charles McIntosh (obituary). *J Obstet Gynaecol Br Emp* 1954; 61: 835–6.

989. Marshall, Charles McIntosh (obituary). *BMJ* 1954; 2: 875–8.

990. Marshall J. On the employment of the heat of electricity in practical surgery. *Archives of the Royal Society of Medicine.* 1827: 221–31.

991. Marston AD. A short survey of the life and work of Joseph Clover. *Med Press* 1946; 226: 455–8.

992. Marston AD. Life and achievements of Joseph Thomas Clover. *Ann R Coll Surg Engl* 1949; 4: 267–80.

993. Martin, August Eduard (obituary). *Trans Am Gynecol Soc* 1934; 59: 353.

994. Martin C. Reminiscences of Lawson Tait. *J Obstet Gynaecol Br Emp* 1921; 28: 117–23.

995. Martin PL, Breese MW (eds) *Trans Pacific Coast Obstet Gynecol Soc* 1969; 37.

996. Martini JA, Bacon DR, Vasdev GM. Edward Tuohy: the man, his needle and its place in obstetric analgesia. *Reg Anesth Pain Med* 2002; 27: 520–3.

997. Marx GF, Katsnelson T. The introduction of nitrous oxide analgesia into obstetrics. *Obstet Gynecol* 1992; 80: 715–18.

998. Marzano DA, Haefner HK. The Bartholin gland cyst: past, present and future. *J Low Genit Tract Dis* 2004; 8: 195–204.

999. Mather GR. *Two Great Scotsmen: The Brothers William and John Hunter*. Glasgow: Maclehose; 1893.

1000. Mathers H, McIntosh T. *Born in Sheffield: A History of the Women's Health Services, 1864–2000*. Barnsley: Wharncliffe Books; 2000.

1001. Mathieu A. The history of hysterectomy. *West Surg Obstet Gynecol* 1934; 42: 1–13.

1002. Matthews ET. R Lawson Tait: his influence on anaesthetic practice. In: Barr AM, Boulton TB, Wilkinson DJ (eds) *Essays on the History of Anaesthesia*: London: Royal Society of Medicine Press Ltd; 1996, pp. 152–6.

1003. Mattingly RF, Thompson JD. *Te Linde's Operative Gynecology*. 6th edn. Philadelphia, PA: JB Lippincott Co; 1985.

1004. Maude A. *Marie Stopes: Her Work and Play*. London: Peter Davies; 1933.

1005. Mayer A. Gustav Adolf Walcher. *Zentralbl Gynäkol* 1935; 59: 2705–6.

1006. Maylard, Alfred Ernest (obituary). *Glasgow Med J* 1947; 28: 337–41.

1007. Maynard A, Chalmers I (eds) Non-Random Reflections on Health Services Research: On the 25th Anniversary of Archie Cochrane's *Effectiveness and Efficiency*. London: BMJ; 1997.

1008. Mayo Clinic. EB Tuohy. In: *Physicians of the Mayo Clinic and the Mayo Foundation*. Minneapolis, MN: University of Minnesota Press; 1937, pp. 1389–90.

1009. Mayo WJ. Sister Mary Joseph (1856–1939): In Memoriam. *St Mary's Alumnae Quarterly* (Rochester, MN) 1939; 23: 6.

1010. McCarl MR. Publishing the works of Nicholas Culpeper, astrological herbalist and translator of Latin medical works in seventeenth-century London. *Can Bull Med Hist* 1996; 13: 225–76.

1011. McClintock A. On the rise of the Dublin school of midwifery; with memoirs of Sir Fielding Ould, and Dr JC Fleury. *Dublin Quart J Med Sci* 1858; 25: 1–20.

1012. McCook A. Sune K Bergström (obituary). *Lancet* 2004; 364: 930.

1013. McCredie J. *Beyond Thalidomide: Birth Defects Explained*. London: RSM Press; 2007.

1014. McDonald E. The diagnosis of early pregnancy: with report of one hundred cases and special reference to the sign of flexibility of the isthmus of the uterus. *Am J Obstet Dis Women Child* 1908; 57: 323–46.

1015. McDonald, Ian Alexander (obituary). *Aust NZ J Obstet Gynaecol* 1990; 20: 96.

1016. McFadyen RE. Thalidomide in America: a brush with tragedy. *Clio Medica* 1976; 11: 79–93.

1017. McGowan SW. Sir James Young Simpson: Bart 150 years on. *Scot Med J* 1997; 42: 185–7.

1018. McGregor DK. *From Midwives to Medicine: The Birth of American Gynecology*. New Brunswick, NJ: Rutgers University Press; 1998.

1019. McIlwaine G. Two wise men. *Br J Obstet Gynaecol* 1985; 92: 113–4.

1020. McIntyre N. Medical statues: Ignac Fülöp Semmelweis (1818–65). *J Med Biog* 2009; 17: 22.

1021. McKay WJS. *The History of Ancient Gynecology.* London: Baillière, Tindall & Cox; 1901.

1022. McKay WJS. *Lawson Tait: His Life and Work.* New York, NY: William Wood and Company; 1922.

1023. McKechnie, RC. William Harvey. *Resuscitation* 2002; 55: 133–6.

1024. McKelvey JL. In memoriam: Robert Otto Meyer (1864–1947). *Trans Am Gynec Soc* 1949; 71: 293.

1025. McLane JW. The Sloane Maternity Hospital. Report on the first series of one thousand successive confinements from January 1st, 1888 to October 1st, 1890. *Am J Obstet* 1891; 24: 385–418.

1026. McLaren A. *A History of Contraception: From Antiquity to the Present Day.* Oxford: Blackwell; 1990.

1027. McLaughlin L. *The Pill, John Rock and the Church: The Biography of a Revolution.* Boston, MA: Little, Brown and Company; 1982.

1028. McMurty LS. Master surgeons of America: Ephraim McDowell. *Surg Gynecol Obstet* 1923; 36: 286–8.

1029. McNay MB, Fleming JEE. Forty years of obstetric ultrasound, 1958–1997. *Ultrasound Med Biol* 1999; 25: 3–56.

1030. Meade RH. *An Introduction to the History of General Surgery.* Philadelphia, PA: WB Saunders Co; 1968, pp. 263.

1031. Medvei VC. *The History of Clinical Endocrinology.* New York, NY: Parthenon Publishing Group; 1993.

1032. Megison, JW. Save the Barton forceps. *Obstet Gynecol* 1993; 82: 313.

1033. Meigs, Joe Vincent (obituary). *J Obstet Gynaecol Br Commonw* 1964; 7: 310–2.

1034. Mengert WF. The origin of the male midwife. *Ann Med Hist* 1932; 4: 453–65.

1035. Mengert WF. *History of the American College of Obstetricians and Gynecologists: 1950–1970.* Chicago, IL: ACOG; 1971.

1036. Menon, Krishna. *J Obstet Gynaecol India* 1975; 25: 25–6.

1037. Menon, Krishna (obituary). *Lancet* 1988; 2: 463.

1038. Mercurio S. *La commare o riccoglitrice.* Venice: Ciotti; 1596.

1039. Merhi ZO, Awonuga AO. The role of uterine fundal pressure in the management of the second stage of labor: a reappraisal. *Obstet Gynecol Surv* 2005; 60: 599–603.

1040. Merrill JA. Cullen's sign: a historical review and report of histologic observations. *Obstet Gynecol* 1958; 12: 317–24.

1041. Mettlere L, Semm KS. Historical profile of Kurt Karl Stephen Semm, born March 23, 1927 in Munich, Germany, resident of Tucson, Arizona, USA since 1996. *J Soc Laparoendo Surg* 2003; 7: 185–8.

1042. Meyer R. A short abstract of a long life: to my friends in the United States of America. *J Hist Med* 1947; 2: 419–50.

1043. Meyer, R. *Autobiography of Dr Robert Meyer.* New York, NY: Henry Schuman; 1949.

1044. Michalas SP. The Pap test: George N. Papanicolaou (1883–1952). A screening test for the prevention of cancer of uterine cervix. *Eur J Obstet Gynecol Reprod Biol* 2000; 90: 135–8.

1045. Michler M. Soranus. In: Gillispie CC (ed.) *Dictionary of Scientific Biography.* New York, NY: Charles Scribner's Sons. 1975; 12: 538–4.

1046. Milian G. Le docteur H. Hallopeau (1842–1919). *Paris Méd* 1919; 32: 135–6.

1047. Miller AH. The origin of the word Anaesthesia. *Boston Med Surg J* 1927; 197: 1218–22.

1048. Miller M. Sir James Young Simpson. *J Obstet Gynaec Br Commonw* 1962; 69: 142–50.

1049. Milne GP. The history of midwifery in Aberdeen. *Aberdeen Univ Review* 1978; 47: 293–303.

1050. Miltenberger GW. Ectopic gestation. In: *Proceedings of the Obstetrical and Gynaecological Society of Baltimore City.* Baltimore, MD: Griffin, Curley & Co; 1890, pp. 3–23.

1051. Minnitt RJ. The history and progress of gas and air analgesia for midwifery. *Proc R Soc Med* 1944; 37: 45–8.

1052. Minnitt, Robert James (obituary). *BMJ* 1974; 1: 464.

1053. Mitchell R. Dr John Clarence Webster (1863–1950): man of two careers. *Can J Surg* 1963; 6: 407–13.

1054. Mitchell RG. The Moro reflex. *Cerebral Palsy Bull* 1960: 2: 135–41.

1055. Mitchinson W. *The Nature of Their Bodies: Women and their Doctors in Victorian Canada.* Toronto: University of Toronto Press; 1991.

1056. Miyazaki FS. The Bonney test: a reassessment. *Am J Obstet Gynecol* 1997; 177: 1322–9.

1057. Moffatt LEF, Hamilton DN, Ledingham IM. To stop his wounds, lest he do bleed to death. *J R Coll Surg Edin* 1985; 30: 73–81.

1058. Moir JC. Marion Sims and the vesico-vaginal fistula: then and now. *BMJ* 1940; 2: 773–8.

1059. Moir JC. Joseph B. DeLee. *J Obstet Gynaecol Br Emp* 1942; 49: 444–6.

1060. Moir JC. November, 1847 and its sequel. *Edin Med J* 1947; 54: 593–610.

1061. Moir JC. The history and present-day use of ergot. *Can Med Assoc J* 1955; 72: 727–34.

1062. Moir JC. Sir JY Simpson: his impact and influence. *J Obstet Gynaecol Br Commonw* 1964; 71: 171–9.

1063. Moir JC. *Munro Kerr's Operative Obstetrics*. 7th edn. London: Baillière, Tindall and Cox; 1964, pp. 858.

1064. Moir JC. The obstetrician bids, and the uterus contracts. *BMJ* 1964; 2: 1025–9.

1065. Moir JC. Edinburgh's obstetrical heritage: some names from the past. *Scot Med J* 1970; 15: 427–32.

1066. Moir JC. Ergot: from 'St Anthony's Fire' to the isolation of its active principle, ergometrine (ergonovine). *Am J Obstet Gynecol* 1974; 120: 291–6.

1067. Moir, John Chassar (obituary). *Lancet* 1977; 2: 1240.

1068. Moir, John Chassar (obituary). *BMJ* 1977; 2: 1551.

1069. Moir, J. The Chassar Moir Maternity Unit. *Montrose Review*. 28 October 1993.

1070. Moll FH, Marx FJ. A pioneer in laparoscopy and pelviscopy: Kurt Semm (1927–2003). *J Endourol* 2005; 19: 269–71.

1071. Monaghan JM. Britain and Europe, the gynaecological oncology connection. In: O'Brien PMS (ed.) *The Yearbook of Obstetrics and Gynaecology*. London: RCOG Press; 1998, pp. 15–22.

1072. Montgomery DW. Hieronymus Fracastorius, the author of the poem called Syphilis. *Ann Med Hist* 1930; 2: 406–13.

1073. Montgomery, William (obituary). *Lancet* 1860; 1: 24.

1074. Monti A. *Antonio Scarpa*. New York, NY: Vigo Press; 1957.

1075. Moore DH. The impact of IC Rubin, MD, on obstetrics and gynecology. *Obstet Gynecol Surv* 1993; 48: 589–90.

1076. Moore W. *The Knife Man: The Extraordinary Life and Times of John Hunter, father of Modern Surgery*. London: Bantam Press; 2005.

1077. Moore W. Botany and birth control. *BMJ* 2012; 345: e7208.

1078. Mörch ET, Major RH. 'Anaesthesia' (early uses of this word). *Curr Res Anesth Analg* 1954; 33: 64–8.

1079. Morris WIC. Brotherly love: an essay on the personal relations between William Hunter and his brother John. *Med Hist* 1959; 3: 20–32.

1080. Morton RS, Hudson MM. The iconography of Girolamo Fracastoro (c.1483–1553). *J Med Biog* 1999; 7: 118-21.

1081. Moschcowitz, Alexis Victor (memoir). *J Mt Sinai Hosp* 1934; 2: 26–7.

1082. Moscucci O. *The Science of Woman: Gynaecology and Gender in England, 1800–1929*. Cambridge: Cambridge University Press; 1990.

1083. Moss SW. Historical perspective: the Stroganoff method for the treatment of eclampsia. *ACOG Clin Rev* 2000; 5: 12–14.

1084. Mouton WG, Bessell JR, Maddem GJ. Looking back to the advent of modern endoscopy: 150th birthday of Maximilian Nitze. *World J Surg* 1998; 22: 1256–8.

1085. Muffly TM, Tizzano AP, Walters MD. The history and evolution of sutures in pelvic surgery. *J R Soc Med* 2011; 104: 107–112.

1086. Muir TW. Vaginal surgery for prolapse. *J Pelvic Med Surg* 2006; 12: 289–305.

1087. Müller, Johannes (obituary). *Med Times Gaz* 1858; 17: 66–8.

1088. Mundé PF. In memoriam: Friedrich Wilhelm von Scanzoni. *Am J Obstet Dis Women Child* 1891; 24: 935–8.

1089. Mundé PF. Dr J. Marion Sims: the father of modern gynaecology. *Med Record* 1894; 46: 514–5.

1090. Mundé PF. John Braxton Hicks. *Gynecol Trans* 1898; 23: 477–80.

1091. Murphy JA. *The College: A History of Queen's College Cork, 1845–1995*. Cork: Cork University Press; 1995.

1092. Murray, R Milne (obituary). *J Obstet Gynaecol Br Emp* 1904; 5: 302–3.

1093. Musacchio JM. *The Art and Ritual of Childbirth in Renaissance Italy*. New Haven, CT: Yale University Press; 1999.

1094. Mutlu S, Scully C. The person behind the eponym: Hulusi Behçet (1889–1948). *J Oral Pathol Med* 1994; 23: 289–90.

1095. Myer JEM. Historical perspective: motherhood and morality: American physicians' attitudes toward birth control. *ACOG Clin Rev* 1996; 1: 14–16.

1096. Nadeau OE, Kampmier OF. Endoscopy of the abdomen. Abdominoscopy: a preliminary study, including a summary of the literature and a description of the technique. *Surg Gynecol Obstet* 1925; 41: 259–72.

1097. Napjus JW. De hoogleeraren in de geneeskunde aan de Hoogeschool en bet Athanaeum te Franeker (1585–1843). *XII. Abraham Cyprianus. Ned tijdschr Geneesk* 1939; 83: 70–8.

1098. Nation EF. Howard Atwood Kelly (1858–1943), urologist. *J Pelvic Surg* 1997; 3: 71–4.

1099. Naylor B. The history of exfoliate cancer cytology. *Univ Mich Med Bull* 1960; 26: 289–96.

1100. Naylor B. The century of cytopathology. *Acta Cytologica* 2000; 44: 709–25.

1101. Neale AV. Was Little right? *Cerebral Palsy Bull* 1958; 1: 23–5.

1102. Needham J. *A History of Embryology*. 2nd edn. Cambridge: Cambridge University Press; 1959.

1103. Neisser, Albert (obituary). *Ztschr farztl Fortbild* 1916; 13: 519.

1104. Neisser, Albert (obituary). *Br J Dermatol* 1916; 28: 320–1.

1105. Nelson DL, Maltby JR. Virginia Apgar: a medical pioneer. *Ann R Coll Phys Surg Can* 2001; 34: 34–8.

1106. Nelson GH. Prostaglandins and reproduction. *Curr Probl Obstet Gynecol* 1980; 4: 4–33.

1107. Neuburger M. British medicine and the old Vienna Medical School. *Bull Hist Med* 1942; 12: 486–528.

1108. Neville, William Cox (obituary). *BMJ* 1904; 2: 1493.

1109. Newson SW. Pioneers in infection control: Ignaz Philip Semmelweis. *J Hosp Infect* 1993; 23: 175–87.

1110. Nicholson M, Fleming J, Spencer I. Hyaline membrane and neonatal radiology: Ian Donald's first venture into imaging research. *Scot Med J* 2005; 50: 35–7.

1111. Nicholson P. Problems encountered by early endoscopists. *Urol* 1982; 19: 114–9.

1112. Noble CP. Treatment of placenta previa: a historical and critical sketch. *Med Surg Rep* 1888; 58: 625–31.

1113. Noble RL. JB Collip, 1893–1965. *J Reprod Fertil* 1966; 11: 167–70.

1114. Noble RL. Memories of James Bertram Collip, 1892–1965. *Biographical Memorirs of Fellows of the Royal Society* 1973; 19: 234.

1115. Norman JM (ed.) *Morton's Medical Bibliography*. 5th edn. Cambridge: Scolar Press; 1991.

1116. Novak E. Life and works of Robert Meyer. *Am J Obstet Gynecol* 1947; 53: 50–64.

1117. Novak, Emil (obituary). *West J Surg Obstet Gynecol* 1957; 65: 107–110.

1118. Nowoczek P. In memoriam: Prof Dr Hans Heidler. *Wein Med Wochenschr* 1955; 42: 855.

1119. Nuland SB. The enigma of Semmelweis: an interpretation. *J Hist Med Allied Sci* 1979; 34: 255–72.

1120. Nuland SB. *The Origins of Anesthesia*. Birmingham: Classics of Medicine Library, Gryphon Editions; 1983.

1121. Nuland SB. *Doctors: The Biography of Medicine*. New York, NY: Vintage Books, Random House Inc; 1989.

1122. Nuland SB. *The Doctors' Plague*. New York, NY: WW Norton & Co; 2003.

1123. Nürnberger L. Albert Döderlein. *München Med Wochenschr* 1942; 89: 107–9.

1124. Oakley A. *The Captured Womb: A History of the Medical Care of Pregnant Women*. Oxford: Basil Blackwell; 1984.

1125. Ober WB, Sciagura C. Leydig, Sertoli, and Reinke: three anatomists who were on the ball. *Pathol Annu* 1981; 16: 1–13.

1126. O'Brien E, Crookshank A, Wolstenholme G. *A Portrait of Irish Medicine*. Swords: Ward River Press Ltd; 1984.

1127. O'Connor JL, Bloom DA. William Bovie and electrosurgery. *Surgery* 1996; 119: 390–6.

1128. O'Donnell CPF, Gibson AT, Davis PG. Pinching, electrocution, raven's beaks, and positive pressure ventilation: a brief history of neonatal resuscitation. *Arch Dis Child Fetal Neonatal Ed* 2006; 91: F369–73.

1129. O'Dowd MJ, Philipp EE. *The History of Obstetrics and Gynaecology*. New York, NY: Parthenon Publishing Group; 1994.

1130. O'Dowd MJ. *The History of Medications for Women*. New York, NY: Parthenon Publishing Group; 2001.

1131. O'Dwyer E. Cutting the cord: an obstetrical odyssey. *J Irish Med Assoc* 1958; 42: 118–23.

1132. O'Grady JP. *Modern Instrumental Delivery*. Baltimore, MD: Williams & Wilkins; 1988.

1133. O'Grady JP, Gimovsky ML, McIlhargie CJ. *Vacuum Extraction in Modern Obstetric Practice*. New York, NY: Parthenon Publishing Group; 1995.

1134. Ojanuga D. The medical ethics of the 'Father of Gynecology', Dr J. Marion Sims. *J Med Ethics* 1993; 19: 28–31.

1135. Old WL. They made surgical history in Virginia. *Va Med* 1981; 108: 273–5.

1136. Old WL, Fitchett CW. *Surgery and surgeons in Virginia, 1607–1995: an historical monograph*. Norfolk, VA: Eastern Virginia Medical School; 1997.

1137. Oleckno WA. Remembering Dr John Snow on the sesquicentennial of his death. *Can Med Assoc J* 2008; 178: 1691–2.

1138. Ollerenshaw R. Dr Hunter's 'Gravid uterus': a bicentenary note. *Med Biol Illustr* 1974; 24: 43–57.

1139. O'Malley CD. The lure of Padua. *Med Hist* 1970; 14: 1–9.

1140. Oppenheimer JM. *New Aspects of John and William Hunter*. New York, NY: Henry Schuman; 1946.

1141. Oppenheimer JM. Karl Ernst Ritter von Baer. In: Gillispie CC (ed.) *Dictionary of Scientific Biography*. New York, NY: Charles Scribner's Sons. 1970; 1: 385–9.

1142. Oppenheimer JM. *Autobiography of Dr Karl Ernst von Baer (English translation).* Canton, MA: Science History Publications; 1987.

1143. O'Rahilly R. Benjamin Alcock, Anatomist. *Ir J Med Sci* 1947; 6: 622.

1144. O'Rahilly R. *Benjamin Alcock: The First Professor of Anatomy and Physiology in Queen's College, Cork.* Oxford: Cork University Press; 1948.

1145. Oriel JD. Emminent venerologists I: Albert Neisser. *Genitourin Med* 1989; 65: 229–34.

1146. Oriel JD. *The Scars of Venus: A History of Venerology.* London: Springer-Verlag; 1994.

1147. Osler W. Oliver Wendell Holmes. *Bull Johns Hopkins Hosp.* 1894; 5: 85–8.

1148. Osler W. Sir Thomas Browne. *BMJ* 1905; 2: 993–8.

1149. Osler W. *An Alabama Student and other Biographical Essays.* London: Oxford University Press; 1908.

1150. O'Sullivan EP. Dr Robert J Minnitt, 1889–1974: a pioneer of inhalational analgesia. *J R Soc Med* 1989; 82: 221–2.

1151. O'Sullivan, JV (obituary). *BMJ* 1976; 1: 590–1.

1152. O'Sullivan, JV (obituary). *Lancet* 1976; 1: 598–9.

1153. Otis EO. The medical achievements of Dr Holmes. *Boston Med Surg J* 1909; 69: 95.

1154. Oudshoorn N. *Beyond the Natural Body: An Archeology of Sex Hormones.* London: Routledge; 1994.

1155. Outwin EL. The development of the modern catheter. *Am Surg Trade Assoc J* 1955; 2: 47–55.

1156. Packard FR. *History of Medicine in the United States.* (Vol. 2) New York, NY: Paul B. Holber Inc; 1932.

1157. Paget S (ed.) *Memoirs and Letters of Sir James Paget.* London: Longmans, Green & Co; 1901.

1158. Pajot, Charles (obituary). *BMJ* 1896; 2: 538.

1159. Palmer AC. Changing practice in obstetrics and gynaecology. *Proc R Soc Med* 1953; 46: 81–5.

1160. Palmer, Raoul (obituary). *Lancet* 1985: 2: 568.

1161. Palmer, Raoul (obituary). *Acta Eur Fertil* 1985; 16: 309–10.

1162. Paneth N. Birth and the origins of cerebral palsy. *N Engl J Med* 1986; 315: 124–6.

1163. Paneth N. Apgar score and risk of cerebral palsy. *BMJ* 2010; 341: 788–9.

1164. Papanicolaou-Kokkori M. *George N. Papanicolaou MD, PhD: Life and Career, the Way to the Pap Test.* New York, NY: Hellenic Medical Society; 2008.

1165. Parker GH. Anthony van Leeuwenhoek and his microscopes. *Sci Monthly* 1933; 37: 434–41.

1166. Parkes AS. The rise of reproductive endocrinology, 1926–1940. *J Endocrinol* 1966; 34: 19–32.

1167. Parkhurst C. *In memoriam: J. Marion Sims.* New York, NY: GP Putnam's Sons, Inc; 1884.

1168. Parry-Jones E. *Kielland's Forceps.* London: Butterworth & Co; 1952.

1169. Parry-Jones E. *Barton's Forceps.* London: Sector Publishing Ltd; 1972.

1170. Partridge HG. History of the obstetric forceps. *Am J Obstet Dis Women Child* 1905; 51: 765–73.

1171. Parvin T. Marmaduke Burr Wright. *Trans Am Gynecol Soc* 1880; 4: 433–7.

1172. Pasquale M, Paulshock BZ. Christian Doppler (1803–1853): an ingenious theory, an important effect. *J Lab Clin Med* 1991; 118: 384–6.

1173. Paul O. Doctor's autobiographies. *J Med Biog* 1997; 5: 102–15.

1174. Pawlik, Karl (obituary). *Mschr f Geburtsch Gynäk* 1914; 11: 684–6.

1175. Pawlik, Karl. In Keene FE (ed.) Album of the Fellows of the American Gynecological Society, 1876–1930. Philadelphia, PA: Wm Dornan; 1930, p. 450.

1176. Peachey GC. Matthew Baillie, MD. *Med Press Circ* 1930; 180: 472–4.

1177. Peachey GC. William Hunter's obstetrical career. *Ann Med Hist* 1930; 2: 476–9.

1178. Pearlman SJ. Bozzini's classical treatise on endoscopy: a translation. *Q Bull North-Western Univ Med School* 1949; 23: 332–54.

1179. Peck HT. On Monsel's salt. *Am J Pharmacol* 1862; 34: 201–4.

1180. Peckham CH. A brief history of puerperal infection. *Bull Hist Med* 1935; 3: 182–90.

1181. Peel J. A century of obstetrics. *The Practitioner.* 1968; 201: 85–90.

1182. Peel J. A historical review of diabetes and pregnancy. *J Obstet Gynaecol Br Cwlth* 1972; 79: 385–95.

1183. Peel J. *The Lives of the Fellows of the Royal College of Obstetricians and Gynaecologists, 1929–1969.* London: William Heinemann; 1976.

1184. Peel J. The Royal College of Obstetricians and Gynaecologists, 1929 to 1979. *Br J Obstet Gynaecol* 1979; 86: 673–92.

1185. Peel J. *William Blair-Bell: Father and Founder.* London: RCOG; 1986.

1186. Peel J. *The Gynaecological Visiting Society 1911–1971.* Dorchester: Dorset Press; 1992.

1187. Peel KR. Reginald Hamlin 1908–1993. In: Studd J (ed.) *The Yearbook of the Royal College of*

Obstetricians and Gynaecologists. London: RCOG Press; 1994, pp. 1–2.

1188. Peller S. Studies on mortality since the Renaissance. *Bull Med Hist* 1943; 13: 427–61.

1189. Peller S. Dr Kasper Blond, 1889–1964 (obituary). *Pirquet Bulletin of Clinical Medicine* 1965; 12: 13–4.

1190. Penfield AJ. The Filshie clip for female sterilization: a review of world experience. *Am J Obstet Gynecol* 2000; 182: 485–9.

1191. Penman WR. William Goodell, MD and the Preston Retreat. *Trans Coll Phys Philadelphia* 1972; 73: 112–9.

1192. Penzias AS, DeCherney AH. History of ectopic pregnancy. In: Stovall TG, Ling FW (eds) *Extrauterine Pregnancy*. New York, NY: McGraw-Hill Inc; 1993, pp. 1–7.

1193. Perkins W. Midwives versus doctors: the case of Louise Bourgeois. *Seventeenth Century* 1988; 3: 135–57.

1194. Perkins W. *Midwifery and Medicine in Early Modern France: Louise Bourgeois*. Exeter: University of Exeter Press; 1996.

1195. Perri AJ, Hsu S. A review of thalidomide's history and current dermatological applications. *Dermatology Online Journal* 9(3): 5. Retrieved 23 December 2016.

1196. Persaud TVN. *Problems of Birth Defects: From Hippocrates to Thalidomide and After*. Baltimore, MD: University Park Press; 1977.

1197. Persaud TVN. *Early History of Human Anatomy*. Springfield, IL: Charles C Thomas; 1984.

1198. Persaud TVN. *A History of Anatomy: The Post-Vesalian Era*. Springfield, IL: Charles C Thomas; 1997.

1199. Petersen W. *Malthus*. Cambridge, MA: Harvard Univ Press; 1979.

1200. Pfannenstiel, Herman J (obituary). *J Obstet Gynaecol Br Emp* 1909; 16: 274.

1201. Pfeffer N. *The Stork and the Syringe: A Political History of Reproductive Medicine*. Cambridge: Polity Press; 1993.

1202. Philip AGS. The evolution of neonatology. *Ped Res* 2005; 58: 799–815.

1203. Phillips MH. The history of the prevention of puerperal fever. *BMJ* 1938; 1: 1–7.

1204. Phillips MH. Percivall Willughby's *Observations in Midwifery*. *J Obstet Gynaecol Br Emp* 1952; 59: 753–62.

1205. Pickrell KL. An inquiry into the history of cesarean section. *Bull Soc Med Hist* 1935; 4: 414–53.

1206. Pijnenborg R. Manipulating human reproduction: a retrospective view on Aldous Huxley's *Brave New World*. *Gynecol Obstet Invest* 2006; 61: 149–54.

1207. Pilcher LS. Tribute to George Ryerson Fowler. *Brooklyn Med J* 1906; 20: 114–7.

1208. Pincock S. David Barker (obituary). *Lancet* 2013; 382: 1170.

1209. Pincus G. *The Control of Fertility*. New York, NY and London: Academic Press; 1965.

1210. Pinkerton JHM. Kergaradec, friend of Laennec and pioneer of foetal auscultation. *Proc R Soc Med* 1969; 62: 477–83.

1211. Pinkerton JHM. Fetal auscultation-some aspects of its history and evolution. *Ir Med J* 1976; 69: 363–8.

1212. Pinkerton JHM. John Creery Ferguson (1802–1865): physician and fetologist. *Ulster Med J* 1981; 50: 10–20.

1213. Pinkerton JHM. Evory Kennedy: a master controversial. *Ir Med J* 1984; 77: 77–81.

1214. Pinto-Carreia C. *The Ovary of Eve: Egg and Sperm and Preformation*. Chicago, IL: University of Chicago Press; 1997.

1215. Pipkin FB. The development of fetal physiology over the 20th century: contribution to obstetric practice. In: O'Brien PMS (ed.) *The Yearbook of Obstetrics and Gynaecology*. London: RCOG Press; 2000, pp. 51–60.

1216. Piscacek, Ludwig (obituary). *Zentralbl Gynäkol* 1932; 56: 2690.

1217. Pitcock CD, Clark RB. From Fanny to Fernand: the development of consumerism in pain control during the birth process. *Am J Obstet Gynecol* 1992; 167: 581–7.

1218. Pitkin RM. Classic articles: Friedman EA. Primigravid labor: a graphic statistical analysis. *Obstet Gynecol* 2003; 101: 216.

1219. Pitkin RM. Classic Articles: McCall ML. Posterior culdeplasty. *Obstet Gynecol* 2003; 101: 625.

1220. Pitkin RM. Classic Articles: Bishop EH. *Pelvic scoring for elective induction*. *Obstet Gynecol* 2003; 101: 846.

1221. Pitkin RM. Classic Articles. Potter EL. *Bilateral absence of ureters and kidneys: a report of 50 cases*. *Obstet Gynecol* 2003; 101: 1159.

1222. Pittinger CB. The anesthetization of Fanny Longfellow for childbirth on April 7, 1847. *Anesth Analg* 1987; 66: 368–9.

1223. Platt WB. Johannes Müller, a university teacher. *Johns Hopkins Hosp Bull* 1896; 7: 16–8.

1224. Playfair WS. Dr Barnes' water bags. *Med Times Gaz* 1869; 2: 392–3.

1225. Plentyl AA, Stone RE. The Bracht maneuver. *Obstet Gynecol Surv* 1953; 8: 313–25.

1226. Pollitzer, Sigmund (obituary). *Arch Dermat Syphil* 1938; 37: 499–503.

1227. Porro, Edoardo (obituary). *J Obstet Gynaecol Br Emp* 1902; 2: 405–7.

1228. Porter IA. *Alexander Gordon, MD of Aberdeen, 1752–1799*. Edinburgh: Oliver & Boyd; 1958.

1229. Porter ML. Dr Lyman Guy Barton, Senior. *NY State J Med* 1945; 45: 1094–6.

1230. Porter R. *The Greatest Benefit to Mankind: A Medical History of Humanity from Antiquity to the Present*. London: Harper Collins Publishers; 1997.

1231. Porter W. Alexander Couvelaire. *Bull Acad Nat Med* 1948; 132: 341–3.

1232. Potter NW. George Ryerson Fowler (obituary) *Buffalo Med J* 1906; 61: 449–56.

1233. Pottiee-Sperry F. The hysterotomotokie or 'Caesarean Birth' of Francois Rousset (Paris 1581). The book of an imposter or that of a precursor? *Hist Sci Med* 1996; 30: 259–68.

1234. Powell JL. Hulka tenaculum and clip. *J Pelvic Surg* 1999; 5: 181–2.

1235. Powell JL. The Uchida sterilization techniques: Hajime Uchida, MD (1921–1996). *J Pelvic Surg* 2001; 7: 128–9.

1236. Powell JL. The Burch procedure: John Christopher Burch (1900–1977). *J Pelvic Surg* 2001; 7: 130–2.

1237. Powell JL. Gilliam's uterine suspension: David Tod Gilliam (1844–1923). *J Pelvic Surg* 2001; 7: 199–200.

1238. Powell JL, Gonzalez JJ. The Breisky–Navratil retractor. *J Pelvic Surg* 2002; 8: 69–71.

1239. Powell JL. Charles Bingham Penrose, MD (1862–1925). *J Pelvic Surg* 2002; 8: 129–30.

1240. Powell JL. Ian Alexander McDonald (1922–1990). *J Pelvic Surg* 2002; 8: 227–8.

1241. Powell JL. Armand Joseph Pereyra, MD (1904–1988) *J Pelvic Surg* 2002; 8: 229–30.

1242. Powell JL. Biographic sketch: Hans Peter Hinselmann, MD (1884–1959). *Obstet Gynecol Surv* 2004; 59: 693–5.

1243. Powell JL. Edward Harry Bishop, MD (1913–1995). *Obstet Gynecol Surv* 2006; 61: 425–6.

1244. Powell JL. Fritz Brenner, MD (1877–1969). *J Pelvic Med Surg* 2007; 13: 43–4.

1245. Powell JL. Richard Wesley Te Linde, MD (1894–1985). *Obstet Gynecol Surv* 2007; 62: 365–6.

1246. Powell JL. John Albertson Sampson MD (1873–1946) *J Pelvic Med Surg* 2008; 14: 209–10.

1247. Powell JL, Brun JL. Leon Monsel (1817–1878) *J Pelvic Med Surg* 2008; 14: 453–4.

1248. Powell JL. Heinrich Martius, MD (1885–1965). *J Pelvic Med Surg* 2009; 15: 157–8.

1249. Poynter FNL. Nicholas Culpeper and his books. *J Hist Med* 1962; 17: 152–67.

1250. Prescott O. *A Dissertation on the Natural History and Medicinal Effects of the Secale Cornutum or Ergot*. Boston, MA: Cummings and Holliard; 1813.

1251. Preston C. *Thomas Browne and the Writing of Early Modern Science*. Cambridge: Cambridge University Press; 2005.

1252. Price JA. The early ovariotomists: pioneers in abdominal surgery. *Ulster Med J* 1967; 36: 1–12.

1253. Priest FO. Dr John Clarence Webster. *Can Med Assoc J* 1951; 64: 351–3.

1254. Pusey WA. *The History and Epidemiology of Syphilis*. Springfield, IL: Charles C Thomas; 1933.

1255. Quattlebaum JK. On Dr George R White. In: *Reminiscences*. Savannah, GA: Georgia Medical Society; 1966, pp. 12–13.

1256. Quecke K. Francois Rousset und die erste Monographie über den Kaiserschnitt. *Centaurus* 1953; 2: 349–63.

1257. Queenan JT. *The Chamberlen's Secret: How a Century of Women Were Robbed of Safe Childbirth*. Lexington, KY: John T Queenan; 2012.

1258. Quétel C. *History of Syphilis*. Baltimore, MD: Johns Hopkins University Press; 1990.

1259. Räber D. *Der Gynäkologe Max Walthard (1867–1933)*. Zurich: Juris Druck; 1991.

1260. Radcliffe W. *The Secret Instrument*. London: Wm Heinemann; 1947.

1261. Radcliffe W. *Milestones in Midwifery*. Bristol: John Wright & Sons Ltd; 1967.

1262. Radel E, Schorr JB. Erythroblastosis fetalis-historical aspects. *Jewish Memorial Hospital Bulletin: Commemorative Issue* 1965; 10: 11–24.

1263. Rae S, Wildsmith J. So just who was James Young Simpson? *Br J Anaesth* 1997; 79: 271–3.

1264. Raju TNK. Soranus of Ephesus: Who was he and what did he do? In: Smith GF, Vidyasagar D (eds) *Historical Review and Recent Advances in Neonatal and Perinatal Medicine* (Vol. 2) New York, NY: Mead Johnson Ltd; 1981, pp. 179–86.

1265. Raju TNK. History of neonatal resuscitation. *Clin Perinatol* 1999; 26: 629–40.

1266. Raju TNK. The Nobel chronicles. 1982: Sune Karl Bergström (b 1916); Bengt Ingemar Sammelsson (b 1934); John Robert Vane (b 1927). *Lancet* 1999; 354: 1914.

1267. Raju TNK. Historical perspectives: perinatal profiles. Sir Joseph Barcroft: the 20th century's renaissance perinatal physiologist. *Neoreviews* 2007; 8: e311–12.

1268. Ramachandran M, Aronson JK. John Marshall's first description of surgical electrosurgery. *J R Soc Med* 2011; 104: 355–60.

1269. Randall CL. Irving White Potter 1868–1956. *Trans Am Assoc Obstet Gynecol* 1956; 67: 227–9.

1270. Randall P, Krogman WM, Jahina S. Pierre Robin and the syndrome that bears his name. *Cleft Palate Journal* 1965; 2: 237–46.

1271. Rathert P, Lutzeyer W, Goddwin WE. Philipp Bozzini (1773–1809) and the lichtleiter. *Urology* 1974; 3: 113–8.

1272. Read, Grantly Dick (obituary). *BM J* 1959; 1: 1625.

1273. Reed CAL. Memorial address on the life and character of Lawson Tait. *JAMA* 1899; 33: 875–80.

1274. Reed J. *The Birth Control Movement in North America: From Private Vice to Public Virtue.* Princeton, NJ: Princeton University Press; 1978.

1275. Reese AB. An epitaph for retrolental fibroplasia. *Am J Ophthalmol* 1955; 40: 267–9.

1276. Reichle HS. Emil Noeggerath (1827–1895). *Ann Med Hist* 1928; 10: 77–84.

1277. Reid DE. In memoriam: Frederick Carpenter Irving. *Trans Am Gynec Soc* 1958; 81: 229–31.

1278. Reid WL. The history, forms and theories of the vaginal speculum. *Glasgow Med J* 1896; 46: 161–73.

1279. Reiss HE. John William Ballantyne 1861–1923. *J Obstet Gynaecol* 2000; 20: 343–6.

1280. Resinelli G. Leonardo Gigli. *Ginecologia* 1908; 5: 193–8.

1281. Retzius, AA (obituary). *Edin Med J* 1861; 6: 777–83.

1282. Reuter MA, Reuter HJ. The development of the cystoscope. *J Urol* 1968; 159: 638–40.

1283. Rey R. *The History of Pain. Translated by LE Wallace, JA Cadden and SW Cadden.* Cambridge, MA: Harvard University Press; 1998.

1284. Rhodes P. The Bartholin family. *J Obstet Gynaecol Br Emp* 1957; 64: 741–3.

1285. Rhodes P. A critical appraisal of the obstetric forceps. *J Obstet Gynaecol Br Emp* 1958; 65: 353–9.

1286. Rhodes P. Edmund Chapman. *J Obstet Gynaecol Br Commonw* 1968; 75: 793–9.

1287. Rhodes P. *Doctor John Leake's Hospital.* London: Davis-Poynter; 1977.

1288. Ricci JV. *One Hundred Years of Gynecology: 1800–1900.* Philadelphia, PA: Blakiston Co; 1945.

1289. Ricci JV. The vaginal speculum and its modifications throughout the ages. In: *Contributions of the Department of Gynaecology of the City Hospital,* New York, NY, 1948–9, pp. 1–55.

1290. Ricci JV, Thom CH, Kron WC. Cleavage planes in reconstructive vaginal surgery. *Am J Surg* 1948; 76: 354–63.

1291. Ricci JV. *The Development of Gynecological Surgery and Instruments.* Philadelphia, PA: Blakiston Company; 1949.

1292. Ricci JV. *The Genealogy of Gynecology: History of the Development of Gynecology Throughout the Ages. 2000 BC–1800 AD.* Philadelphia, PA: Blakiston Co; 1972.

1293. Richards W, Parbrook GA, Wilson J. Stanislav Klikovich (1853–1910): pioneer of nitrous oxide and oxygen analgesia. *Anaesthesia* 1976; 31: 933–40.

1294. Richardson AC. The rectovaginal septum revisited: Its relationship to rectocele and its importance in rectocele repair. *Clin Obstet Gynecol* 1993; 36: 976–83.

1295. Richardson BW. The life of John Snow, MD: a memoir. In: *Snow J. Chloroform and Other Anaesthetics: Their Action and Administration.* London: John Churchill; 1858, pp. 1–64.

1296. Riddle JM. *Contraception and Abortion from the Ancient World to the Renaissance.* Cambridge: Harvard University Press; 1992.

1297. Riddle JM. *Eve's Herbs: A History of Contraception and Abortion in the West.* Cambridge: Harvard University Press; 1997.

1298. Rigby Edward. *Letters from France in 1789.* London: Longmans, Green & Co; 1880.

1299. Riordan HD. *Medical Mavericks. Vol. II.* Wichita, KA: Bio-communications Press; 1989.

1300. Risdon W. *Robert Lawson Tait.* London: Murray, Edwards & Co Ltd; 1967.

1301. Ritgen, Ferdinand von (obituary). *Monatschr Geburtsk Frauenkrankh* 1867; 29: 443–63.

1302. Robb H. Remarks on the writings of Louise Bourgeois. *Johns Hopkins Hospital Bulletin* 1893; 4: 75–81.

1303. Robb H. Madame Boivin. *Johns Hopkins Hospital Bulletin* 1894; 4: 1–10.

1304. Robb H. The writings of Mauriceau. *Johns Hopkins Hospital Bulletin* 1895; 6: 51–7.

1305. Robb-Smith AHT. John Hunter's private press. *J Hist Med* 1970; 25: 262–9.

1306. Robb-Smith AHT. Morgagni and English medicine. In: *Proceedings of the XXIII International Congress of the History of Medicine.* London: Wellcome Institute for the History of Medicine; 1974, pp. 18–31.

1307. Roberts ADG, Baskett TF, Calder AA, Arulkumaran S. William Smellie and William Hunter: two great obstetricians and anatomists. *J R Soc Med* 2010; 103: 205–6.

1308. Roberts S. *Sir James Paget: The Rise of Clinical Surgery*. London: Royal Society of Medicine Services Ltd; 1989.

1309. Robertson WH. *An Illustrated History of Contraception*. Park Ridge, NJ: Parthenon Publishing Group; 1990.

1310. Robin, Pierre (obituary). *Rev Stomat* 1950; 51: 120.

1311. Robinson J. *Tom Cullen of Baltimore*. London: Oxford University Press; 1949.

1312. Robinson V. Guillaume Benjamin Duchenne. *Med Life* 1929; 36: 287–306.

1313. Robson M, Murphy M, Byrne F. Quality assurance: the 10-group classification system (Robson classification), induction of labour and caesarean delivery. *Int J Gynecol Obstet* 2015; 131: s23–7.

1314. Rock JA, Johnson TRB, Woodruff JD (eds). *The Department of Obstetrics and Gynecology. The Johns Hopkins University School of Medicine: The First 100 years*. Baltimore, MD: Johns Hopkins University Press; 1991.

1315. Rock JA, Warshaw JR. The history and future of operative laparoscopy. *Am J Obstet Gynecol* 1994; 170: 7–11.

1316. Rock, John (obituary). *New York Times*. 5 December 1984.

1317. Rodin AE. *The Influence of Matthew Baillie's Morbid Anatomy*. Springfield, IL: Charles C Thomas; 1973.

1318. Rodin AE. The influence of Matthew Baillie on disease concepts. In: *Proceedings of the XXIII International Congress of the History of Medicine*. London: Wellcome Institute for the History of Medicine; 1974, pp. 69–71.

1319. Roediger E. Der Frankfurter Arzt Philipp Bozzini, der Erfinder des Lichtleiters, 1773–1809. *Medizinhistorisches Journal* 1972; 7: 204–17.

1320. Roger H. Le professeur JA Sicard: sa vie et son oeuvre. *Hist Méd* 1955; 5: 61–77.

1321. Rogers FJ. William Hannah and the Hannah portrait. *J Med Biog* 1993; 1: 48–51.

1322. Rolleston H. Medical eponyms. *Ann Med Hist* 1937; 9: 1-12.

1323. Romero R. A profile of Emanuel A. Friedman. *Am J Obstet Gynecol* 2016; 215: 413–14.

1324. Romm S. The persons behind the name: Charles Bingham Penrose. *Plastic Reconstruct Surg* 1982; 70: 397–9.

1325. Roos CA. Physicians to the Presidents, and their patients: a biobibliography. *Bull Med Library Assoc* 1961; 49: 296–302.

1326. Rose E. Fitz-Hugh, Thomas (obituary). *Trans Assoc Am Phys*, 1964; 19–21.

1327. Rose J. *Marie Stopes and the Sexual Revolution*. London: Faber and Faber; 1992.

1328. Rosenberg J. In memoriam: Carl Siegmund Franz Credé. *Am J Obstet Dis Women Child* 1892; 25: 780–2.

1329. Rosenkranz G. The early days of Syntex. *Chemical Heritage* 2004; 23: 2–12.

1330. Rothschuh KE. *History of Physiology*. New York, NY: Robert E Kreiger Publishing Co; 1973.

1331. Rubin A, Rubin SC. IC Rubin: a fertile mind in the field of infertility. *J Pelvic Surg* 1997; 3: 9–10.

1332. Rucker MP. John Peter Mettauer: early southern gynecologist. *Ann Med Hist* 1938; 10: 38.

1333. Rucker MP, Rucker EM. A librarian looks at cesarean section. *Bull Hist Med* 1942; 132–48.

1334. Rucker MP. Silver sutures. *Bull Hist Med* 1950; 24: 190–2.

1335. Rudloff V, Ludwig H. Jewish gynecologists in Germany in the first half of the twentieth century. *Arch Gynecol Obstet* 2005; 272: 245–60.

1336. Rushman GB, Davies NJH, Atkinson RS. *A Short History of Anaesthesia: The First 150 Years*. Oxford: Butterworth-Heinemann; 1996.

1337. Russell KF. *British Anatomy 1525–1800: A Biography*. Melbourne: Melbourne University Press; 1963.

1338. Sakula A. *Royal Society of Medicine London: Portraits, Painting and Sculptures*. London: RSM Press, 1988.

1339. Sakula A. Sir Henry Dale (1875–1968) *J Med Biog* 1995; 3: 98.

1340. Sakula A. Joseph Clover, FRCS (1825–1882). *J Med Biog* 2004 12: 201.

1341. Saling E. Roberto Caldeyro-Barcia (obituary). *J Perinat Med* 1997; 25: 9–10.

1342. Samarrae K. Puerperal inversion of the uterus, with reference to pregnancy following Spinelli's operation. *J Obstet Gynaecol Br Emp* 1965; 72: 426–9.

1343. Sampson JA. Little biographies: VII. Fallopius, 1533–1563. *Albany Med Ann* 1906; 27: 496–9.

1344. Sandor J, Ballagi F, Nagy A, Rakoczi I. A needle-puncture that helped change the world of surgery: homage to János Veres. *Surg Endosc* 2000; 14: 201–2.

1345. Sanger, Margaret (obituary). *New York Times*. 7 September 1966.

1346. Sänger, Max (obituary). *BMJ* 1903; 1: 229.

1347. Sänger, Max (obituary). *J Obstet Gynaecol Br Emp* 1903; 3: 292–4.

1348. Satran R. Augusta Dejerine-Klumpke. *Ann Int Med* 1974; 80: 260–4.

1349. Saunders N, Patterson C. Can we abandon Naegele's rule? *Lancet* 1991; 337: 600–1.

1350. Saylan T. Life story of Dr Hulusi Behçet. *Yonsei Med J* 1997; 38: 327–32.

1351. Schachner A. *Ephraim McDowell: Father of Ovariotomy and Founder of Abdominal Surgery.* Philadelphia, PA and London: JB Lippincott Co; 1921.

1352. Schadewaedt H. Albert Ludwig Siegmund Neisser. In: Gillispie CC (ed.) *Dictionary of Scientific Biography.* New York, NY: Charles Scribner's Sons; 1974, pp. 17–9.

1353. Schifrin BS, Longo LD. William John Little and cerebral palsy: a reappraisal. *Eur J Obstet Gynecol Reprod Biol* 2000; 90: 139–44.

1354. Schiller, Walter (obituary). *Chicago Sun Times.* 5 May 1960.

1355. Schindler C. Max Madlener. *München Med Wochnschr* 1938; 85: 65–6.

1356. Schmitz HE. In memoriam: Rudolph Wieser Holmes (1870–1953). *Trans Am Gynec Soc* 1953; 76: 233–5.

1357. Schorr MR. Needles: some points to think about. *Part II. Anesth Analgesia* 1966; 45: 514–19.

1358. Schuchardt, Karl (obituary). *Deutsche Med Wochenschr* 1901; 27: 883.

1359. Schumann EA. John Montgomery Baldy, 1860–1934. *Gynecol Trans* 1935; 60: 339–42.

1360. Schumann EA. In memoriam: Milton Lawrence McCall 1911–1963. *Trans Am Gynec Soc* 1964; 87: 171–4.

1361. Schutte H, Herman JR. Philipp Bozzini (1773–1809). *Invest Urol* 1972; 9: 447–8.

1362. Scott JA. Concerning the Fothergill pictures at the Pennsylvania Hospital. *Univ Penn Med Bull* 1904; 16: 338–93.

1363. Scott JC, Hunt AB, Keys TE. A note on William Hunter's monograph The Anatomy of the Human Gravid Uterus. *Mayo Clin Proc* 1964; 39: 197–204.

1364. Scott WA. The development of the cystoscope: from 'Lichtleiter' to fiber optics. *Invest Urol* 1969; 6: 657–61.

1365. Sedlacek TV. Development and implementation of colposcopy in the United States. *J Pelvic Surg* 1998; 4: 57–61.

1366. Semm K, Giese KP. Ernst Gräfenberg: the life and work of the specialist of Kiel on the hundredth anniversary of his birth on 26 September 1881. *Int J Fertil* 1983; 28: 141–8.

1367. Semm K, Weichart-von Hassel M. (eds) *Kiel University Hospital of Gynecology and Michaelis School of Midwifery: Its Contributions to Gynecology from 1805 to 1985.* Alpendruck; 1985.

1368. Semm K. Gustav Adolf Michaelis (1798–1848). *Zentrabl fur Gynäkol* 1988; 110: 1234–42.

1369. Senior A. Friedrich Berthold Reinke (1862–1919): brilliant yet troubled anatomist. *J Laryngol Otol* 2015; 129: 1053–7.

1370. Senn N. The early history of vaginal hysterectomy. *Chicago Med Rec* 1895; 8: 333–49.

1371. Setchell BP. The contributions of Regnier de Graaf to reproductive biology. *Eur J Obstet Gynecol* 1974; 4: 1–13.

1372. Shah M. Premier chirurgien du roi: the life of Ambroise Paré (1510–1590). *J R Soc Med* 1992; 85: 292–4.

1373. Shampo MA. Modern midwifery: Hendrik van Deventer to the present. *J Pelvic Surg* 1996; 2: 334–6.

1374. Shampo MA, Kyle RA. Sune Bergström: Nobel Prize for prostaglandin studies. *Mayo Clin Proc* 1998; 73: 462–4.

1375. Shampo MA. Ambroise Paré: father of modern surgery. *J Pelvic Surg* 1998; 4: 186–8.

1376. Shampo MA. Hermann Johan Pfannenstiel and the Pfannenstiel incision. *J Pelvic Surg* 1998; 4: 312–4.

1377. Shampo MA. George Papanicolaou: the 'pap-smear'. *J Pelvic Surg* 2000; 6: 174–7.

1378. Shampo MA. Landsteiner, Wiener, and Levine: the story of blood groups. *J Pelvic Surg* 2000; 6: 232–5.

1379. Shampo MA. Margaret Sanger: pioneer in the birth control movement. *J Pelvic Surg* 2000; 6: 307–9.

1380. Shampo MA. Tests, signs, and indications of pregnancy. *J Pelvic Surg* 2001; 7: 133–5.

1381. Shampo MA. The pill: its history and development (the 40th anniversary). *J Pelvic Surg* 2001; 7: 196–81.

1382. Shampo MA. Howard A. Kelly: pioneer American surgeon. *J Pelvic Surg* 2001; 7: 324–6.

1383. Shampo MA. Friedrich Trendelenburg: the Trendelenburg position. *J Pelvic Surg* 2001; 7: 327–9.

1384. Shampo MA. The world's first 'test-tube baby': gynecologist Steptoe and physiologist Edwards. *J Pelvic Surg* 2002; 8: 120–2.

1385. Shapiro SM. Ina May Gaskin and the battle for at-home births. *New York Times Magazine.* 23 May 2012.

1386. Sharp J. *The Midwives Book: On the Whole Art of Midwifry Discovered. Edited by Elaine Hobby*. Oxford: Oxford University Press; 1999.

1387. Shaw AB. *Norfolk and Norwich Medicine: A Retrospect*. Norwich: Norwich Medico-Chirurgical Society; 1992.

1388. Shaw AB. Sir Thomas Browne, physician and man of letters, with an account of his skull. *J Med Biog* 1993; 1: 230–5.

1389. Shaw PA. The history of cervical screening: the Pap test. *J Soc Obstet Gynaecol Can* 2000; 22: 110–14.

1390. Shaw WF. Archibald Donald. *J Obstet Gynaecol Br Emp* 1937; 44: 527–35.

1391. Shaw WF. The Manchester operation for genital prolapse. *J Obstet Gynaecol Br Emp* 1947; 54: 632–5.

1392. Shaw WF. The birth of a College. *J Obstet Gynaecol Br Emp* 1950; 57: 875–89.

1393. Shaw WF. Charles Clay: the father of ovariotomy in England. *J Obstet Gynaecol Br Emp* 1952; 58: 930–40.

1394. Shaw WF. The College: its past, present and future. *J Obstet Gynaecol Br Emp* 1954; 61: 557–66.

1395. Shaw WF. *Twenty-Five Years: The Story of the Royal College of Obstetricians and Gynaecologists, 1929–1954*. London: J & A Churchill Ltd; 1954.

1396. Sheehan, Harold Leeming (obituary). *BMJ* 1988; 297: 1465.

1397. Sheffey IC. The earlier history and transition period of obstetrics and gynecology in Philadelphia. *Ann Hist Med* 1940; 2: 215–24.

1398. Shelley WB, Crissey JT. *Classics in Clinical Dermatology with Biographical Sketches. Second Printing*. Springfield, IL: Charles C Thomas; 1970.

1399. Shephard DAE. John Snow and research. *Can J Anaesth* 1989; 36: 224–41.

1400. Shephard DAE. *John Snow: Anaesthetist to a Queen and Epidemiologist to a Nation. A Biography*. Chapel Hill, NC: Professional Press; 1995.

1401. Shephard DAE, Baskett TF. John Snow and resuscitation. *Resuscitation* 2001; 49: 3–7.

1402. Shepherd JA. *Spencer Wells, The Life and Work of a Victorian Surgeon*. Edinburgh: E & S Livingstone Ltd; 1965.

1403. Shepherd JA. *Simpson and Syme of Edinburgh*. Edinburgh: E & S Livingstone; 1969.

1404. Shepherd JA. *Lawson Tait, the Rebellious Surgeon*. Lawrence, KA: Coronado Press; 1980.

1405. Shirodkar VN. *Contributions to Obstetrics and Gynaecology*. Edinburgh and London: E & S Livingstone Ltd; 1960.

1406. Shirodkar, Vithal Nagesh (obituary). *J Obstet Gynaecol India* 1971; 21: 261–3.

1407. Siddal AC. Bloodletting in American obstetric practice, 1800–1945. *Bull Hist Med* 1980; 54: 101–10.

1408. Siebold EGJ de. *Essai d'une Histoire de l'Obstétricie*. Vol. 2. Paris: G. Steinheil; 1891.

1409. Siegler AM. *Hysterosalpingography*. 2nd edn. New York, NY: Medcom Press; 1974, pp. 1–4.

1410. Siegler AM, Grunebaum A. The 100th anniversary of tubal sterilsation. *Fertil Steril* 1980; 34: 610–13.

1411. Sigerist HE, Soranus of Ephesus. In: *The Great Doctors: A Biographical History of Medicine*. New York, NY: Wm Norton & Co; 1933.

1412. Sigerist HE. Developments and trends in gynecology. *Am J Obstet Gynecol* 1941; 42: 714–22.

1413. Silverberg SG. Arias-Stella phenomenon in spontaneous and therapeutic abortion. *Am J Obstet Gynecol* 1972; 112: 777–80.

1414. Simmer HH. On the history of hormonal contraception I. Ludwig Haberlandt and his concept of 'hormonal sterilization'. *Contraception* 1970; 1: 3–27.

1415. Simmer HH. Robert Tuttle Morris (1857–1945): a pioneer in ovarian transplants. *Obstet Gynecol* 1970; 35: 314–28.

1416. Simmer HH. On the history of hormonal contraception II. Otto Fellner and estrogens as antifertility hormones. *Contraception* 1971; 3: 1–20.

1417. Simmons JG. *Doctors and Discoveries: Lives that Created Today's Medicine*. Boston, MA: Houghton Mifflin Company; 2002.

1418. Simmons SF, Hunter J. *William Hunter, 1718–1783: A Memoir*. Glasgow: University of Glasgow Press; 1983.

1419. Simpson AR. Introductory lecture on the Ninth International Medical Congress and American gynaecology. *BMJ* 1887; 2: 977–82.

1420. Simpson AR. The invention and evolution of the midwifery forceps. *Scot Med Surg J* 1900; 7: 465–95.

1421. Simpson JY, *Anaesthetic Midwifery: Report on its Early History and Progress*. Edinburgh: Sutherland and Knox; 1848.

1422. Simpson JY. The funeral of Sir James Simpson. *BMJ* 1870; 1: 526.

1423. Simpson, James Young (obituary). *BMJ* 1870; 1: 505–7.

1424. Simpson M. *Simpson the Obstetrician*. London: Victor Gollancz; 1972.

1425. Sims JM. *The Story of My Life*. New York, NY: Da Capo Press; 1968.(Republication of 1st edn, 1884).

1426. Sinclair WJ. *Semmelweis: His Life and His Doctrine.* Manchester: Manchester University Press; 1909.

1427. Singleton HM. Historical perspective: the lesser known Dr Sims. *ACOG Clin Rev* 2009; 14: 13–16.

1428. Skene, Alexander (obituary). *Proc Conn St Med Soc* 1901; 5: 276–9.

1429. Skene, Alexander Johnston Chalmers (obituary). *Am J Obstet Dis Women Child* 1900; 42: 712–4.

1430. Skippen M, Kirkup J, Maxton RM, McDonald SW. The chain saw: a Scottish invention. *Scot Med J* 2004; 49: 72–5.

1431. Skolnick AA. Apgar quartet plays perinatologist's instruments. *JAMA* 1997; 277: 1939–40.

1432. Slater SD, Dow DA (eds) *The Victoria Infirmary of Glasgow, 1890–1990. A Centenary History.* Glasgow: Victoria Infirmary; 1990.

1433. Slater SD. Alfred Ernest Maylard, 1855–1947: Glasgow surgeon extraordinaire. *Scot Med J* 1994; 39: 86–90.

1434. Slemans JM. *John Whitridge Williams: Academic Aspects and Bibliography.* Baltimore, MD: Johns Hopkins Press; 1935.

1435. Smibert J. Centenary of antenatal care. *Aust Fam Physician* 1978; 9: 1083–4.

1436. Smith, Albert (obituary). *Buffalo Med Surg J* 1886; 25: 329.

1437. Smith, Albert (obituary). *New Orleans Med Surg J* 1886; 13: 664.

1438. Smith M. Summer outing to Norwich. *J R Soc Med* 1996; 89: 297–8.

1439. Smith WDA. A history of nitrous oxide and oxygen anaesthesia. Part 1A: the discovery of nitrous oxide and oxygen. *Br J Anaesth* 1972; 44: 297–304.

1440. Smith WDA. *Under the Influence: A History of Nitrous Oxide and Oxygen Anaesthesia.* London: MacMillan Publishers Ltd; 1982.

1441. Smith YR, Haefner HK. Vulvar lichen sclerosus: pathophysiology and treatment. *Am J Clin Dermatol* 2004; 5: 105–25.

1442. Smithells, Richard Worthington (obituary). *BMJ* 2002; 325: 445.

1443. Smyly W. De la kraurosis vulvae, par Breisky (Revue des Journaux). *L'Union Med* 1885; 40: 452.

1444. Snow J. *On Chloroform and Other Anaesthetics: Their Action and Administration.* London: John Churchill; 1858. Also published in: The Classics of Obstetrics and Gynecology Library. New York, NY: Gryphon Editions; 1993 (facsimile).

1445. Snow SJ. John Snow, MD (1813–1858). Part I: a Yorkshire childhood and family life. *J Med Biog* 2000; 8: 27–31.

1446. Snow SJ. John Snow, MD (1813–1858). Part II: becoming a doctor – his medical training and early years of practice. *J Med Biog* 2000; 8: 71–7.

1447. Snow SJ. *Operations Without Pain: The Practice and Science of Anaesthesia in Victorian Britain.* Basingstoke: Palgrave Macmillan; 2006.

1448. Soferman N. Professor Joseph G Asherman. *Harefuah* 1969; 76: 32–5.

1449. Solinas A, Classen M. Phillip Bozzini: a true pioneer of endoscopy. *Int J Gastroenterol* 1985; 17: 43–5.

1450. Sonntag E. Hegar's sign of pregnancy. *Am J Obstet Dis Women Child* 1892; 26: 145–51.

1451. Souchon E. Reminiscences of Dr J Marion Sims in Paris. *Am J Obstet Dis Women Child* 1895; 31: 297.

1452. Sourkes T. *Nobel Prize winners in Medicine and Physiology, 1901–1965.* London: Abelard-Schuman ;1967.

1453. Spalding P. *The History of the Medical College of Georgia.* Athens, GA: University of Georgia Press; 1987.

1454. Sparkman RS. The woman in the case, Jane Todd Crawford, 1763–1842. *Ann Surg* 1979; 189: 529–45.

1455. Sparkman RS (ed.) *The Southern Surgical Association: The First 100 years, 1887–1987.* Philadelphia, PA: JB Lippincott Co; 1989.

1456. Speert H. Gabriele Fallopio and the Fallopian tubes. *Obstet Gynecol* 1955; 6: 467–70.

1457. Speert H. James Douglas and the peritoneal cul-de-sac. *Surg Gynecol Obstet* 1955; 101: 495–501.

1458. Speert H. Alfred Hegar: Hegar's sign and dilators. *Obstet Gynecol* 1955; 6: 679–83.

1459. Speert H. Friedrich Krukenberg and ovarian tumors. *Cancer* 1955; 8: 869–71.

1460. Speert H. Cloquet's Node, Basset's operation and cancer of the vulva. *Cancer* 1955; 8: 1083–6.

1461. Speert H. Giovanni Battista Morgagni and the hydatids of Morgagni. *Am J Clin Path* 1955; 25: 1341–8.

1462. Speert H. Champetier de Ribes, James Ditmars Vorhees and their metreurynters. *Bull Sloane Hosp for Women* 1956; 2: 13–20.

1463. Speert H. Martin Naboth and cervical cysts. *Fertil Steril* 1956; 7: 66–70.

1464. Speert H. Alfred Spalding and his sign of fetal death in utero. *Bull Sloane Hosp for Women* 1956; 2: 109–14.

1465. Speert H. Fritz Brenner and Brenner tumours of the ovary. *Cancer* 1956; 9: 217–21.

1466. Speert H. John Braxton Hicks, bipolar version, and the contractions of the pregnant uterus. *J Obstet Gynaecol Br Emp* 1956; 63: 268–71.

1467. Speert H. John Clarence Webster, John Montgomery Baldy and their operation for uterine retroversion. *Surg Gynecol Obstet* 1956; 102: 377–80.

1468. Speert H. Edmund Brown Piper and his forceps for the aftercoming head. *Surg Gynecol Obstet* 1956; 103: 367–70.

1469. Speert H. Reinier de Graaf and the Graafian follicles. *Obstet Gynecol* 1956; 7: 582–8.

1470. Speert H. Thomas Wharton and the jelly of the umbilical cord. *Obstet Gynecol* 1956; 8: 380–2.

1471. Speert H. Ernst Wertheim and his operation for uterine cancer. *Cancer* 1956; 9: 859–65.

1472. Speert H. Alexander Skene and the paraurethral ducts. *J Obstet Gynaecol Br Emp* 1956; 63: 908–10.

1473. Speert H. Léon Le Fort and his operation for uterine prolapse. *Surg Gynecol Obstet* 1957; 104: 121–4.

1474. Speert H. Friedrich Trendelenburg and the Trendelenburg position. *Surg Gynecol Obstet* 1957; 105: 114–9.

1475. Speert H. Francois Mauriceau and his maneuver in breech delivery. *Obstet Gynecol* 1957; 9: 371–6.

1476. Speert H. Caspar Bartholinus and the vulvovaginal glands. *Med Hist* 1957; 1: 355–8.

1477. Speert H. Alexandre Couvelaire and utero-placental apoplexy. *Obstet Gynecol* 1957; 9: 740–3.

1478. Speert H. Carl Siegmund Credé, placental expression and the prevention of neonatal ophthalmia. *Obstet Gynecol* 1957; 10: 335–9.

1479. Speert H. Obstetrical-Gynaecological eponyms: James Young Simpson and his obstetric forceps. *J Obstet Gynaecol Br Emp* 1957; 64: 744–9.

1480. Speert H. *Obstetrics and Gynecologic Milestones: Essays in Eponymy*. New York, NY: MacMillan Co; 1958.

1481. Speert H. IC Rubin, a gynecologic eponym. *J Mt Sinai Hosp* 1958; 25: 221–8.

1482. Speert H. Vasili Vasilievich Strogonov and his eclamptic regimen. *Obstet Gynecol* 1958; 11: 234–9.

1483. Speert H. Edoardo Porro and caesarean hysterectomy. *Surg Gynecol Obstet* 1958; 106: 245–50.

1484. Speert H. *The Sloane Hospital Chronicle*. Philadelphia, PA: FA Davis; 1963.

1485. Speert H. *Obstetrics and Gynaecology in America: A History*. Chicago, IL: American College of Obstetricians and Gynecologists; 1980.

1486. Speert H. *Obstetrics and Gynecology: A History and Iconography*. 2nd edn. San Francisco, CA: Norman Publishing; 1994.

1487. Speert H. Memorable medical mentors: John Whitridge Williams (1866–1931). *Obstet Gynecol Surv* 2004; 59: 311–18.

1488. Speert H. Memorable medical mentors: Thomas S. Cullen (1868–1953). *Obstet Gynecol Surv* 2004; 59: 557–63.

1489. Speert H. Memorable Mentors: X. Richard Wesley Te Linde (1894–1989) *Obstet Gynecol Surv* 2005; 60: 143–6.

1490. Speert H. Memorable medical mentors: Emil Novak (1884–1957). *Obstet Gynecol Surv* 2005; 60: 273–8.

1491. Speert H. Memorable medical mentors XIII. Willard M. Allen (1904–1993). *Obstet Gynecol Surv* 2005; 60: 621–4.

1492. Speert H. Memorable medical mentors: Isidor C. Rubin (1883–1958). *Obstet Gynecol Surv* 2007; 62: 77–81.

1493. Speiser P, Smekal FG. *Karl Landsteiner (English translation R. Rickett)*. Vienna: Verlag Brüder Hollinek; 1975.

1494. Spencer HR. William Harvey, obstetric physician and gynaecologist. *Lancet* 1921; 2: 837–42.

1495. Spencer HR. *The History of British Midwifery from 1650 to 1800*. London: John Bale, Sons & Danielsson; 1927.

1496. Spencer HR. The history of ovariotomy. *Proc R Soc Med* 1934; 27: 49–56.

1497. Spencer HR. The history of ovariotomy. In: Cope, Z (ed.) *Sidelights of the History of Medicine*. London: Butterworths & Co; 1957, pp. 188–99.

1498. Speroff L. *A Good Man: Gregory Goodman Pincus*. Parkland: Arrix Publishing Inc; 2009.

1499. Spiegelberg, Otto (obituary). *Am J Obstet Dis Women Child* 1882; 15: 445–8.

1500. Spiller WG. Madame Degerine-Klumpke. *Arch Neur* 1928; 20: 193–4.

1501. Spinelli, Pier Guiseppe (obituary). *La Riforma Medica* 1929; 45: 1162.

1502. Spink MS, Lewis GL. *Albucasis. On Surgery and Instruments. A Definitive Edition of the Arab Text with English Translation and Commentaries*. Berkeley, CA: University of California Press; 1973.

1503. Spitzbart H. Otto Küstner (1848–1931). *Zentralbl Gynäkol* 1985; 107: 322–4.

1504. Stahlman MT. Assisted ventilation in newborn infants. In: Smith GF, Vidyasagar D (eds) *Historical Review and Recent Advances in Neonatal and Perinatal Medicine*. Vol. II. New York, NY: Mead Johnson Ltd; 1981.

1505. Stallworthy JA. Surgery of endometrial cancer in the Bonney tradition. *Ann R Coll Surg Engl* 1971; 48: 293–305.

1506. Stallworthy J. John Chassar Moir (1900–1977) *Trans Am Gynec Soc* 1978; 101: 183.

1507. Stanley GFG. John Clarence Webster: the laird of Shediac. *Acadiensis* 1973; 3: 51–71.

1508. Stark JN (ed.) *An Obstetric Diary of William Hunter, 1762–1765*. Glasgow: Alex MacDougall; 1908.

1509. Starr D. *Blood: An Epic History of Medicine and Commerce*. New York, NY: Harper Collins; 2000.

1510. Stegman SJ. Commentary :the cutaneous punch. *Arch Dermatol* 1982; 118: 943–4.

1511. Stein JB. Jan Palfyn. *Med Rec NY* 1913; 83: 47–55.

1512. Stellato TA. History of laparoscopic surgery. *Surg Clin North Am* 1992; 72: 997–1002.

1513. Stephens T, Brynner R. *Dark Remedy: The Impact of Thalidomide and Its Revival as a Vital Medicine*. Cambridge, MA: Perseus Publishing; 2001.

1514. Steptoe, Patrick Christopher (obituary). *Lancet* 1988; 1: 782.

1515. Steptoe, Patrick Christopher (obituary). *BMJ* 1988; 296: 1135.

1516. Sterpellone L. *Instruments for Health: From Origins to Yesterday*. Rome: Farmitabia Carlo Erba; 1986.

1517. Steudel J. Johannes Peter Muller. In: Gillispie CC (ed.) *Dictionary of Scientific Biography*. New York, NY: Charles Scribner's Sons. 1974, pp. 567–74.

1518. Stewart DB, Williams JG. Historical perspective. Bleeding and purging: a cure for puerperal fever? *J Hosp Infection* 1996; 34: 81–6.

1519. Still GF. *The History of Paediatrics*. London: Dawsons of Pall Mall; 1965.

1520. Stirrat GM. The bundle of life: the placenta in ancient history and modern sciences. In: O'Brien PMS (ed.) *The Yearbook of Obstetrics and Gynaecology*. London: RCOG Press; 1998, pp. 1–14.

1521. Stofft H. Kergaradec et Antoine Dugès. *Histoire des Sciences Médicales* 1983; 3: 15.

1522. Stofft H. Une présentation de l'épaule négligée en 1825. *Histoire des Sciences Médicales* 1984; 4: 331–42.

1523. Stofft H. Newborn's apparent death (1781–1806) through the work of François Chaussier. *Hist Sci Med* 1997; 31: 341–9.

1524. Stokes MA. Sister Mary Joseph's nodule. *Irish Med J* 1993; 86: 86.

1525. Stolley PD, Lasky T. *Investigating Disease Patterns: The Sciences of Epidemiology*. New York, NY: Scientific American Library; 1995.

1526. Stonehouse J. *Idols to Incubators: Reproduction Theory Through the Ages*. London: Searlet Press; 1994, pp. 62–76.

1527. Stovin GHT. *Gas and Air Analgesia in Midwifery*. London; Stopes Press Ltd; 1945.

1528. Strassmann P. Zum andenken an Alfred Duhrssen. *Zentralbl Gynäkol* 1934; 58: 146–52.

1529. Strassmann P. In memoriam: Dr August Martin (1847–1934) *Trans Am Assoc Obstet Gynecol Abd Surg* 1937; 55: 293–6.

1530. Stratmann L. *Chloroform: The Quest for Oblivion*. Stroud: Sutton Publishing; 2003.

1531. Stringer MD. *Eponyms in Surgery and Anatomy of the Liver, Bile Ducts and Pancreas*. London: RSM Press; 2009.

1532. Studdiford WE. William Edgar Caldwell, 1880–1943. *Am J Obstet Gynecol* 1944; 68: 305–8.

1533. Sturmdorf, Arnold (obituary). *JAMA* 1934; 103: 1871.

1534. Sudhoff K. *Essays in the History of Medicine*. New York, NY: Medical Life Press; 1926.

1535. Sudrania OP. Letter to editor. Kurt Semm: a laparoscopic crusader. *J Min Access Surg* 2007; 3: 115.

1536. Sureau C. Historical perspectives: forgotten past, unpredictable future. *Clin Obstet Gynaecol* 1996; 10: 167–84.

1537. Sureau C. In memoriam: Roberto Caldeyro-Barcia. *J Gynecol Obstet Biol Reprod* 1997; 26: 453–4.

1538. Sutton C. 150 years of hysterectomy: from Charles Clay to laparoscopic hysterectomy. In: Studd J (ed.) *The Yearbook of the Royal College of Obstetricians and Gynaecologists*. London: RCOG Press; 1994, pp. 29–39.

1539. Sutton C. Hysterectomy: a historical perspective. In Wood C, Maher PJ (eds) *Clin Obstet Gynaecol* 1997; 11: 1–22.

1540. Sykes WS. *Essays on the First Hundred Years of Anaesthesia*. London: Churchill-Livingstone; 1960.

1541. Szabo I, Laszlo A. Veres needle: in memoriam of the 100th birthday anniversary of Dr János Veres, the inventor. *Am J Obstet Gynecol* 2004; 191: 352–3.

1542. Tacchi D, Lind T. In defence of the Stein–Leventhal syndrome. *J Obstet Gynaecol Br Commonw* 1968; 75: 322–6.

1543. Tait HP, Wallace AT. Dr William Smellie and his library at Lanark, Scotland. *Bull Hist Med* 1952; 26: 403–20.

1544. Tait L. An address on the present aspect of antiseptic surgery. *BMJ* 1890; 2: 728–32.

1545. Tait, Lawson (obituary). *BMJ* 1899; 1: 1561–4.

1546. Tait, Lawson (obituary). *JAMA* 1899; 33: 875–80.

1547. Tait SAS, Tait JF. *A Quartet of Unlikely Discoveries*. London: Athena Press; 2004.

1548. Talbert LM. The assisted reproductive technologies: an historical overview. *Arch Pathol Lab Med* 1992; 116: 320–2.

1549. Talbott JH. Fracastorius. In: *A Biographical History of Medicine*. New York, NY: Grune and Stratton; 1970, pp. 44–70.

1550. Tan SY. Antoni van Leeuwenhoek (1632–1723): father of microscopy. *Singapore Med J* 2003; 44: 557–8.

1551. Tancer ML. Vesicouterine fistula: a review. *Obstet Gynecol Surv* 1986; 41: 743–53.

1552. Tancer ML. Robert Lawson Tait, FRCS, Edinburgh and England: Pioneer Surgeon. *J Pelvic Surg* 1997; 3: 237–9.

1553. Tanner, James Mourilyan 1920–2010 (obituary). *Ann Hum Biol* 2011; 38: 243–6.

1554. Tanner JM. *A History of the Study of Human Growth*. Cambridge: Cambridge University Press; 1981.

1555. Tansey EM, Christie DA (eds) *Looking at the Unborn: Historical Aspects of Obstetric Ultrasound. Wellcome Witnesses to Twentieth Century Medicine. Vol. 5*. London: Wellcome Trust; 2000.

1556. Tansey EM. Medicines and men: Burroughs, Wellcome and Co, and the British drug industry before the Second World War. *JR Soc Med* 2002; 95: 411–6.

1557. Tarolli J. First ladies in medicine in Michigan. *Medicine at Michigan* 2000; 2: 1–14.

1558. Taussig FJ. The story of prenatal care. *Am J Obstet Gynecol* 1937; 34: 731–9.

1559. Taylor CR. The intrauterine bougie and Voorhees bag today. *Am J Obstet Gynecol* 1958; 76: 553–7.

1560. Taylor CW. Lawson Tait: a grateful pupil of James Young Simpson. *J Obstet Gynaecol Br Commonw* 1965; 72: 165–71.

1561. Taylor ES. *History of the American Gynecological Society, 1876–1981 and American Association of Obstetricians and Gynecologists, 1888–1981*. St Louis, MO: CV Mosby; 1985.

1562. Taylor HC. In memoriam: Robert Latou Dickinson, 1861–1950. *Trans Ann Gynec Soc* 1951; 74: 259–61.

1563. Taylor HC. In memoriam: Howard Carman Moloy (1903–1953). *Trans Am Gynec Soc* 1953; 76: 237–8.

1564. Taylor HC. The origin and evolution of the journals of obstetrics and gynaecology. *Obstet Gynecol Surv* 1965; 20: 382–402.

1565. Taylor PJ. Asherman's syndrome revisited. *J Soc Obstet Gynaecol Can* 1990; 12: 47–8.

1566. Taylor RW. Arthur Joseph Wrigley (obituary). St Thomas' Hospital Gazette 1984, p. 31.

1567. Teacher JH. *Catalogue of the Anatomical and Pathological Preparations of Dr William Hunter in the Hunterian Museum, University of Glasgow*. 2 vols. Glasgow: James MacLehase; 1900.

1568. Te Linde RW. In memoriam: Thomas Stephen Cullen (1868–1953). *Trans Am Gynec Soc* 1953; 76: 227–9.

1569. Te Linde RW. Thomas Stephen Cullen. *Am J Obstet Gynecol* 1953; 66: 462–4.

1570. Te Linde RW. Howard Atwood Kelly. *Am J Obstet Gynecol* 1954; 68: 1203–11.

1571. Te Linde RW. Looking forward. *Obstet Gynecol* 1983; 62: 395–6.

1572. Temkin O. *Soranus' Gynecology*. Baltimore, MD: Johns Hopkins University Press, Soft Shell Books Edition; 1991.

1573. Tentler LW. *Catholics and Contraception: An American History*. Ithaca, NY: Cornell University Press; 2004.

1574. Thiery M. High amniotomy and the Drew Smythe catheter. *Eur J Obstet Gynecol Reprod Biol* 1988; 29: 87–91.

1575. Thiery M. Obstetric forceps and vectis: the roots. *Acta Belg Hist Med* 1992; 5: 4–20

1576. Thiery M. Intrauterine contraception: from silver ring to intrauterine contraceptive implant. *Eur J Obstet Gynecol Reprod Biol* 2000; 90: 145–52.

1577. Thin R. *College Portraits: Matthews Duncan*. Edinburgh: Oliver and Boyd; 1927.

1578. Thomas AN. *Doctor Courageous: The Story of Dr Grantly Dick Read*. New York, NY: Harper & Brothers; 1957.

1579. Thomas H. Anesthésie á la reine. *Am J Obstet Gynecol* 1940; 40: 340–6.

1580. Thomas KB. James Douglas of the Pouch, 1675–1742. *BMJ* 1960; 1: 1649–50.

1581. Thomas KB. *James Douglas of the Pouch and his pupil William Hunter*. London: Pitman Medical Publishing Co; 1964.

1582. Thomas KB. The Clover/Snow Collection. *Anaesthesia* 1972; 27: 436–49.

1583. Thomas KB. The great anatomical atlases. *Proc R Soc Med* 1974; 67: 223–32.

1584. Thomas KB. *The Development of Anaesthetic Apparatus*. Oxford: Blackwell Scientific Publications; 1975.

1585. Thomas TA. Self-administered inhalation analgesia in obstetrics. In: *The History of Anaesthesia.* In: Atkinson RS, Boulton TB (eds) London: Royal Society of Medicine Services and Parthenon Publishing Group; 1989, pp. 295–8.

1586. Thomas TG. A century of American medicine, 1776–1876 III. Obstetrics and Gynaecology. *Am J Med Sci* 1876; 72: 133–70.

1587. Thompson B, Fraser C, Hewitt A, Skipper D. *Having a First Baby: Experiences in 1951 and 1985 Compared.* Aberdeen: Aberdeen University Press; 1989.

1588. Thompson CJS. *The History and Evolution of Surgical Instruments.* New York, NY: Schuman's; 1942.

1589. Thompson PW. Joseph Clover Centenary Lecture: 'Out of the nettle . . .'. *Ann R Coll Surg Eng* 1983; 65: 14–17.

1590. Thoms H. Gordon of Aberdeen. *Am J Obstet Gynecol* 1928; 15: 229–33.

1591. Thoms H. John Stearns and pulvis parturiens. *Am J Obstet Gynecol* 1931; 22: 418–23.

1592. Thoms H. Walter Channing and etherization in childbirth. *Anaesthesia Analgesia* 1932; 11: 1–4.

1593. Thoms H. Samuel Bard, the author of the first textbook on obstetrics published in America. *Am J Obstet Gynecol* 1932; 23: 115–21.

1594. Thoms H. *Chapters in American Obstetrics.* Baltimore, MD: Charles C Thomas; 1933.

1595. Thoms H. *Classical Contributions to Obstetrics and Gynecology.* Baltimore, MD: Charles C Thomas; 1935.

1596. Thoms H. Hugh Lennox Hodge: a master mind in obstetrical science. *Am J Obstet Gynecol* 1937; 33: 886–92.

1597. Thoms H. The American obstetric heritage: an inspiration in teaching obstetrics. *Obstet Gynecol* 1956; 8: 648–53.

1598. Thoms H. *Our Obstetric Heritage:The Story of Safe Childbirth.* Hamden, CT: Shoe String Press Inc; 1960.

1599. Thomsen RJ. *An Atlas of Intrauterine Contraception.* New York, NY: McGraw-Hill; 1982.

1600. Thomsen RJ, Rayl DL. Dr Lippes and his loop: four decades in perspective. *J Reprod Med* 1999; 44: 833–6.

1601. Thomson SC. The Great Windmill Street School. *Bull Hist Med* 1942; 12: 377–91.

1602. Thomson SC. The surgeon-anatomists of Great Windmill Street School. *Bull Soc Med Hist (Chicago)* 1943; 5: 55–75.

1603. Thorburn AL. Alexandre Francois Donné, 1801–1878, discoverer of trichomosis vaginalis and of leukaemia. *Br J Vener Dis* 1974; 50: 377–80.

1604. Thornton JL. A biographical sketch of James Hobson Aveling (1828–1892). In: Aveling JH (ed.) *English Midwives: Their History and Prospects.* Reprint of 1872 edition. London: Hugh Elliott Ltd; 1967.

1605. Thornton JL, Want PC. The Royal College of Obstetricians and Gynaecologists. *St Bartholomew's Hospital J* 1973; 77: 36–9.

1606. Thornton JL, Want PC. William Hunter's 'The Anatomy of the Human Gravid Uterus'. 1774–1974. *J Obstet Gynaecol Br Cwlth* 1974; 81: 1–10.

1607. Thornton JL, Want PC. Artist versus engraver in William Hunter's 'Anatomy of the Human Gravid Uterus'. 1774. *Med Biol Illustration* 1974; 24: 137–9.

1608. Thornton JL, Want PC. William Harvey (1578–1657), 'Father of British Obstetrics', and his friend Percival Willughby (1596–1685). *Br J Obstet Gynaecol* 1978; 85: 241–5.

1609. Thornton JL. *Jan Van Rymsdyk: Medical Artist of the Eighteenth Century.* Cambridge: Oleander Press; 1982.

1610. Thornton JL, Reeves C. *Medical Book Illustration: A Short History.* Cambridge: Oleander Press; 1983.

1611. Thorp JM, Short LP, Bowes WA. The Mueller–Hillis maneuver: can it be used to predict dystocia? *Obstet Gynecol* 1993; 82: 519–22.

1612. Thulesius O. *Nicholas Culpeper, English Physician and Astrologer.* London: MacMillan; 1992.

1613. Thulesius O. Nicholas Culpeper, father of English midwifery. *JR Soc Med* 1994; 87: 552–6.

1614. Tietze C, Lewit S. *Intra-uterine Contraception Devices. International Conference Series No. 54.* Amsterdam: Excerpta Medica Foundation; 1962.

1615. Tobias G, Sands RP, Bacon DR. Continuous spinal anesthesia: a continuous history? *Reg Anesth Pain Med* 1999; 24: 453–7.

1616. Tobin CE. Benjamin JA. Anatomical and surgical restudy of Denonvilliers' fascia. *Surg Gynecol Obstet* 1945; 80: 373–88.

1617. Tobyn G. *Culpeper's Medicine. A Practice of Western Holistic Medicine.* Shaftesbury: Element Books Ltd; 1997.

1618. Todman D. Edoardo Porro (1842–1902) and the development of caesarean section: a reappraisal. *Internet J Gynecol Obstet* 2006; 7: 2.

1619. Todman D. Childbirth in ancient Rome: from traditional folklore to obstetrics. *Aust NZ J Obstet Gynaecol* 2007; 47: 82–5.

1620. Todman D. Medical Memorial: Edoardo Porro (1842–1902). *J Med Biog* 2008; 16: 143.

1621. Torpin R. (obituary). *Augusta Chronicle.* 7 February 1976.

1622. Torres J, Riopelle A. History of colposcopy in the United States. *Clin Obstet Gynecol* 1993; 20: 1–5.

1623. Tovell HMM. In memoriam: Albert Herman Aldridge. *Trans Am Gynec Soc* 1984: 67–8.

1624. Tovey LA. The contribution of antenatal anti-D prophylaxis to the reduction of the morbidity and mortality in Rh hemolytic disease of the newborn. *Plasma Ther Transfus Technol* 1984; 5: 99–104.

1625. Tovey LA. Haemolytic disease of the newborn and its prevention. *BMJ* 1990; 300: 313–6.

1626. Tovey LA. Towards the conquest of Rh haemolytic disease: Britain's contribution and the role of serendipity. *Oliver Memorial Lecture. Transfusion Med* 1992; 2: 99–109.

1627. Towler J, Bramell J. *Midwives in History and Society.* London: Croom Helm; 1986.

1628. Trendelenburg F. *Medical Classics* 1940; 4: 922–88.

1629. Trent JC. Obstetrics and Gynecology in America II. Samuel Bard 1742–1821. *North Carolina Med J* 1947; 8: 95–7.

1630. Trent JC. Obstetrics and Gynecology in America III. John Stearns 1770–1848. *North Carolina Med J* 1947; 8: 177–8.

1631. Trolle D. *The History of Caesarean Section.* Copenhagen: Reitzel Booksellers; 1982.

1632. Trout HH. The 'Scotch-Irish' of the Valley of Virginia, and their influence on medical progress in America. *Ann Med Hist* 1938; 10: 71–82, 162–8.

1633. Tubbs RS, Gribben WB, Loukas M. Franz Kasper Hesselbach (1759–1816): anatomist and surgeon. *World J Surg* 2008; 32: 2527–9.

1634. Tucker, Erwin (obituary). *Boston Med Surg J* 1902; 146: 297.

1635. Turk JL. Leonard Colebrook: the chemotherapy and control of streptococcal infections. *J R Soc Med* 1994; 87: 727–8.

1636. Turner E. Bibliographie de François Rousset. *Ann Gynecol* 1880; 14: 1–25.

1637. Turner, Henry H (obituary). *J Clin Endocrinol Metab* 1971; 32: 1–2.

1638. Ulrich U. Das gynäkologische Erbe. Karl Schuchardt zum 90 Todestag. *Zentralbl Gynäkol* 1992; 114: 326–8.

1639. Underwood EA. Medicine and science in the writings of Smollett. *Proc R Soc Med* 1937; 30: 961–74.

1640. Ustun C. A famous Turkish dermatologist, Dr Hulusi Behçet. *Eur J Dermatol* 2002; 12: 469–70.

1641. Uyttenbroeck F. *Past and Present of Radical Surgery in Gynecological and Mammary Cancerology.* Leuven: Peeters; 1987.

1642. Valentine MT. *Biography of Ephraim McDowell, MD.* New York, NY: McDowell Publishing Co; 1897.

1643. Van de Warker E. J Marion Sims. *Trans Am Gynecol Soc* 1884; 9: 398.

1644. Van Dongen PWJ, DeGroot ANJ. History of ergot alkaloids from ergotism to ergometrine. *Eur J Obstet Gynec Reprod Biol* 1995; 60: 109–16.

1645. Vander Veer A. Some personal observations on the work of Lawson Tait. *Am J Obstet Dis Women Child* 1885; 28: 673–88.

1646. Viana O, Vozza F. *L'Obstetrica e la ginecologia in Italia.* Milan: Società Italiana di Ostetricia e Ginecologia; 1933.

1647. Viets HR. Safe deliverance. *N Engl J Med* 1943; 228: 170–1.

1648. Viets HR. Walter Channing (1785–1876) pioneer in obstetric anesthesia. *North Carolina Med J* 1947; 8: 418–9.

1649. Viets HR. Guillaume Duchenne. *Bull NY Acad Med* 1948; 24: 772–83.

1650. Vilos GA. The history of the Papanicolaou smear and the odyssey of George and Andromache Papanicolaou. *Obstet Gynecol* 1998; 91: 479–83.

1651. Virchow R. Johann Müller, the physiologist: a eulogy pronounced in the hall of the University of Berlin. (Translated by AM Adam) *Edin Med J* 1858; 4: 452–63, 527–44.

1652. Vogel JP, Betran AP, Vindevoghel N. Use of the Robson classification to assess caesarean section trends in 21 countries: a secondary analysis of two WHO multicountry surveys. *Lancet Glob Health* 2015; 3: e260–70.

1653. Wagenknecht E (ed.) *Mrs Longfellow: Selected Letters and Journals of Fanny Appleton Longfellow (1817–1861).* New York, NY: Longmans, Green & Co; 1956, pp. 129–30.

1654. Wahl FA. Zum Kristellerschen handgriff. *Arch für Gynäkol* 1932;149:58–62.

1655. Wall C. Nicholas Culpeper. *Lancet* 1933; 1: 673.

1656. Wall LL. Dr George Hayward (1791–1863): a forgotten pioneer of reconstructive pelvic surgery. *Int Urogynecol J* 2005; 16: 330–3.

1657. Wallis F. Piety and prejudice. *Can Med Assoc J* 1997; 156: 1549–51.

1658. Walsh JJ. *History of Medicine in New York.* (Vol. 5) New York, NY: National Americana Society, Inc; 1919, p. 467.

1659. Wangensteen OH, Wangensteen SB. *The Rise of Surgery: From Empiric Craft to Scientific Discipline.* Folkstone: Dawson; 1978.

1660. Ward GG. Marion Sims and the origin of modern gynecology. *Bull NY Acad Med* 1930; 12: 93–8.

1661. Ward GG. In memoriam: William Blair-Bell, 1871–1936. *Tran Am Gynecol Soc* 1936; 61: 369–72.

1662. Ward OC. Down's 1864 case of Prader-Willi syndrome: a follow-up report. *J R Soc Med* 1997; 90: 694–6.

1663. Ward OC. *John Langdon Down, 1828–1896: A Caring Pioneer.* London: Royal Society of Medicine Press; 1998.

1664. Wardrop J. Biographical sketch of the late Dr *Baillie. Edinb Med Surg J* 1824; 21: 220–6.

1665. Warkany J. Congenital malformations in the past. *J Chron Dis* 1959; 10: 84–96.

1666. Waserman M. Sir James Y Simpson and London's 'conservative and so curiously prejudiced' Dr Ramsbotham. *BMJ* 1980; 1: 158–61.

1667. Wasserman, August von (obituary). *Klin Wochenschr* 1925; 4: 902.

1668. Waszynski E. Kristeller's procedure: expression fetus, its genesis and contemporary application. *Ginekol Pol* 2008; 79: 297–300.

1669. Watson IA (ed.) *Physicians and Surgeons of America.* Concord: Republican Press Association; 1896.

1670. Watson MC. An account of an obstetrical practice in Upper Canada. *Can Med Assoc J* 1939; 40: 181–8.

1671. Watson P. *Ideas: A History from Fire to Freud.* London: Weidenfeld and Nicolson; 2005.

1672. Waugh M. The Viennese contribution to venerology. *Br J Vener Dis* 1977; 53: 247–51.

1673. Weber B. Dr James M. Tanner, an expert in how children grow, is dead at 90. *New York Times.* 23 August 2010.

1674. Webster A. Threefold cord of religion, science and literature in the character of Sir Thomas Browne. *BMJ* 1982; 285: 1801–2.

1675. Webster WS. Teratogen update: congenital rubella. *Teratology* 1998; 58: 13–23.

1676. Weese WH. A brief history of colposcopy. *J Reprod Med* 1976; 16: 209–13.

1677. Wegmann A, Gluck R. The history of rhesus prophylaxis with anti-D. *Eur J Pediatrics* 1996; 155: 835–8.

1678. Weiden RMF van der, Hoogsteder WJ. A new light upon Hendrik Van Deventer (1651–1724): identification and recovery of a portrait. *J R Soc Med* 1997; 90: 567–9.

1679. Wells WA. *A Doctor's Life of John Keats.* New York, NY: Vantage Press; 1959.

1680. Wertheim, Ernst (obituary). *Wein Med Wochenschr* 1920; 70: 409–12.

1681. Wertheim, Ernst (obituary). *BMJ* 1920; 1: 455–6.

1682. Wertz RW, Wertz DC. *Lying-In: A History of Childbirth in America.* London: Collier Macmillan Publishers; 1977.

1683. West MJ, Irvine LM. The eponymous Dr James Marion Sims MD, LLD (1813–1883) *J Med Biog* 2015; 23: 35–45.

1684. Westman A. Professor Bernhard Zondek on the occasion of his sixtieth birthday. *Acta Endocrinol* 1951; 7: 1–5.

1685. Whalen FX, Bacon DR, Smith HM. Inhaled anaesthetics: an historical overview. *Best Pract Res Clin Anaesthesiol* 2005; 19: 323–30.

1686. White AB. Gregory Goodwin Pincus (1903–1967) *Endocrinology* 1968; 82: 651–4.

1687. White DN. Johan Christian Doppler and his effect: a brief history. *Ultrasound Med Biol* 1982; 8: 583–91.

1688. White H. An introduction to Thomas Browne (1605–1682) and his connections with Winchester College. *J Med Biog* 1998; 6: 120–2.

1689. White, Priscilla (obituary). *Boston Globe.* 21 Dec 1989.

1690. Whitfield CR. Rhesus disease: success but unfinished business. In: O'Brien PMS (ed.) *The Yearbook of Obstetrics and Gynaecology.* London: RCOG Press. 2000, pp. 161–80.

1691. WHO. Robson Classification Implementation Manual. Geneva: World Health Organization; 2017.

1692. WHO. Statement on Caesarean Section Rates. Geneva: World Health Organization; 2017.

1693. Widdess JDH. The beginnings of medical microscopy in Ireland. *Irish J Med Sci* 1948; 280: 668–78.

1694. Wikström-Haugen I. *Proceedings: Second Symposium, European Association of Museums of History of Medical Sciences.* London: Wellcome Foundation; 1984, pp. 105–7.

1695. Wilkinson DJ. Benjamin Pugh and his air-pipe. In: Barr AM, Boulton TB, Wilkinson DJ (eds) *Essays on the History of Anaesthesia.* London: Royal Society of Medicine Press Ltd; 1996, pp. 1–3.

1696. Willett, John Abernethy (obituary). *BMJ* 1932; 2: 176.

1697. Willett, John Abernethy (obituary). *Lancet* 1932; 1: 1071.

1698. Williams AN, Williams J. 'Proper to the duty of a chirurgeon': Ambroise Paré and sixteenth century paediatric surgery. *J R Soc Med* 2004; 97: 446–9.

1699. Williams G. The Addis Ababa Fistula Hospital: an holistic approach to the management of patients with vesicovaginal fistulae. *J R Coll Surg Edinb Irel* 2007; 5: 54–7.

1700. Williams JW. A sketch of the history of obstetrics in the United States up to 1860. In: Dohrn P. (ed.) *Geschichte der Geburtshülfe der Neuzeit.* Erste Abtheilung. Tübingen; 1903, pp. 193–264.

1701. Williams, John Whitridge (obituary). *J Obstet Gynaecol Br Emp* 1932; 39: 100–8.

1702. Williams PF. A book review: Samuel Bard's 'A Compendium of the Theory and Practice of Midwifery'. *Am J Obstet Gynecol* 1955; 70: 701–10.

1703. Williams TI. *A Biographical Dictionary of Scientists.* London: John Wiley and Sons; 1969.

1704. Willis AM. John Peter Mettauer. *Surg Gynecol Obstet* 1926; 43: 235–6.

1705. Willius FA, Keys TE. *Cardiac Classics.* St Louis, MO: CV Mosby Co; 1941.

1706. Willocks J, Calder AA. The Glasgow Royal Maternity Hospital 1834–1984. 150 years of service in a changing obstetric world. *Scot Med J* 1985; 30: 247–54.

1707. Willocks J. Ian Donald and the birth of obstetric ultrasound. In: Nielson JP, Chambers SE (eds) *Obstetric Ultrasound.* New York, NY: Oxford University Press; 1993, pp. 1–18.

1708. Willocks J, Barr W. *Ian Donald: A Memoir.* London: RCOG Press; 2004.

1709. Willson JR. The conquest of cesarean section-related infections: a progress report. *Obstet Gynecol* 1988; 72: 519–32.

1710. Wilson A. *The Making of Man-Midwifery: Childbirth in England 1660–1770.* London: UCL Press; 1995.

1711. Wisenhaan PF. Hendrik van Deventer (1651–1724). In: Houtzager HL, Lammes FB (eds) *Obstetrics and Gynaecology in the Low Countries: A Historical Perspective.* Zeist: Medical Forum International; 1996.

1712. Witkowski GJ. *Histoire des accouchements chez tous les peuples.* Paris: Steinheil; 1887.

1713. Wolfe RJ. *The First Operation Under Ether.* Boston, MA: Boston Medical Library in the Francis A Countway Library of Medicine; 1993.

1714. Wolstenholme G. (ed.) *The Royal College of Physicians of London: Portraits.* London: J & A Churchill Limited; 1964.

1715. Wolstenholme G, Kerslake JF. (eds) *The Royal College of Physicians of London: Portraits. Catalogue II.* Amsterdam: Elsevier; 1997.

1716. Wood C, Suitters B. *The Fight for Acceptance: A History of Contraception.* Aylesbury: Medical and Technical Publishing Co; 1970.

1717. Wood C, Trounson AO. Historical perspective of IVF. In: Trounson AO, Gardner DK (eds) *Handbook of In Vitro Fertilization.* 2nd edn. Boca Raton, FL: CRC Press; 2000, pp. 1–14.

1718. Wood M. Eponymous biliary tract surgery. *Am J Surg* 1979; 138: 746–54.

1719. Wood Library-Museum. Chaussier laryngeal tube. www.woodlibrarymuseum.org/museum/item/934/chaussier-laryngeal-tube.

1720. Woodruff JD. Richard Wesley Telinde (1894–1989) *Trans Am Gynecol Obstet Soc* 1991; 9: xciii.

1721. Woods GE. The early history of infantile cerebral palsy. In: *Infantile Cerebral Palsy.* Bristol: Clinical Press ; 1994, pp. 15–18.

1722. Woollam CHM. Joseph T. Clover (1825–1882). *Curr Anaesth Crit Care* 1994; 5: 53–61.

1723. Woolley B. *The Herbalist, Nicholas Culpeper and the Fight for Medical Freedom.* London: Harper Collins Publishers; 2004.

1724. Word BH, Montgomery HA, Baden WF, Walker T. Vaginal approach to anterior paravaginal repair: alternative techniques. In: Baden WF, Walker T. (eds) *Surgical Repair of Vaginal Defects.* Philadelphia, PA: JB Lippincott; 1992, pp. 196–207.

1725. Word, Samuel Buford (obituary). *Birmingham Post-Herald* (Alabama). 5 January 1971.

1726. Word, Samuel Buford (obituary). *The Alabama MD.* 1971; 7: 3.

1727. Wright P. Sune K Bergström (obituary). *The Guardian.* 18 August 2004.

1728. Wright-StClair RE. The history of mutilating obstetric operations. *NZ Med J* 1963; 62: 468–70.

1729. Wrigley, Arthur (obituary). *BMJ* 1984; 288: 156–7.

1730. Writer D. Epidural analgesia for labor. *Anesthesiol Clin North Am* 1992; 10: 59–83.

1731. Wulf K. The history of fetal heart rate monitoring. In: Künzel W (ed.) *Fetal Heart Rate Monitoring.* Berlin: Springer-Verlag; 1985.

1732. Wynbrandt J, Ludman MD. *The Encyclopedia of Genetic Disorders and Birth Defects.* New York, NY: Facts on File; 1991.

1733. Wynn RM. In memoriam: Elizabeth M. Ramsey (1906–1993). *Placenta* 1994; 15: x–xi.

1734. Young JH. *Caesarean Section: The History and Development of the Operation from Earliest Times.* London: HK Lewis & Co Ltd; 1944.

1735. Young JH. John Braxton Hicks (1823–1897). *Med Hist* 1960; 4: 153–62.

1736. Young JH. James Blundell, 1790–1878; experimental physiologist and obstetrician. *Med Hist* 1964; 8: 159–69.

1737. Young M. Classics revisited. Researches on prenatal life by Sir Joseph Barcroft. *Placenta* 1992; 13: 607–12.

1738. Young RH. History of gynecological pathology. *Int J Gynecol Path* 1996; 15: 181–6.

1739. Zacharin RF. *Obstetric Fistula.* New York, NY: Springer-Verlag; 1988.

1740. Zacharin RF. A history of obstetric vesicovaginal fistula. *Aust NZ J Surg* 2000; 70: 851–4.

1741. Zallen DT, Christie DA, Tansey EM (eds). *The Rhesus Factor and Disease Prevention. Wellcome Witnesses to Twentieth Century Medicine. Vol. 22.* London: Wellcome Trust; 2005.

1742. Zanobio B. Girolamo Fracastoro. In: Gillispie CC (ed.) *Dictionary of Scientific Biography.* New York, NY: Charles Scribner's Sons, 1972, pp. 104–7.

1743. Zanobio B. Enrico Sertoli. In: Gillispie CC (ed.) *Dictionary of Scientific Biography.* New York, NY: Charles Scribner's Sons. 1975, pp. 319–20.

1744. Zimmerman DR. *Rh: The Intimate History of a Disease and its Conquest.* New York, NY: Macmillan Publishing; 1973.

1745. Zimmerman LM, Howell KM. History of blood transfusion. *Ann Med Hist* 1932; 4: 415–33.

1746. Zimmerman LM, Veith I. *Great Ideas in the History of Surgery.* Baltimore, MD: Williams and Wilkins, pp. 386–93.

1747. Zinsser F. Emil Noeggerath. *München Med Wochenschr* 1927; 74: 1677.

1748. Zipursky A. The rise and fall of Rh disease. In: Smith GF, Vidyasagar D (eds) *Historical Review and Recent Advances in Neonatal and Perinatal Medicine (Vol. 1).* New York, NY: Mead Johnson Ltd; 1981, pp. 99–106.

1749. Zollinger RM. David Tod Gilliam. *Surg Gynecol Obstet* 1930; 51: 873–5.

1750. Zondek, B. An interview. *J Reprod Fert* 1966; 12: 3–19.

1751. Zuck D. Joseph Thomas Clover (1825–1882). In: Matthew HCG, Harrison, B (eds) *Dictionary of National Biography.* Oxford: Oxford University Press; 2004.

1752. Zuspan FP. Edith Potter (1901–1993) *Trans Am Gyne Obstet Soc* 1995; 13: xxxvii.

Index